Interprofessional Practice in Pharmacy

Interprofessional Practice in Pharmacy

Featuring Illustrated Case Studies

Joseph A. Zorek, PharmD, BCGP
Director, Linking Interprofessional Networks for Collaboration
Office of the Vice President for Academic, Faculty, and Student Affairs
Associate Professor, School of Nursing
University of Texas Health Science Center at San Antonio
San Antonio, Texas

New York   Chicago   San Francisco   Athens   London   Madrid   Mexico City
Milan   New Delhi   Singapore   Sydney   Toronto

1 2 3 4 5 6 7 8 9   DSS   25 24 23 22 21 20

ISBN 978-1-260-46242-5
MHID 1-260-46242-0

This book was set in MinionPro by MPS Limited.
The editors were Michael Weitz and Peter J. Boyle.
The production supervisor was Catherine H. Saggese.
The text was designed by Mary McKeon.
Project management was provided by Rishabh Gupta, MPS Limited.

This book is printed on acid-free paper.

Cataloging-in-publication data for this book is on file at the Library of Congress.

McGraw Hill books are available at special quantity discounts to use as premiums and sales promotions or for use in corporate training programs. To contact a representative, please visit the Contact Us pages at www. mhprofessional.com.

To my daughters Anna and Marie,
whose love of graphic novels inspired this book.

Contents

About the Author

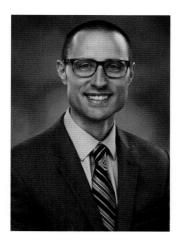

Joseph A. Zorek is an educator, pharmacist, and Fulbright scholar. To the latter, Joe attributes his enduring interest in people occupying different spaces in society whose collaborations, while neither easy nor seemingly natural, are necessary to achieve great things. It is this passion for intersections that led Joe to interprofessional practice and education, a field devoted to improving healthcare delivery by building mutual respect, trust, and understanding across the health professions.

Joe earned his bachelor's degree in psychology at the University of Iowa alongside certification in secondary social studies education. After several years of teaching at this level, Joe pivoted to healthcare by earning his doctorate degree from the University of Illinois at Chicago College of Pharmacy and completing a 2-year residency at Texas Tech University Health Sciences Center School of Pharmacy in Amarillo, Texas. Joe's passion for education led to a faculty position at the University of Wisconsin–Madison School of Pharmacy, where he was promoted, first to Director of Interprofessional Education, then to Associate Professor, based on the strength of his research, teaching, and service record.

Joe is the recipient of several accolades, including the Rufus A. Lyman Award and a Baldwin Award, both of which annually recognize the best articles published in the *American Journal of Pharmaceutical Education* and the *Journal of Interprofessional Care*, respectively. His work exploring the regulatory environment in health professions education has been widely cited, including within prestigious venues such as the *New England Journal of Medicine* and reports from the National Academy of Medicine. Joe represented the National Center for Interprofessional Practice and Education on a collaborative project with the Health Professions Accreditors Collaborative, which resulted in the co-authored *Guidance on Developing Quality Interprofessional Education for the Health Professions*, a national consensus guideline.

Joe currently serves as Director of the Quality Enhancement Plan, *Linking Interprofessional Networks for Collaboration (LINC)*, at the University of Texas Health Science Center at San Antonio. LINC seeks to advance interprofessional education across five schools and numerous educational programs by building consensus within, and facilitating collaborations amongst, key stakeholder groups; this includes academic administrators, faculty, staff, and students. In addition to this role, Joe is proud to be walking the interprofessional talk as a tenured faculty member in nursing, where he teaches advanced pharmacotherapeutics to graduate nursing students and strives to elevate health professions education through creative and impactful scholarship.

Contributors

Susanne G. Barnett, PharmD, BCPS
Associate Professor and
Co-Director of Interprofessional Education
Pharmacy Practice Division
School of Pharmacy
University of Wisconsin–Madison
Madison, Wisconsin
Chapter 8

Jessica M. Bergsbaken, PharmD, BCPPS
Clinical Pharmacist in Pediatrics
Department of Pharmacy
University of Wisconsin Health
Madison, Wisconsin
Chapter 6

Ana F. Bienvenida, PharmD
PGY-2 Resident in Emergency Medicine
University of Wisconsin Health
Madison, Wisconsin
Chapter 10

Monica C. Bogenschutz, PharmD, BCPS, BCPPS
Pharmacy Coordinator in Pediatrics
Department of Pharmacy
University of Wisconsin Health
Madison, Wisconsin
Chapter 6

Barbara F. Brandt, PhD, EdM, FNAP
Director
National Center for Interprofessional Practice and Education
University of Minnesota
Minneapolis, Minnesota

Professor
Department of Pharmaceutical Care and Health Systems
College of Pharmacy
University of Minnesota
Minneapolis, Minnesota
Chapter 1

Robert M. Breslow, BSPharm, RPh
Associate Professor Emeritus
Pharmacy Practice Division
School of Pharmacy
University of Wisconsin–Madison
Madison, Wisconsin
Chapter 7

Melgardt M. de Villiers, BPharm, MSc, PhD, PgDip
Professor, Vice Dean and Associate Dean for Academic Affairs
Pharmaceutical Sciences Division
School of Pharmacy
University of Wisconsin–Madison
Madison, Wisconsin
Chapter 2

John M. Dopp, PharmD, MS
Associate Professor and Vice Chair
Pharmacy Practice Division
School of Pharmacy
University of Wisconsin–Madison
Madison, Wisconsin
Chapter 5

Jeffrey T. Fish, PharmD, BCCCP
Clinical Pharmacist in Critical Care
Department of Pharmacy
University of Wisconsin Health
Madison, Wisconsin

Adjunct Clinical Assistant Professor
Pharmacy Practice Division
School of Pharmacy
University of Wisconsin–Madison
Madison, Wisconsin
Chapter 11

Casey E. Gallimore, PharmD, MS
Associate Professor and
Co-Director of Interprofessional Education
Pharmacy Practice Division
School of Pharmacy
University of Wisconsin–Madison
Madison, Wisconsin
Chapter 12

David R. Hager, PharmD, BCPS
Director of Clinical Pharmacy Services
Department of Pharmacy
University of Wisconsin Health
Madison, Wisconsin

Adjunct Clinical Associate Professor
Pharmacy Practice Division
School of Pharmacy
University of Wisconsin–Madison
Madison, Wisconsin
Chapter 15

Kimberly Harrison, PharmD
Pharmacy Coordinator in Medication Systems and
Operations
Department of Pharmacy
University of Wisconsin Health
Madison, Wisconsin
Chapter 13

Mary S. Hayney, PharmD, MPH, FCCP, BCPS
Professor
Pharmacy Practice Division
School of Pharmacy
University of Wisconsin–Madison
Madison, Wisconsin
Chapter 4

Tyler Ho, PharmD, BCACP
Outpatient Pharmacy Coordinator
Department of Pharmacy
University of Wisconsin Health
Madison, Wisconsin
Chapter 2

Paul R. Hutson, PharmD, MS, BCOP
Professor
Pharmacy Practice Division
School of Pharmacy
University of Wisconsin–Madison
Madison, Wisconsin
Chapter 9

Mara A. Kieser, MS, RPh
Professor and Assistant Dean for Experiential Education
Pharmacy Practice Division
School of Pharmacy
University of Wisconsin–Madison
Madison, Wisconsin
Chapter 7

Karen J. Kopacek, MS, BPharm
Associate Professor and Associate Dean for Student Affairs
Pharmacy Practice Division
School of Pharmacy
University of Wisconsin–Madison
Madison, Wisconsin
Chapter 5

Sarah E. Kubes, PharmD, BCPPS
Clinical Assistant Professor
Pharmacotherapy Division
College of Pharmacy
University of Texas at Austin
Austin, Texas

Adjoint Clinical Assistant Professor
Department of Pediatrics
Joe R. and Teresa Lozano Long School of Medicine
University of Texas Health Science Center at San Antonio
San Antonio, Texas

Clinical Pharmacist in Pediatrics
Department of Pharmacotherapy and Pharmacy Services
University Health System
San Antonio, Texas
Chapter 6

Laurel M. Legenza, PharmD, MS
Assistant Scientist and Interim Director of Global Health
Social and Administrative Sciences Division
School of Pharmacy
University of Wisconsin–Madison
Madison, Wisconsin
Chapter 14

Amanda Margolis, PharmD, MS, BCACP
Assistant Professor
Pharmacy Practice Division
School of Pharmacy
University of Wisconsin–Madison
Madison, Wisconsin
Chapter 3

Beth A. Martin, PhD, MS, RPh
Professor and Chair
Pharmacy Practice Division
School of Pharmacy
University of Wisconsin–Madison
Madison, Wisconsin
Chapter 4

Rebecca Moote, PharmD, MSc, BCPS
Clinical Associate Professor and Assistant Head
Pharmacotherapy Division
College of Pharmacy
University of Texas at Austin
Austin, Texas

Adjoint Clinical Associate Professor
Department of Medicine
Joe R. and Teresa Lozano Long School of Medicine
University of Texas Health Science Center at San Antonio
San Antonio, Texas

Clinical Pharmacist in General and Hospital Medicine
Department of Pharmacotherapy and Pharmacy Services
University Health System
San Antonio, Texas
Chapter 1

Cameron L. Ninos, PharmD, BCOP
Clinical Pharmacist in Oncology
Department of Pharmacy
University of Wisconsin Health
Madison, Wisconsin
Chapter 9

Denise L. Walbrandt Pigarelli, PharmD, BC-ADM, RPh
Associate Professor
Pharmacy Practice Division
School of Pharmacy
University of Wisconsin–Madison
Madison, Wisconsin
Chapter 3

Andrea L. Porter, PharmD
Associate Professor and
Director of Pharmacotherapy Laboratories
Pharmacy Practice Division
School of Pharmacy
University of Wisconsin–Madison
Madison, Wisconsin
Chapter 5

Edward C. Portillo, PharmD, BCACP
Assistant Professor
Pharmacy Practice Division
School of Pharmacy
University of Wisconsin–Madison
Madison, Wisconsin
Chapter 2

Trisha M. Seys Rañola, PharmD, CDE, BCGP
Clinical Assistant Professor and
Assistant Director of Global Health
Pharmacy Practice Division
School of Pharmacy
University of Wisconsin–Madison
Madison, Wisconsin
Chapter 14

Warren E. Rose, PharmD, MPH, FCCP, FIDSA
Associate Professor of Pharmacy and Medicine
Pharmacy Practice Division
School of Pharmacy
University of Wisconsin–Madison
Madison, Wisconsin
Chapter 8

Steve Rough, MS, RPh, FASHP
Senior Vice President
Visante, Inc.
Madison, Wisconsin
Chapter 15

Daniel J. Ruhland, PharmD
Clinical Pharmacist in Informatics
Department of Pharmacy
University of Wisconsin Health
Madison, Wisconsin
Chapter 13

Valerie A. Schend, PharmD, RPh
Lecturer and Clinical Instructor
Pharmacy Practice Division
School of Pharmacy
University of Wisconsin–Madison
Madison, Wisconsin
Chapter 3

Chloe R. Schmidt, PharmD
PGY-2 Resident in Critical Care
Department of Pharmacy
University of Wisconsin Health
Madison, Wisconsin
Chapter 11

Natalie S. Schmitz, MPA, PharmD, PhD
Assistant Professor
Pharmacy Practice Division
School of Pharmacy
University of Wisconsin–Madison
Madison, Wisconsin
Chapters 13 & 14

Christine A. Sorkness, PharmD, RPh
Distinguished Professor of Pharmacy and Medicine
Pharmacy Practice Division
School of Pharmacy
University of Wisconsin–Madison
Madison, Wisconsin
Chapter 3

Eva M. Vivian, PharmD, MS, PhD, BC-ADM, FADCES
Professor
Pharmacy Practice Division
School of Pharmacy
University of Wisconsin–Madison
Madison, Wisconsin
Chapter 4

Cody J. Wenthur, PharmD, PhD
Assistant Professor
Pharmacy Practice Division
School of Pharmacy
University of Wisconsin–Madison
Madison, Wisconsin
Chapter 12

Emily M. Zimmerman, PharmD, BCPS, BCCCP
Clinical Pharmacist in Emergency Medicine
Department of Pharmacy
University of Wisconsin Health
Madison, Wisconsin
Chapter 10

Joseph A. Zorek, PharmD, BCGP
Director, Linking Interprofessional Networks for Collaboration
Office of the Vice President for Academic, Faculty and Student Affairs
Associate Professor, School of Nursing
University of Texas Health Science Center at San Antonio
San Antonio, Texas
Chapters 1–15

Reviewers

Amie Taggart Blaszczyk, PharmD, BCGP, BCPS, FASCP
Associate Professor and Division Head of Geriatrics and Pediatrics
Department of Pharmacy Practice
School of Pharmacy
Texas Tech University Health Sciences Center
Dallas/Fort Worth, Texas
Chapter 7

Noelle RM Chapman, PharmD, BCPS, FASHP
Vice President of Pharmacy Operations
Advocate Aurora Health
Oak Lawn, Illinois
Chapter 15

Michelle E. Condren, PharmD, BCPPS, AE-C, CDE, FPPA
Professor of Pediatrics and Vice Chair for Research
School of Community Medicine
University of Oklahoma
Tulsa, Oklahoma
Chapter 6

Jennifer L. Engen, PharmD, BCCCP
Critical Care Pharmacist
Legacy Health
Portland, Oregon
Chapter 11

Eric H. Gilliam, PharmD, BCPS
Associate Professor
Department of Clinical Pharmacy
Skaggs School of Pharmacy & Pharmaceutical Sciences
University of Colorado Anschutz Medical Campus
Aurora, Colorado
Chapter 10

Gloria R. Grice, PharmD, BCPS, FNAP
Professor and Interim Chair
Department of Pharmacy Practice
Assistant Dean for Curriculum and Assessment
St. Louis College of Pharmacy
St. Louis, Missouri
Chapter 4

Elizabeth B. Hirsch, PharmD
Assistant Professor
Department of Experimental and Clinical Pharmacology
College of Pharmacy
University of Minnesota
Minneapolis, Minnesota
Chapter 8

Eric J. MacLaughlin, PharmD, FASHP, FCCP, BCPS
Professor and Chair
Department of Pharmacy Practice
Jerry H. Hodge School of Pharmacy
Texas Tech University Health Sciences Center
Amarillo, Texas
Chapter 5

Marina Maes, PharmD, BCPS, BCACP
Assistant Professor
Pharmacy Practice Division
School of Pharmacy
University of Wisconsin–Madison
Madison, Wisconsin
Chapter 3

Lisa M. Meny, PharmD
Professor and Coordinator of Accreditation and Assessment
Department of Pharmacy Practice
College of Pharmacy
Ferris State University
Big Rapids, Michigan
Chapter 2

Cynthia L. Raehl, PharmD, FASHP, FCCP
Grover E. Murray Professor
Department of Pharmacy Practice
Jerry H. Hodge School of Pharmacy
Texas Tech University Health Sciences Center
Amarillo, Texas
Chapter 7

Ivan A. Reveles, PharmD, MS, BCOP
Pharmacist Manager
Department of Investigational Drug Section
University of Texas Health San Antonio MD Anderson
Cancer Center
San Antonio, Texas

Adjoint Clinical Assistant Professor
Pharmacotherapy Division
College of Pharmacy
University of Texas at Austin
Austin, Texas
Chapter 9

Sarah P. Shrader, PharmD, BCPS
Professor and Director of Interprofessional Education
Department of Pharmacy Practice
School of Pharmacy
University of Kansas
Lawrence, Kansas
Chapter 1

Susan M. Stein, DHEd, MS, BS Pharm, FNAP, FOSHP, RPh
Professor Emeritus
School of Pharmacy
Pacific University
Hillsboro, Oregon

Managing Member
Susan M. Stein Consulting, LLC
Astoria, Oregon
Chapter 14

Orly Vardeny, PharmD, MS, FHFSA
Core Investigator
Center for Care Delivery and Outcomes Research
Minneapolis Veterans Affairs Health Care System
Minneapolis, Minnesota

Associate Professor
School of Medicine
University of Minnesota
Minneapolis, Minnesota
Chapter 5

Cody J. Wenthur, PharmD, PhD
Assistant Professor
Pharmacy Practice Division
School of Pharmacy
University of Wisconsin–Madison
Madison, Wisconsin
Chapters 9 & 13

Foreword

Interprofessional Practice in Pharmacy: Featuring Illustrated Case Studies by Joseph A. Zorek and contributors is a creative and engaging resource to support the education of prospective and future pharmacists. Rooted in a case study method described by the author as "an innovative educational art form inspired by graphic novels and comic strips," we believe it will be a well-received educational approach for current and future generations of learners. To our knowledge, the educational format of this book is unique not only for pharmacy education but also for the education of other health professionals.

Surveys in the United States and other countries have demonstrated that many people identify the pharmacist's role in healthcare primarily as the distributor of prescription medications in the community pharmacy setting. As such, pharmacy educators find it important to expose prospective and current pharmacy students to the broad range of expanding roles and career choices for pharmacists, including their valuable contributions to patient and public health. Chapters of the book focus on issues germane to locations of practice (e.g., community, primary care, emergency medicine, critical care), specialty care (e.g., cardiology, oncology, mental health, pediatrics, geriatrics), and other relevant topics (e.g., prevention and wellness, population health, technology, administration). Current and well-referenced educational reading material related to a chapter topic are presented to the reader, with the incorporation of illustrated case studies that not only call for application of the chapter content to real-world issues but also simultaneously expose the reader to roles pharmacists play well beyond drug distribution.

Of note, consistent with the title of the book, the first chapter focuses on interprofessional practice in pharmacy and sets the stage for illustrated case studies that demonstrate real-world examples of the role and contributions of the pharmacist in team-based care. The widely accepted definition of interprofessional education (IPE) is when learners from two or more professions learn about, from and with each other. While not a new concept, interprofessional learning to equip health professionals to advance team-based care has grown markedly over the last decade. The Interprofessional Education Collaborative (IPEC) was established in 2009 by leaders from six associations of health professional education, including the American Association of Colleges of Pharmacy. The IPEC *Core Competencies for Interprofessional Collaborative Practice*[1] and multiple faculty and leadership development programs offered by the collaborative have contributed to significant expansion of interprofessional learning that has equipped contemporary graduates for team-based care. Over this same period, specialized accreditation agencies have strengthened the emphasis on interprofessional learning in national standards, encouraged by an analogous network known as the Health Professions Accreditors Collaborative (HPAC). Recently, HPAC partnered with the National Center for Interprofessional Practice and Education to provide the field with *Guidance on Developing Quality Interprofessional Education for the Health Professions*, which was co-authored by Dr. Zorek.[2] The illustrated case studies throughout this book help bring the role of the pharmacists on healthcare teams to life, and they reinforce the shared vision for health professional education and practice espoused by IPEC, HPAC, and the National Center.

Based on our combined knowledge of the Doctor of Pharmacy curricula in the accredited pharmacy colleges and schools in the United States, we can see a variety of uses by faculty for *Interprofessional Practice in Pharmacy: Featuring Illustrated Case Studies*. Exposure to the book, its contents, and purpose during orientation sessions for new classes will provide important insight for students to what their curriculum will prepare them to do, as well as open their eyes to new and important pharmacy career choices. For example, informing the students during orientation that preparation of students to be "team ready" at graduation is an accreditation requirement will provide early appreciation of the purpose and importance of the IPE they will participate in. The illustrated cases will offer educational material for practice simulation laboratories and help prepare students for their introductory pharmacy practice experiences. Moreover, the book will help final-year students be better prepared for advanced pharmacy practice experiences and to guide their selection of elective rotations that the text has exposed them to. Faculty from various health professions can use the illustrated cases to plan together their IPE activities, with the opportunity to extend the cases and have students role-play different scenarios. Finally, we believe the quality of the content of the reading material and the illustrated case studies will be valuable for the continuing professional development of pharmacists in practice.

Dr. Zorek may not have set out to create a learning resource that has the potential to fill so many roles, addressing educational needs ranging from prospective pharmacy students to practicing professionals, yet that is what we have found in our review. Furthermore, the potential for this book to stimulate and support interprofessional learning is substantial. As strong proponents of IPE for team-based care, we look forward to observing the use of this resource by faculty and students within pharmacy and throughout the health professions. As team-based care continues to grow, the public served by these teams will be the ultimate beneficiaries.

Lucinda Maine, PhD, RPh
Executive Vice President and Chief Executive Officer
American Association of Colleges of Pharmacy
Co-Founder, Interprofessional Education Collaborative

Peter H. Vlasses, PharmD, DSc (Hon.), FCCP
Executive Director Emeritus
Accreditation Council for Pharmacy Education
Convener, Health Professions Accreditors Collaborative

REFERENCES

1. Interprofessional Education Collaborative. (2016). Core competencies for interprofessional collaborative practice: 2016 update. Washington, DC: Interprofessional Education Collaborative.

2. Health Professions Accreditors Collaborative. (2019). Guidance on developing quality interprofessional education for the health professions. Chicago, IL: Health Professions Accreditors Collaborative.

Preface

While I could not have known it at the time, the seeds for this book were sown the moment I decided to leave my career as a high school social studies teacher. Having already experienced what felt like a false start, I made it my personal mission as a pharmacy student to learn as much as possible about this profession. In search of a career path that would sustain me, I read every book I could and met with a dizzying number of pharmacists doing things I had no idea pharmacists did.

This process taught me incredible lessons. First, the profession of pharmacy is expansive. This book highlights a piece of that expanse, but certainly does not cover it all. Second, pharmacists' knowledge and expertise generate unbelievable value for society. Medications are the most widely used tool in healthcare, with a projected 5 billion prescriptions soon to be filled annually in the United States alone. The ubiquity of medications is perhaps only matched by the dangers their inappropriate or suboptimal use pose, which pharmacists are uniquely qualified to mitigate. Lastly, pharmacy is in the midst of a major transformation. For most of our history, pharmacists have practiced in siloes, often isolated from the work of other health professionals. Such isolation is slowly becoming a relic of the past as the value of pharmacists' contributions to interprofessional teams is becoming readily apparent.

A primary goal of this book is to expose current and prospective pharmacy students to these lessons, with the hope that doing so early in their careers will help them achieve their goals and fulfill their potential. If this book prevents a single career U-turn akin to mine, I would consider it a success. It would be even better if a prospective student who had written off pharmacy based on commonly held misperceptions was inspired by this book to become a pharmacist. Perhaps best of all would be if educators in other health professions use this book to teach their students about the work and value of pharmacists. This would accelerate the already rapid trend of incorporating pharmacists into healthcare teams.

To appreciate fully the impact of interprofessional practice in pharmacy, one must not only see it, but also be able to contextualize it. Hence, this book combines visual and written strategies. Each chapter opens with a general background of a particular topic or area of pharmacy practice, which includes a description of pharmacists' roles, other health professionals with whom they collaborate, and real-world examples of pharmacists in action. Next, illustrated case studies inspired by graphic novels and comic strips—but by no means funny—dig deeper into specific areas or issues. Characters communicate through dialogue boxes with inner ruminations displayed as thought bubbles, and clues embedded throughout facilitate engagement with the material. A detailed essay follows each illustrated case study, filling in holes and highlighting knowledge and skills required for pharmacists to succeed in each area.

This book would not have been possible without the strong support of several key individuals. Chief among these is my wife, Liz, who encouraged me to pursue this idea and single-handedly held down the fort to create the time and space needed to bring the book to life, much of which took place during a quarantine. That is a debt I doubt I will be able to repay. Without the support of Michael Weitz and Peter Boyle at McGraw Hill, and Steve Swanson at the University of Wisconsin–Madison, this project would still be sitting as an archived art exhibit somewhere in the bowels of Rennebohm Hall. As it relates to the art, George Folz masterfully breathed life and emotion into the characters and worlds envisioned. Of course, a book like this is only possible when lots of smart people pull together in the same direction; that said, I am grateful for the hard work and persistence of all contributors. Finally, I would be remiss if I did not acknowledge the efforts of our reviewers, whose constructive criticisms and advice significantly improved the book.

Joseph A. Zorek
San Antonio, Texas, November 2020

CHAPTER 1

Interprofessional Practice in Pharmacy

Featuring the Illustrated Case Study "Breakdown"

Authors
Rebecca Moote, Barbara F. Brandt, & Joseph A. Zorek

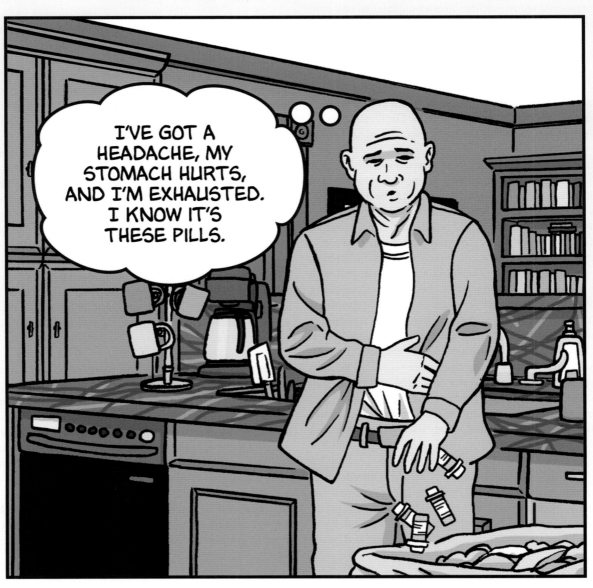

Illustration by George Folz, © 2019 Board of Regents of the University of Wisconsin System

BACKGROUND

Pharmacy practice is, by its very nature, interprofessional. Pharmacists who practice in hospitals, clinics, community pharmacies, and elsewhere collaborate on a regular basis with an array of other health professionals. As medication experts, they advocate for the safe and effective use of medications on behalf of patients, families, and caregivers, often with a focus on minimizing costs to make improvements in health outcomes possible. Such advocacy requires an impressive depth of knowledge about medications and medication use, which is built upon a solid foundation of topics taught in Doctor of Pharmacy (PharmD) curricula ranging from biochemistry, medicinal chemistry, and pharmacology to pharmacotherapy, patient safety, and pharmacy law.[1] To work effectively with other health professionals in a team environment, pharmacists must be knowledgeable about other team members' capabilities and contributions to patient care. Additionally, they must possess strong interpersonal and communication skills. This chapter will explore the landscape of interprofessional practice, the unique roles and responsibilities pharmacists play as members of interprofessional teams, and the impact of pharmacists' contributions to team-based care on health outcomes.

The World Health Organization defines interprofessional practice as:

> When multiple health workers from different professional backgrounds work together with patients, families, carers, and communities to deliver the highest quality of care.[2]

For context, the term *caregiver,* as opposed to carer, is more commonly used in the United States. It is important to note that this definition of interprofessional practice has been endorsed and adopted throughout the United States, and it is an expectation that all PharmD students will be adequately prepared for success in this area prior to graduation.[1] Such preparation is called interprofessional education, which involves individuals from two or more professions learning about, from, and with each other to develop knowledge, skills, and attitudes conducive to effective teamwork to improve health outcomes.[2–4] Emphasis on interprofessional practice and education, thus, is not unique to pharmacy. In fact, it is a national movement that has been embraced throughout the health professions on both the educational and practice sides of the healthcare sector.[5–10] What is unique to pharmacy, however, is the education and training of pharmacists. As medication experts on the team, pharmacists are uniquely prepared to advocate for the safe and effective use of one of the most important and widely used tools to improve health.

Nearly 80% of all medical treatments in the United States involve the use of medications.[11] By 2021, it is estimated that approximately 5 billion prescriptions will be filled each year.[12] Many different types of health professionals, referred to as prescribers, order medications to treat patients and write prescriptions for them to take at home; this includes dentists, nurse practitioners, physicians, and physician assistants across countless specialty areas of practice. State laws and regulations dictate who has the authority to prescribe medications, including which types of medications can be prescribed by whom.[13] In some states, this authority has been granted to pharmacists for specific medications or within specific practice settings.[14,15] It is common for patients to see multiple prescribers who are not directly coordinating their efforts.[16–18] Further complicating the situation, it is also common for patients to fill their prescriptions at multiple pharmacies and potentially in multiple states.[19] Such complexities raise the potential for patients to experience a host of serious medication-related problems, including incorrect doses, drug-drug and drug-food interactions, duplicate therapy, side effects and adverse drug events, and inappropriate polypharmacy. For in-depth discussions of adverse drug events and polypharmacy, readers are encouraged to explore the illustrated cases "Support" in Chapter 3 Primary Care and "Burden" in Chapter 7 Geriatrics, respectively.

Pharmacists are key partners in addressing medication-related problems, and this is not trivial work. Medication-related problems cost the US healthcare system between $100 and $289 billion each year.[20] This book is replete with examples of pharmacists contributing their expertise to the identification, prevention, and correction of such problems, working directly with patients, families, and caregivers and via close collaboration with other health professionals in a variety of settings. One of the most common problems pharmacists work to address is medication non-adherence, which occurs when patients are unable or neglect to take their medications as prescribed.[20] Suboptimal medication adherence is a major contributor to excess healthcare utilization. It has been associated with worsening of existing health conditions, the emergence of new health conditions, increased hospitalizations, and even death. The opening illustrated case of this book, "Breakdown" (below), intentionally features medication non-adherence as a mechanism to highlight how central addressing this particular problem is to interprofessional practice in pharmacy. The illustrated case "Holistic" in Chapter 4 Prevention & Wellness further explores this complexity through the lens of medication access issues; specifically, a patient's inability to afford a lifesaving medication.

Interprofessional practice is best represented when health professionals within a team demonstrate mutual respect for one another and value the expertise and contributions of each team member.[21] Teams that work collaboratively seek common goals and work together to identify and overcome problems that arise.[22] Effective teams maintain open communication, make decisions collectively, distribute credit for good outcomes, and share responsibility for failures.[21]

The collaborative potential within teams of health professionals is influenced by many factors.[23] Perhaps the most important of these is the practice setting itself, which dictates the types of health professionals present and the resources available to support interprofessional practice. In hospital settings, for example, teams of health professionals routinely work together in real-time through an activity called rounding, whereby members of the interprofessional team visit patients together. Rounding teams discuss the patient's clinical status and care plan in collaboration with the patient, family, and/or caregiver(s).[21,23,24] In long-term care facilities, also called nursing homes, teams may schedule interprofessional meetings in which they evaluate patient treatments and outcomes.[24,25] Other settings, such as primary care or specialty care clinics, traditionally have less health professionals physically present. Community pharmacies, meanwhile, typically have no other health professionals physically present. In these settings, technologies (e.g., fax machines, telephones, smartphones, electronic health records) are leveraged to facilitate interprofessional practice through written and verbal means. Those interested in technologies used to advance teamwork are encouraged to read Chapter 13 Technology and the illustrated cases "Integrated" and "Innovator."

Significant barriers and challenges to fully implementing robust interprofessional teamwork throughout the US healthcare system exist.[26] Individual professional cultures and identities can be fraught with stereotypes and biases, leading to attitudes and perceptions that may undermine interprofessional practice. Negative attitudes and perceptions can cause friction and unproductive hierarchical power dynamics within teams.[23,24,26] Importantly, however seemingly entrenched, such complications have proven responsive to interprofessional education interventions.[27] As such, they also serve as valuable fodder for authentic and meaningful interprofessional learning activities intended to train students and clinicians. Adding another layer of complexity, the architectural design of health facilities can also serve as an impediment to interprofessional practice; for example, workspaces that promote segregation like nursing stations and physician workrooms.[24] Hospital pharmacies further highlight this conundrum. Often located in basements, they physically separate pharmacists from patients and other health professionals. Fortunately, in spite of this architectural separation, hospital pharmacy practice models have evolved around physical barriers to bring pharmacists into closer proximity with patients and their interprofessional teammates.[28]

Despite these barriers and challenges, significant progress over several decades, particularly as it relates to educational transformation, portend a future where health professionals of all stripes will learn and practice together to the advantage of patients and our healthcare system.[5-7] A concerted effort to transform interprofessional clinical learning environments has been underway for several years, which promises to further solidify these advances.[7,10] The National Academy of Medicine, then called the Institute of Medicine, released a series of reports two decades ago that generated intense momentum for interprofessional practice and education.[29-32] Experts who authored these reports called for wholesale transformation of health

professions education to advance a vision where patients would receive the care they deserved, and health professionals would lean on one another's unique knowledge and skills to make that happen. While much work remains, this vision is coming to fruition, and pharmacists have proven themselves to be willing and able partners and teammates.

Role of Pharmacists within Interprofessional Teams

Broadly speaking, pharmacists take responsibility for the safe and effective use of medications on interprofessional teams and the identification, prevention, and correction of medication-related problems. It is important to note that, when using the term *medication,* pharmacists refer to all substances that are used to produce a physiologic effect in a person or animal. This definition encompasses much more than prescription medications; it also includes non-prescription (i.e., over-the-counter) medications, vitamins, supplements, herbals, vaccines, and complementary or alternative medications. This responsibility leads to a multitude of roles and professional activities, perhaps the most important being educating patients and advocating for their needs. While additional professional activities are common across practice settings, others are unique to the locations and teams within which a pharmacist practices. Table 1-1 provides a list of common contributions pharmacists make to interprofessional teams.

As described in Table 1-1, pharmacists' roles and professional activities extend beyond acquiring and dispensing medications for patients. More than half of medication-related problems are characterized as inadequate therapy; that is, for a variety of reasons, the patient is on the wrong medication, the wrong dose, or alternative/additional therapy is needed.[12] Because of their unique, advanced study of medications and their clinical knowledge, pharmacists have the expertise to address these issues and help patients achieve their health goals. Pharmacists work in collaboration with other health professionals to deliver comprehensive medication management.[33]

Comprehensive medication management is defined as:

> The standard of care that ensures each patient's medications are individually assessed to determine that each medication is appropriate for the patient, effective for the medical condition, safe given the comorbidities and other medications being taken, and able to be taken by the patient as intended.[34]

Comprehensive medication management includes evaluating the appropriateness of therapy based on the patient's diagnosis and goals of care. Pharmacists consider allergies, drug-drug interactions, side effect risks, cost of the medication, and ability of the patient to take the medication as indicated. Pharmacists also evaluate patient data to ensure that the medications are dosed appropriately based on patient parameters such as weight, age, and kidney and liver function. They will also determine

Table 1-1. Common Roles and Professional Activities of Pharmacists on Interprofessional Teams	
Professional Activity	**Description**
Verification of medication orders and prescriptions	Review medication orders and prescriptions for indication (i.e., approved usage), safety, and accuracy and work with prescribers to correct identified issues
Optimize drug selection	Recommend preferred drug therapy based on expert-developed guidelines or clinical trial data, while incorporating patient-specific factors
Optimize drug dosing	Recommend changes to drug dosages based on best available evidence from the published literature, as well as patient-specific factors such as kidney and liver function
Prevent adverse drug events	Identify and avoid drug-drug and drug-food interactions, as well as drug allergies/intolerances
Educate patients, families, caregivers, and health professionals	Provide medication counseling regarding side effects and how to take medications, answer drug information questions, and provide education for other health professionals
Monitor patient response to medications for safety and effectiveness	Recommend dose adjustments or different medications based on changes in kidney and liver function, laboratory data, and/or patient-reported side effects or adverse drug events (dizziness, confusion, medication-induced falls, etc.)
Ensure access to medications	Address insurance and cost barriers, utilize medication assistance programs, and navigate drug shortages

Table 1-2. Examples of Health Professionals Who Collaborate with Pharmacists		
Care coordinators	Health informaticists	Physician assistants
Community health workers	Medical assistants	Physicians
Dental hygienists	Medical laboratory scientists	Psychologists
Dentists	Nurse practitioners	Respiratory therapists
Dietitians/Nutritionists	Nurses	Social workers
Emergency medical service professionals	Occupational therapists	Speech-language pathologists
Genetic counselors	Physical therapists	Veterinarians

appropriate monitoring and follow-up to assess patient response for safety and efficacy.[33] Additionally, pharmacists are a valuable drug information resource for the interprofessional team and can provide education to the team on medication-related topics.

This book is replete with examples of impactful interprofessional practice in pharmacy across a broad range of healthcare settings. Importantly, each chapter includes an in-depth explanation of pharmacists' roles within interprofessional teams practicing in specific areas (e.g., primary care, cardiology, pediatrics, geriatrics, infectious diseases, oncology, emergency medicine, and critical care). Readers are encouraged to review the Table of Contents for practice areas of interest and to read these dedicated chapters for more information.

Other Health Professionals Who Collaborate with Pharmacists

Pharmacists collaborate with a wide range of health professionals.[21,22] They work with aforementioned prescribers—dentists, nurse practitioners, physician assistants, physicians, and veterinarians—to optimize prescribing and monitor medications to achieve improved outcomes.[35,36] They work closely with nurses in a variety of settings; in the hospital, they determine safe medication administration practices. Nurses often consult pharmacists to determine if two intravenous medications can be given at the same time, how fast they can be administered, and what monitoring should be completed. Pharmacists may work with dietitians to individualize nutrition orders for patients, especially for nutrition given intravenously (termed *parenteral nutrition*). Pharmacists may work with large collaborative teams in both a hospital and primary care setting to provide services for specific groups of patients; examples of health professionals they interact with include physical therapists, occupational therapists, social workers, and care coordinators.[37,38] Additionally, specialty settings such as end-of-life or hospice care create unique and meaningful interprofessional opportunities for pharmacists to work with chaplains, psychologists, and a host of different therapists.[39] Table 1-2 provides examples of health professionals with whom pharmacists may collaborate.

Impact of Pharmacists on Interprofessional Teams

The ultimate goal of interprofessional practice has expanded in recent years from the Triple Aim to the Quadruple Aim; that is, improvements in the patient experience of care, population health outcomes, and health professionals' satisfaction with their work, while reducing healthcare costs.[40] In light of this recent shift, there has not been overwhelming evidence that interprofessional practice can impact Quadruple Aim outcomes.[21,41,42] However, evidence is growing.[22] Specifically, studies have demonstrated that interprofessional teams with pharmacists embedded have improved medication-related outcomes in multiple settings, including primary care, prison clinics, and nursing homes.[21,22] In a primary care setting, pharmacists worked collaboratively with physicians and nurse practitioners to optimize medication use, which resulted in improved control of patients' blood pressure, blood glucose, and cholesterol levels.[35,36,43–46] A similarly composed interprofessional team demonstrated positive impact on blood glucose management in patients with diabetes in a prison system.[47] In Swedish nursing homes, pharmacists organized monthly interprofessional meetings with physicians, nurses, and nursing assistants to evaluate safe and appropriate medication use for residents, which resulted in decreased use of unsafe medications.[25]

Studies such as these represent an important trend that interprofessional practice in pharmacy has a positive impact on meaningful outcomes in healthcare. Additional published examples of pharmacists' contributions to team-based care, including associated impact on health outcomes and patient care, are summarized in the next section. These summaries demonstrate that interprofessional practice in pharmacy can reduce healthcare costs, improve chronic disease state management, and improve adherence to evidence-based recommendations for care.

INTERPROFESSIONAL PHARMACY PRACTICE IN ACTION

Cost Savings Galore

A group of researchers evaluated the impact of interprofessional practice in pharmacy on patient outcomes and health services utilization.[43] Six hospitals and 22 patient-centered medical homes (PCMHs) participated. PCMHs are patient-centered models of care with one prescriber coordinating a team of health professionals to ensure that the patient receives comprehensive and integrated care.[48] Pharmacists were incorporated into already established interprofessional teams, which consisted of care coordinators, medical assistants, nurse practitioners, nurses, and physicians. Pharmacists contributed across the entire spectrum of patient care, from hospital admission and discharge to follow-up visits in clinics and prescription pick-up.[49] Medication care plans for patients taking four or more medications were developed for patients prescribed two or more new medications for chronic conditions, including heart failure, diabetes, high blood pressure, asthma, chronic lung disease, high cholesterol, and depression. A total of 2480 patients received this pharmacist-augmented interprofessional care, which was compared to a "usual care group" that did not include embedded pharmacists. Interprofessional teams that included pharmacists produced significant improvements in blood pressure, diabetes, and cholesterol control compared to teams without a pharmacist. Hospitalizations decreased in the pharmacist group, and cost savings of the program reached $2619 per patient, which equated to over $5 million in savings. The return on investment, after accounting for the cost of embedding pharmacists on the interprofessional teams, was an impressive 504%.

Faster and Better

High blood pressure affects nearly half of adults in the United States. Left untreated, this can lead to strokes, heart attacks, and kidney disease. Of patients treated for high blood pressure, less than 50% reach their blood pressure goal. A group of researchers evaluated the time it took to reach blood pressure goals for uninsured patients when seen by an interprofessional team that included nurses, pharmacists, and physicians in an inner-city, safety-net clinic.[36] Pharmacists provided comprehensive medication management and initiated medication therapy for uncontrolled patients under an agreement with the physicians (i.e., they acted as prescribers). After 1 year, blood pressure control was analyzed and compared between the group of patients who saw the interprofessional team versus those who did not. Patients who were cared for by the interprofessional team that included pharmacists met their blood pressure goal after 36 days; for those who did not see this team, it took 259 days. At the end of the year, 80% of patients were controlled in the group that received interprofessional care compared to 44% in the usual care group. Readers are encouraged to explore Chapter 5 Cardiology for more details on the impact of interprofessional pharmacy practice in this area.

High Impact for Complex Care

Multiple myeloma is the second most common blood cancer.[50] Treatment for this cancer is complex due to oncology (i.e., cancer) medications that are both expensive and strictly regulated to ensure their safe use.[51] Many other types of medications are also used to prevent complications from treatment and to prolong survival, and these regimens are often complicated. For example, treatment of multiple myeloma can lead to reduced bone density, bone fractures, and disability. As a result of this complexity, including the number of medications needed to provide comprehensive care, medication non-adherence is a real challenge in this patient population. One cancer center created a clinic for patients with multiple myeloma that emphasized interprofessional practice between hematologists (physicians who specialize in treating blood diseases) and oncology pharmacists.[50] Each patient was seen separately by a hematologist and an oncology pharmacist, who then met to develop an interprofessional care plan. Pharmacy services included medication-related education, comprehensive medication management, monitoring patient adherence and treatment-related toxicity, supportive care management, and navigation of insurance approvals to facilitate access to medications. After 1 year, patient outcomes were compared to the previous year, which did not include such interprofessional collaboration. Results demonstrated significant improvement in adherence to supportive medications and vaccines. Delays obtaining oncology medications were decreased in the interprofessional group from 15 to 7 days, and the start time of medications to prevent bone disease was shortened from 97 to 5 days. Readers are encouraged to explore Chapter 9 Oncology for more details on the impact of interprofessional pharmacy practice in this area.

BECOMING A PHARMACIST

The PharmD is considered an entry-level degree; meaning, all pharmacists entering the profession must earn this degree from a program accredited by the Accreditation Council for Pharmacy Education (ACPE) in order to obtain a license to practice.[52] The vast majority of PharmD programs require 4 years to complete, while some offer accelerated options whereby students can complete their degree in 3 years.[52] Application to pharmacy school typically requires 2 to 4 years of prerequisite undergraduate coursework.[53] Many students enter pharmacy school after earning a bachelor's degree, and some pharmacy schools require this for consideration. As of 2020, there were 143 accredited PharmD programs in the United States.[52] ACPE has placed a strong emphasis on interprofessional education and preparation for interprofessional teamwork, and all current students can expect this in their program.[1] About one-third of pharmacy school graduates elect to pursue additional training via postgraduate residencies.[54] Residencies provide pharmacists with advanced clinical training that prepares them to provide direct patient care in a variety of settings, with additional opportunities to advance knowledge and skills specific to interprofessional practice. Residency programs are competitive; in 2020, 63% of applicants who applied to first-year residency programs successfully matched.[54] Additional training and certifications are available in a number of specialty practice areas.[55] More information on these options is available within chapters throughout this book dedicated to these specialty practice areas.

BREAKDOWN: An Illustrated Case Study

Original story by Jamie M. Hess, Kari R. Hirvela, Paula Jarzemsky, Scott M. Mead, & Joseph A. Zorek
Adaptation by Rebecca Moote & Joseph A. Zorek
Illustrations by George Folz, © 2019 Board of Regents of the University of Wisconsin System

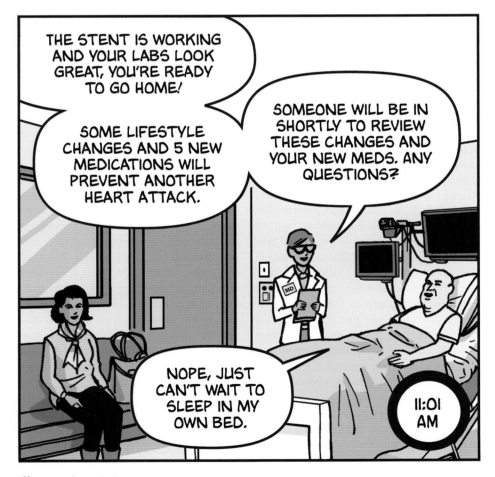

Illustration 1-1

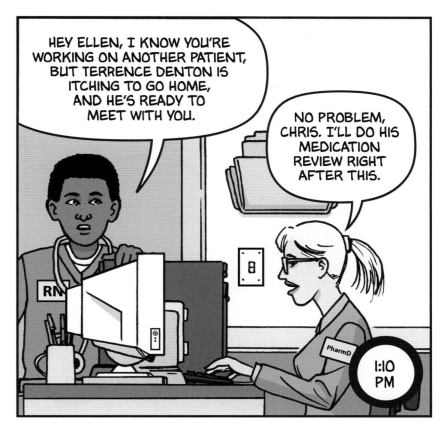

Illustration 1-2

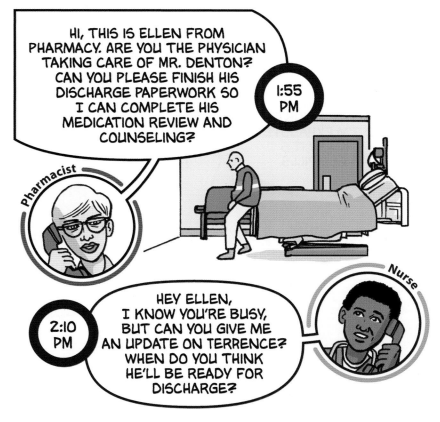

Illustration 1-3

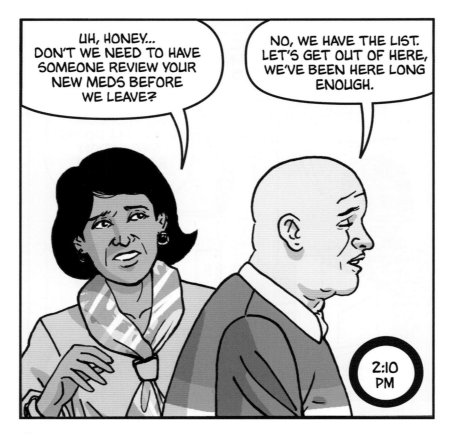

Illustration 1-4

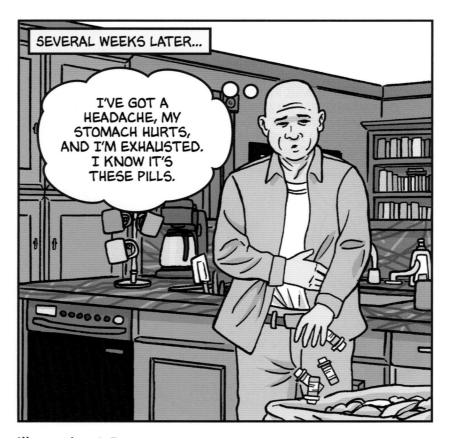

Illustration 1-5

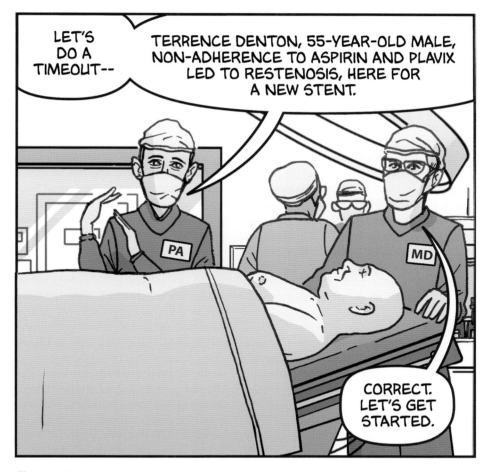

Illustration 1-6

Thoughts on "Breakdown"

The main character in the illustrated case "Breakdown" is Terrence Denton, a middle-aged man diagnosed with an acute myocardial infarction (MI), more commonly known as a heart attack. Mr. Denton underwent an emergency procedure called percutaneous coronary intervention (PCI) to treat this condition by restoring blood flow to his heart. After PCI, several medications are critically important to maintain adequate blood flow, protect the heart, and prevent a repeat MI. Unfortunately, Mr. Denton stopped his medications due to intolerable side effects and incomplete knowledge about their importance, which resulted in a second hospitalization and repeat PCI. A crucial missed opportunity for medication education by Dr. Ellen Ericson, a cardiology pharmacist, was a contributing factor. Due to delays caused by breakdowns in interprofessional teamwork, Mr. Denton left the hospital before Ellen was able to educate him about his medications. This unfortunate series of events nearly cost Mr. Denton his life.

Heart disease is the leading cause of death in the United States.[56] Shockingly, a new MI occurs about every 40 seconds in America.[56] It is estimated that over half of patients who experience a first MI will have a repeat episode, like Mr. Denton, and that approximately 15% of these patients will die as a result.[56]

Heart disease has a significant impact on the US healthcare system, with associated costs totaling nearly $220 billion annually. MI is one of the most expensive contributors to this figure, with annual costs estimated at $12 billion.[56]

An acute MI is a medical emergency requiring hospitalization and specialized care.[57] MIs are the most severe manifestation of coronary artery disease, which presents as blockage in the arteries that supply the heart with the oxygen-rich blood it needs to function.[58] The medical terms *cardiac* and *coronary* refer to the heart. Blockages are caused by the buildup of plaques inside the coronary arteries, which may accumulate over time due to uncontrolled high blood pressure, high cholesterol, diabetes, and smoking.[59] MI occurs when one of these plaques ruptures or erodes, leading to clot formation inside the coronary artery and blockage of blood flow.[57] If the blockage is not corrected, the patient could experience cardiac arrest and die as a result. Those interested in a more in-depth exploration of heart disease and pharmacists' contributions to the management of high blood pressure are encouraged to read Chapter 5 Cardiology and the illustrated case "Underlying Cause." For more information on diabetes, see the illustrated cases "Holistic" in Chapter 3 Primary Care, "Screen" in Chapter 4 Prevention & Wellness, and "Type 1" in Chapter 11 Critical Care. The illustrated case

"Change Talk" in Chapter 4 Prevention & Wellness provides a detailed description of the health effects of nicotine-containing products (e.g., cigarettes, vaping devices) and a pharmacist-led cessation intervention.

The illustrated case "Breakdown" begins after Mr. Denton's first PCI. While not shown, his backstory involved the onset of sharp chest pain that radiated to his left arm and back, as well as feelings of weakness and difficulty breathing that led his wife to call 9-1-1. Such complaints represent the cardinal symptoms of acute MI.[57] Emergency medical service (EMS) professionals attempted to stabilize Mr. Denton at his home by giving him oxygen, aspirin, and a drug called nitroglycerin, which is a potent vasodilator; meaning, it causes blood vessels, like Mr. Denton's blocked coronary artery, to open up.[60] They also used an electrocardiogram (ECG) to evaluate the electrical activity of Mr. Denton's heart, which indicated that he was having a severe heart attack that typically requires emergency PCI. As a result, Mr. Denton was quickly transported to the emergency department of a local hospital.

A clot that blocks all blood flow from a coronary artery causes a more severe heart attack. It also appears on an ECG with characteristic markings called ST-segment elevations; hence, this type of MI is called ST-segment elevation MI, or STEMI.[57] Partial blockage causes a less severe heart attack without ST-segment elevation in the ECG, which leads to a diagnosis of non-STEMI, also called NSTEMI. For patients who arrive to the emergency department on their own, or otherwise without the benefit of an EMS-administered ECG, emergency department staff seek to obtain an ECG reading and bloodwork within 10 minutes.[57,61] Those with STEMI receive PCI, like Mr. Denton, while those with NSTEMI are further evaluated and monitored. A protein called troponin is measured from the patient's bloodwork. During an MI, the heart muscles leak this protein. Patients with NSTEMI have troponin levels measured every 6 hours to observe trends. Results of the ECG and troponin tests, combined with other assessments, determine the patient's care plan.

Restoring blood flow to the heart is the primary goal in the treatment of MI.[57] This is termed *coronary reperfusion*. Patients who receive PCI, like Mr. Denton, have this procedure done in a cardiac catheterization lab (i.e., cath lab). About 34% of hospitals in the United States contain a cath lab.[62] The goal is to have patients in the cath lab in less than 90 minutes from first medical contact.[61] Specialty-trained physicians called interventional cardiologists perform PCIs, during which they use imaging tools and special dyes inserted into the patient's blood to locate the exact blockage site in the heart. Under sedation, a thin, flexible tube called a catheter is placed in a vein and routed to the heart. Dye is injected into the vein and the interventional cardiologist takes real-time images of blood flow through the heart, revealing the location of the blockage.

To restore blood flow, a stent is then placed at the site of the blockage. A stent is a wire mesh tube that pushes the blockage against the sides of the artery, holding it in place and allowing blood to once again pass through.[63] Some stents are coated with a drug that slowly releases (i.e., drug-eluting stent, or DES) to prevent reactions between blood and the stent that might lead to a new clot. DESs are the most common stents used and have lower rates of stent clots, repeat MI, and cardiac arrest.[57] Failure of a stent like this is called restenosis. In Illustration 1-1, Mr. Denton's physician excitedly reports that the DES placement was successful. Success rates are high with PCIs and patients can leave the hospital as quickly as 3 days after the procedure.[57]

As mentioned above, the risk of experiencing a second MI is high. Fortunately, there are several known strategies for reducing this risk.[59] These include lifestyle modifications, cardiac rehabilitation, annual influenza vaccination, and several medications. Prior to leaving the hospital, patients should receive education on lifestyle modifications such as smoking cessation, diet, and exercise.[57,61] Management of diabetes, cholesterol, and blood pressure will also help reduce the risk of a recurrent event. Patients should be referred for cardiac rehabilitation as well as follow-up appointments with a cardiologist.[57] Readers interested in cardiac rehabilitation are encouraged to explore the illustrated case "Educator" in Chapter 5 Cardiology.

Medications are vitally important in the prevention of recurrent MI, and patients should receive thorough counseling and education on how these work, and also what steps should be taken to troubleshoot common and/or serious side effects. The stakes are quite high; not only are patients at risk of a second MI, but they are also at risk of developing heart failure. Heart failure is the impairment of the heart to fill or pump blood.[64] Because the heart muscle is damaged during a MI, this damage can result in heart failure during the MI or afterwards. Medication therapy is focused on preventing both a second MI and the development of heart failure. Illustration 1-1 reveals that Mr. Denton will leave the hospital on five different medications, all of which have been shown to reduce a second MI and death in patients with a history of MI.[65-69] Evidence-based medication therapy for patients with a history of MI, described in detail in Table 1-3,[61] include the following combination:

1) Two antiplatelet agents;
2) A beta-blocker (BB);
3) An angiotensin-converting enzyme inhibitor (ACEI) or an angiotensin receptor blocker (ARB); and
4) A statin.

Illustration 1-2 depicts an exchange between Ellen and Chris Evans, Mr. Denton's nurse. Chris and Ellen are part of the cardiology team, working in collaboration with physicians, a social worker, and physical and occupational therapists. Ellen and Chris are coordinating their efforts, trying to figure out how to incorporate Mr. Denton's hospital discharge activities into the work they are both doing on behalf of other patients. Chris' comment about Mr. Denton "itching to go home" sets the stage for the time pressures and mounting frustrations that foreshadow trouble later in the case. Prior to leaving the hospital, cardiology pharmacists like Ellen perform several important

Table 1-3. Categories and Examples of Medications Commonly Used to Prevent Recurrent Myocardial Infarction

Category	Medication Examples*	Physiologic Effect
Beta-blockers	▪ carvedilol (Coreg) ▪ metoprolol (Lopressor, Toprol)	Block beta-receptors in the heart, causing decreases in heart rate, force of heart muscle pumping, and blood pressure
Angiotensin-converting enzyme (ACE) inhibitors	▪ benazepril (Lotensin) ▪ captopril (Capoten) ▪ enalapril (Vasotec) ▪ lisinopril (Prinivil, Zestril) ▪ quinapril (Accupril) ▪ ramipril (Altace)	Prevent formation of angiotensin II, a hormone that constricts blood vessels and increases body fluid volume through its impact on the kidney; blocking angiotensin II stops these effects, which reduces blood pressure and chronic changes in the heart that lead to heart failure
Angiotensin-receptor blockers (ARBs)	▪ candesartan (Atacand) ▪ losartan (Cozaar) ▪ valsartan (Diovan)	Block angiotensin II receptors, preventing the angiotensin II hormone from exerting its negative effects on blood pressure and heart remodeling as stated above for ACE inhibitors
Antiplatelets	▪ aspirin ▪ clopidogrel (Plavix) ▪ prasugrel (Effient) ▪ ticagrelor (Brilinta)	Prevent platelets from forming clots
HMG-CoA reductase inhibitors**	▪ atorvastatin (Lipitor) ▪ rosuvastatin (Crestor)	Decrease cholesterol and the formation of coronary artery plaques

* Medication examples presented in alphabetical order as "generic name (Brand Name)."

** More commonly referred to as "statins."

functions. As it relates to Mr. Denton, Ellen, a trusted member of the team, will begin by ensuring that he has been prescribed the appropriate regimen of five medications mentioned above, and that each is dosed appropriately. Next, she will check these medications against others he may take to confirm the absence of drug-drug interactions. Perhaps the most important step is the one that was missed in this case; namely, medication education. Had she had the opportunity, Ellen would have sat down with Mr. and Mrs. Denton to review educational materials, taught them how each drug works, what side effects to look out for, and how to react if a side effect or adverse drug event is experienced. The goal is to empower patients with knowledge, promote medication adherence and patient safety, and to prevent poor health outcomes. Unfortunately, Ellen was having an unusually busy day. A pharmacist called in sick and Ellen was covering an additional group of patients. This extra workload contributed to a breakdown in her typical workflow. As a result, as depicted throughout the illustrated case, Ellen was being pulled in multiple directions.

Thorough patient education upon discharge has been shown to improve medication adherence and may decrease hospital readmissions and death in patients who recently experienced an MI.[18,70] Knowing how to react to side effects or adverse drug events is not trivial. One in five patients discharged from the hospital will experience an adverse event, and over 70% of these are related to medications.[71] Taken in combination, as recommended, BBs and ACEIs can lead to excessive blood pressure lowering, which can lead to a host of side effects.[72,73] While dual antiplatelet therapy is critical to prevent clots and protect stents, it can also lead to excessive bleeding.[61] Patients need to know the signs and symptoms of bleeding that require medical attention, as well as what to do if they experience an injury; for example, a fall that results in head trauma.

Inefficiencies in coordination between Ellen, Chris, and Mr. Denton's physician begin to show in Illustration 1-3. Here, it is revealed that 45 minutes have elapsed since Chris first shared with Ellen Mr. Denton's strong desire to be discharged. And it has been nearly 3 hours since Mr. Denton's physician set the expectation in Illustration 1-1 that his discharge would happen quickly. Illustration 1-3 reveals that Ellen was waiting on discharge paperwork from Mr. Denton's physician, which she needs to be completed in order to finish his medication review and prepare medication education materials. Like Ellen and Chris, Mr. Denton's physician likely intended to complete this, but then had her attention pulled in a different direction from any number of potential competing responsibilities, emergencies, and/or distractions. Fifteen minutes after Ellen's call with Mr. Denton's physician, Chris' call to Ellen depicted at the bottom of Illustration 1-3 reveals that Ellen has yet to complete her tasks. Meanwhile, in Illustration 1-4, Mr. Denton's frustration has reached a tipping point, and he is preparing to leave the hospital for home.

Illustrations 1-3 and 1-4 take place during a critically important time in Mr. Denton's hospital stay, referred to as a transition of care. Upon his return home, Mr. Denton will be scheduled for a series of follow-up medical appointments, including with a cardiologist, a primary care provider, and a cardiac rehabilitation program. This transition of care period, and more specifically the discharge process immediately prior to it, is a pivotal point for pharmacist involvement and strong team communication.[61] Effective discharge planning should be completed early and interprofessionally. It should also include follow-up planning, focused education sessions with the patient and their family/caregivers, and distribution of the follow-up plan with the patient's primary care provider.[18] Social workers, nurses, physicians, and pharmacists should have early discussions on what procedure Mr. Denton was having, what his living situation is, and what barriers to treatment he might have, as examples. High-performing hospitals utilize an interprofessional approach to the discharge process and education for patients with MI.

Stopping evidence-based medications for MI shortly after discharge has been associated with negative health outcomes, including recurrent MI, heart failure, and death.[61,74] Patients must receive medication counseling prior to discharge to ensure they understand how important medications are to prevent these outcomes. In addition to covering each medication's purpose, and common and/or serious adverse effects, the consequences of non-adherence to medications should also be directly addressed at this time. Had he not left the hospital prior to meeting with Ellen, Mr. Denton would have learned strategies to address the side effects he ultimately experienced, as well as how dangerous stopping these medications would be. That is not to say that Mr. Denton's poor outcome was his fault. He has every right to be frustrated, upset, scared about the future, and just plain ready to get home. Many patients do not like being in the hospital. They do not sleep well and they feel constantly poked and prodded. Patients experience increased stress and anxiety in the hospital.[75] It is important for the interprofessional team to recognize these feelings as they can have a direct and deleterious impact on patient care and health outcomes.

The American Heart Association and the American College of Cardiology Foundation recommend improved communication among the healthcare team providing care for MI patients.[58] National patient safety standards specifically include effective communication among physicians, pharmacists, and nurses to ensure comprehensive care.[76] They also draw attention to the need to address medication reconciliation and careful transitions between care settings. Hospitals that do not implement these safety standards may be penalized for avoidable hospital readmissions.[61,77] Failure to meet these standards can affect a hospital's reimbursement for services as well as its accreditation status, both of which are vitally important to the function of a hospital.[78] Providing the right medications to MI patients at discharge is considered a core requirement.[77]

In Illustration 1-5, Mr. Denton's thoughts reveal his struggles with headache, stomach pain, and fatigue. These represent common side effects of the combination of medications prescribed for patients with a history of MI. Fatigue is a common side effect of BBs.[72] Stomach upset is a common side effect of antiplatelet therapy.[79,80] Headache could be caused by one of the antiplatelets, by the BB, or the ACEI.[72,73,80] Mr. Denton considered these side effects to be severe enough to warrant stopping the medications. Because he did not have the appropriate medication counseling regarding the significant benefit of these medications on his cardiac health, he judged the negative side effects to outweigh any perceived benefit.

Unfortunately, this decision is not uncommon. Discontinuation rates for MI medications 1 month after discharge can be as high as 30% and can result in increased mortality.[74] Mr. Denton stopped all of his medications with the outcome of having a second MI due to restenosis of the stent. Illustration 1-6 shows Mr. Denton in the cath lab getting ready to receive a second PCI to open the stent that has failed. This specific complication is most likely due to stopping his antiplatelet therapy. The antiplatelet regimen of aspirin and clopidogrel together decreases the risk of restenosis.[81] Stopping these medications led to an emergent, life-threatening complication. It can be inferred, as well, that Mr. Denton did not have an established relationship with a community pharmacist. This is unfortunate, as a community pharmacist could have helped to troubleshoot the side effects he experienced and work with Mr. Denton's prescribers to optimize his medication regimen. Those interested in further exploring how Mr. Denton might have benefited from such a relationship are encouraged to read Chapter 2 Community Pharmacy and the illustrated cases "Organized Chaos" and "Breathe."

Acute MI is a life-threatening heart condition that requires prompt and effective clinical intervention. Once stabilized, it is critical for patients to take several medications that have been shown to prevent recurrent events and negative downstream health effects, such as the development of heart failure. The importance of cardiology pharmacists ensuring the safe and effective use of medications during this period cannot be overstated. Furthermore, the days immediately following an acute MI can be understandably difficult for patients, and teams of health professionals must effectively coordinate their efforts to minimize the stress, frustration, and confusion that can jeopardize patients' health. The illustrated case "Breakdown" demonstrates a series of unintentional and unfortunate events that draw attention to issues with interprofessional teamwork and communication that nearly resulted in the loss of life. The experience of Mr. Denton in this illustrated case highlights that when it comes to health, interprofessional teamwork is as serious as a heart attack.

DISCUSSION QUESTIONS FOR "BREAKDOWN"

1. In Illustration 1-1, Mr. Denton is told that someone will be in shortly to educate him on lifestyle changes and medications. What are some reasons that might explain why Mr. Denton's physician chose not to name a specific health professional in this situation?

2. What steps do you think this hospital might employ to ensure that situations like Mr. Denton's do not recur?

3. This illustrated case is titled "Breakdown." Where do you think the primary breakdown in interprofessional teamwork occurred? What factors led to this breakdown? How could it have been avoided?

4. Mr. Denton waited roughly 3 hours before leaving the hospital without completing the full discharge process. Think about your own experience with hospital care, or that of a family member. Reflecting on this experience, does Mr. Denton's decision seem understandable or inexcusable to you? Why?

5. Refer back to Table 1-2. If you could pick one health professional from this list to incorporate into Mr. Denton's interprofessional team, who would it be, and why?

CHAPTER SUMMARY

- Pharmacists practice in collaboration with an array of health professionals and serve as medication experts, advocating for the safe and effective use of medications on behalf of patients, families, and caregivers.

- Interprofessional practice, defined by the World Health Organization and endorsed throughout the United States, occurs when multiple health workers from different professional backgrounds work together with patients, families, caregivers, and communities to deliver the highest quality of care.

- There is growing evidence that interprofessional teams with pharmacists embedded have improved medication-related outcomes in multiple healthcare settings.

- The ultimate goal of interprofessional practice is to improve the patient experience of care, population health outcomes, and health professionals' satisfaction with their work, while reducing healthcare costs.

- Heart disease is the leading cause of death in the United States, and a leading contributor to hospitalizations.

- Myocardial infarctions, commonly referred to as heart attacks, are a life-threatening manifestation of heart disease that results in a medical emergency requiring complex, coordinated, interprofessional care.

- Pharmacists' contributions to the interprofessional care of patients who have experienced a myocardial infarction involve optimizing medication selection and dosing, preventing drug-drug interactions and other adverse drug events, and educating patients on their medications in order to empower them with knowledge, promote adherence and patient safety, and prevent poor health outcomes.

- For patients who experience life-altering health events requiring hospitalization, the discharge process represents a pivotal time period, and interprofessional practice in pharmacy is vitally important to optimize health outcomes.

REFERENCES

1. Accreditation Council for Pharmacy Education. *Accreditation Standards and Key Elements for the Professional Program in Pharmacy Leading to the Doctor of Pharmacy Degree. Standards 2016.* Chicago, IL: Accreditation Council for Pharmacy Education; 2015.
2. World Health Organization (WHO). *Framework for Action on Interprofessional Education and Collaborative Practice.* Geneva: World Health Organization; 2010. Available at http://www.who.int/hrh/resources/framework_action/en/. Accessed May 30, 2020.
3. Interprofessional Education Collaborative. *Core Competencies for Interprofessional Collaborative Practice: 2016 Update.* Washington, DC: Interprofessional Education Collaborative; 2016.
4. Health Professions Accreditors Collaborative. *Guidance on Developing Quality Interprofessional Education for the Health Professions.* Chicago, IL: Health Professions Accreditors Collaborative; 2019.
5. Interprofessional Education Collaborative. Available at https://www.ipecollaborative.org/. Accessed May 17, 2020.
6. Health Professions Accreditors Collaborative. Available at https://healthprofessionsaccreditors.org/. Accessed May 17, 2020.
7. National Center for Interprofessional Practice and Education. Available at https://nexusipe.org/. Accessed May 17, 2020.
8. National Academy of Medicine. Available at https://nam.edu/. Accessed May 17, 2020.
9. National Academies of Practice. Available at https://www.napractice.org/. Accessed May 17, 2020.
10. National Collaborative for Improving the Clinical Learning Environment. Available at https://www.ncicle.org/. Accessed May 17, 2020.
11. How pharmacists can improve our nation's health. Centers for Disease Control and Prevention Public Health Grand Rounds. Available at https://www.cdc.gov/grand-rounds/pp/2014/20141021-pharmacist-role.html. Accessed May 7, 2020.
12. American College of Clinical Pharmacy. Comprehensive medication management in team-based care. Available at www.accp.com/docs/positions/misc/CMM%20Brief.pdf. Accessed May 9, 2020.
13. National Conference of State Legislatures. Scope of practice archive database. Available at https://www.ncsl.org/research/health/scope-of-practice-overview.aspx. Accessed May 23, 2020.
14. American Pharmacists Association Foundation and American Pharmacists Association. Consortium recommendations for advancing pharmacists' patient care services and collaborative practice agreements. *J Am Pharm Assoc.* 2013;53:e132-e141.
15. American Pharmacists Association Foundation. Collaborative practice agreements (CPA) and pharmacists' patient care services. Available at https://www.aphafoundation.org/collaborative-practice-agreements. Accessed May 23, 2020.
16. Enthoven AC. Integrated delivery systems: the cure for fragmentation. *Am J Manag Care.* 2009;15:S284-S290.
17. van Leijen-Zeelenberg JE, van Raak AJ, Duimel-Peeters IG, et al. Interprofessional communication failures in acute care chains: how can we identify the causes? *J Interprof Care.* 2015;29:320-330.
18. Cherlin EJ, Curry LA, Thompson JW, et al. Features of high quality discharge planning for patients following acute myocardial infarction. *J Gen Intern Med.* 2012;28:436-443.
19. Marcum ZA, Driessen J, Thorpe CT, Gellad WF, Donohue JM. Impact of multiple pharmacy use on medication adherence and drug-drug interactions in older adults with Medicare Part D. *J Am Geriatr Soc.* 2014;62:244-252.
20. Viswanathan M, Golin CE, Jones CD, et al. Interventions to improve adherence to self-administered medications for chronic diseases in the United States: a systematic review. *Ann Intern Med.* 2012;157:785-795.
21. Reeves S, Pelone F, Harrison R, Goldman J, Zwarenstein M. Interprofessional collaboration to improve professional practice and healthcare outcomes. *Cochrane Database Syst Rev.* 2017;22(6):CD000072.
22. Lutfiyya MN, Chang LF, McGrath C, Dana C, Lipsky MS. The state of the science of interprofessional collaborative practice: a scoping review of the patient health-related outcomes based literature published between 2010 and 2018. *PLoS One.* 2019;14(6):e0218578.
23. Uhlig PN, Doll J, Brandon K, et al. Interprofessional practice and education in clinical learning environments: frontlines perspective. *Acad Med.* 2018;93:1441-1444.

24. Dow A. *Handbook of Interprofessional Practice: A Guide for Interprofessional Education and Collaborative Care.* Dubuque, IA: Kendall Hunt; 2018.

25. Schmidt I, Claesson CB, Westerholm B, Nilsson LG, Svarstad BL. The impact of regular multidisciplinary team interventions on psychotropic prescribing in Swedish nursing homes. *J Am Geriatr Soc.* 1998;46:77-82.

26. Brandt B, Kitto S, Cervero RM. Untying the interprofessional gordian knot: the National Collaborative for Improving the Clinical Learning Environment. *Acad Med.* 2018;93:1437-1440.

27. Reeves S, Perrier L, Goldman J, Freeth D, Zwarenstein M. Interprofessional education: effects on professional practice and healthcare outcomes (update). *Cochrane Database Syst Rev.* 2013;28:CD002213.

28. Elenbass RM, Worthen DB. Transformation of a profession: an overview of the twentieth century. In: *Clinical Pharmacy in the United States: Transformation of a Profession.* Lenexa, KS: American College of Clinical Pharmacy; 2009:131-165.

29. Institute of Medicine. *Educating for the Health Team: Report of the Conference on the Interrelationship of Educational Programs for Health Professions.* Washington, DC: National Academy of Sciences; 1972.

30. Institute of Medicine. *To Err Is Human: Building a Safer Health System.* Washington, DC: National Academies Press; 1999.

31. Institute of Medicine. *Crossing the Quality Chasm: A New Health System for the 21st Century.* Washington, DC: National Academies Press; 2001.

32. Institute of Medicine. *Health Professions Education: A Bridge to Quality.* Washington, DC: National Academies Press; 2003.

33. American College of Clinical Pharmacy. Standards of practice for clinical pharmacists. *Pharmacotherapy.* 2014;34(8):794-797.

34. Murphy JE, Liles AM, Bingham AL, et al. Interprofessional education: principles and application. an update from the American College of Clinical Pharmacy. *J Am Coll Clin Pharm.* 2018;1:e17-e28.

35. Anderegg MD, Gums TH, Uribe L, Coffey CS, James PA, Carter BL. Physician-pharmacist collaborative management: narrowing the socioeconomic blood pressure gap. *Hypertension.* 2016;68:1314-1320.

36. Dixon DL, Sisson EM, Parod ED, Van Tassell BW, Nadpara PA, Carl D, Dow A. Pharmacist-physician collaborative care model and time to goal blood pressure in the uninsured population. *J Clin Hypertens.* 2018; 20:88-95.

37. Arana M, Harper L, Qin H, Mabrey J. Reducing length of stay, direct cost, and readmissions in total joint arthroplasty patients with an outcomes manager-led interprofessional team. *Orthop Nurs.* 2017;36:279-284.

38. Shrader S, Jernigan S, Nazir N, Zaudke J. Determining the impact of an interprofessional learning in practice model on learners and patients. *J Interprof Care.* 2018;13:1-8.

39. Who's who in a palliative care team. Available at https://www. betterhealth.vic.gov.au/health/servicesandsupport/whos-who-in-a-palliative-care-team. Accessed May 17, 2020.

40. Bodenheimer T, Sinsky C. From triple to quadruple aim: care of the patient requires care of the provider. *Ann Fam Med.* 2014;12:573-576.

41. Brandt B, Lutfiyya MN, King JA, Chioreso C. A scoping review of interprofessional collaborative practice and education using the lens of the triple aim. *J Interprof Care.* 2014;28(5):393-399.

42. Cox M, Cuff P, Brandt B, Reeves S, Zierler B. Measuring the impact of interprofessional education on collaborative practice and patient outcomes. *J Interprof Care.* 2016;30(1):1-3.

43. Matzke GR, Moczygemba LR, Williams KJ, Czar MJ, Lee WT. Impact of a pharmacist-physician collaborative care model on patient outcomes and health services utilization. *Am J Health Syst Pharm.* 2018;75:1039-1047.

44. Sisson EM, Dixon DL, Kildow DC, Van Tassell BW, Carl DE, Varghese D, Electricwala B, Carroll NV. Effectiveness of a pharmacist-physician team-based collaboration to improve long-term blood pressure control at an inner-city safety-net clinic. *Pharmacotherapy.* 2016;36:342-347.

45. Ledford JL, Hess R, Johnson FP. Impact of clinical pharmacist collaboration in patients beginning insulin pump therapy: a retrospective and cross-sectional analysis. *J Drug Assess.* 2013:19:81-86.

46. Nagelkerk J, Thompson ME, Bouthillier M, et al. Improving outcomes in adults with diabetes through an interprofessional collaborative practice program. *J Interprof Care.* 2018;32:4-13.

47. Bingham JT, Mallette JJ. Federal Bureau of Prisons clinical pharmacy program improves patient A1C. *J Am Pharm Assoc.* 2016;56(2):173-177.

48. Primary Care Collaborative. Patient-centered medical home: what is a patient-centered medical home (PCMH). Available at https://www.pcpcc.org/resource/patient-centered-medical-home-what-patient-centered-medical-home-pcmh. Accessed May 17, 2020.

49. Matzke GR, Czar M, Lee W, et al. Improving health of at risk rural patients: a collaborative care model. *Am J Health Syst Pharm.* 2016;73:1760-1768.

50. Sweiss K, Wirth SM, Sharp L, et al. Collaborative physician-pharmacist-managed multiple myeloma clinic improves guideline adherence and prevents treatment delays. *J Oncol Pract.* 2018;14:e674-e682.

51. Kumar SK, Vij R, Noga SJ, et al. Treating multiple myeloma patients with oral therapies. *Clin Lymphoma Myeloma Leuk.* 2017;17:243-251.

52. Accreditation Council for Pharmacy Education. Available at https://www.acpe-accredit.org/. Accessed May 4, 2020.

53. American Association of Colleges of Pharmacy. Pharmacy school admission requirements 2019–2020. Available at https://www.aacp.org/sites/default/files/2019-12/psar-19-20-table-6.pdf. Accessed May 9, 2020.

54. American Society of Health-System Pharmacists. Resident matching program. Available at http://natmatch.com/ashprmp/stats/2020applstats.pdf. Accessed May 7, 2020.

55. Board of Pharmacy Specialties. Available at https://www.bpsweb.org/. Accessed May 17, 2020.

56. Benjamin EJ, Muntner P, Alonso A, et al. Heart disease and stroke statistics-2019 update: a report from the American Heart Association. *Circulation.* 2019;139(10):e56-e528.

57. Anderson JL, Morrow DA. Acute myocardial infarction. *N Engl J Med.* 2017;376:2053-2064.

58. Reed GW, Rossi JE, Cannon CP. Acute myocardial infarction. *Lancet.* 2017;389:197-210.

59. Smith SC Jr., Benjamin EJ, Bonow RO, et al. AHA/ACCF secondary prevention and risk reduction therapy for patients with coronary and other atherosclerotic vascular disease: 2011 update: a guideline from the American Heart Association and American College of Cardiology Foundation endorsed by the World Health

Federation and the Preventive Cardiovascular Nurses Association. *J Am Coll Cardiol*. 2011:58:2432-2446.

60. Nitroglycerin [package insert]. Detroit, MI: Parke-Davis; 2018.

61. O'Gara PT, Kushner FG, Ascheim DD, et al. 2013 ACCF/AHA guideline for the management of ST-elevation myocardial infarction: a report of the American College of Cardiology Foundation/American Heart Association Task Force on Practice Guidelines. *J Am Coll Cardiol*. 2013;61:e139-e228.

62. Shah RU, Henry TD, Rutten-Ramos S, Gaberich RF, Tighiouart M, Bairey Merz CN. Increasing percutaneous coronary interventions for ST-segment elevation myocardial infarction in the United States: progress and opportunity. *JACC Cardiology Interv*. 2015;8:139-146.

63. Heart and Stroke Foundation of Canada. Percutaneous coronary intervention (PCI or angioplasty with stent). Available at https://www.heartandstroke.ca/heart/treatments/surgery-and-other-procedures/percutaneous-coronary-intervention. Accessed May 16, 2020.

64. Mosterd A, Hoes AW. Clinical epidemiology of heart failure. *Heart*. 2007;93:1137-1146.

65. Yusuf S, Zhao F, Mehta SR, Chrolavicius S, Tognoni G, Fox KK, and the Clopidogrel in Unstable Angina to Prevent Recurrent Events Trial Investigators. Effects of clopidogrel in addition to aspirin in patients with acute coronary syndromes without ST-segment elevation. *N Engl J Med*. 2001;345:494-502.

66. Steinhubl SR, Berger PB, Mann JT 3rd, et al, and the CREDO Investigators. Clopidogrel for the reduction of events during observation. Early and sustained dual oral antiplatelet therapy following percutaneous coronary intervention: a randomized controlled trial. *JAMA*. 2002;288:2411-2420.

67. Freemantle N, Cleland J, Young P, Mason J, Harrison J. Beta blockade after myocardial infarction: systematic review and meta regression analysis. *BMJ*. 1999;318:1730-1737.

68. Pfeffer MA, Braunwald E, Moyé LA, et al; the SAVE Investigators. Effect of captopril on mortality and morbidity in patients with left ventricular dysfunction after myocardial infarction: results of the Survival and Ventricular Enlargement Trial. *N Engl J Med*. 1992;327:669-677.

69. Cannon CP, Braunwald E, McCabe CH, et al. Intensive versus moderate lipid lowering with statins after acute coronary syndromes. *N Engl J Med*. 2004;350:1495-1504.

70. Schnipper JL, Kirwin JL, Cotugno MC, et al. Role of pharmacist counseling in preventing adverse drug events after hospitalization. *Arch Intern Med*. 2006;166:565-571.

71. American Pharmacists Association and American Society of Health-System Pharmacists. Improving care transitions: optimizing medication reconciliation. *J Am Pharm Assoc*. 2012;52(4):e43-e52.

72. Toprol-XL (metoprolol succinate) [package insert]. Parsippany, NJ: New American Therapeutics; 2016.

73. Prinivil (lisinopril) [package insert]. Kenilworth, NJ: Merck Sharp & Dohme Corp; 2019.

74. Ho PM, Spertus JA, Masoudi FA. Impact of medication therapy discontinuation on mortality after myocardial infarction. *Arch Intern Med*. 2006;166:1842-1847.

75. Baldwin KM, Spears MJ. Improving the patient experience and decreasing patient anxiety with nursing bedside report. *Clin Nurse Spec*. 2019;33:82-89.

76. National Quality Forum. Safe practices for healthcare 2010 update. Available at http://qualityforum.org/projects/safe_practices_2010.aspx. Accessed May 17, 2020.

77. Jneid H, Addison D, Bhatt DL, et al. 2017 AHA/ACC clinical performance and quality measures for adults with ST-elevation and non–ST-elevation myocardial infarction: a report of the American College of Cardiology/American Heart Association Task Force on Performance Measures. *Circ Cardiovasc Qual Outcomes*. 2017;10:e000032.

78. Mansukhani RP, Bridgeman MB, Candelario D, Eckert LJ. Exploring transitional care: evidence-based strategies for improving provider communication and reducing readmissions. *P T*. 2015;40:690-694.

79. Aspirin [package insert]. Mississauga, ON: Bayer Inc.; 2017.

80. Plavix (clopidogrel) [package insert]. Princeton, NJ: Bristol-Myers Squibb Sanofi Pharmaceuticals; 2019.

81. Chen ZM, Jiang LX, Chen YP, et al. Addition of clopidogrel to aspirin in 45,852 patients with acute myocardial infarction: randomised placebo-controlled trial. *Lancet*. 2005;366:1607-1621.

CHAPTER 2

Community Pharmacy

Featuring the Illustrated Case Studies "Organized Chaos," "Transformation," & "Breathe"

Authors

Edward C. Portillo, Tyler Ho, Melgardt M. de Villiers, & Joseph A. Zorek

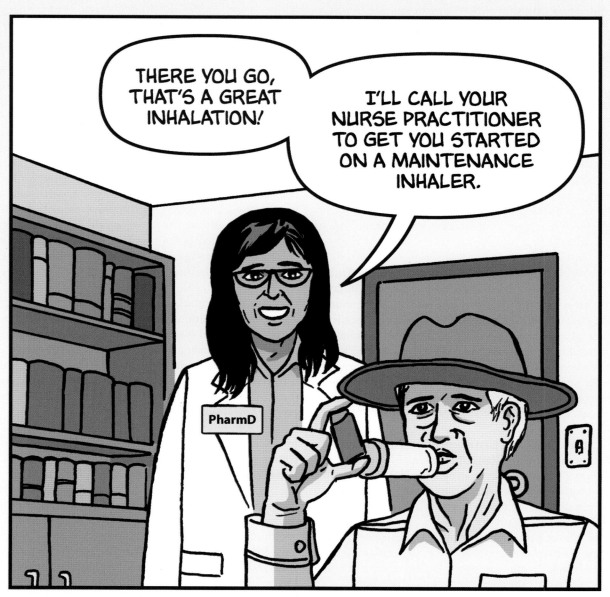

Illustration by George Folz, © 2019 Board of Regents of the University of Wisconsin System

BACKGROUND

Community pharmacists are the most accessible of all health professionals, a distinction that has led some to dub this segment of pharmacy the "face of neighborhood healthcare."[1-5] The positive impact that community pharmacists have on their patients and communities is evident and widespread within small towns and large cities alike.[2,6-10] Community pharmacists promote patient health and well-being by ensuring appropriate, safe, and effective medication use.[11] The role of pharmacists in community practice settings continues to expand well beyond the dispensing of prescription medications; this includes health screenings, medication therapy monitoring and management programs, vaccine administration (i.e., immunizations), and medication compounding services all tailored to the needs of individual patients and the communities within which they live.[12-14] Readers interested in health screenings and immunizations are encouraged to explore the illustrated cases "Screen" and "Mobilized," respectively, in Chapter 4 Prevention & Wellness, while those interested in compounding are referred to the illustrated case "Transformation" later in this chapter.

Community pharmacists practice in a diverse array of workplace settings that promote high accessibility to the public. Compared to other health professionals who may provide services by appointment and based on insurance coverage, community pharmacists are often positioned in public spaces such as grocery stores, large chain pharmacies, and independently owned drug stores.[15-17] It is somewhat unique that in the same grocery store where consumers shop for their bananas and bread, they can also quickly consult with a highly trained health professional without appointment, proof of insurance, or payment. This accessibility, where anyone can discuss medication-related questions on their schedule and at their convenience, places community pharmacists on the front lines of healthcare delivery.[18]

There are roughly 310,000 licensed pharmacists in the United States, with over 40% of these individuals practicing in community pharmacy settings.[9,19] Thirty-five percent of community pharmacies are independently owned, while 37% are considered larger chain pharmacy corporations. Another 14% of pharmacies are located in supermarkets and 14% are positioned within large retail stores.[19] Regardless of practice setting, community pharmacists serve the public as medication experts capable of providing comprehensive services to ensure the safe and effective use of medications.[8,20]

The impact that community pharmacists have on patient health and wellness cannot be overstated. In the United States, 4.1 billion prescriptions were filled at pharmacies in 2017 alone.[21] This equates to nearly one in two Americans having reported using a prescription drug in the past 30 days.[22] Among patients aged 60 to 79, prescription medication use increases even further with nearly 84% of patients having filled a recent prescription medication.[23] The vast majority of these prescriptions are filled at local pharmacies, with over 90% of prescriptions treating chronic conditions.[24,25] The ability to treat these conditions, such as heart disease and diabetes, with prescription medications has resulted in improved patient outcomes and increased longevity for our population as a whole.[26,27]

Community pharmacists also play a pivotal role ensuring the right patient receives the right drug, at the right dose, administered through the right route, and at the right time.[28] Medical errors are the third-leading cause of death in the United States, and medication errors constitute a large portion of these; specifically, roughly 1.3 million Americans are injured annually by medications.[29,30] To minimize the significant risk of medication error-induced harm, community pharmacists must consider the unique characteristics of each individual patient and their medications to evaluate risks and identify opportunities to improve patient well-being.[31] Through this process, community pharmacists have the opportunity to form meaningful, long-term relationships with patients, helping them ensure the appropriateness of their medications to minimize the risk of adverse drug events.[27]

Community Pharmacists' Contributions to Interprofessional Health Teams

Opportunities for community pharmacists to serve patients through innovative approaches in collaboration with other health professionals are plentiful, and many have been well described. Many of these evaluations demonstrate how the integration of pharmacists within care teams improves patient outcomes.[32] Community pharmacists have taken a lead role in the provision of medication therapy management (MTM) services, which involve focused visits between patients and pharmacists to advance effective medication use, opportunities for health behavior change (i.e., lifestyle improvements), and needed interventions and referrals to improve patients' overall well-being.[8] MTM services have been applied to help improve patient adherence to medications, and to help with management of chronic health conditions such as high blood pressure, elevated cholesterol, and diabetes, among others.

Community pharmacists often generate the most complete list of patients' medications, especially if patients are seen by multiple prescribers and specialists. Through MTM programs, a comprehensive medication review (CMR) helps to ensure patients have an accurate medication list.[8] The community pharmacist is then able to discuss potential interventions and referrals from these MTM visits with other health professionals on the interprofessional team.

In addition to evaluating for appropriate medication use, community pharmacists are heavily engaged in public health initiatives. All states have integrated pharmacists in providing vaccination services, and community pharmacists have taken the lead in administration of vaccines to improve public health.[33] As of 2018, immunizations were offered at 73% of community pharmacies nationwide, and these vaccinations have led to reduced death from diseases ranging from influenza and pneumonia to tetanus, diphtheria, and pertussis.[33,34] Pharmacists leverage legally binding, collaborative practice agreements with prescribers, mostly physicians, to provide immunizations to their patients.[35] In 40 states, pharmacists with appropriate training are able to administer injectable medications in addition to vaccines. Such activities lend themselves well to collaboration with prescribers for documentation and coordination of injection administration.[36,37] Pharmacists also often administer vaccinations outside of the pharmacy at health and wellness fairs, community events, and schools in collaboration with other health professionals to protect the community from vaccine-preventable illnesses.

COMMUNITY PHARMACISTS IN ACTION

Wellness within the Community Pharmacy

High blood pressure and elevated cholesterol both increase the risk for cardiovascular disease, which leads to one death every 39 seconds.[38] Unfortunately, blood pressure remains uncontrolled in 50% of the 68 million patients with a diagnosis of hypertension. Similarly, cholesterol readings remain elevated in close to 66% of the 71 million patients in the United States with dyslipidemia. Community pharmacists trained to serve the public as wellness coaches in 11 Missouri community pharmacies aimed to change these disheartening statistics.[39] Community pharmacist wellness coaches engaged with patients every 1 to 2 months to improve cholesterol, hypertension, diabetes, or weight management. Patients received a health screening at the beginning of this intervention, and completed sessions in a private room within the community pharmacy with their pharmacist coach. These sessions lasted up to 60 minutes in length and resulted in statistically significant improvements in cholesterol levels and diastolic blood pressure. Fasting blood glucose readings in diabetic patients also significantly improved, which has been shown to additionally reduce risk of poor cardiovascular outcomes.[39]

This evaluation is unique in that wellness care occurred on-site at the community pharmacy, and community pharmacists used point-of-care testing (POCT) devices to provide patients with quick access to their health data. POCT facilitates quicker decision-making by allowing completion of laboratory tests at the locations where patients receive healthcare rather than in laboratories. This provides the opportunity for quick, patient-centered decision-making to improve health, including through maximizing medication use, without delay waiting for test results.[40] In the spirit of interprofessional teamwork, this team of community pharmacist wellness coaches developed a process to share POCT results with the other members of the healthcare team to speed care coordination, promote the team-based approach, and demonstrate the critical role of pharmacists within this team.[39]

Pharmacists Fight COVID-19 Pandemic

Coronavirus Disease 2019 (COVID-19), caused by the deadly virus SARS-CoV-2, generated widespread disruption to the lives of people across the globe, with sweeping closures of schools and universities, businesses, and mass cancellations of domestic and international travel in an attempt to stave off the spread of this deadly disease.[41-43] As life began to abruptly change for so many people, urgent plans needed to be made to slow the rampant spread of COVID-19, and the need for testing large numbers of patients emerged.[44] Community pharmacies embedded within the fabric of neighborhoods across the United States sprung into action. Walmart, CVS Health, Walgreens, and Target began collaborating with the White House to determine how best to leverage their stores and pharmacies to increase access to, and speed of, COVID-19 testing.[45] As COVID-19 became a national emergency, community pharmacists continued to serve as the lifeline for patients needing just-in-time care.[46,47] Community pharmacists and pharmacies served on the front line of this global pandemic and provided care to patients through effective triaging of patients with symptoms and answered medication questions. Community pharmacists also coordinated with prescribers' offices to increase the supply of medications dispensed for patients at risk for medication shortages.[47]

The engagement of pharmacists to serve patients during national and global health emergencies is clear, and will likely only continue to increase. The American Society of Health System Pharmacists (ASHP) has released guidance urging lawmakers to swiftly expand community pharmacists' abilities to administer vaccinations, complete POCT, initiate time-sensitive antiviral therapies, and increase opportunities for pharmacist reimbursement for caring for patients with infectious diseases.[48] Through the COVID-19 pandemic, the critical role of community pharmacists has demonstrated the need for increased pharmacist involvement in coordination and planning for emergency responses.[48] For an additional example of pharmacists engaged in an emergency response, see the illustrated case "Mobilized" in Chapter 4 Prevention & Wellness.

BECOMING A COMMUNITY PHARMACIST

The Doctor of Pharmacy (PharmD) degree is required for entry-level community pharmacy practice.[49] This involves completion of 3 to 4 years of professional training at a college or school of pharmacy accredited by the Accreditation Council for Pharmacy Education (ACPE). After receiving a PharmD degree, applicants must pass a national licensure exam called the North American Pharmacist Licensure Examination (NAPLEX) as well as a Multistate Pharmacy Jurisprudence Examination (MPJE) to demonstrate expertise in federal and state laws governing pharmacy practice.[50,51]

Additional opportunities are available for PharmD graduates to gain advanced training in community pharmacy practice, including postgraduate year 1 (PGY-1) residency training programs in community pharmacy.[52] These residencies are typically 1 year in length and provide participants with advanced training that includes direct mentorship by community pharmacists in leadership endeavors, development and implementation of patient care services, and teaching opportunities, among other activities. The experience gained during this year of training is often considered equal to 3 to 5 years of practice experience.

For pharmacists who desire additional credentialing to demonstrate expertise, the Board of Pharmacy Specialties (BPS) has designated a program for becoming a Board Certified Ambulatory Care Pharmacist (BCACP).[53] Written examination for this certification is available to actively licensed individuals who have graduated from an ACPE-accredited pharmacy program (or its international equivalent), and have either (a) completed 4 years of practice experience with at least 50% of time focused on described ambulatory care content; (b) completed a PGY-1 residency, plus 2 years of practice experience with at least 50% of time focused on ambulatory care content; or (c) completed a PGY-2 residency in ambulatory care pharmacy. After passing the BCACP examination, individuals are certified to use the BCACP credential for a period of 7 years, with recertification contingent upon either (a) earning 100 hours of continuing education credit provided by a BPS-approved entity, or (b) passing a 100-item recertification examination administered by BPS.

As community pharmacy practice evolves, community pharmacists must stay up to date on advancement of new therapies and opportunities to improve patient care.[54] Many national pharmacy associations exist to provide support for this information, including the National Community Pharmacist Association (NCPA) and the American Pharmacists Association (APhA).[55,56] Through attending national meetings, engaging in workgroups emphasizing specific areas of community practice, and maintaining up-to-date knowledge of emerging areas of care, community pharmacists remain well-positioned as widely accessible health professionals equipped to make widespread positive impact.

ORGANIZED CHAOS: An Illustrated Case Study

Story by Tyler Ho & Joseph A. Zorek
Illustrations by George Folz, © 2019 Board of Regents of the University of Wisconsin System

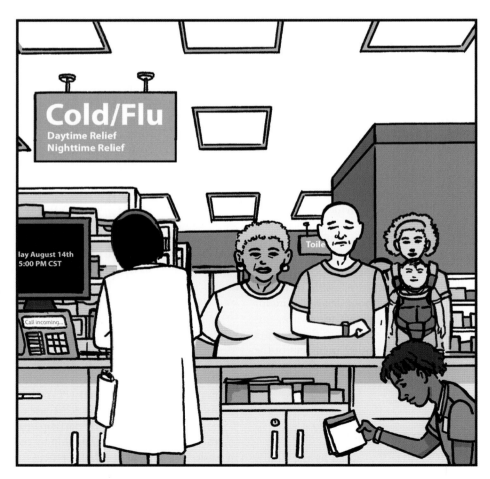

Illustration 2-1

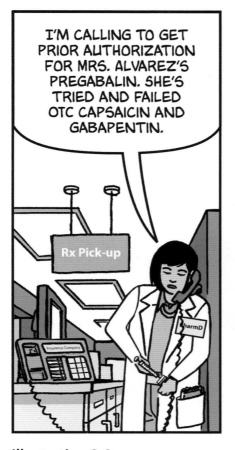
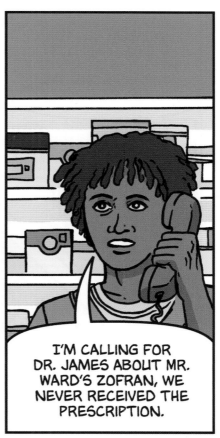

Illustration 2-2

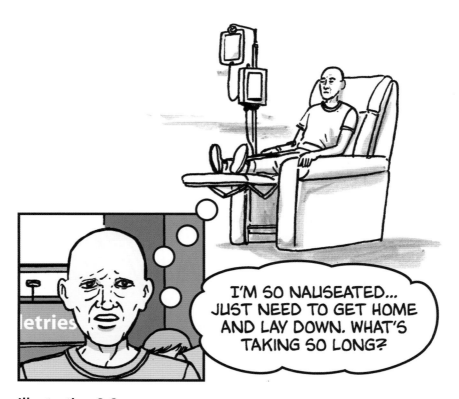

Illustration 2-3

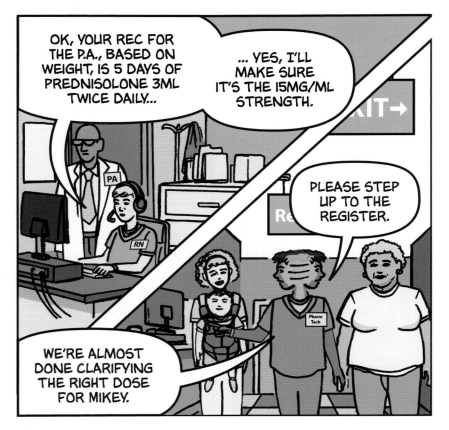

Illustration 2-4

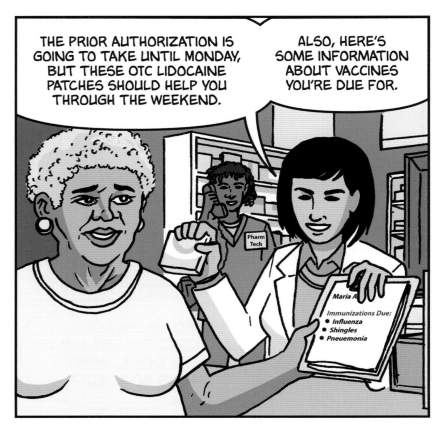

Illustration 2-5

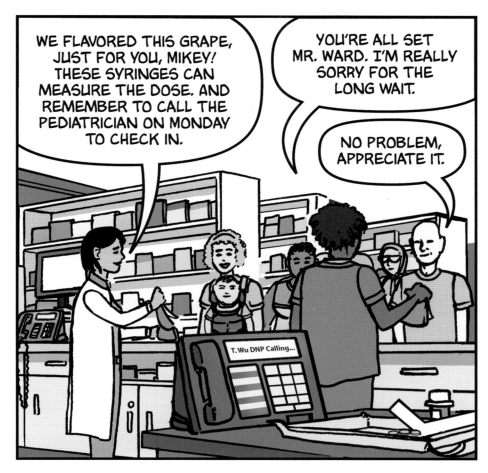

Illustration 2-6

Thoughts on "Organized Chaos"

The ubiquity of community pharmacies conceals their complexity.[57] Hidden by an unassuming appearance, with drive-thru windows and walk-up counters, community pharmacies stand as one of the most critical and important pillars of the US healthcare system. The economic impact of community pharmacies, and community pharmacists by proxy, is staggering. In 2017, it was estimated that the top three community pharmacy retail chains (CVS, Walgreens, and Walmart) accounted for $138 billion in revenue.[22] The same report highlighted that over 4 billion prescriptions were filled in 2017, directly impacting the lives and health of nearly 200 million Americans. The ease with which everyday Americans can access the knowledge and skills of their community pharmacist surely drives this value; in fact, one study showed that patients see their pharmacist up to 10 times more frequently than they see their primary care physician.[58] Another study showed that 90% of Americans live within 2 miles of a community pharmacy.[9] Opportunities for frequent contact that result from this combination of proximity and accessibility perhaps explain why pharmacy is consistently rated among the most trusted professions.[59]

Community pharmacists' roles are dynamic and complex, requiring an impressive breadth of skills and depth of knowledge. A core function of all community pharmacists is to serve as a liaison between patients, prescribers (e.g., physicians, physician assistants, nurse practitioners, and dentists), and payers (e.g., insurance companies). This involves negotiating and advocating on behalf of patients. It is the community pharmacist who stands as the last health professional between a patient and a serious drug interaction, or a child and a miscalculated dose. It is the community pharmacist who must deliver difficult news from insurers; for example, that a needed medication is not covered and, thus, the patient will have to pay the full price out-of-pocket. And it is the community pharmacist who, while calling the child's physician to correct the miscalculated dose and the insurer to figure out a cost-effective option, must also establish an alternative medication supply for a drug that has been recalled, or might be unavailable due to a shortage. While these activities are challenging, they also create opportunities to help patients and families, and are professionally rewarding.

The illustrated case "Organized Chaos" attempts to capture as much of this complexity as possible during a typical day in a community pharmacy. This pharmacy, run by a pharmacist (white coat) with support from a pharmacy technician (green scrubs), is a hub of interprofessional practice. The pharmacy technician shown in Illustration 2-2 is calling an oncology (i.e., cancer) clinic to obtain a prescription from a physician on behalf of a patient, Mr. Ward (Illustration 2-3). Meanwhile, Illustration 2-4 depicts a telephone exchange between the pharmacist, a nurse, and a physician assistant at a pediatrician's office in order to correct the dose of an oral steroid, prednisolone, to treat an asthma exacerbation of a 15-month-old child named Mikey. While Illustration 2-6 brings closure for Mr. Ward and Mikey, an incoming call from a nurse practitioner (i.e., DNP, Doctor of Nursing Practice) introduces an unknown opportunity for the pharmacist to improve medication use and health outcomes through interprofessional practice. Readers interested in learning more about the role of oncology pharmacists are encouraged to explore the illustrated cases "Compromising" and "Compassion" in Chapter 9 Oncology. For more information on asthma and pharmacists' roles helping patients/families manage this condition, see the illustrated case "Swish" in Chapter 3 Primary Care.

As the last line of defense for the safe and effective use of medications, and often the first opportunity for patients to vent, community pharmacists require a diverse set of skills. They must be able to maintain a razor-sharp focus on fine details while balancing multiple tasks and distractions, as the placement of a decimal point on a prescription order can mean the difference between the right dose and an overdose.[60] Having learned Mikey's weight from his mother, the pharmacist intervenes in Illustration 2-4 to ensure he receives the right dose.

Much of the work community pharmacists do to ensure effective and safe medication use takes place behind the counter, out of view, and under time constraints/pressure. The illustrated case "Organized Chaos" is set on a Friday afternoon at 5:00 p.m. to capture this dynamic, with a line of patients queuing just as doctor's offices are about to close for the weekend. For Mr. Ward, it appears that the oncology clinic has sent the electronic prescription order for his anti-nausea medication ondansetron (Zofran) to the wrong pharmacy, or accidentally under the wrong patient's name. As the pharmacy technician works to address this, the pharmacist works to obtain clearance for Mrs. Alvarez to obtain the correct drug. She has lived with type 2 diabetes for many years. Unfortunately, this has left her with a condition called diabetic neuropathy, which is caused by nerve damage that manifests as painful stinging, tingling, or burning, typically beginning in the feet or lower legs.[61] Having just recently turned 65, Mrs. Alvarez receives prescription coverage through Medicare Part D, and there are certain conditions that must be met for her to obtain the new medication prescribed by her physician called pregabalin (Lyrica). Illustration 2-2 shows the pharmacist working through these conditions with the Part D insurance company. For more information on type 2 diabetes, see the illustrated cases "Holistic" and "Screen" in Chapter 3 Primary Care and Chapter 4 Prevention & Wellness, respectively. Readers interested in prescription insurance coverage are encouraged to explore the illustrated case "Relapse" in Chapter 14 Population Health.

The incredible accessibility of community pharmacies has real consequences for workflow. The pharmacist and technician in "Organized Chaos" are operating primarily in a reactionary mode; that is, they are solving problems that likely would have been unknown to them just a few hours before. At any given time, community pharmacists must be prepared for their time and attention to get pulled in any number of different directions, including responsibilities to meet the performance metrics of employers.[62] They must be flexible, capable of multitasking, and able to communicate effectively with patients, their staff, and other health professionals. Community pharmacists also proactively perform professional activities to optimize patients' health and avoid medication errors. This includes offering vaccinations and CMRs.[63] This book is replete with CMR examples; for more information on this topic, as well as examples of community pharmacists providing CMRs, readers are encouraged to explore the illustrated cases "Breathe" in this chapter and "Barriers" in Chapter 12 Mental Health.

Vaccinations to protect against infections such as influenza (i.e., the flu) highlight one example of community pharmacist proactivity. Standing at the end of the line in Illustration 2-1, behind Mikey's mother, is a patient preparing for his freshman year of college who has an appointment to receive his second meningitis B vaccine (MenB). While the pharmacist is on the phone helping Mrs. Alvarez obtain pregabalin, she can be seen drawing up this patient's vaccine into a syringe for administration. Later, in Illustration 2-5, Mrs. Alvarez receives guidance and advice about three vaccines she is scheduled to receive, based on age or other indications. These vaccines are the annual influenza (offered to all patients over 6 months old) and the pneumococcal and shingles (offered to patients over 65). State laws dictate specific vaccines pharmacists can administer, as well as other parameters such as age requirements.[64] Many insurers, including Medicare and Medicaid, cover some or all costs of vaccines administered in community pharmacies.[65] Importantly, community pharmacists have improved vaccination rates across the United States.[66] For more information on MenB and other types of vaccinations, see the illustrated case "Mobilized" in Chapter 4 Prevention & Wellness.

In order to prepare for an unpredictable workflow, it is essential for community pharmacists to have good management skills. For example, training, scheduling, and conducting performance evaluations of staff, such as pharmacy technicians, is vital to success. Equally important is the maintenance of accurate pill counts for inventory purposes and documentation processes, like those required for controlled substances dispensed. Readers interested in the interface of community pharmacy and controlled substance use/misuse are encouraged to explore the illustrated case "Gasping" in Chapter 12 Mental Health.

Community pharmacy staffing models may vary widely depending on services offered and prescription volume, among other factors.[67] This is complicated by variability in state laws that govern pharmacy practice; for example, the number of pharmacy technicians who can work under the supervision of a licensed pharmacist at any given time.[68] As seen in Illustration 2-1, this pharmacy has one pharmacist and one pharmacy technician working closely together, which is a common arrangement for many sites with a lower volume of prescription sales. As prescription volume and the complexity of services provided grow, the pharmacy may choose to expand the number of staff assisting the pharmacist.

The core roles of pharmacy technicians include preparing prescriptions, submitting insurance claims, and communicating with patients and providers.[69] Pharmacy technicians are the lifeblood of any community pharmacy and the key to success and efficiency. Technician roles are expanding at many sites as pharmacists take on more nontraditional tasks such as offering vaccinations and CMRs, as described above. National credentialing programs have been created in recent years to support the professional development and training of pharmacy technicians. One credential, called the "Certified Pharmacy Technician," or CPhT for short, is offered by the Pharmacy Technician Certification Board (PTCB) and the National Healthcareer Association (NHA).[70] Many pharmacies require CPhT credentialing for technicians to perform advanced duties, which studies show are overwhelmingly welcomed by technicians.[71,72] Students preparing for application to pharmacy school are encouraged to gain pharmacy technician experience in any pharmacy setting.[73,74]

Another essential duty of a community pharmacist is inventory management, as the satisfaction of patients and financial health of the business depend on having medications available when they are needed. Pharmacists must keep shelves stocked with essential medications while maintaining fiscally responsible inventory levels.[75] This task is complicated by differences in the value of medications, which can range from pennies per pill to over $60,000 per month of therapy.[76]

Drug shortages and recalls are prime examples of the barriers pharmacists face when trying to keep medications in stock. Shortages occur when a medication is out of stock at a pharmacy's wholesaler, often with no resolution date in sight.[77] This can lead to delays in patients receiving necessary treatments, or may necessitate changing a patient's therapy to a different medication that may be less effective or, in some cases, more expensive.[78] Drug recalls, on the other hand, are a safety mechanism in place to ensure the public is not exposed to defective or dangerous medications.[79] Recent recalls include commonly used medications such as those designed to lower blood pressure and reduce heartburn, both of which have been found to be contaminated by a potential carcinogenic (i.e., cancer-causing) substance.[80,81] Those interested in learning more about drug shortages are encouraged to read the illustrated case "Interconnected" in Chapter 14 Population Health.

Community pharmacists perform critically important functions for society. On any given day, in any given city, a patient with a prescription can walk into any given pharmacy, with no advance warning, and walk out with medication in hand *and*, if they desire, personalized advice from a medication expert with a doctorate degree. The community pharmacist, working with one or more pharmacy technicians, would have squeezed this patient into their workflow and troubleshot any number of potential issues, mostly out-of-sight and unbeknownst to the patient. The illustrated case "Organized Chaos" attempts to capture a day in the life of a busy community pharmacy doing just that. In the span of about an hour, the pharmacist and pharmacy technician collaborate with one another, as well as a physician, physician assistant, nurse practitioner, nurse, and insurance company, to (1) prevent a pediatric overdose, (2) administer a vaccine, (3) acquire an anti-nausea medication for a patient who just completed a round of chemotherapy, and (4) advocate for a patient to obtain a medication capable of controlling pain from diabetic neuropathy. To grasp the magnitude of community pharmacists' impact on the US healthcare system, one need only multiply the individual positive effects captured in "Organized Chaos" by the billions of outpatient prescriptions filled annually.[22]

DISCUSSION QUESTIONS FOR "ORGANIZED CHAOS"

1. When examining the skills associated with high-quality community pharmacy practice, multitasking and communication were highlighted. What other skills or characteristics do you think might help a community pharmacist succeed?

2. The accessibility of community pharmacists was emphasized as an important benefit to patients and communities. What services beyond dispensing medications can you imagine a community pharmacist might perform to leverage this accessibility and improve health outcomes?

3. In Illustration 2-3, a patient who recently completed a chemotherapy session is shown thinking to himself, "What's taking so long?" Clearly exhausted and feeling ill, it is unclear what, if anything, the pharmacist or pharmacy technician did to accommodate his needs. What could, or should, they have done in this situation?

4. The expanding role of pharmacy technicians was touched upon in this example. How might requiring national certification and the expansion of pharmacy technician roles and responsibilities impact the practice of community pharmacy?

5. The illustrated case "Organized Chaos" attempted to capture the fast pace, pressure, and challenges that are typical in community pharmacies. What was your reaction to these aspects of the case? What are potential positives and negatives associated with a work environment like this?

TRANSFORMATION: An Illustrated Case Study

Story by Melgardt M. de Villiers & Joseph A. Zorek
Illustrations by George Folz, © 2019 Board of Regents of the University of Wisconsin System

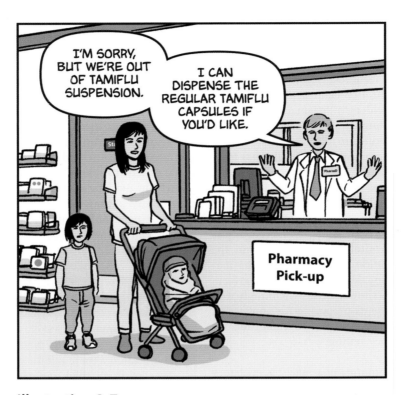

Illustration 2-7

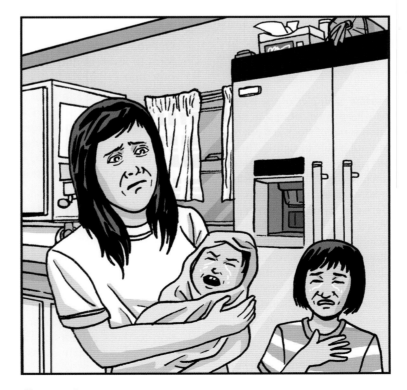

Illustration 2-8

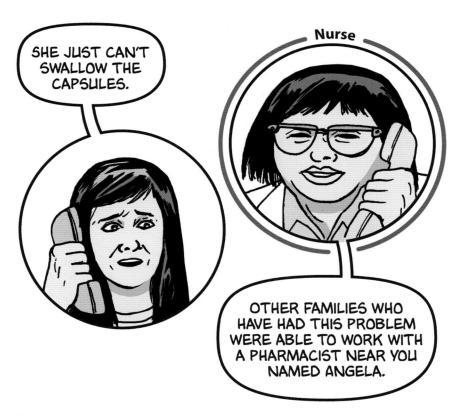

Illustration 2-9

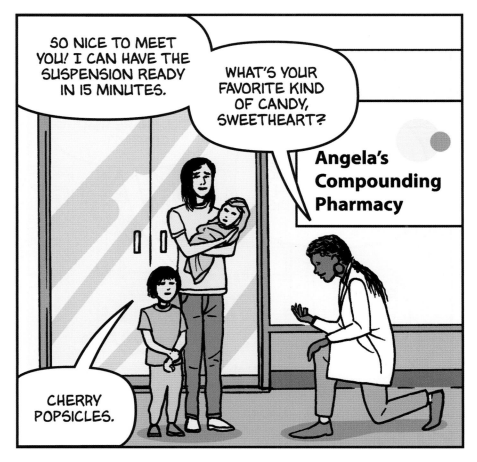

Illustration 2-10

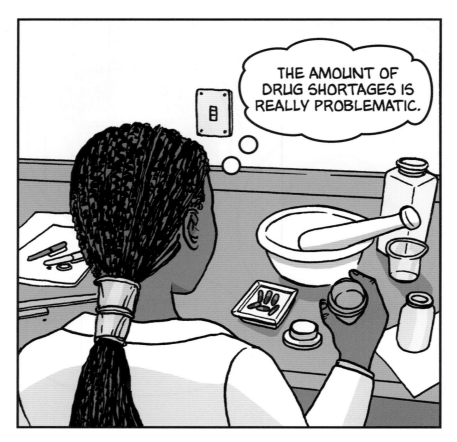

Illustration 2-11

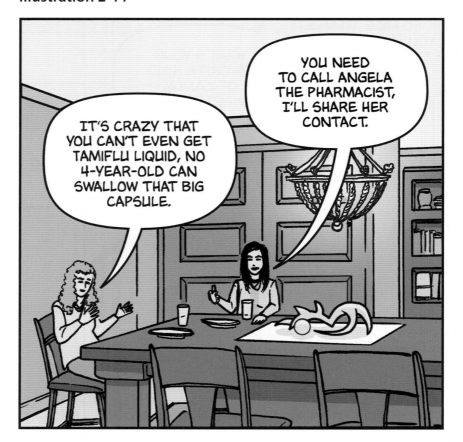

Illustration 2-12

Thoughts on "Transformation"

The illustrated case "Transformation" explores the value and importance of compounding pharmacy within healthcare in the United States. While not explicitly stated, the focus on oseltamivir (Tamiflu) implies that the family featured in this case is dealing with influenza (i.e., the flu). Oseltamivir is an antiviral medication commercially available in capsule and suspension (i.e., liquid) form that is approved by the US Food and Drug Administration (FDA) for the treatment of acute, uncomplicated influenza in patients who are older than 2 weeks and whose symptoms have been present for less than 48 hours.[82] The community pharmacist in Illustration 2-7, perhaps inexperienced dealing with young children, offers an ill-advised solution to a shortage of oseltamivir suspension. While not explicitly stated, part of the mother's stress depicted in Illustration 2-8 stems from her fear that the 48-hour window mentioned above was closing. Fortunately, the nurse at the pediatrics clinic (Illustration 2-9) was able to connect her to a pharmacy that specializes in compounding (Illustration 2-10). The value and impact of this compounding pharmacy becomes evident in Illustration 2-12.

Compounding is defined as the preparation of medicines for a specific patient.[83] Often, this involves the transformation of a medicine from one formulation to another; hence, the title of this illustrated case. Although it has been an integral part of the profession of pharmacy since antiquity, over the last 100 years, with the growth of manufacturing and the pharmaceutical industry, there has been a significant decline in compounding by pharmacists. Estimates vary on the number of compounded prescriptions dispensed by pharmacies. A 1994 survey of US pharmacies showed that less than 1% dispensed compounded prescriptions.[84] In 2002, the FDA estimated that roughly 250 million compounded prescriptions were dispensed in the United States per year, or between 1% and 8% of total prescriptions dispensed.[85] However, since 2002, there has been a growth in compounding.[86] Some attribute this trend to the rising popularity of personalized medicine, whereby health professionals are placing a greater emphasis on treating diseases based on the needs and unique characteristics of individual patients.[86] Commercially available medications do not always meet these needs; in those instances, a compounded medication may be the best solution. The Alliance for Pharmacy Compounding (APC) estimates that around 7500 of the roughly 56,000 pharmacies in the United States specialize in compounding. Some 3000 of these pharmacies make sterile products, which are described in greater detail below.[87]

A 2002 US Supreme Court decision addressed the application of federal law to pharmacy compounding.[88] In this decision, the government asserted that three substantial interests underlie the FDA Modernization Act of 1997: (1) preserving the effectiveness and integrity of the FDA's new drug approval process and the protection of the public health it provides; (2) preserving the availability of compounded drugs for patients who, for particular medical reasons, cannot use commercially available products approved by the FDA; and (3) achieving the proper balance between those two competing interests. This decision expanded the traditional definition and application of compounding. Justice Sandra Day O'Connor, writing the majority opinion for the Court, described compounding as "… a process by which a pharmacist or doctor combines, mixes, or alters ingredients to create a medication tailored to the needs of an individual patient." Illustration 2-11 provides an example. This decision, in particular the ideas of altering ingredients and placing compounding outside the oversight of the FDA, are major reasons why compounding on a larger scale has become a growing business model for many pharmacies in the last two decades.

Notwithstanding, the need for compounding is real because many patients have unique health needs that off-the-shelf, manufactured medications cannot meet. The ability to provide personalized medications in this manner, prescribed by licensed providers and prepared by trained, licensed pharmacists, often are the only solutions for patients. This means that a compounding pharmacist, working closely with a prescriber, can prepare customized medications that meet the individual needs of patients such as children, older adults, and even animals. Some of the most compelling reasons for compounding, including examples to highlight each, are included in Table 2-1.[87]

Table 2-1. Common Reasons Highlighting the Necessity and Importance of Compounding Pharmacy

Reason	Description
Shortage or commercial product unavailable	As shown in the oseltamivir example above, the pharmacist can compound the liquid oseltamivir medicine using capsules.
Allergy to commercial product	When the patient is allergic to certain preservatives, dyes, or binders in available off-the-shelf medications, the pharmacist can prepare a medication that does not contain these ingredients. Examples include some food dyes (tartrazine or FD&C yellow #5), lactose (in people who have lactose intolerance), wheat, barley, or rye derivatives (in people who have celiac sprue or gluten sensitivity), cornstarch (in people who have a corn allergy), and more.
Custom dosage needed	Many patients require tailored dosage strengths. For example, the dose for an infant or child can be smaller than that of an adult.
Increase adherence	Patients do not prefer some dosage forms. These include injections and suppositories. Preparing an oral dosage form with the same medicine can increase adherence.
Difficulty swallowing commercial product	Many patients cannot swallow larger capsules or tablets. Preparing a liquid dosage form will help these patients.
Commercial product unpalatable	Children have well-developed sensory systems for detecting tastes and smells which could make them reject unpalatable medications. Adding a pleasant flavor such as bubble gum may help induce children to consume a medicine.

Although not extensive, Table 2-1 demonstrates why some valuable medications are available only via compounding. Several cases provide additional real-world context to highlight the importance of compounding. *The Wall Street Journal* reported in 2011 that the FDA started to notice a short supply of oseltamivir (Tamiflu) oral suspension used by children and patients who have difficulty swallowing capsules, or when lower doses than available in the commercial capsules are required.[89] The agency said at the time that the liquid was on back order, but that supplies remained at distributors, wholesalers, and pharmacies. This incident led to a proliferation in the compounding of oseltamivir suspension from capsules.

Another report highlighted the importance of technique on the stability of compounded products.[90] Generally speaking, the term *"stability"* refers to whether a compounded product will remain in its desired formulation or whether it will, over time, separate out into its constituent parts. When a pharmacist mixes finely grounded tablets into a "suspension vehicle" (i.e., a liquid) to create a product that can more easily be swallowed, for example, the number of tablets is carefully chosen so that the final suspended product contains the correct concentration. The stability is critical because the finely grounded drug needs to mix evenly and stay mixed evenly so that each dose is accurate and consistent. In one report, researchers utilized the same amount of finely grounded drug, but varied the type of suspension vehicle and the amount of agitation (i.e., mixing), and then tested the stability of each preparation at different points in time. The results of this study broadened the number of suspension vehicles capable of producing stable suspensions and provided clarity in terms of optimal compounding technique to decrease the variability of doses. This study is significant because the use of this suspension in infants and neonates requires particular attention to stability and potential toxicity.

Another study highlighted that the thyroid replacement drug levothyroxine (Synthroid) may cause allergies or sensitivities in people who have lactose intolerance (it contains lactose).[91] These concerns led to the development of compounded formulations without lactose, which allowed lactose-allergic or -intolerant patients to take a medication vital to their health. Subsequently, a commercially available, lactose-free formulation came on the market.

In pharmacy practice, the difference between sterile and nonsterile compounding is more nuanced than most people typically understand. Sterile compounded medications are intended to be used as injections, infusions, or applications to the eye. Because the risks of infection from using injectable medications are higher, they must be prepared following very strict quality standards established by the United States Pharmacopeia (USP).[89] These standards for compounding sterile products may require a large capital investment for equipment, testing, training, and maintenance. The tasks performed during sterile compounding are completed using an approach called "aseptic technique," which minimizes the risks of contamination by pathogens, such as bacteria, viruses, or fungi. Nonsterile medications include the production of solutions, suspensions, ointments, creams, powders, suppositories, capsules, and tablets.

It is important to note that federal and state laws and regulations dictate what compounding pharmacists can and cannot do.[92,93] Under federal law, for example, pharmacists may not compound a medication for which there is a commercially available, FDA-approved product. Compounding activities must be, in other words, complementary to manufacturing. As soon as a compounding pharmacy begins to act like a manufacturer, it becomes subject to associated manufacturing laws and regulations.[92] A good rule of thumb differentiating compounding pharmacy from manufacturing is based on scale; the former is typically performed in service of a single patient (or animal), while the latter is focused on mass production and distribution. The exemption to these general rules is when the FDA-approved product labeling, for example oseltamivir (Tamiflu) suspension prepared from capsules, allows for compounding.

Rapid changes in technology and/or methodology used to produce and furnish drug products to patients has been associated with challenges in the pharmaceutical industry, in the practice of pharmacy, and in federal and state regulatory bodies.[94] A prime example is the development that led to regulators putting greater scrutiny on compounding pharmacies following incidents linked to poor oversight by State Boards of Pharmacy. This led to the FDA dividing pharmacies into two sectors: 503A and 503B. Compounding pharmacies under 503B are those with outsourcing facilities that may manufacture large batches with or without prescriptions to be sold to healthcare facilities for office use only.

At a minimum, all pharmacies and pharmacists, including compounding pharmacies, are licensed and strictly regulated by State Boards of Pharmacy. Additionally, the FDA has authority over some aspects of compounded prescriptions.[95] Compounded drugs are not FDA-approved. This means that the FDA does not review these drugs to evaluate their safety, effectiveness, or quality before they reach patients. However, Congress passed the Drug Quality and Security Act (DQSA) in 2013, which provided legal clarification regarding human drug compounding. Since DQSA implementation, the FDA has worked diligently to issue policy documents to provide important guidance to compounding pharmacists and pharmacies.[95] In order to comply with regulations, compounding pharmacists rely on standards established by the USP.[92] Established in 1820, the USP began publishing its compendium of standards in conjunction with the National Formulary (NF). Standards established within USP-NF must be integrated into the day-to-day practice of pharmacy compounding and are mandated in most states.

The USP is a scientific non-profit organization that sets public standards for identity, strength, quality, and purity of medicines. USP standards are recognized in various provisions of the federal Food, Drug and Cosmetic Act (FDCA) and in laws, regulations, and policies promulgated by states.[87] These standards are enforced by the FDA, states, and other oversight organizations. The FDCA specifically references and mandates USP standards for compounding. USP standards are recognized in Section 503A of the 1997 Food and Drug Administration Modernization Act, which states that a compounder must use bulk drug substances and ingredients that comply with the standards of an applicable USP–NF monograph, if a monograph exists, and the USP chapter on pharmacy compounding. The guidance specifically references USP General Chapter <795> Pharmaceutical Compounding—Nonsterile Preparations, USP General Chapter <797> Pharmaceutical Compounding—Sterile Preparations, and USP General Chapter <800>, a new standard developed by USP that establishes practice and quality standards of hazardous drugs to minimize exposure to hazardous drugs within healthcare settings.[86]

The USP does its work through a Compounding Expert Committee that is composed of 18 members representing a variety of disciplines including healthcare practitioners, many of them pharmacists, who have expertise in sterile and nonsterile compounding, veterinary compounding, aseptic technique, microbiology, environmental engineering, and analytical testing. Additionally, 10 government liaisons participate in the Compounding Expert Committee, including 7 representatives from the FDA and 3 representatives from the US Centers for Disease Control and Prevention.[87]

In addition to FDA oversight, state pharmacy regulatory bodies are responsible for oversight of the practice of pharmacy. Almost all states have laws, regulations, or policies specific to compounding.[88] Based on the 2016 National Association of Boards of Pharmacy (NABP) Survey of Pharmacy Law, at least 87% of state boards of pharmacy either require full compliance with USP General Chapter <797> or incorporate it into their state regulations in some way.[95] For the state boards that do not have such requirements, most have regulations pending or consider it as a standard of practice.[84] Additionally, the NABP Model Pharmacy Act/Rules, which provide boards of pharmacy with model language that may be used when developing state laws or board rules, incorporates USP General Chapters <795> and <797>.[84]

Several nonprofit agencies also provide oversight through accreditation processes. For example, PTCB recently launched the PTCB Certified Compounded Sterile Preparation Technician Program.[96] BPS, described earlier in this chapter, also offers certification in Compounded Sterile Preparations Pharmacy.[88] Accreditation and certification processes like these are important, as they help ensure that sterile preparations meet the clinical needs of patients. Certified pharmacists and pharmacy technicians also ensure that quality, safety, and environmental control requirements in all phases of preparation, storage, transportation, and administration remain in compliance with established standards, regulations, and professional best practices. Currently, there are more than 400 Board Certified Sterile Compounding Pharmacists and over 700,000 Certified Compounding Technicians.[96]

Recent events involving mistakes made by compounding pharmacies highlight the need for greater understanding of the differences between FDA-approved drugs and pharmacy-compounded preparations.[88] It would seem that compounding accidents and incidents should be a rarity in the 21st century. Surely, with frequent news media stories of accidents and well-researched and widely distributed reports, such as the Institute of Medicine's *To Err Is Human*, there should be a heightened awareness of potential problems concerning patient safety. According to the drug safety project published by the Pew Charitable Trust there were 69 reported compounding errors or potential errors that were associated with more than 1418 adverse events, including 114 deaths, from 2001 to 2017.[97] Furthermore, especially since the early 1990s, there has been increased activity in published standards of practice, guidelines, and federal guidance plus a great variety of readily available information on acceptable techniques, processes, and formulations.[99] Unfortunately, problems with unacceptable compounded preparations continue to be reported.

One reason for these unacceptable practices is that some pharmacies have seized upon a burgeoning business opportunity to expand their activities beyond the scope of traditional pharmacy compounding.[100] Examples of improper compounding include making products containing drugs that have not been approved for use in the United States or have been removed by the FDA for safety reasons, large-scale production of compounded medications without prescriptions, and creating very similar (essentially copies of) FDA-approved drugs.[100] Errors have occurred in such settings, and these are not trivial; some even leading to patients dying. A 2013 tragedy highlighted risks associated with improper compounding of sterile products. In this case, contaminated steroid injections caused serious infections and other injuries in at least 753 patients and resulted in at least 76 patient deaths.[101]

As the old saying goes, accidents do happen. That said, society has entrusted the profession of pharmacy with ensuring the safe use of medications, and even one compounding error is too many. In analyzing cases of compounding errors, a variety of reasons emerge.[102] While most incidents are truly accidents, many cases described in the media show that pursuit of increased profits contributes to errors.[101] However, even more cases show that there was either inadequate training or lack of knowledge of the accepted standards, while other times the pharmacist is aware of the guidelines, but thinks that the standards are too stringent and/or too costly and disregards them. Mathematical, weighing and measuring, ingredient selection, or compounding procedure errors are also common. Often these mistakes could have been avoided by using well-documented procedures, independent colleague verification, and/or the triple check systems that are encouraged by the FDA, NABP, and USP.[83,84,92]

In summary, traditional pharmacy compounding plays a valuable role in providing access to medications for individuals with unique medical needs, which cannot be met with a commercially available product. This is highlighted in the illustrated case "Transformation," where a compounding pharmacist creates a suspension in order for a child to be able to take a needed medication. Such activities require knowledge, skill, and incredible attention to detail. As with every other area of pharmacy practice, before embarking on a new or specialty area of practice, such as compounding nonsterile and sterile products, the pharmacist should read and study available literature, guidelines, and standards. Pursuit of additional training and certification, obtaining information from a variety of professional organizations and governmental agencies, and use of both basic science knowledge and critical thinking skills to make good judgments, always in the best interests of the patient, is critical.[92] Lastly, although pharmacists should be reimbursed for the act of compounding, they should avoid compounding as a way to increase profits.[103]

BREATHE: An Illustrated Case Study

Story by Edward C. Portillo & Joseph A. Zorek
Illustrations by George Folz, © 2019 Board of Regents of the University of Wisconsin System

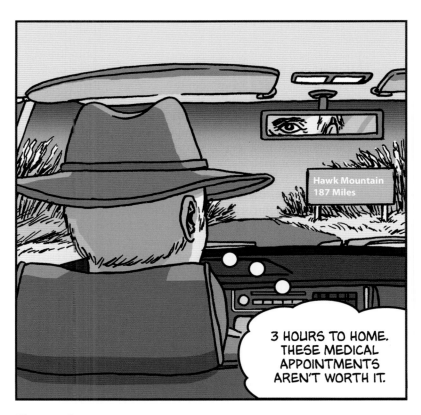

Illustration 2-13

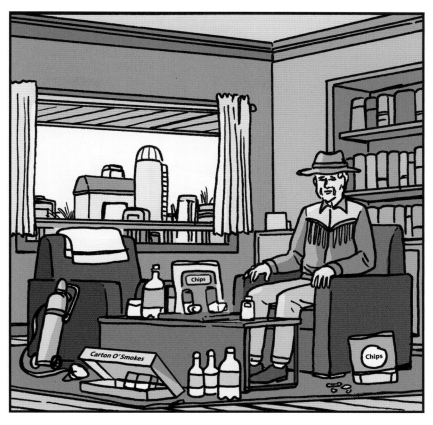

Illustration 2-14

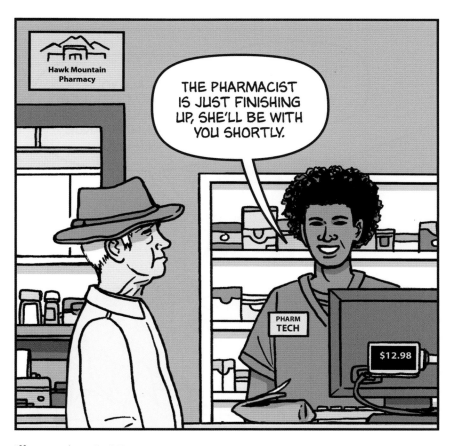

Illustration 2-15

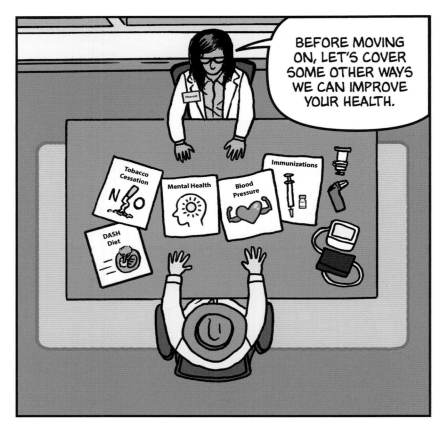

Illustration 2-16

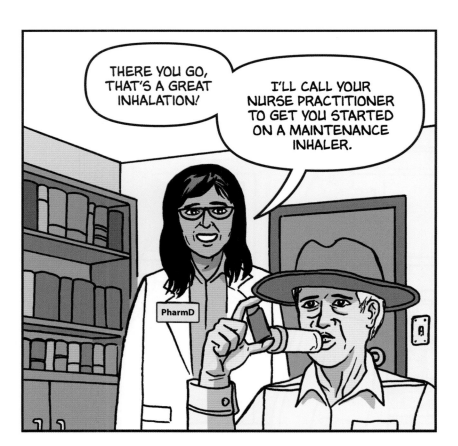

Illustration 2-17

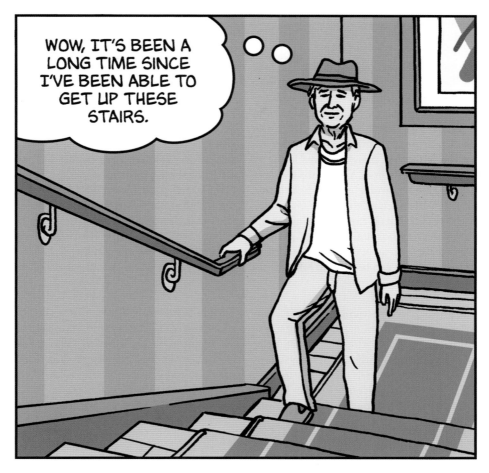

Illustration 2-18

Thoughts on "Breathe"

Community pharmacists practicing in rural areas of the United States serve an essential role in promoting healthcare access for patients. In rural communities, providing patients with comprehensive care in a timely manner is critical, as patients are often sicker, poorer, and older than their urban counterparts.[104,105] In fact, patients living in rural America are more likely to die from the five leading causes of death (heart disease, stroke, cancer, unintentional injury, and chronic lower respiratory disease) than patients living in urban settings.[106] Importantly, as it relates to the value of community pharmacists working in rural communities, many of these deaths have been reported as preventable. By increasing access to care and collaborating interprofessionally with other health professionals, as demonstrated in the illustrated case "Breathe," pharmacists working in rural areas can make a positive impact on the lives of patients living in their communities.

Defining "rural" can be challenging, as the definitions of "rural" versus "urban" can vary widely depending on how population density and geographic land mass are classified. The fact that there is not one universally accepted definition to classify rural

America likely reflects the rich diversity and unique attributes of each rural community across the country.[107] According to US Census statistics, nearly 60 million people live in rural areas, which is close to 19% of the US population. With such a large rural population, it can be expected that each rural community will have unique healthcare needs. Still, trends do exist in rural populations when compared to their urban counterparts. Eleven percent of adolescents living in the most rural counties smoke, for example, compared to 5% for adolescents living in central counties of large metro areas.[108] Smoking is the most important risk factor for chronic respiratory conditions, many of which are associated with higher death rates in rural areas. Disparities in health insurance coverage also exist in rural communities, where 12.3% of Americans are uninsured compared to 10.1% in mostly urban counties.[109] This pattern also holds true for prescription drug coverage through Medicare Part D, a federal program designed to provide prescription drug coverage to patients 65 years of age or older.[110,111]

Community pharmacists are well positioned to help improve the health of patients living in rural communities. In fact, the vast majority of Americans live within 5 miles of their community pharmacy, making the community pharmacist one of the most accessible healthcare practitioners for patients in both urban and rural communities.[112] The illustrated case "Breathe" highlights the challenges patients experience in such settings, as well as the benefits that can be reaped through partnership with pharmacists. Illustration 2-13 introduces readers to the main character of the case, an elderly patient driving home from a medical visit with a whopping 187 miles remaining to get home. Unfortunately, driving long distances to receive medical care is a reality for many patients living in rural communities. Twenty-five percent of Americans living in rural areas report being unable to receive needed healthcare, 45% of whom blamed either distance or difficulty in obtaining an appointment as barriers.[113] This is not surprising, as the average drive time to the nearest hospital for rural patients is double that of those in urban areas, while the distance to receive specialty healthcare services can be several hours from home.[114]

A national shortage of physicians practicing in rural communities contributes to the challenges many patients face receiving care in rural areas.[105] While 20% of the US population lives in rural communities, only 9% of physicians practice there. By the year 2030, there is expected to be a shortage of more than 100,000 physicians in the United States, and this shortage is likely to impact rural communities disproportionately.[115,116]

In addition to the looming physician shortage, there is a clear need for more community pharmacists to practice in rural areas.[117] A number of community pharmacies, and in particular independently owned community pharmacies, have closed in rural communities since 2003.[118] In fact, 630 rural communities in the United States that previously had access to a local community pharmacy no longer do as a result of closures. This statistic is alarming considering community pharmacy closures negatively impact patient access to critically needed medications and the professional services of pharmacists, whose accessibility and knowledge have earned the public's trust.[119] As a result, patients living in rural America, many of whom demonstrate the greatest need for healthcare, may experience the most significant barriers to care.[104] The healthcare workforce shortage in rural communities becomes even more significant for professions requiring greater years of education and training. For example, the number of pharmacists per 10,000 patients is 6.4 in rural areas compared to 8.8 in urban communities.[117] The number of dentists per 10,000 patients is 3.6 in rural areas compared to 5.9 in urban communities. Many rural communities are considered to be Health Professional Shortage Areas (HPSAs), which is a federal designation indicating a geographic, population, or facility-based healthcare workforce shortage.[120] In fact, 62.9% of all designated primary medical HPSAs are in rural communities. For more information on how medication access issues can result in poor health outcomes, readers are encouraged to explore the illustrated cases "Holistic" in Chapter 3 Primary Care and "Opportunities" in Chapter 15 Administration.

While a dwindling rural workforce may seem discouraging, the opportunity for community pharmacists practicing in rural areas to positively impact patients is clear. Owning an independent community pharmacy in these settings is one such opportunity. In fact, independent pharmacies make up 52% of all community pharmacies in rural areas, and there are still nearly 7500 independently owned rural pharmacies across the United States.[121] These pharmacists serve a critical role, and in many cases are the only pharmacy access point in the community they serve.[122] As a result, pharmacists in these settings are making a demonstrable difference in the lives of patients;[20] examples include provision of essential health services, such as screening for chronic disease states, monitoring disease progression, and even prescribing medications in collaboration with physicians.[12,123,124] Given the shortage of primary care providers in rural areas, the opportunity for community pharmacists to provide such critical health services has arguably never been greater.

The illustrated case "Breathe" attempts to capture and contextualize much of the information provided above. Illustration 2-14, for example, shows a patient who would clearly benefit from pharmacy services. An oxygen tank and carton of cigarettes on the floor and inhalers on the coffee table provide the first clues that this patient may suffer from chronic obstructive pulmonary disease (COPD), a chronic and progressive lung condition characterized by shortness of breath, coughing, wheezing, and excessive production of mucus.[125] The prevalence of COPD in rural communities is two times higher than in urban ones.[126] Chronic respiratory disease, and most predominately COPD, is the third largest killer in the United States, and over 15.3 million patients have been diagnosed with COPD.[125,127] Just to provide some perspective on how many people are impacted by this disease, there are only four states in the United States with populations higher than 15 million: California, Texas, Florida, and New York. The most common cause of COPD is cigarette, pipe, and cigar use, which also happens to be the leading cause of preventable death in the United States.[127,128]

Illustration 2-14 also draws attention to other factors influencing the main character's overall well-being. There are bags of potato chips and bottles of soda in the room in Illustration 2-14. This was an intentional effort to highlight the lack of food retailers in many rural communities and, in effect, lack of access to healthy, affordable food that many patients face in remote parts of the United States.[130] For more information on food insecurity and other nonmedical factors that influence health, readers are encouraged to explore the illustrated cases "Screen" in Chapter 4 Prevention & Wellness and "Unsung Hero" in Chapter 14 Population Health.

To understand what causes COPD symptoms, it is helpful to review the basic anatomy of the lungs, which is described in the asthma-based illustrated case "Swish" in Chapter 3 Primary Care. COPD symptoms are caused by chronic airway inflammation, which leads to cough, mucus production, and damage to millions of small air sacs called alveoli. Oxygen from the air we breathe is exchanged for carbon dioxide, a waste product of metabolism, within the alveoli, which is a critical function for our health and ability to breathe normally.[129] COPD, thus, can dramatically impact a person's life, resulting in reduced activity and inability to work.[131] Activities most people take for granted, such as walking or climbing stairs, are reported as difficult for more than one in three adults with COPD.

When COPD symptoms acutely worsen, and they often do, patients experience what is termed a *COPD exacerbation*. Acute COPD exacerbations can be deadly, costly, and have a long-lasting impact on patients' quality of life.[132] The average cost of a COPD exacerbation has been shown to be as high as $7100.[133] Furthermore, the mortality rate has been shown to be 26.2% within 1 year of a COPD exacerbation; meaning, one in four patients who experience a COPD exacerbation will die within 1 year of the event. After a COPD exacerbation, patients' lungs, and in effect their quality of life, may permanently worsen.[134] While COPD considered in isolation is serious, patients with COPD also experience significant comorbidities (i.e., additional health issues) including anxiety, depression, heart disease, lung cancer, diabetes, and poor bone health, among others.[135] Illustration 2-16 highlights the importance of managing these conditions, as well, with the pharmacist providing critical education to the patient.

Fortunately, medication therapy is available for patients to improve COPD symptoms and overall well-being. Many of the medication options are delivered through specially designed inhalers, which are delivery devices that allow for medication distribution directly to the lungs. The challenge, however, is that patients may use their inhalers incorrectly to administer medications, and as a result do not receive the benefit they could from their medications.[136] In fact, evaluations have demonstrated error rates in inhaler use by patients ranging from 50% to 65%.[136,137] This is especially unfortunate considering the out-of-pocket cost many patients pay for their COPD medications, which can reach nearly $1200 per year.[138] There are additional options to facilitate medication delivery into the lungs, including nebulizer systems that create a mist for inhalation and small, tube-like devices called spacers that can be used with some inhalers to improve medication delivery.

Medications for COPD treatment can be divided into two broad categories: (1) rescue medications and (2) maintenance medications. Rescue medications help to open up the patient's airways, and are used to treat COPD symptoms at the time they occur. Maintenance medications are taken on a regularly scheduled basis (i.e., every day) to help reduce future symptoms from occurring. Patients with COPD are often prescribed both rescue and maintenance medications together to improve COPD symptom control and reduce the risk of COPD exacerbations. Many of these medications are included in Table 2-2. In addition to the products mentioned in Table 2-2, options also exist that combine medications from multiple categories into one inhaler. These combination products minimize the need for patients to use multiple maintenance inhalers for COPD control.

Fortunately for this patient, an independent community pharmacy recently opened in his home town (Illustration 2-15). Hawk Mountain Pharmacy is equipped with a private consultation room, as shown in Illustration 2-16, and is owned by a pharmacist who is passionate about the holistic care of her patients. This is demonstrated in the consultation that takes place in Illustration 2-17, which includes extensive education beyond just answering questions about the COPD inhaler the patient came to Hawk Mountain Pharmacy to fill. The pharmacist also demonstrates a willingness and ability to advocate for her patient with other health professionals to improve medication use through interprofessional practice, as depicted in Illustration 2-17.

There are many examples of rural pharmacists who serve their patients in a similar manner. A group of five rural community pharmacies in Arizona, for example, provided health promotion and prevention services for patients with diabetes and/or hypertension.[139] Services provided included health screenings, such as blood glucose testing with education on diet and exercise similar to the illustrated case "Screen" in Chapter 4 Prevention & Wellness, diabetic foot examinations as shown in the illustrated case "Holistic" in Chapter 3 Primary Care, and blood pressure evaluations as demonstrated in the illustrated case "Underlying Cause" in Chapter 5 Cardiology. The rural pharmacists in Arizona also provided vaccinations and evaluation of appropriate medication use.[139] Collectively, this group provided over 1000 health promotion interventions and more than 200 medication-related interventions to 517 patients. Importantly, improvements in participating patients' blood glucose readings were demonstrated.

Another example of community pharmacists making a positive impact on the health of patients living in rural areas took place in Mississippi, where 13 community pharmacists across nine counties completed comprehensive MTM services.[140] Broadly speaking, comprehensive MTM services involve pharmacists meeting individually with patients to complete a full review of medications for various conditions and to develop a care plan with recommendations made to resolve identified concerns. Community pharmacists in this project identified and resolved nearly 1500 drug-related problems in 468 patients across the state. Specific high-impact interventions of these rural pharmacists included addition of needed medications, optimization of medication doses, and improvement of medication nonadherence. Indeed, the continued dissemination and evaluation of such innovative service models is a promising opportunity to enhance rural healthcare delivery.

In the illustrated case "Breathe," the Hawk Mountain pharmacist makes several important interventions similar to those provided in the Arizona and Mississippi examples above. For example, she identifies that her patient is missing a maintenance inhaler, a key component of quality, evidence-based treatment

Table 2-2. Categories and Examples of Medications Commonly Used in the Treatment of Chronic Obstructive Pulmonary Disease

Category	Medication Examples[*]	Physiologic Effects
Short-acting beta-2 agonists (SABAs)	▪ albuterol (ProAir, Proventil, Ventolin) ▪ levalbuterol (Xopenex)	Relax the muscles surrounding the airways
Long-acting beta-2 agonists (LABAs)	▪ indacaterol (Arcapta Neohaler) ▪ olodaterol (Striverdi Respimat) ▪ salmeterol (Serevent Diskus)	
Short-acting muscarinic antagonists (SAMAs)	▪ ipratropium (Atrovent HFA)	Allow for airway opening by inhibiting the action of acetylcholine[**]
Long-acting muscarinic antagonists (LAMAs)	▪ aclidinium (Tudorza Pressair) ▪ glycopyrrolate (Seebri Neohaler) ▪ tiotropium (Spiriva Respimat, Spiriva Handihaler) ▪ umeclidinium (Incruse Ellipta)	
Short-acting muscarinic antagonist/Short-acting beta-2 agonist combination product (SAMAs/SABAs)	▪ ipratropium/albuterol (Combivent Respimat)	Allow for airway opening by inhibiting the action of acetylcholine[**] while also relaxing the muscles surrounding the airways
Long-acting muscarinic antagonist/Long-acting beta-2 agonist combination products (LAMAs/LABAs)	▪ glycopyrrolate/formoterol (Bevespi Aerosphere) ▪ glycopyrrolate/indicaterol (Utibron Neohaler) ▪ tiotropium/olodaterol (Stiolto Respimat) ▪ umeclidinium/vilanterol (Anoro Ellipta)	Allow for airway opening by inhibiting the action of acetylcholine[**] while also relaxing the muscles surrounding the airways
Inhaled corticosteroid/Long-acting beta-2 agonist combination products (ICS/LABAs)	▪ budesonide/formoterol (Symbicort MDI) ▪ fluticasone/salmeterol (Advair Diskus, Wixela Inhub) ▪ fluticasone/vilanterol (Breo Ellipta)	Reduce inflammation, airway swelling, and mucous production while also allowing for airway opening by inhibiting the action of acetylcholine[**]
Inhaled corticosteroid/Long-acting muscarinic antagonist/Long-acting beta-2 agonist combination product	▪ fluticasone/umeclidinium/vilanterol (Trelegy Ellipta)	Reduce inflammation, airway swelling, and mucous production while allowing for airway opening by inhibiting the action of acetylcholine[**] and relaxing the muscles surrounding the airways

[*] Medication examples presented in alphabetical order as "generic name (Brand Name)."

[**] Acetylcholine is a neurotransmitter (i.e., a chemical messenger) that causes narrowing of the airways.

for COPD (see Table 2-2).[141] Addition of a maintenance inhaler is intended to reduce symptoms of COPD, as well as reduce the risk of future COPD flare-ups. In addition, the patient's inhaler technique is reviewed to ensure effective medication delivery. The importance of this intervention cannot be overstated, as it is reported that two-thirds of patients with COPD do not use their inhalers correctly.[136] In other words, roughly 65% of the patients prescribed optimal treatment of COPD, who are motivated and willing to use COPD inhalers, do not benefit from their use because poor technique prevents delivery of the active ingredients into the lungs. The pharmacist in "Breathe" recognizes this problem, and she provides guidance and coaching, along with a spacer device, to help the patient get the medication where it needs to go. For more information on inhaler technique, including the use of spacer devices, see the illustrated case "Swish" in Chapter 3 Primary Care.

Arguably, the most critical element of the Hawk Mountain pharmacist's work is her ability to connect with other members of the interprofessional team (e.g., nurses, physicians, social workers). The patient in "Breathe," who is frustrated and disheartened by difficulties associated with distant medical visits (Illustration 2-13), is able to get one-on-one attention from a knowledgeable, skilled health professional who holds the trust of other members of the interprofessional team and, as a result, is able to advocate on his behalf to maximize the efficacy of medication therapies available. This community pharmacist contacts the patient's prescriber to discuss proposed changes to his medications; a successful intervention that, coupled with proper inhalation technique, leads to marked improvements in the patient's condition as evidenced by Illustration 2-18.

Illustration 2-18 highlights the full impact of the Hawk Mountain pharmacist. It is here that a change in the patient's demeanor is observed from one of frustration, or even despair, to hope. The patient, who by virtue of circumstance was a victim of limited healthcare access and suboptimal medication treatment, is able to walk up the stairs in his home for the first time in years without experiencing shortness of breath from COPD symptoms. The interventions implemented by the community pharmacist have been effective. Perhaps more important still, a patient with multiple chronic conditions has now discovered an additional member of the interprofessional team, his community pharmacist, who is eager to provide support.

DISCUSSION QUESTIONS FOR "BREATHE"

1. In Illustration 2-13, the main character in the illustrated case "Breathe" is shown driving 3 hours to receive medical care for his COPD management. If he were to experience an acute COPD exacerbation, with severe shortness of breath, what options do you think he would have to receive treatment for his symptoms? Would driving himself to the nearest hospital be a good option?

2. In Illustration 2-16, the pharmacist is shown providing extensive education to help the main character improve his overall health and well-being. It is unlikely, however, that she will be able to address all of the patient's healthcare needs in one visit. What additional health-related items do you think the pharmacist might follow up about in a subsequent visit?

3. In Illustration 2-17, we learn that the main character was not using a maintenance medication for his COPD symptoms, which was likely contributing to his poor breathing. What are some reasons you can think of that might explain this lack of a key medication? Moving forward, what barriers might he face with adherence to this maintenance inhaler?

4. In Illustration 2-18, the main character is shown expressing relief that he can now walk up his stairs comfortably. How might this accomplishment influence his ability to continue improving his overall health?

5. In the illustrated case "Breathe," the patient drove to his local pharmacy for an in-person visit with the pharmacist. What other technologies might a pharmacist consider to provide timely medication therapy management services to patients in their community? How might these approaches impact the quality of care provided?

CHAPTER SUMMARY

- Community pharmacists are incredibly accessible front-line health professionals who make themselves, and their expert guidance and advice on medications, available to patients without need for appointment, insurance, or payment.

- Community pharmacy practice continues to expand well beyond dispensing of medications to include patient-centered care initiatives such as health screenings, point-of-care testing, medication therapy management, and administration of vaccinations and injectable medications.

- There is a clear role for community pharmacists to serve as patient advocates through negotiations with prescribers and payers to promote safe, effective care at the lowest possible cost.

- There has been a resurgence in community pharmacy compounding to support personalized medicine, customized patient dosage needs, improvements in medication tolerability, increased medication adherence, and to combat medication shortages.

- Community pharmacists play a critical role in the care of rural patient populations, who are on average older, sicker, and poorer compared to their urban counterparts.

- In rural areas, independently owned community pharmacies represent a large portion of pharmacy practice settings and often may serve as the only pharmacy access point.

- The community pharmacist is at the heart of neighborhoods across the United States, and is a health professional with tremendous visibility, knowledge, trust, and opportunity to improve the lives of patients across the country.

ACKNOWLEDGMENT

The authors would like to acknowledge Vince Wartenweiler, Doctor of Pharmacy student at the University of Wisconsin–Madison School of Pharmacy in Madison, Wisconsin, for his assistance in managing in-text citations and the reference section for this chapter.

REFERENCES

1. Pharmacy Is Right For Me. 5 ways pharmacists are helping people live healthier lives. Available at https://pharmacyforme.org/2018/12/05/5-ways-pharmacists-help-people-live-healthier/. Accessed March 5, 2020.

2. Maine LL. Pharmacists on the frontline of healthcare. Available at http://www.thesullivanalliance.org/cue/blog/pharmacists-on-the-frontline-of-healthcare.html. Accessed March 5, 2020.

3. Yee M. Community pharmacy. *Pharm J.* 2012;288(7708-7709):670.

4. Melton BL, Lai Z. Review of community pharmacy services: what is being performed, and where are the opportunities for improvement? *Integr Pharm Res Pract.* 2017;6:79-89.

5. World Health Organization. The role of the pharmacist in the health care system: report of a WHO consultative group, New Delhi, India, 13–16 December 1988; report of a WHO meeting, Tokyo, Japan, 31 August–3 September 1993. Available at https://apps.who.int/iris/handle/10665/59169. Accessed May 30, 2020.

6. Longo KG. Top ways pharmacists' roles are changing. Available at https://www.drugtopics.com/article/top-ways-pharmacists'-roles-are-changing. Accessed March 5, 2020.

7. Gale R. In patient safety efforts, pharmacists gain new prominence. *Health Aff.* 2018;37(11):1726-1729.

8. Centers for Disease Control and Prevention. Community pharmacists and medication therapy management. Available at https://www.cdc.gov/dhdsp/pubs/guides/best-practices/pharmacist-mtm.htm. Accessed March 12, 2020.

9. Qato DM, Zenk S, Wilder J, Harrington R, Gaskin D, Alexander GC. The availability of pharmacies in the United States: 2007–2015. *PLoS One.* 2017;12(8):e0183172.

10. San-Juan-Rodriguez A, Newman TV, Hernandez I, et al. Impact of community pharmacist-provided preventive services on clinical, utilization, and economic outcomes: an umbrella review. *Prev Med.* 2018;115:145-155.

11. Spears T. Community pharmacists play key role in improving medication safety. Available at https://www.

pharmacytimes.com/publications/issue/2010/november2010/communitypharmacists_medsafety. Accessed March 9, 2020.

12. American Public Health Association. The role of the pharmacist in public health. Available at https://www.apha.org/policies-and-advocacy/public-health-policy-statements/policy-database/2014/07/07/13/05/the-role-of-the-pharmacist-in-public-health. Accessed May 31, 2020.

13. Minnesota Department of Health. Pharmacists—a prescription for healthy communities. Available at https://www.health.state.mn.us/diseases/cardiovascular/tools/pharmacist.html. Accessed March 3, 2020.

14. LaVito A. CVS to open 1,500 HealthHUB stores over next two years. Available at https://www.cnbc.com/2019/06/04/cvs-to-add-healthhub-stores-drugstore-announces-ahead-of-investor-day.html. Accessed May 30, 2020.

15. Holmes E, Dubois S. National Community Pharmacists Association 2017 Digest. Available at http://www.ncpa.co/pdf/digest/2017/2017-digest-lr.pdf. Accessed March 15, 2020.

16. Dalton K, Byrne S. Role of the pharmacist in reducing healthcare costs: current insights. *Integr Pharm Res Pract*. 2017;6:37-46.

17. Ofri D. A doctor's guide to a good appointment. Available at https://www.nytimes.com/guides/well/make-the-most-of-your-doctor-appointment. Accessed March 15, 2020.

18. California Pharmacists Association. Pharmacist 101: behind the white coat. Available at https://cpha.com/about/pharmacist-101-behind-the-white-coat/. Accessed March 9, 2020.

19. United States Bureau of Labor Statistics. Pharmacists: occupational outlook handbook. Available at https://www.bls.gov/oes/2018/may/oes291051.htm. Accessed March 3, 2020.

20. Dubois S, Mu C. National Community Pharmacists Association 2016 Digest. Available at http://www.ncpa.co/pdf/digest/2016/2016-ncpa-digest-spon-cardinal.pdf. Accessed March 15, 2020.

21. Kehrer JP, Eberhart G, Wing M, Horon K. Pharmacy's role in a modern health continuum. *Can Pharm J*. 2013;146(6):321-324.

22. National Association of Chain Drug Stores. NACDS Chain Member Fact Book, 2018–2019. Available at https://www.nacds.org/wp-content/uploads/2019/05/2018_ChainDrugFactbook.pdf. Accessed May 30, 2020.

23. United States Bureau of Labor Statistics. Occupational employment statistics. Available at https://www.bls.gov/oes/2018/may/oes291051.htm. Accessed May 30, 2020.

24. Hales CM, Servais J, Martin CB, Kohen D. Prescription drug use among adults aged 40–79 in the United States and Canada. NCHS Data Brief No. 347. 2019:1-8.

25. Brown MT, Bussell JK. Medication adherence: WHO cares? *Mayo Clin Proc*. 2011;86(4):304-314.

26. Centers for Disease Control and Prevention. About chronic diseases. Available at https://www.cdc.gov/chronicdisease/about/index.htm. Accessed March 11, 2020.

27. Neiman AB, Ruppar T, Ho M, et al. CDC grand rounds: improving medication adherence for chronic disease management—innovations and opportunities. *Am J Transplant*. 2018;18(2):514-517.

28. Federico F. The five rights of medication administration. Available at http://www.ihi.org/resources/Pages/ImprovementStories/FiveRightsofMedicationAdministration.aspx. Accessed March 12, 2020.

29. Agency for Healthcare Research and Quality. The pharmacist's role in medication safety. Available at https://psnet.ahrq.gov/primer/pharmacists-role-medication-safety#. Accessed March 12, 2020.

30. World Health Organization. WHO launches global effort to halve medication-related errors in 5 years. Available at https://www.who.int/news-room/detail/29-03-2017-who-launches-global-effort-to-halve-medication-related-errors-in-5-years. Accessed March 12, 2020.

31. Makary MA, Daniel M. Medical error—the third leading cause of death in the US. *BMJ*. 2016;353:i2139.

32. Carroll AE. The unsung role of the pharmacist in patient health. Available at https://www.nytimes.com/2019/01/28/upshot/pharmacists-drugs-health-unsung-role.html. Accessed May 30, 2020.

33. MacDonald JV. State laws and vaccination services. Available at https://www.drugtopics.com/article/state-laws-and-vaccination-services. Accessed May 30, 2020.

34. Centers for Disease Control and Prevention. Birth to 18 years immunization schedule. Available at https://www.cdc.gov/vaccines/schedules/hcp/imz/child-adolescent.html. Accessed March 13, 2020.

35. Association of State and Territorial Health Officials. Pharmacy legal toolkit. Available at https://www.astho.org/Infectious-Disease/Pharmacy-Legal-Toolkit/. Accessed March 13, 2020.

36. Thompson CA. Scope of practice in Wisconsin expands to drug product administration. *Am J Heal Pharm*. 2016;73(18):1380-1381.

37. Bonner L. Beyond vaccines: pharmacists improve patient access to injectable medications. *Pharm Today*. 2018;24(2):34-37.

38. Centers for Disease Control and Prevention. High blood pressure and cholesterol: out of control. Available at https://www.cdc.gov/vitalsigns/cardiovasculardisease/index.html. Accessed May 30, 2020.

39. DiDonato KL, May JR, Lindsey CC. Impact of wellness coaching and monitoring services provided in a community pharmacy. *J Am Pharm Assoc*. 2013;53(1):14-21.

40. Florkowski C, Don-Wauchope A, Gimenez N, Rodriguez-Capote K, Wils J, Zemlin A. Point-of-care testing (POCT) and evidence-based laboratory medicine (EBLM)—does it leverage any advantage in clinical decision making? *Crit Rev Clin Lab Sci*. 2017;54(7-8):471-494.

41. Gilberston D. Travel ban aftershocks: American, United, Delta slashing Europe flights. Available at https://www.usatoday.com/story/travel/airline-news/2020/03/12/coronavirus-europe-travel-ban-fallout-airlines-cancel-more-flights/5031305002/. Accessed March 15, 2020.

42. World Health Organization. Coronavirus disease (COVID-19) advice for the public. Available at https://www.who.int/emergencies/diseases/novel-coronavirus-2019/advice-for-public. Accessed March 15, 2020.

43. Reuters. Coronavirus deprives nearly 300 million students of their schooling: UNESCO. Available at https://www.nytimes.com/reuters/2020/03/05/world/europe/05reuters-health-coronavirus-education.html?searchResultPosition=7. Accessed March 15, 2020.

44. McCoy K. Coronavirus test component is in short supply. Available at https://www.usatoday.com/story/news/2020/03/11/coronavirus-covid-19-response-hurt-by-shortage-testing-components/5013586002/. Accessed March 15, 2020.

45. Goldstein A, McGinley L, Abutaleb Y. Trump says he will partner with private sector to expand coronavirus testing but details are sketchy. Available at https://www.washingtonpost.com/health/under-heavy-fire-trump-administration-takes-steps-to-expand-coronavirus-testing/2020/03/13/f86b481e-6525-11ea-acca-80c22bbee96f_story.html. Accessed March 15, 2020.

46. Walgreens. Our response to COVID-19. Available at https://news.walgreens.com/our-stories/covid-19-response.htm. Accessed March 15, 2020.

47. CVS Health. CVS Health announces additional COVID-19 resources focused on patient access. Available at https://cvshealth.com/newsroom/press-releases/cvs-health-announces-additional-covid-19-resources-focused-patient-access. Accessed March 15, 2020.

48. American Society of Health-System Pharmacists. Pharmacy readiness for coronavirus disease 2019 (COVID-19): recommendations for state policymakers. Available at https://www.ashp.org/-/media/assets/advocacy-issues/docs/Pharmacy-Readiness-for-Coronavirus-Disease-2019-COVID-19-STATE.ashx?la=en&hash=6420DD319DEF9C0C008B161D36615C8E3229532B. Accessed March 15, 2020.

49. Kowarski I. How to become a pharmacist. Available at https://www.usnews.com/education/best-graduate-schools/articles/2019-07-22/how-to-get-into-pharmacy-school-and-become-a-pharmacist. Accessed March 15, 2020.

50. National Association of Boards of Pharmacy. NAPLEX. Available at https://nabp.pharmacy/programs/naplex/. Accessed March 15, 2020.

51. National Association of Boards of Pharmacy. MPJE. Available at https://nabp.pharmacy/programs/mpje/. Accessed March 15, 2020.

52. American Pharmacists Association. Is a postgraduate year 1 community pharmacy residency program right for you? Available at https://www.pharmacist.com/sites/default/files/files/09-479%20PharmResidBrochure_LR.pdf. Accessed March 15, 2020.

53. Board of Pharmacy Specialties. Ambulatory care pharmacy. Available at https://www.bpsweb.org/bps-specialties/ambulatory-care/#1517747142312-7425fd17-dd471517779729021. Accessed March 15, 2020.

54. Schroeder MN. Staying up-to-date as a new practitioner. Available at https://www.pharmacist.com/article/staying-date-new-practitioner?is_sso_called=1. Accessed March 15, 2020.

55. National Community Pharmacists Association. Available at https://ncpa.org/. Accessed March 15, 2020.

56. American Pharmacists Association. Available at https://www.pharmacist.com/. Accessed March 15, 2020.

57. Duong, C. Can retail pharmacies run like fast food restaurants? Available at https://www.pharmacytimes.com/contributor/catherine-duong-pharmd-candidate/2016/09/can-retail-pharmacies-run-like-fast-food-restaurants. Accessed May 30, 2020.

58. Tsuyuki RT, Beahm NP, Okada H, Al Hamarneh YN. Pharmacists as accessible primary health care providers: review of the evidence. *Can Pharm J*. 2018;151(1):4-5.

59. National Association of Chain Drug Stores. Pharmacists rank second again among Gallup's most trusted professionals. Available at https://www.nacds.org/news/pharmacists-rank-second-again-among-gallups-most-trusted-professionals/. Accessed May 30, 2020.

60. Billstein-Leber M, Carrillo CJD, Cassano AT, Moline K, Robertson JJ. ASHP guidelines on preventing medication errors in hospitals. *Am J Health Syst Pharm*. 2018;75(19):1493-1517.

61. American Diabetes Association. Neuropathy. Available at https://www.diabetes.org/diabetes/complications/neuropathy. Accessed May 30, 2020.

62. Gabler E. How chaos at chain pharmacies is putting patients at risk. Available at https://www.nytimes.com/2020/01/31/health/pharmacists-medication-errors.html. Accessed February 6, 2020.

63. Took RL, Liu Y, Kuehl PG. A study to identify medication-related problems and associated cost avoidance by community pharmacists during a comprehensive medication review in patients one week post hospitalization. *Pharmacy*. 2019;7(2):51.

64. Milenkovich N. The community pharmacist as a provider of immunizations. Available at https://www.pharmacytimes.com/publications/supplements/2019/November2019/the-community-pharmacist-as-a-provider-of-immunizations. Accessed May 30, 2020.

65. Centers for Disease Control and Prevention. Vaccine information for adults. Available at https://www.cdc.gov/vaccines/adults/pay-for-vaccines.html. Accessed May 30, 2020.

66. Isenor JE, Edwards NT, Alia TA, et al. Impact of pharmacists as immunizers on vaccination rates: a systematic review and meta-analysis. *Vaccine*. 2016; 34(47):5708-5723.

67. Doucette WR, Rippe JJ, Gaither CA, Kreling DH, Mott DA, Schommer JC. Influences on the frequency and type of community pharmacy services. *J Am Pharm Assoc*. 2017;57(1):72-76.

68. Malacos K. Pharmacy technician regulation. Available at https://www.pharmacytimes.com/publications/issue/2016/June2016/Pharmacy-Technician-Regulation. Accessed January 10, 2020.

69. United States Bureau of Labor Statistics. Pharmacy technicians: occupational outlook handbook. Available at https://www.bls.gov/ooh/healthcare/pharmacy-technicians.htm. Accessed May 30, 2020.

70. Alkhateeb FM, Shields KM, Broedel-Zaugg K, Bryan A, Snell J. Credentialing of pharmacy technicians in the USA. *Int J Pharm Pract*. 2011;19(4):219-227.

71. Miller RF, Cesarz J, Rough S. Evaluation of community pharmacy tech-check-tech as a strategy for practice advancement. *J Am Pharm Assoc*. 2018;58(6):652-658.

72. Boughen M, Sutton J, Fenn T, Wright D. Defining the role of the pharmacy technician and identifying their future role in medicines optimisation. *Pharmacy*. 2017;5(4):40.

73. University of Minnesota College of Pharmacy. Become a strong applicant. Available at https://www.pharmacy.umn.edu/degrees-and-programs/doctor-pharmacy/admissions/become-strong-applicant. Accessed January 10, 2020.

74. University of North Carolina Eshelman School of Pharmacy. Who we look for. Available at https://pharmacy.unc.edu/academics/the-pharmd/applicants/. Accessed January 10, 2020.

75. U.S. Pharmacist. Five key tips to improve inventory management. Available at https://www.uspharmacist.com/article/five-key-tips-to-improve-inventory-management. Accessed May 30, 2020.

76. Rexaline S. The 5 most expensive drugs in US: what you should know. Available at https://finance.yahoo.com/news/5-most-expensive-drugs-us-205657840.html. Accessed May 30, 2020.

77. American Society of Health System Pharmacists. Current drug shortages. Available at https://www.ashp.org/Drug-Shortages/Current-Shortages. Accessed May 30, 2020.

78. Ventola CL. The drug shortage crisis in the United States: causes, impact, and management strategies. *P T.* 2011;36(11): 740-757.

79. United States Food and Drug Administration. Drug recalls. Available at https://www.fda.gov/drugs/drug-safety-and-availability/drug-recalls. Accessed May 30, 2020.

80. Demler TL. FDA update on recent voluntary ARB drug recalls. Available at https://www.uspharmacist.com/article/fda-update-on-recent-voluntary-arb-drug-recalls. Accessed May 30, 2020.

81. Alltucker K. Zantac is prescribed 15 million times a year. So how did it become a potential cancer risk? Available at https://www.theadvertiser.com/story/news/health/2019/11/07/how-did-zantac-become-potential-cancer-risk-fda-wants-find-out/2509043001/. Accessed May 30, 2020.

82. Oseltamivir [package insert]. Foster City, CA: Gilead Sciences; 2012.

83. United States Food and Drug Administration. Human drug compounding. Available at https://www.fda.gov/drugs/guidance-compliance-regulatory-information/human-drug-compounding. Accessed May 30, 2020.

84. National Association of Boards of Pharmacy Good Compounding Practices Applicable to State Licensed Pharmacies. National Association of Boards of Pharmacy, Park Ridge, IL; 2001:151.

85. Subramaniam V, Sokol G, Zenger V, et al. Survey of drug products compounded by a group of community pharmacies: findings from a Food and Drug Administration study. *J Clin Pharmacol.* 2002;42(9):1031-1050.

86. Global Market Insights, Inc. US compounding pharmacies market trends statistics report 2025 with focus on top players. Available at https://www.openpr.com/news/1555675/u-s-compounding-pharmacies-market-trends-statistics-report-2025-with-focus-on-top-players-absolute-pharmacy-b-braun-medical-baxter-cantrell-drug-company-central-compounding-center-clinigen-group-dougherty-s-pharmacy-fagron-fresenius-kabi-ic.html. Accessed May 30, 2020.

87. Alliance for Pharmacy Compounding. Available at www.https://a4pc.org/. Accessed May 30, 2020.

88. O'Connor SD, and Supreme Court of the United States. *U.S. Reports: Thompson v. Western States Medical Center, 535 US 357.* Available at https://www.loc.gov/item/usrep535357/. Accessed May 30, 2020.

89. Murphy M. Pharmacies turn Tamiflu to liquid. Available at https://www.wsj.com/articles/SB10001424052748704506004576174760531649934. Accessed May 30, 2020.

90. Helin-Tanninen M, Autio K, Keski-Rahkonen P, Naaranlahti T, Järvinen K. Comparison of six different suspension vehicles in compounding of oral extemporaneous nifedipine suspension for paediatric patients. *Eur J Hosp Pharm.* 2012;19:432-437.

91. Cellini M, Santaguida MG, Gatto I, et al. Systematic appraisal of lactose intolerance as cause of increased need for oral thyroxine. *J Clin Endocrinol Metab.* 2014;99(8):1454-1458.

92. United States Pharmacopeial Convention. Compounding standards. Available at https://www.usp.org/compounding. Accessed May 30, 2020.

93. National Association of Boards of Pharmacy. Model pharmacy act/rules. Available at https://nabp.pharmacy/publications-reports/resource-documents/model-pharmacy-act-rules/. Accessed May 30, 2020.

94. United States Food and Drug Administration. Registered outsourcing facilities. Available at https://www.fda.gov/drugs/human-drug-compounding/registered-outsourcing-facilities. Accessed May 30, 2020.

95. United States Food and Drug Administration. Compounding laws and policies. Available at https://www.fda.gov/drugs/human-drug-compounding/compounding-laws-and-policies. Accessed May 30, 2020.

96. Pharmacy Technician Certification Board. CPhT statistics and data. Available at https://www.ptcb.org/history/chpt-statistics-and-data. Accessed May 30, 2020.

97. Pew Charitable Trusts. US illnesses and deaths associated with compounded medications or repackaged medications: 2001–2017. Available at https://www.pewtrusts.org/en/research-and-analysis/data-visualizations/2017/us-illnesses-and-deaths-associated-with-compounded-medications-or-repackaged-medications. Accessed May 30, 2020.

98. Board of Pharmacy Specialties. Compounded sterile preparations pharmacy. Available at https://www.bpsweb.org/bps-specialties/compounded-sterile-preparations-pharmacy/. Accessed May 30, 2020.

99. United States Government Accountability Office. Drug compounding: FDA has taken steps to implement compounding law, but some states and stakeholders reported challenges. Available at https://www.gao.gov/products/GAO-17-64. Accessed May 30 2020.

100. Gudeman J, Jozwiakowski M, Chollet J, Randell M. Potential risks of pharmacy compounding. *Drugs R D.* 2013;13(1):1-8.

101. Bidgood J. Pharmacist gets 9-year prison term in deadly meningitis outbreak. Available at https://www.nytimes.com/2017/06/26/us/pharmacy-meningitis-deaths-steroids-crisis.html. Accessed May 30, 2020.

102. Elder DL. General guidelines for preparing compounded drug products. In: *A Practical Guide to Contemporary Pharmacy Practice and Compounding.* 4th ed. Alphen an den Rijn, South Holland, Netherlands: Wolters Kluwer; 2018:141-155.

103. McPherson T, Fontane P, Iyengar R, Henderson R. Utilization and costs of compounded medications for commercially insured patients, 2012–2013. *J Manag Care Spec Pharm.* 2016;22(2):172-181.

104. Kelleher KJ, Gardner W. Out of sight, out of mind—behavioral and developmental care for rural children. *N Engl J Med.* 2017;376(14):1301-1303.

105. Rosenblatt RA, Hart LG. Physicians and rural America. *West J Med.* 2000;173(5):348-351.

106. Moy E, Garcia MC, Bastian B, et al. Leading causes of death in nonmetropolitan and metropolitan areas—United States, 1999–2014. *MMWR Surveill Summ.* 2017;66(1):1-8.

107. United States Department of Agriculture Economic Research Service. What is rural? Available at https://www.ers.usda.gov/topics/rural-economy-population/rural-classifications/what-is-rural.aspx. Accessed May 30, 2020.

108. Meit M, Knudson A, Gilbert T, et al. The 2014 update of the rural-urban chartbook. Available at https://ruralhealth.und.edu/projects/health-reform-policy-research-center/pdf/2014-rural-urban-chartbook-update.pdf. Accessed May 30, 2020.

109. United States Census Bureau. Health insurance in rural America. Available at https://www.census.gov/library/stories/2019/04/health-insurance-rural-america.html. Accessed May 30, 2020.

110. Jonk YC, O'Connor H, Casey M, Moscovice I. Comparing rural and urban Medicare Part D enrollment patterns and prescription drug coverage rates. University of Minnesota Rural Health

Research Center. Available at http://rhrc.umn.edu/wp-content/files_mf/may2013partdpolicybrief.pdf. Accessed May 30, 2020.

111. Medicare.gov. Drug coverage (Part D). Available at https://www.medicare.gov/drug-coverage-part-d. Accessed May 30, 2020.

112. Fredrick J. By the numbers: how community pharmacists measure up. Available at https://drugstorenews.com/pharmacy/numbers-how-community-pharmacists-measure#close-olyticsmodal. Accessed May 30, 2020.

113. National Public Radio. The struggle to hire and keep doctors in rural areas means patients go without care. Available at https://www.npr.org/sections/health-shots/2019/05/21/725118232/the-struggle-to-hire-and-keep-doctors-in-rural-areas-means-patients-go-without-c. Accessed May 30, 2020.

114. Pew Research Center. How far do urban, suburban and rural Americans live from a hospital? Available at https://www.pewresearch.org/fact-tank/2018/12/12/how-far-americans-live-from-the-closest-hospital-differs-by-community-type/. Accessed May 30, 2020.

115. Mann S. Research shows shortage of more than 100,000 doctors by 2030. Available at https://www.aamc.org/news-insights/research-shows-shortage-more-100000-doctors-2030. Accessed May 30, 2020.

116. Sharma S. The need to serve rural America. *Biotechnol Healthc.* 2010;7(4):24-25.

117. National Center for Health Workforce Analysis. Distribution of US health care providers residing in rural and urban areas. Available at https://www.ruralhealthinfo.org/assets/1275-5131/rural-urban-workforce-distribution-nchwa-2014.pdf. Accessed May 30, 2020.

118. Esposito L. Rural pharmacies are closing: where does that leave patients? Available at https://health.usnews.com/health-care/patient-advice/articles/2018-10-17/rural-pharmacies-are-closing-where-does-that-leave-patients. Accessed May 30, 2020.

119. Crossley K. Public perceives pharmacists as some of the most trusted professionals. Available at https://www.pharmacytimes.com/publications/career/2019/CareersWinter19/public-perceives-pharmacists-as-some-of-the-most-trusted-professionals. Accessed May 30, 2020.

120. Health Resources & Services Administration. Health Professional Shortage Areas (HPSAs). Available at https://bhw.hrsa.gov/shortage-designation/hpsas. Accessed May 30, 2020.

121. Shambaugh-Miller MD, Vanosdel N, Mueller KJ. Reliance on independently owned pharmacies in rural America. *Rural Policy Brief.* 2007;(PB2007-6):1-4.

122. National Community Pharmacists Association. United States House of Representatives Energy & Commerce Committee Subcommittee on Health Hearing on the CMS Proposed Medicare Part D Rule. Available at http://www.pbmwatch.com/uploads/8/2/7/8/8278205/ncpa-statement-ec-health-subcommittee-part-d.pdf. Accessed May 30, 2020.

123. Scott DM, Strand M, Undem T, Anderson G, Clarens A, Liu X. Assessment of pharmacists' delivery of public health services in rural and urban areas in Iowa and North Dakota. *Pharm Pract.* 2016;14(4):836.

124. Goode J-V, Owen J, Page A, Gatewood S. Community-based pharmacy practice innovation and the role of the community-based pharmacist practitioner in the United States. *Pharmacy.* 2019;7(3):106.

125. Centers for Disease Control and Prevention. Basics about COPD. Available at https://www.cdc.gov/copd/basics-about.html. Accessed May 30, 2020.

126. Croft JB, Wheaton AG, Liu Y, et al. Urban-rural county and state differences in chronic obstructive pulmonary disease—United States, 2015. *MMWR Morb Mortal Wkly Rep.* 2018;67(7):205-211.

127. American Lung Association. Learn about COPD. Available at https://www.lung.org/lung-health-and-diseases/lung-disease-lookup/copd/learn-about-copd/how-serious-is-copd.html. Accessed May 30, 2020.

128. Centers for Disease Control and Prevention. Smoking & tobacco use: fast facts. Available at https://www.cdc.gov/tobacco/data_statistics/fact_sheets/fast_facts/index.htm. Accessed May 30, 2020.

129. National Heart, Lung, and Blood Institute (NHLBI). COPD. Available at https://www.nhlbi.nih.gov/health-topics/copd. Accessed January 19, 2020.

130. Rural Health Information Hub. Rural hunger and access to healthy food. Available at https://www.ruralhealthinfo.org/topics/food-and-hunger. Accessed May 30, 2020.

131. Centers for Disease Control and Prevention. Living with COPD. Available at https://www.cdc.gov/features/copd/index.html. Accessed May 30, 2020.

132. Celli BR, Barnes PJ. Exacerbations of chronic obstructive pulmonary disease. *Eur Respir J.* 2007;29(6):1224-1238.

133. Guarascio AJ, Ray SM, Finch CK, Self TH. The clinical and economic burden of chronic obstructive pulmonary disease in the USA. *Clinicoecon Outcomes Res.* 2013;5(1):235-245.

134. Miravitlles M, Ferrer M, Pont À, et al. Effect of exacerbations on quality of life in patients with chronic obstructive pulmonary disease: a 2 year follow up study. *Thorax.* 2004;59(5):387-395.

135. Cavaillès A, Brinchault-Rabin G, Dixmier A, et al. Comorbidities of COPD. *Eur Respir Rev.* 2013;22(130):454-475.

136. Navaie M, Ganapathy V, Cho-Reyes S, Celli B, Dembe K, Yeh K. Inhalation device technique errors among patients with obstructive lung diseases using metered-dose inhalers: a systematic review and meta-analysis of US studies. *Chest.* 2018;154(4):784A-785A.

137. Duarte-De-Araújo A, Teixeira P, Hespanhol V, Correia-De-Sousa J. COPD: misuse of inhaler devices in clinical practice. *Int J Chron Obstruct Pulmon Dis.* 2019;30(14):1209-1217.

138. Tseng CW, Yazdany J, Dudley RA, et al. Medicare Part D plans' coverage and cost-sharing for acute rescue and preventive inhalers for chronic obstructive pulmonary disease. *JAMA Intern Med.* 2017;177(4):585-588.

139. Johnson M, Jastrzab R, Tate J, et al. Evaluation of an academic-community partnership to implement MTM services in rural communities to improve pharmaceutical care for patients with diabetes and/or hypertension. *J Manag Care Spec Pharm.* 2018;24(2):132-141.

140. Ross LA, Bloodworth LS. Patient-centered health care using pharmacist-delivered medication therapy management in rural Mississippi. *J Am Pharm Assoc.* 2012;52(6):802-809.

141. Global Initiative for Chronic Obstructive Lung Disease. Global strategy for the diagnosis, management, and prevention of chronic obstructive pulmonary disease. Available at https://goldcopd.org/wp-content/uploads/2019/11/GOLD-2020-REPORT-ver1.0wms.pdf. Accessed May 30, 2020.

CHAPTER 3

Primary Care

Featuring the Illustrated Case Studies "Support," "Swish," & "Holistic"

Authors

Amanda Margolis, Denise L. Walbrandt Pigarelli, Valerie A. Schend, Christine A. Sorkness, & Joseph A. Zorek

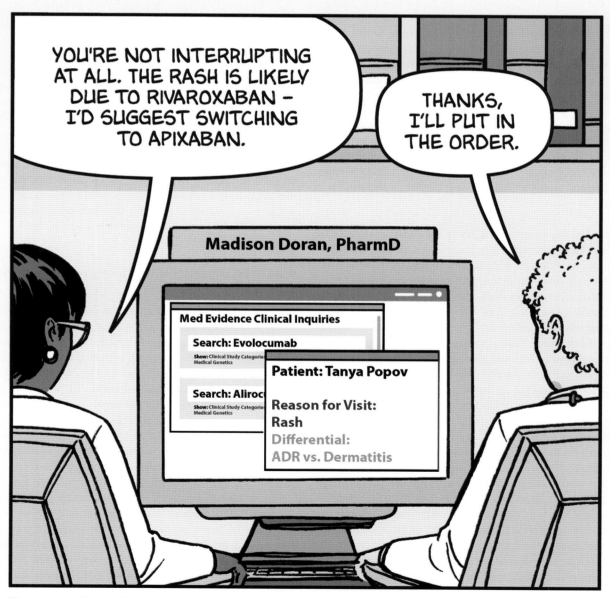

Illustration by George Folz, © 2019 Board of Regents of the University of Wisconsin System

BACKGROUND

Practice settings in healthcare are frequently categorized as inpatient or outpatient based on whether care is being delivered/received inside or outside of a hospital. Primary care clinics represent the foundation, or hub, of outpatient healthcare services. Interprofessional teams within primary care take responsibility for the entirety of a patient's health and well-being. This includes directly managing acute illnesses and chronic conditions unless they are severe or uncommon.[1-4] For severe acute illnesses and uncommon diagnoses, specialists are needed, and the primary care team steps into a coordination role, making referrals to, or recommendations for consultation with, appropriate providers.[3,5] Sometimes these referrals are to specialty outpatient providers (e.g., cardiology, rheumatology, urology clinics), while other situations require referral for urgent or emergency care.

Importantly, primary care teams continue to coordinate with other providers in referral situations, which allows them to advocate for the overall healthcare needs of patients when multiple specialty providers become involved. After urgent or emergent situations are addressed, patients then transition back into the care of the primary care team. Another key feature of primary care is the provision of preventive health services, including helping patients stay up-to-date on immunizations and health promotion such as improving lifestyle (e.g., diet, exercise, smoking cessation).[2] Primary care teams also conduct recommended screenings to identify health issues early in the course of a disease before severe consequences emerge. For more information on lifestyle and prevention efforts by pharmacists, readers are encouraged to explore the illustrated cases "Change Talk," "Screen," and "Mobilized" in Chapter 4 Prevention & Wellness.

The four pillars of primary care delivery include first-contact care, continuous care, comprehensive care, and care coordination.[2,6] Primary care providers are often the first contact patients have with the healthcare system.[3] From there, the primary care team attempts to provide continuous care; meaning, care delivered by the same team. This allows the patient, as well as their family and community, to establish relationships with healthcare providers and other health professionals.[2,7] From a pharmacy perspective, the term *provider* is generally reserved for health professionals who are legally empowered to write prescriptions or order medications, such as physicians, physician assistants, nurse practitioners, and dentists; in some states, pharmacists are also granted limited prescribing authority as well. The ability of patients to develop trusting relationships with primary care providers and other health professionals on the team through repeated encounters promotes patient-centered care. Common conditions managed by primary care teams include high blood pressure, upper respiratory infections, depression, anxiety, back pain, arthritis, dermatitis, ear infection, diabetes, and cough.[1] Lastly, primary care teams coordinate the overall health plan for patients to ensure the recommendations from specialists, as well as the conditions that the primary care team is managing, are safe and comprehensive.[2] Without this coordination, patient care can become fragmented

and lead to confusion, medical and medication errors, duplicative care, and/or unmet needs.[5]

There are several types of primary care teams. These teams are typically differentiated by the types of patients they serve, usually depending on age, and sometimes sex. Examples include family medicine, internal medicine, pediatrics, geriatrics, and obstetrics and gynecology (OB/GYN).[8] See the illustrated case "Burden" in Chapter 7 Geriatrics for an example of a primary care team focused on older adults. Most patients see their primary care team in an outpatient clinic; however, patients can also be seen by home-based primary care teams.[3] Regardless of the specific clinic or location, all primary care teams serve as the main contact and coordinator for their patients within the healthcare system by following the four pillars of primary care.

Members of the Interprofessional Primary Care Team

The interprofessional team-based model of care is prevalent in primary care settings.[2,4,6,7,9-14] Most of these teams are led by physicians; however, a growing number, especially in rural settings, are being led by nurse practitioners or physician assistants.[2] The composition of teams varies within different settings, but the following health professionals are often involved in primary care teams: behavioral health providers (e.g., counseling psychologists), dietitians/nutritionists, medical assistants, nurses, nurse practitioners, pharmacists, physicians, physician assistants, and social workers, as well as administrative staff (e.g., schedulers or receptionists).[4,7] The team-based approach, often involving the physical colocation of different health professionals to facilitate coordination, communication, and shared decision making, is adopted to improve health outcomes of individual patients and populations (i.e., groups of patients with common ailments such as diabetes, high blood pressure, or depression), patient satisfaction, and health professionals' job/career satisfaction.[4,7]

Role of Pharmacists within Interprofessional Primary Care Teams

Primary care pharmacists contribute to improved health outcomes and patient satisfaction by maximizing the safe and effective use of medications. The core professional roles in this setting include assisting providers with evidence-based drug selection, monitoring for and troubleshooting medication side effects, and improving medication adherence by educating patients about both prescription and over-the-counter medications.[14-16] Primary care pharmacists contribute to the development and implementation of services (i.e., targeted interventions) aimed at improving patient care; some well-known examples include annual wellness visits, medication therapy management, transitions of care, population health management, and medication education for patients and other health professionals.[4,13,17] Pharmacists in primary care spend the majority of their time engaging in direct patient care.[14] This care can be delivered through in-person clinic appointments, telephone calls, or video conferencing.[13,14,18] Appointments between patients and pharmacists can be used to supplement the care from primary care providers between visits or can take place in conjunction with those visits.[9,19,20]

Readers are encouraged to explore the illustrated cases below, as well as "Underlying Cause," "Educator," and "Empowerment" in Chapter 5 Cardiology for examples of in-person clinic appointments. Those interested in visits completed via video conferencing should read the illustrated case "Wounded" in Chapter 8 Infectious Diseases, while those who would benefit from an example of a pharmacist utilizing other technologies, including smart devices and virtual reality, to contribute to the interprofessional care of patients should explore the illustrated case "Innovator" in Chapter 13 Technology.

Pharmacists in the primary care setting can have a profound impact on the medication management and health of their patients.[21] Common interventions made by primary care pharmacists include stopping unnecessary medications, initiation of new medications, and dose adjustments.[15,20] In an evaluation of primary care medication therapy management appointments, pharmacists identified an average of four medication-related problems and resolved an average of two problems per appointment.[15] The most common problem resolved was the need for an additional medication. Similarly, in the Veterans Health Administration (VA), clinical pharmacists made approximately 1.6 interventions per patient care encounter for a variety of health conditions including anticoagulation, diabetes, mental health, and high blood pressure.[22] A variety of health outcomes have demonstrated improvement following pharmacist interventions. Many health systems, for example, have successfully improved metrics of diabetes management through pharmacist interventions.[17,20,23,24] Impressively, integration of primary care pharmacists across 25 clinics in the Netherlands yielded a 30% decrease in medication-related hospitalizations.[25] Kaiser Permanente of Colorado, meanwhile, observed a 30% increase in the proportion of patients with blood pressure at goal/target following the introduction of primary care pharmacists into their clinics.[14]

Currently, pharmacists are able to prescribe and adjust medications, order labs, and/or make referrals through legal agreements with providers.[26,27] These agreements are often called collaborative practice agreements, and they focus on specific health conditions, management of specific medications, and refill authorization.[28] Health conditions where use of collaborative practice agreements is common by primary care pharmacists include anticoagulation, diabetes, hyperlipidemia, and high blood pressure management.[14] There has been a concerted effort over many years to expand prescriptive authority to pharmacists.[29]

Incorporation of primary care pharmacists into care delivery models also increases patients' access to care. Pharmacists in this setting decrease provider workload and open additional appointments for patients with more complex or acute needs who require provider attention.[12,30] One way pharmacists add value is through medication titration and monitoring in between provider appointments, essentially extending the time between provider appointments while ensuring medication

safety and effectiveness.[13,19] Another way pharmacists alleviate time pressures for the primary care team is by answering drug information questions. As medication experts, pharmacists are most efficient in answering medication-related questions from both patients and providers.[30] Access to health resources and medications can also improve when primary care pharmacists are given the responsibility of managing medication refills.[9] Pharmacists in this role ensure that appropriate labs are drawn and assessments are completed in a timely manner to safely renew medications.[31]

In addition to direct patient care, primary care pharmacists also assist primary care teams in population health management initiatives. According to the National Association of Community Health Centers, population health management is "management of health and outcomes for subpopulations, such as the population of patients served by a health center."[32] As stated above, other common subpopulations within a primary care practice include patients who share the same health condition (e.g., diabetes, high blood pressure, depression). Pharmacists review these populations as a whole, exploring, for example, the average blood pressure of all patients with a high blood pressure diagnosis. Individuals not meeting blood pressure goals are identified by pharmacists and interventions are made to improve their health.[33] Examples of pharmacist-led population health management initiatives include ensuring appropriate medication use among patients with cardiovascular disease,[34] checking blood pressure and initiating medications among patients overdue for blood pressure evaluations,[35] and titrating medication doses for patients with diabetes.[36] These initiatives can be implemented to minimize health costs, address patient care needs, and improve quality measures.[33,37]

PRIMARY CARE PHARMACISTS IN ACTION

Mental Health Integration into Primary Care

Following Operation Enduring Freedom, Operation Iraqi Freedom, and Operation New Dawn, approximately 1 million new veterans initiated care with the (VA) health system.[11] Over half of the patients newly seeking care with the VA were suffering from a mental health condition, primarily posttraumatic stress disorder, depression, and anxiety. This influx of patients created a need for additional mental health services within the VA. One way the South Texas Veterans Healthcare System increased access to care for patients with mental health concerns was to offer mental health services integrated into primary care. Importantly, this included partnering with a clinical pharmacy specialist. These pharmacists were able to see patients with uncomplicated mental health conditions, and they were empowered to prescribe and adjust dosing for antidepressants, medications for nightmares, certain non-habit-forming medications for anxiety, and sleep aids. Patients who did not respond or whose conditions were deemed complex were referred to a mental health specialist. While under the care of a pharmacist, 77% of patients achieved a response or remission from their mental health condition. The pharmacists were able to maintain 90% of their patients in primary care, which increased the availability of mental health specialists for patients who required a higher level of care.

Stopping Unnecessary Medications

Proton pump inhibitors (PPIs) are a class of medications used to decrease stomach acid production.[38] PPIs are used for a number of gastrointestinal conditions including heartburn symptoms; however, PPIs are not recommended to be used for long periods of time due to adverse effects such as increased risk of bone fractures, pneumonia, and kidney disease. Unfortunately, despite the potential for serious complications, PPIs are often overprescribed and they are not discontinued in a timely manner. To address this problem, primary care pharmacists at the Bethesda Family Medicine Clinic in St. Paul, Minnesota started a PPI tapering service for their patients.[39] The PPI taper slowly decreased patients' doses until the PPI was able to be discontinued without recurrence of heart burn symptoms. Patients initially met with the pharmacist the same day they were in clinic to see their primary care provider for patient convenience. During the appointment, the patient received education on the taper and the pharmacist ordered supportive medication to manage potential symptoms during the PPI taper. There was also at least one follow-up appointment with the pharmacist recommended to the patient. Eighty-six percent of the patients who saw a pharmacist as part of this service were able to discontinue their PPI within 8 weeks.

Decreasing Opioid Use

The opioid epidemic of misuse, overuse, and death from opioid overdose has been well documented.[40] Many health systems have developed interventions to decrease opioid use in an effort to keep patients safe. Pharmacists in primary care have contributed meaningfully to these efforts. At Virginia Mason Medical Center in Seattle, Washington, pharmacists collaborated with other members of the interprofessional team to better serve patients who use opioid medications.[10] These pharmacists worked closely with physicians in the clinic to start nonopioid pain medications, decrease opioid doses and use, and ensure that urine drug screenings and medication agreements between patients and providers were completed. A substantial decrease in opioid use among patients who worked with the pharmacist was observed. Additionally, pharmacists initiated nonopioid medications during nearly 20% of appointments, increased urine drug screenings by 55%, and increased documentation of medication agreements by roughly 150%. The addition of primary care pharmacists increased the clinic's compliance with best practices for opioid management and significantly decreased the wait time for patients to see a provider. Overall, primary care pharmacists contributed meaningfully to medication safety for patients who used opioid medications. Readers are encouraged to explore the illustrated case "Gasping" in Chapter 12 Mental Health for a more detailed discussion of opioids.

BECOMING A PRIMARY CARE PHARMACIST

Most primary care pharmacists are empowered to order and adjust prescriptions for patients as part of their medication management duties, generally through collaborative practice agreements with providers. Prescribing and monitoring medications typically requires additional training beyond the Doctor of Pharmacy (PharmD) degree. Many health systems require a postgraduate year 1 (PGY-1) residency and may also require a postgraduate year 2 (PGY-2) residency in ambulatory care.[14] During an ambulatory care residency, pharmacists get additional training in managing health conditions often seen in primary care and other population health activities.

Many primary care pharmacists become board certified either due to their employers' requirements or for career advancement purposes.[14] The most common board certification that primary care pharmacists obtain is the Board Certified Ambulatory Care Pharmacist (BCACP) certification offered by the Board of Pharmacy Specialties (BPS).[41] Individuals eligible to take the BCACP exam must have a current, active license to practice pharmacy and have at least one of the following: (1) at least 4 years of practice delivering patient care in an ambulatory care outpatient setting, (2) completion of a PGY-1 residency and 1 additional year of experience practicing in ambulatory are, or (3) completion of a PGY-2 residency in ambulatory care pharmacy. Once a pharmacist passes the BCACP exam and is certified, the certification lasts for 7 years. Recertification can be achieved by either passing a recertification exam or completing 100 hours of BPS-approved continuing education credits prior to the expiration of the certification.

SUPPORT: An Illustrated Case Study

Story by Amanda Margolis & Joseph A. Zorek
Illustrations by George Folz, © 2019 Board of Regents of the University of Wisconsin System

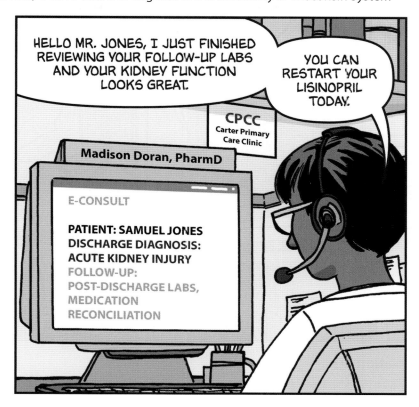

Illustration 3-1

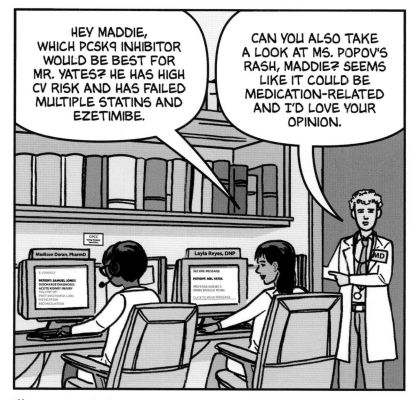

Illustration 3-2

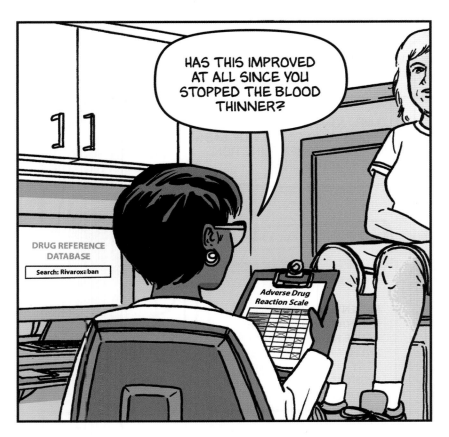

Illustration 3-3

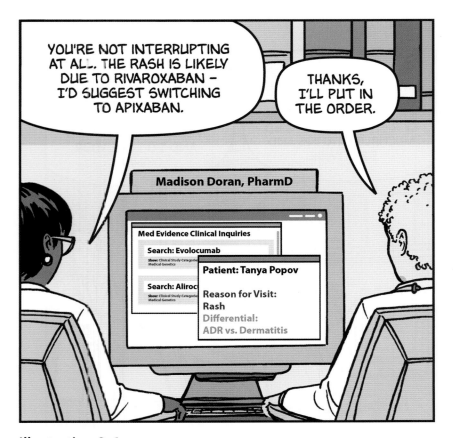

Illustration 3-4

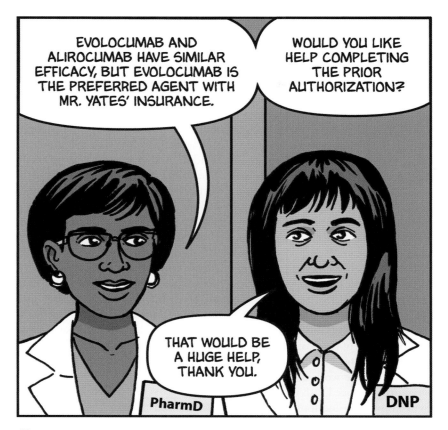

Illustration 3-5

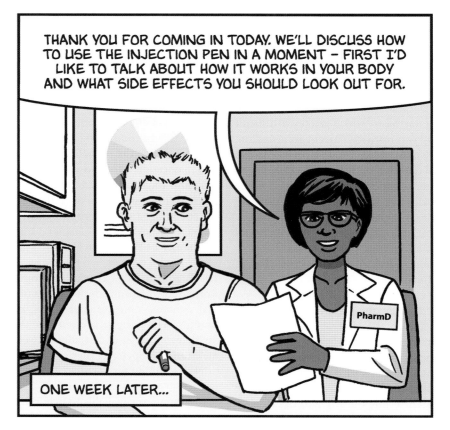

Illustration 3-6

Thoughts on "Support"

The illustrated case "Support" highlights a range of professional activities performed by Dr. Madison "Maddie" Doran, a primary care pharmacist employed by the Carter Primary Care Clinic. Told mostly over the course of a single day, "Support" touches upon some of the most timely and important scenarios encountered in contemporary primary care pharmacy; these include evidence-based decision making, the identification and mitigation of adverse drug reactions, and the critical role of patient engagement and education to ensure the safe and effective use of medications.

Perhaps one of the most important types of support Maddie provides to this interprofessional primary care team is her understanding of the evidence upon which the safe and effective use of medications is based. Coupled with her clinical judgment, this provides Maddie an opportunity to contribute expertise that fills a well-defined need in the clinic. In Illustration 3-2, the nurse practitioner is shown leaning on Maddie's knowledge and skills to help select the best medication option in a relatively new, and thus less well understood, class of medications to treat high cholesterol. Simultaneously, and later in Illustrations 3-3 and 3-4, Maddie is shown supporting the work of a physician who is suspicious of a potential drug-induced rash in one of his patients by leveraging available knowledge and tools.

Evidence-based medicine combines the best available research, the clinician's clinical judgment, and the patient's preference to determine an individual patient's care plan.[42] The most valuable source of evidence is a randomized controlled trial (RCT). Broadly speaking, an RCT compares one medication to another to determine the efficacy and safety of medications.[43,44] By randomizing the study participants to which medication they will receive, as many variables as possible which could impact efficacy and safety are kept consistent between the groups to determine the clinical effect of the medication.[45] A high volume of data is published on a regular basis, which makes it difficult for health professionals to keep up with current information. Systematic reviews combine multiple RCTs into a single analysis to answer a specific clinical question.[46] This allows clinicians to review the body of literature, as opposed to a single RCT, while providing a high level of evidence. In Illustration 3-5, Maddie shares her conclusions from a high-quality systematic review comparing the two medications of interest: evolocumab and alirocumab.[47] In this systematic review, the cardiovascular outcomes from 39 RCTs were included, giving a stronger level of evidence than a single RCT can offer.

In the absence of RCTs and systematic reviews, observational research may be extrapolated to the clinical scenario.[48,49] In observational research, patients and their health team determine the medication and health plan; the investigator does not assign the medication or intervention.[50] This makes it harder to determine causality compared to an RCT. A case report is one type of observational research. While the strength of evidence for a case report is low, they describe a detailed account of the treatment and outcomes in a single patient and are particularly useful for rare diseases or adverse drug reactions (ADR) and may generate ideas which lead to further research.[51]

Pharmacists utilize literature and other sources of information to make evidence-based recommendations to the interprofessional primary care team.[52,53] The majority of clinical questions can be answered using a tertiary resource.[54] Tertiary resources summarize and catalog information from primary resources (e.g., RCTs, observational studies). Throughout "Support," Maddie is shown using a drug reference database. Databases, like this fictitious one, are perhaps the most common form of tertiary resources utilized in contemporary health. Common examples include the commercial products Lexicomp and Micromedex.[55,56] In addition to data from primary sources, these tertiary resources include information from US Food and Drug Administration–approved package inserts, which contain details such as approved indications and doses, as well as brief summaries of the mechanism of action, drug interactions, and adverse effects.[54] Another type of tertiary resource is a compilation of narrative reviews written by experts. These reviews cover the basics of disease states, as well as treatment recommendations from guidelines. UpToDate and Pharmacist Letter are two commonly used commercial products in this category.[57,58]

Pharmacists use a five-step process to apply evidence-based medicine in practice.[59] Table 3-1 provides an example of how Maddie would have used these steps in "Support," in combination with actual evidence from the published literature, to determine an appropriate medication recommendation plan for Mr. Yates, the nurse practitioner's patient depicted in Illustrations 3-2, 3-5, and 3-6.

While Maddie is able to use RCTs and systematic reviews to help guide her recommendations related to Mr. Yates, she must use a lower level of evidence in support of the physician's request. Specifically, a patient named Ms. Popov has presented to Carter Primary Care Clinic with a potential ADR. Pharmacists in many patient care settings assist with the identification of ADRs.[14,60,61] In completing these assessments, generally the task is to determine the probability, or likelihood, that the medication in question is the causative agent. Fortunately, there are criteria and tools available to help with these ADR assessments. For additional examples of ADRs and possible ADRs, readers are encouraged to explore the illustrated cases "Swish" in this chapter, "Innovator" in Chapter 13 Technology, and "Relapse" in Chapter 14 Population Health.

The Bradford Hill Criteria is a commonly referenced framework used when considering issues of probability and causation that contains nine principles (i.e., criteria).[62,63] However, the Bradford Hill Criteria is often applied more broadly, including the determination of causality between an adverse effect and a medication.[64] Specific criteria are presented in Table 3-2 with a brief description for context.

Several tools are available to help pharmacists and other health professionals determine whether a patient complaint can be attributed to an ADR. These are referred to in the published

Table 3-1. Evidence-Based Decision Making Applied to the Case of Mr. Yates in "Support"

Step	Description	Application to Mr. Yates' Case
Ask	A question such as "What medication is best to lower cholesterol" is too broad to conduct a meaningful literature search. Therefore, the first step is to narrow the clinical question.	Maddie would frame the question as "In patients who have failed statin therapy, how does the rate of cardiovascular events using evolocumab compare to alirocumab?"
Acquire	Identification and retrieval of randomized controlled trials and systematic reviews. PubMed is a commonly used search and indexing system to identify and retrieve literature.	Maddie uses the search terms "evolocumab" and "alirocumab" in a database to retrieve dozens of studies. Fortunately, there are also systematic reviews which include both agents.
Appraise	Determination of the quality of evidence available. Focuses on the internal validity of the research, or whether a reader believes a cause-and-effect relationship has been established.	Maddie identifies high-quality randomized controlled trials in her search. However, there are no direct head-to-head comparisons of evolocumab to alirocumab and an indirect analysis is needed.
Apply	Answers the clinical question. The pharmacist combines the evidence with their own clinical experience and patient preference to determine and implement the patient care plan.	In reviewing the available evidence, Maddie learns that there is not a meaningful difference in the rate of cardiovascular events or cardiovascular death when using evolocumab compared to using alirocumab; however, Mr. Yates' insurance prefers evolocumab over alirocumab.
Assess	Follow-up and determination of whether the patient care plan worked.	Maddie educates Mr. Yates on the use of evolocumab, and she will continue to follow up with him to ensure the drug is working and/or to make adjustments as needed.

literature as causality assessment tools, or CATs. Several well-known CATs exist and have been studied; for example, ALDEN, Naranjo, and Liverpool.[64,65] The Naranjo Adverse Drug Reaction Probability Scale (i.e., the Naranjo scale) is one of the most well-known tools pharmacists use.[66] Several Naranjo scale questions link to Bradford Hill Criteria and assist clinicians in systematically collecting information to determine the likelihood that a specific medication caused a specific adverse reaction. There are a number of recently published case reports using the Naranjo scale to determine the likelihood that an ADR was caused by a medication for a specific patient. Examples include nightmares caused by metformin, a medication for diabetes;[67] acute pancreatitis caused by mirtazapine, an antidepressant;[68] and a rash caused by topiramate, an anti-seizure drug.[69] In all of these cases, the ADR was atypical and received a high score on the Naranjo scale indicating the medication was probably causal of the adverse reaction.

As depicted in Illustration 3-3, Ms. Popov has a mild rash on her left lower extremity. While not explicitly stated, the computer monitor in Illustration 3-3 hints that Maddie has already completed an exploration of the literature to guide her evidence-based recommendation to the physician. When reporting safety outcomes, RCTs in the published literature often include tables of adverse reactions reported by patients who participate in the studies, and these tables serve as a common source of evidence that pharmacists utilize. When an adverse reaction is not experienced by RCT participants, pharmacists turn to observational research, and case reports in particular. It can be assumed that Maddie was unable to identify rash as an ADR in RCTs during her database search of rivaroxaban, the "blood thinner" (i.e., anticoagulant) in question, because she is employing an ADR scale. This scale is a fictitious tool to provide a visual example of how ALDEN, Naranjo, and Liverpool would be put to use. Also not shown is that Maddie's literature search uncovered two case reports of rash closely following initiation of rivaroxaban.[70,71] Both case reports scored high on the Naranjo scale, indicating that the rash was likely caused by the drug. Maddie is shown using the ADR scale in Illustration 3-3 to generate an additional piece of evidence upon which to base her recommendation to the physician in Illustration 3-4.

Beyond supporting prescribers' efforts to select the best medication possible for patients, or to help troubleshoot ADRs, primary care pharmacists play a critical role engaging and educating patients on the safe and effective use of medications. Intentionally, the illustrated case "Support" opens with Maddie engaged in this type of professional activity to emphasize its importance. Illustration 3-1 depicts a transitions of care (TOC) telephone call between Maddie and a patient recently discharged from the hospital, who is now adjusting back to his regular life and routine at home. These transitions often involve changes to patients' medication regimens.

The following TOC definition is promoted by the World Health Organization:

> Transitions of care refers to the various points where a patient moves to, or returns from, a particular physical location or makes contact with a health care professional for the purposes of receiving health care. This includes transitions between home, hospital, residential care settings and consultations with different health care providers in out-patient facilities.[72]

Table 3-2. Bradford Hill Criteria Applied to Assessment of Adverse Drug Reactions

Criteria	Description	Application to Adverse Drug Reactions
Strength	The larger the correlation (or mathematical association) between an exposure and an outcome, the more likely the exposure caused the outcome.	When there is a larger likelihood of the ADR[*] among individuals taking the medication compared to individuals not taking the medication, there is evidence the medication may be causing the ADR.
Consistency	Repeated observation of the association between an exposure and an outcome in different settings and studies strengthens the likelihood of causation.	An ADR described in multiple reports involving the same medication is more likely to be causative.
Specificity	When only individuals with one specific exposure develop the outcome, that exposure is likely to be causal.	Less applicable for ADRs
Temporality	An exposure needs to come first in order to cause an outcome.	The medication needs to be taken before the ADR in order for the medication to cause the ADR.
Biological gradient	Evidence for causation is present when individuals with higher amounts of the exposure are more likely to develop the outcome.	When a higher dose of the medication has a higher rate of the ADR, it is more likely the ADR is due to the medication. While often this is the case, this criteria does not always hold true for ADRs.
Plausibility	There is a biological reason that the exposure causes the outcome.	A rational explanation, rooted in physiology, exists for why the medication might have induced the ADR.
Coherence	The potential cause-and-effect relationship between the exposure and outcome should make sense based on other knowledge.	When considering alternative explanations for the ADR, if none are present it is more likely that the medication caused the ADR.
Experiment	When the exposure is manipulated, often removed, the risk for developing the outcome decreases.	When the medication is stopped, the ADR diminishes or resolves. This is not always possible depending on the ADR.
Analogy	Clinicians may be more accepting of causality between an exposure and outcome if a similar exposure also causes the outcome.	If a similar medication has been shown to produce the same ADR, it is more likely that the medication in question is responsible for the ADR.

[*] ADR = Adverse Drug Reaction

Unfortunately, following the transition from hospital to home, readmissions to the hospital within 30 days are common.[73] These preventable events are difficult on patients and costly. Rates of 30-day readmissions vary by age, insurance, diagnosis, and procedures. However, one report demonstrated that approximately 10% of patients aged 1 to 64 with private insurance were readmitted to the hospital within 30 days. The readmission rate for adults 65 and older was 21%. Preventable hospitalizations ranged in cost from $6000 to $14,000 per readmission. Given the frequency and associated costs, primary care teams have developed services and appointments to minimize the risk of readmission.[74-76]

Many TOC programs target patients at the highest risk for readmission, such as patients with heart failure or older adults.[16,73,75,77] Activities incorporated into TOC programs include review of the hospitalization and discharge plan with the patient, lab monitoring as needed, coordination of referrals and follow-up appointments, ensuring medication lists are accurate and up-to-date (i.e., medication reconciliation), and providing education to patients.[74] In Illustration 3-1, Maddie is shown performing common TOC services, including lab monitoring, medication reconciliation, and patient education.[16,74,75] While resource intense, these TOC primary care programs have the potential to be impactful; for example, one program reported a 38.7% decrease in readmissions among patients who received the service.[75] Patient education to facilitate the safe and effective use of medications is a common professional activity performed by primary care pharmacists outside the scope of TOC programs, as well, as depicted in Illustration 3-6.

Pharmacists in primary care settings have established themselves as an integral part of the interprofessional team. Their expertise is leveraged to improve the care of patients in multiple ways; among the most common, as shown in the illustrated case "Support," are evidence-based decision-making, the identification and mitigation of adverse drug reactions, and one-on-one interactions with patients, either in person, via telephone, or over secured video, to ensure the safe and effective use of medications. Contributing their expert knowledge and skills to the interprofessional team, in both direct and indirect patient care roles, further enhances the reach, impact, and value of primary care pharmacists.

1. Given all of the changes, such as new medications and medical instructions, that take place at hospital discharge, it is not surprising that misuse of medications by patients once they are home is common. How do you think this impacts the rate of readmission following hospital discharge?

2. Have you, or someone you know, ever experienced a side effect to a medication? What about a reaction to something else, such as a food allergy? How did you know what caused the reaction? Apply the Bradford Hill Criteria to this experience. Which criteria applied? Which did not?

3. Think of a time you used data or a resource to inform a decision. How did you find the information? How did you know the information was accurate? How did the information influence your decision?

4. Illustration 3-5 describes a prior authorization, which is a request to an insurance company to use a specific medication. Pharmacists often assist in preparing, reviewing, and approving prior authorizations. Why do you think a pharmacist might be involved in this process?

5. Pharmacists in primary care often deliver direct patient care using non-scheduled phone or video calls in between face-to-face appointments. Thinking about your own experience with the healthcare system as a patient, or perhaps the experience of a relative, what examples can you think of where this modality of pharmacist intervention might have been useful?

SWISH: An Illustrated Case Study

Story by Christine A. Sorkness, Valerie A. Schend, & Joseph A. Zorek
Illustrations by George Folz, © 2019 Board of Regents of the University of Wisconsin System

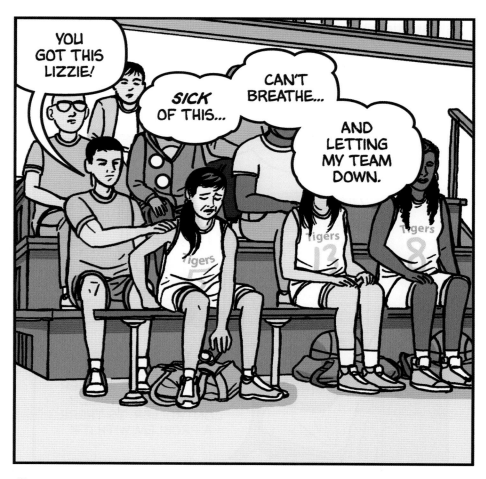

Illustration 3-7

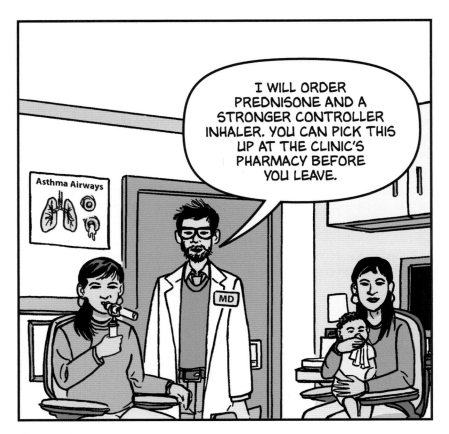

Illustration 3-8

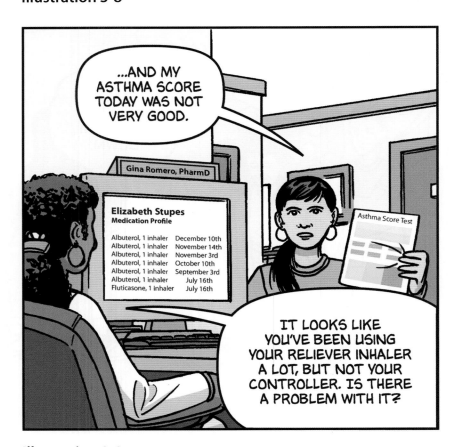

Illustration 3-9

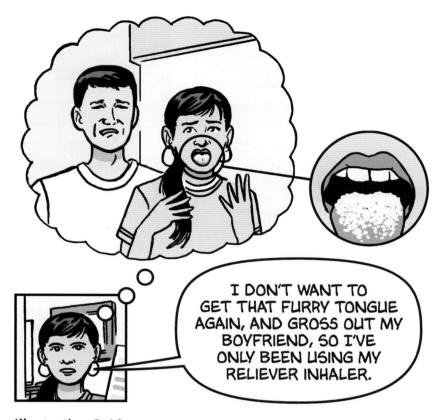

Illustration 3-10

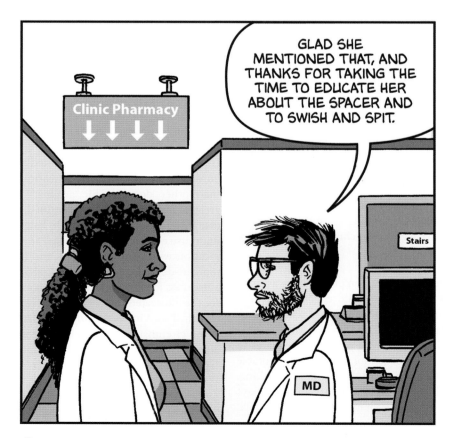

Illustration 3-11

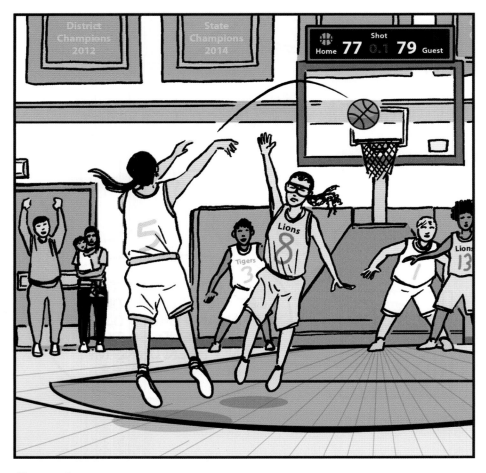

Illustration 3-12

Thoughts on "Swish"

The illustrated case "Swish" highlights common struggles experienced by children and adolescents with asthma. The main character, Lizzie, is depicted as a teenager who plays several roles; she's an athlete and teammate (Illustrations 3-7 and 3-12), a girlfriend (Illustrations 3-7 and 3-10), and a daughter and sister (Illustration 3-8). Transcending all of this is the fact that Lizzie lives with asthma, a common chronic condition that impacts all facets of her life.

In the United States, more than 25 million people have asthma, including 7.7% of adults and 8.4% of children.[78] Almost one-half of children with asthma miss at least 1 day of school annually due to an asthma exacerbation, and a child with asthma generally misses 3 to 5 days per school year.[79] This equates to roughly 14 million missed days of school each year attributable to asthma.[80] The impact of asthma on adults is similarly striking; for example, a typical adult with asthma will miss roughly 6 days of work per year, whereas an adult with more severe asthma will miss an average of 13 working days per year.[79] In 2007, it was estimated that asthma costs in the United States totaled more than $56 billion, with the annual cost per person averaging $3259.[80,81]

Risk factors for asthma include family history (i.e., a relative has asthma) and existing allergies or eczema, also referred to as atopic dermatitis.[82,83] Unfortunately, Black and Hispanic populations in the United States experience a greater burden of asthma and poorer asthma-related health outcomes than other demographic groups.[84] Several reasons for this greater burden have been identified, including socioeconomic disparities, less access to health, language and literacy barriers, underuse of asthma medications, and distrust or poor communication with health providers and healthcare systems.[84] For a more in-depth exploration of social factors that influence health outcomes, formally referred to as social determinants of health, see the illustrated case "Unsung Hero" in Chapter 14 Population Health. Those interested in the impact of language barriers and living circumstances on health are encouraged to explore the illustrated cases "Barriers" in Chapter 12 Mental Health and "Screen" in Chapter 4 Prevention & Wellness, respectively.

Asthma is characterized by narrowing of the airways and difficulty breathing.[82,83] While rudimentary, the "Asthma Airways" poster displayed in Illustration 3-8 highlights the root causes. The image on the left-hand side displays the trachea carrying air from the oral cavity into the chest, then branching into the right and left lungs. These branches are called primary bronchi. The primary bronchi continue to branch as they penetrate deeper into each lung, first into secondary bronchi, then into tertiary bronchi. With each branch, the diameter of the bronchi decreases; hence, the space available for air to pass through decreases. In asthma, as depicted on the right-hand side of the poster, bronchoconstriction (airway narrowing), airway wall thickening, increased mucus, and inflammation restrict the ability of air to flow through these bronchi to fill the lungs.

Bronchoconstriction refers to the tightening of the bronchial muscles, while inflammation refers to swelling and increased mucus production within the bronchi.[82,83] When combined, these changes in the airways make it difficult for patients with asthma to breathe.[83] Specific symptoms include wheezing, shortness of breath, chest tightness, and cough.[82,83] While some people with asthma have only one of these symptoms, others may experience multiple symptoms. Difficulty breathing might occur every day (i.e., persistent asthma), on occasion (i.e., intermittent asthma), or only when exposed to certain stimuli referred to as "triggers." Asthma also causes activity limitations and attacks (flare-ups) that sometimes require urgent care and may be fatal.

Asthma triggers can vary. Common triggers include exercise (especially in cold weather), upper respiratory viral infections, allergens at home or work, stress, and irritants.[78,84] For Lizzie, it is possible that increased exercise during basketball season is contributing to her worsening asthma symptoms. Equally likely is a viral infection. Illustration 3-8 shows Lizzie's mother wiping the nose of her younger sibling, who can have anything from the common cold to influenza. Illustration 3-7 shows that Lizzie is under pressure to perform at a high level, and that her inability to do so is causing stress that may be contributing to her symptoms.

While not explicitly tied to "Swish," additional triggers such as allergens and irritants are worthy of discussion. Allergens, such as ragweed, trees, grasses, house dust mites, furry or feathered pets, molds, and cockroaches are known triggers.[82,83] Asthma exacerbations may be due to outdoor exposure to allergens or when visiting a home or other building with pet dander, molds, or cockroaches. Irritants, on the other hand, represent a broad category of triggers that range from smoke/aerosols from tobacco, e-cigarette, or tetrahydrocannabinol (THC) products to environmental exposures such as ozone, cleaning chemicals, and vehicle exhaust. Irritants can be found in old buildings with poor ventilation, damp places with mold, or even outdoors on days with poor air quality. These irritants can cause breathing problems for everyone, but people with asthma are at greater risk.

Vaping has become a major public health issue. Reports about the dangers associated with vaping appear regularly in both the lay press (newspapers, magazines, and television) and medical literature.[85-88] E-cigarette, or vaping, product use-associated lung injury (EVALI) is the official term used by the US Centers for Disease Control and Prevention (CDC) to describe injuries caused by vaping, including those associated with the use of THC-containing products. Particles from e-cigarettes are deposited in the lungs of users and bystanders (i.e., secondhand smoke/aerosols).[89] Some of the chemicals and substances found in e-cigarette aerosols are nicotine, propylene glycol, glycerin, flavorings (e.g., diacetyl), volatile organic compounds, formaldehyde, other cancer-causing chemicals, and heavy metals (e.g., tin, lead, nickel). THC products may contain vitamin E acetate, plant oils, and petroleum distillates.

The CDC has stated that e-cigarette use is unsafe for kids, teens, and young adults.[89] Furthermore, evidence suggests that use of e-cigarettes may lead to smoking traditional cigarettes.[90] Vaping has been linked to increased asthma symptoms in smokers with asthma, and in people with asthma exposed to secondhand smoke/aerosols.[91] EVALI symptoms include shortness of breath, fever, cough, vomiting, diarrhea, headache, dizziness, and chest pain.[92] Reported EVALI cases due to e-cigarettes have resulted in hospitalization, intubation (i.e., mechanical breathing assistance), asthma exacerbations, and lung transplants.[85-87] Several deaths have been attributed to EVALI, as well. Taken together, the well-documented EVALI complications pose serious risks for people with and without asthma alike.[89,90,92]

Pharmacists, like Dr. Gina Romero in "Swish," play an important role helping patients and other health professionals minimize asthma risk and control asthma symptoms by maximizing the use of medications (Illustrations 3-9 and 3-11). The pharmacist's assessment begins with a comprehensive review of asthma symptoms, because medication selection is driven by their frequency and severity.[82,83] While symptoms can vary daily, a pattern has been established linking asthma severity to three factors: use of reliever inhalers, nighttime awakenings, and impact on daily activities. Using these markers, the current state of a patient's asthma is categorized into one of four "Steps:" Step 1, intermittent asthma; Step 2, persistent mild asthma; Step 3, persistent moderate asthma; or Step 4, persistent severe asthma (see Table 3-3). Pharmacists and other members of the interprofessional team use this approach, often called "Step Therapy," to manage asthma and select the best treatment options.

Asthma attacks can be severe, leading to hospitalizations and even death; importantly, using the right asthma medication can prevent these negative outcomes.[82,83] With effective treatment and good asthma control, people with asthma can live normal, productive lives. A variety of asthma medications are used to accomplish two broad goals: (1) relieving asthma symptoms when they occur, and (2) preventing asthma symptoms from occurring. Medications to quickly alleviate symptoms are referred to as "reliever," "quick-relief," or "rescue" medications, while those used to prevent symptoms and inflammation are referred to as "controller" medications. Table 3-4 includes common asthma reliever and controller medications.

One important contribution pharmacists make to the interprofessional care of asthma patients is in self-management skills training, which pharmacists provide to both patients and

Table 3-3. Categorization of Asthma Based on Symptom Frequency and Severity

Step	Step 1: Intermittent	Step 2: Persistent Mild	Step 3: Persistent Moderate	Step 4: Persistent Severe
Description	**Well Controlled**	**Partly Controlled**	**Not Well Controlled**	**Uncontrolled**
Symptom frequency and severity	▪ Not very often; occurs with viral illness or trigger exposure	▪ Using reliever therapy more often ▪ Waking up at night because of asthma ▪ Able to participate most of the time in daily activities	▪ Using reliever therapy on a daily basis ▪ Waking up at night regularly because of asthma ▪ Unable to participate in many daily activities	▪ Using reliever therapy throughout the day ▪ Waking up most nights due to asthma ▪ Unable to participate in most daily activities

Table 3-4. Categories and Examples of Medications Commonly Used to Treat Asthma

Category	Medication Examples[*]	Physiologic Effect
Inhaled reliever: bronchodilators	▪ albuterol (ProAir, Proventil, Ventolin) ▪ levalbuterol (Xopenex)	Relax the muscles surrounding the airways, usually within 5–10 minutes
Oral reliever: corticosteroids	▪ methylprednisolone ▪ prednisolone ▪ prednisone	Reduce inflammation, airway swelling, and excess mucous production, typically within 1–3 days
Inhaled controller: corticosteroids	▪ beclomethasone (QVar) ▪ budesonide (Pulmicort) ▪ ciclesonide (Alvesco) ▪ fluticasone (Flovent, ArmonAir, Arnuity) ▪ mometasone (Asmanex)	Reduce inflammation, airway swelling, and mucous production, typically over 7–10 days
Oral controller: leukotriene modifiers	▪ montelukast (Singulair)	Decrease airway inflammation and relax the muscles surrounding the airways
Inhaled combined reliever/controller: corticosteroids and bronchodilators	▪ budesonide/formoterol (Symbicort) ▪ fluticasone/salmeterol (Advair, AirDuo, Wixela) ▪ fluticasone/vilanterol (Breo) ▪ mometasone/formoterol (Dulera)	See individual physiologic effect descriptions above for inhaled relievers (bronchodilators) and inhaled controllers (corticosteroids)

[*] Medication examples presented in alphabetical order as "generic name (Brand Name)."

families.[82,83] These activities include providing information about asthma medications and usage; teaching inhaler skills; motivating patients toward adherence with prescribed medications; aiding self-monitoring of symptoms and/or peak flows; providing regular medication review; and contributing to the creation of written asthma action plans (AAPs).

It is essential that an AAP is developed and shared with key individuals involved in the care of a child or adolescent with asthma (e.g., parents, school nurse, childcare providers, teachers, coaches). An AAP is a written plan with instructions on daily medication use, as well as how and when to step up asthma therapy for worsening or increasing symptoms. AAPs consist of three "Zones": Green Zone, "Go," when all is good and controller medications should continue to be used as prescribed; Yellow Zone, "Caution," when symptoms are starting to increase and asthma treatment needs to be adjusted (i.e., stepped up); and Red Zone, "Danger," when symptoms are more severe, warranting increased reliever use and seeking medical attention.

Health professionals use published guidelines to diagnose and assess asthma to best achieve management goals of risk reduction and symptom control.[82,83] The interprofessional team applies these guidelines, along with an asthma score generated by one of several validated surveys/questionnaires (e.g., Asthma Control Test, or ACT) to determine which medications would be preferred.[93-97] Surveys used to produce asthma scores contain a range of questions that ask patients about asthma symptoms and control over the last 1 to 4 weeks, and some can be used for patients as young as 4 years of age with adult involvement.[95] These surveys can help identify changes in symptoms, including subtle changes that may go underrecognized (Illustration 3-9).

Illustration 3-9 takes place at the clinic pharmacy, where Lizzie has gone to pick up new asthma prescriptions following her physician visit. Lizzie shares with Gina the results of her "Asthma Score Test," which demonstrates a worsening of her asthma consistent with increased symptom frequency and severity. While not explicitly shown, during this encounter Gina would have also attempted to improve Lizzie's adherence through encouragement, updated Lizzie's AAP, and even explored preventive measures such as administering Lizzie's annual influenza vaccine if needed.[98]

Through the course of their regular medication reviews, pharmacists often uncover clues to inadequate disease control or progression. A good example of this is shown in Illustration 3-9, where Gina discovers that Lizzie has not been refilling her fluticasone inhaler after reviewing her prescription records using the pharmacy's tracking software. Fluticasone is an inhaled corticosteroid classified as a controller (see Table 3-4). Regular use of a controller inhaler has been shown to decrease the number of asthma exacerbations, as well as the need for additional medications, like prednisone, that are taken orally and have systemic effects, meaning they impact the entire body, not just the lungs (Table 3-4). Those interested in other examples of pharmacists uncovering clues to maximize medication use are encouraged to explore the illustrated cases "Burden" and "Sleuth" in Chapter 7 Geriatrics.

One might wonder why Lizzie's physician would order a step-up controller if her worsening condition was attributable to simply not using her current controller already prescribed. While not shown in Illustration 3-8, the backstory for this full encounter involved Lizzie responding untruthfully when asked about this, so as not to disappoint her physician or her mother. Further questioning by Gina in Illustrations 3-9 and 3-10 identified the real reason for Lizzie's non-adherence; namely, her unwillingness to risk a repeated episode of candidiasis, a side effect caused by fluticasone use that she considers repulsive and embarrassing. Importantly, candidiasis can be treated and subsequently prevented. For a more detailed discussion of adherence and the impact/consequences of non-adherence, readers are encouraged to explore the illustrated case "Opportunities" in Chapter 15 Administration.

Candidiasis is a yeast (*Candida albicans* fungus) infection commonly referred to as thrush when it occurs in the mouth or throat.[99] Everyone has candida in their mouth, along with other kinds of naturally occurring, non-harmful microorganisms like bacteria. However, candida can overgrow and cause symptoms such as white, creamy, cottage cheese–like patches on the tongue and inner cheeks (Illustration 3-10), the roof of the mouth, gums or tonsils, and the back of the throat. It is mostly painless but sometimes causes redness, soreness, burning, or a cottony feeling in the mouth.

Inhaled corticosteroid-induced candidiasis arises through its disturbance of the natural balance between these oral microorganisms, coupled with a weakened immunity in specific patient populations (e.g., HIV/AIDS, chemotherapy or radiation treatment for cancer, organ transplantation).[100] Instruction on good inhaler technique can help prevent this adverse effect, which Gina provided to Lizzie after learning the true reason for her non-adherence (Illustration 3-11). Examples of good inhaler technique include coordinated inhalation timed with drug release if not using a spacer, use of a spacer when available, and swishing/gargling with water and spitting after use.

Pharmacists also monitor asthma patients for other adverse effects or side effects due to medications. Bronchodilators can cause jitteriness, excitation, or chest palpitations; leukotriene modifiers might cause strange dreams, behavioral changes, or mild flu-like symptoms; and inhaled corticosteroids can cause a sore throat, candidiasis, hoarse voice, or cough. Inhaled corticosteroids may also reduce growth velocity, especially if prescribed at high doses in younger children.

The illustrated case "Swish" highlights the potential burden of asthma faced by an adolescent female, Lizzie, and the need to identify the patient's own goals regarding asthma and its treatment. In Lizzie's case, her goals include reduction in her symptoms that are uncomfortable, troubling, frightening, and limiting activities; playing basketball and competing with her team; and being managed by medications that control asthma without causing side effects she considers "gross." Fortunately, Lizzie's goals can be achieved via open communication and partnerships between the pharmacist, other health professionals, and her family to develop and implement the most effective asthma management plan possible.

DISCUSSION QUESTIONS FOR "SWISH"

1. Illustration 3-8 shows Lizzie receiving a treatment to help her breathe better. What medication do you think she is receiving, and why? Refer to Table 3-4 for support, if needed.

2. In Illustrations 3-9 and 3-10, we learn that Lizzie is not taking her controller medication as prescribed because she fears an adverse effect. Besides adverse effects, what are some other reasons a person might not take their medication(s) as prescribed?

3. We learn in Thoughts on "Swish" that Lizzie did not share the truth about her fluticasone use, or lack thereof, with her mother or physician. What is your reaction to this situation?

4. Imagine that Lizzie, out of fear of being caught in a lie, asked Gina not to tell her mother or physician the truth. How would you respond if you were Gina in this situation?

5. We encounter two health professionals in "Swish," a pharmacist and a physician. Can you think of other health professionals who may also be involved in the care of patients with asthma? What are their roles and/or contributions to the interprofessional team?

HOLISTIC: An Illustrated Case Study

Story by Denise L. Walbrandt Pigarelli & Joseph A. Zorek
Illustrations by George Folz, © 2019 Board of Regents of the University of Wisconsin System

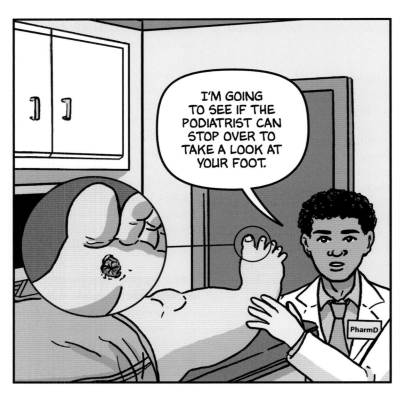

Illustration 3-13

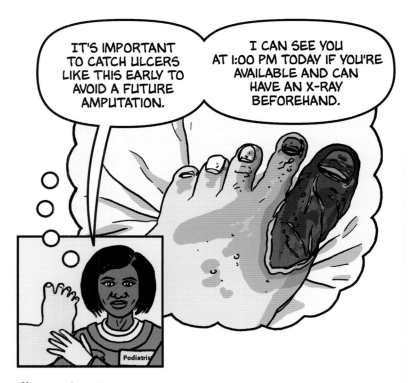

Illustration 3-14

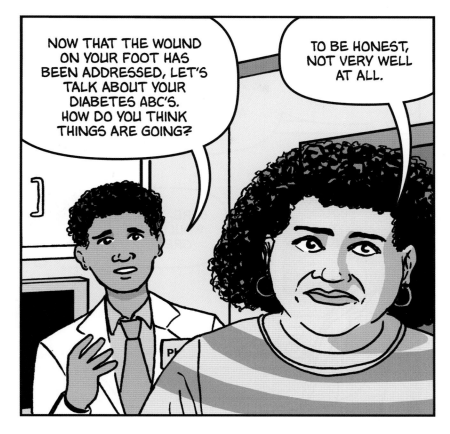

Illustration 3-15

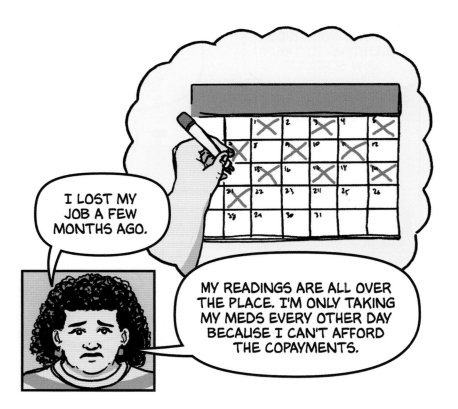

Illustration 3-16

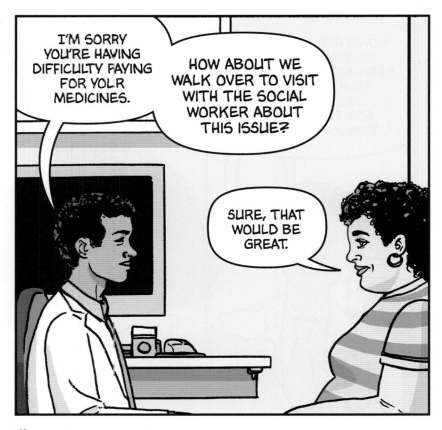

Illustration 3-17

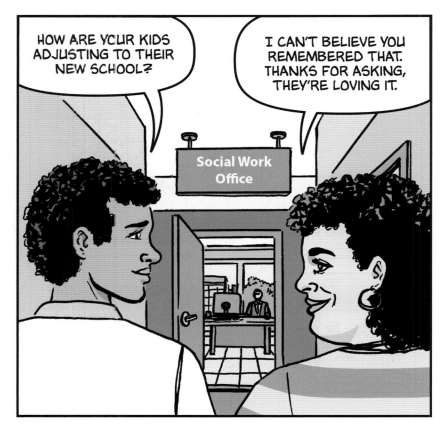

Illustration 3-18

Thoughts on "Holistic"

The illustrated case "Holistic" presents a person with diabetes who is experiencing a complication of a chronic health condition discovered during a visit with a primary care pharmacist (Illustration 3-13). The pharmacist connects the person to needed immediate care with another health professional (Illustration 3-14), as well as uncovers life and self-care aspects related to the development of the complication (Illustrations 3-15 and 3-16). The patient-pharmacist trust relationship (Illustrations 3-17 and 3-18) and an additional interprofessional connection (Illustration 3-18) are also highlighted.

Diabetes mellitus occurs when blood glucose is too high because the body is not able to appropriately use food for energy.[101] This can be the result of the pancreas making too little or no insulin at all as in type 1 diabetes, or it can be due to incorrect processing of food by the body as in type 2 diabetes. Type 1 and type 2 are the most common kinds of diabetes; other categories of diabetes include gestational diabetes (which may affect pregnant women) and several other less common types. Insulin is an important hormone (i.e., a substance produced by one part of the body that impacts how cells, tissues, or organs in other parts of the body function). It was first used as a medication in 1922 and has since become an indispensable tool to improve health outcomes for people with diabetes.[102] This includes multiple types of insulin that are frequently used in combination with one another (e.g., short- and long-acting insulin taken at different times of the day), and according to patient preferences (e.g., insulin syringe versus pen). See Table 3-5 for more details.

As of 2018, 34.1 million people in the United States had diabetes, which represented about 10.5% of the population.[103] Official diabetes diagnoses totaled 26.8 million, with an estimated 7.3 million Americans undiagnosed; meaning, having diabetes but without an official confirmation from a health professional. This latter group accounted for 21.4% of adults who actually had diabetes in 2018, which is a staggering figure that highlights the importance of community engagement and outreach efforts. As people age, they are more likely to develop diabetes; 26.8% of Americans 65 years or older had diabetes in 2018. Diabetes is more common among Asians, non-Hispanic Blacks, and Hispanics than for non-Hispanic Whites. Type 2 accounts for about 90% to 95% of people who have diabetes. For additional background information on diabetes, including the importance of community engagement and health screenings, readers are encouraged to explore the illustrated case "Screen" in Chapter 4 Prevention & Wellness.

When diabetes is not managed well or has affected a person for a long time, serious complications can occur. Such complications comprised a substantial portion of the estimated $327 billion spent in the United States in 2017 for diabetes care, which included both direct and indirect costs.[104] Acute or short-term complications for people with diabetes include hypoglycemia (i.e., low blood glucose) and hyperglycemia (i.e., high blood glucose). Hypoglycemia occurs when blood glucose falls below 70 mg/dL and is classified into three

levels.[105] Level 1 is blood glucose between 54 mg/dL to less than 70 mg/dL; level 2 is blood glucose less than 54 mg/dL; level 3 is any low glucose event which requires assistance from another person. Sulfonylureas and insulins, two categories of diabetes medications (see Table 3-5), are commonly associated with hypoglycemic events. When hypoglycemia happens, a person can experience sudden symptoms of sweating, hunger, vision or mood changes, or feeling shaky or dizzy. Immediate treatment is critical to prevent glucose values from decreasing further, which can cause severe symptoms such as difficulty speaking, drowsiness, seizures, unconsciousness, or even death. Treatment of hypoglycemia in a person who is awake and able to swallow usually involves eating or drinking 15 g of fast-acting, carbohydrate-containing substances such as glucose tablets or gels (which are available over-the-counter in pharmacies), four ounces of fruit juice or sugar-containing soda, or one tablespoon of sugar or honey. Hypoglycemia episodes should be reported to a member of the person's interprofessional team in order to determine the cause and to create a plan to prevent future episodes.

Acute hyperglycemia lasting for at least several hours can also be a dangerous situation.[106] Symptoms of hyperglycemia may include increased thirst, hunger, and urination. Additionally, a person may have difficulty concentrating, and they may feel weak. When hyperglycemia occurs, the interprofessional team should be contacted for management instructions. If hyperglycemia is severe enough, a person with diabetes may develop a life-threatening condition called diabetic ketoacidosis (mostly occurs in people with type 1 diabetes) or hyperglycemic hyperosmolar non-ketotic syndrome (typically occurs in people with type 2 diabetes). For additional information about diabetic ketoacidosis, see the illustrated case "Type 1" in Chapter 11 Critical Care.

Chronic or long-term diabetes complications typically begin after a person has diabetes for several years and can affect much of a person's body, from the brain and eyes all the way down and through the body to the feet. Stroke is a diabetes-related complication that is life-threatening, which results when blood flow to the brain is limited or blocked.[107] Stroke risk is 1.5 times higher in people with diabetes than the general population. Sadly, 16% of people with diabetes who are older than 65 will die from stroke.[107,108] Eye problems represent another serious complication from long-term diabetes, such as diabetic retinopathy, glaucoma, cataracts, and even blindness.[109] It is recommended to have eyes examined routinely by eye care professionals and to keep blood glucose and blood pressure well managed to limit the effects of diabetic eye disease. Diabetes may also affect a person's mouth and oral health. Serious inflammation of the gums may be associated with periodontitis, which may include easy bleeding, gums that retreat from normal position and expose more of the teeth, bad breath, and teeth that are loose or move from their usual position.[110] People with diabetes who have periodontitis may have more challenges in managing their blood glucose values, and, conversely, elevated blood glucose values may be associated with periodontitis. Additionally, thrush, an

Table 3-5. Categories and Examples of Medications Commonly Used to Treat Diabetes

Category	Medication Examples[*]	Physiologic Effect
Oral agents		
Alpha-glucosidase inhibitor	▪ acarbose (Precose) ▪ miglitol (Glyset)	Slows digestion of complex carbohydrates in the small intestine
Biguanide	▪ metformin (Glucophage)	Decreases liver glucose production and intestinal glucose absorption; increases tissue insulin sensitivity
DPP-4 Inhibitor[**]	▪ alogliptin (Nesina) ▪ linagliptin (Tradjenta) ▪ saxagliptin (Onglyza) ▪ sitagliptin (Januvia)	Increases incretins which slow glucagon release from the pancreas, decrease stomach emptying, and increase insulin secretion
Meglitinide	▪ nateglinide (Starlix) ▪ repaglinide (Prandin)	Stimulates insulin release from the pancreas
Sulfonylurea	▪ glimepiride (Amaryl) ▪ glipizide (Glucotrol) ▪ glyburide (Diabeta)	Stimulates insulin release from the pancreas
Thiazolidinedione	▪ pioglitazone (Actos) ▪ rosiglitazone (Avandia)	Increases tissue insulin sensitivity
SGLT2 inhibitor[***]	▪ canagliflozin (Invokana) ▪ dapagliflozin (Farxiga) ▪ empagliflozin (Jardiance) ▪ ertugliflozin (Steglatro)	Prevents reabsorption of glucose in the kidney and increases glucose elimination in the urine
Injectable agents		
GLP-1 receptor agonist[****]	▪ dulaglutide (Trulicity) ▪ exenatide (Byetta, Bydureon) ▪ liraglutide (Victoza) ▪ lixisenatide (Adlyxin) ▪ semaglutide (Ozempic)	Stimulates pancreatic insulin release after eating, decreases glucagon secretion from the pancreas, slows stomach emptying, acts in the brain to decrease appetite
Insulin: U-100 rapid-acting[*****]	▪ aspart (NovoLog) ▪ glulisine (Apidra) ▪ lispro (Humalog)	Facilitates glucose uptake into cells so glucose can be used for energy
Insulin: U-100 short-acting	▪ human regular (Humulin R, Novolin R)	
Insulin: U-100 intermediate-acting	▪ human NPH (Humulin N, Novolin N)	
Insulin: U-100 long-acting	▪ degludec (Tresiba) ▪ detemir (Levemir) ▪ glargine (Basaglar, Lantus)	

[*] Medication examples presented in alphabetical order as "generic name (Brand Name)."

[**] DPP-4: dipeptidyl peptidase 4.

[***] SGLT2: sodium-glucose transport protein 2.

[****] GLP-1: glucagon-like peptide 1.

[*****] U-100: 100 units per milliliter.

oral fungal infection in the mouth, as well as dry mouth in general, can be problematic for people with diabetes.

The heart and kidneys can also be affected by diabetes. At least 68% of people older than 65 will die from heart complications, and adults with diabetes are two to four times more likely to die from heart disease than people without diabetes.[108] The kidneys, which perform the vital function of filtering and cleaning the blood, can be damaged by diabetes and lead to

decreased filtration functionality over time. Chronic kidney disease affects 20% to 40% of people with diabetes and may eventually cause complete kidney failure.[111] Patients with diabetes can limit these and other chronic diabetes-related complications by optimizing blood pressure, blood glucose, and cholesterol management according to evidence-based guidelines under the direction of the interprofessional primary care team. Additionally, some medications in the SGLT2 inhibitor and GLP-1 receptor agonist categories (see Table 3-5) have shown great benefit in preventing or limiting heart and kidney damage and are now considered preferred agents to use for people with these conditions.[112]

Autonomic neuropathy occurs when the nerves that control digestion, blood pressure and heart rate, and bowel and bladder function are damaged.[113] People with long-term diabetes are at risk for slowed and/or altered food passage through the stomach and intestines, which is caused by autonomic neuropathy. This condition is called gastroparesis and can cause symptoms of bloating or nausea after eating a normal amount of food, feeling full after just a few bites of a meal, or experiencing ongoing diarrhea or constipation. Gastroparesis not only causes discomfort, but it presents challenges to coordinate the timing and action of medications, including insulin, as related to the passage and digestion of foods. The bladder and genitals may also be affected by autonomic neuropathy. Urinary incontinence and urine retention in the bladder can occur, and urine retention is a risk factor for bladder infections. Erectile dysfunction and decreased sexual arousal may develop over time, and these conditions may impact quality of life.

Chronic diabetes complications may include foot problems that are related to poor blood flow; changed or decreased nerve sensation; dry, peeling, or cracked foot skin; calluses; and ulcers.[114] Several of these factors are affected by blood pressure, blood glucose, and smoking, as well as decreased blood flow to the lower legs and feet. If foot ulcers do not heal, bacterial infections can occur, leading to tissue necrosis (i.e., death) as depicted in the thought bubble in Illustration 3-14. Such infections are difficult to treat, since poor blood flow hinders antibiotics from reaching the site of infection. Those interested in learning more about infections and antibiotics are encouraged to read the illustrated cases "Wounded" and "Superinfection" in Chapter 8 Infectious Diseases. Unfortunately, up to 24% of foot infections in people with diabetes will require amputation to prevent the spread of infection, which is associated with increased risk of death.[115] Pharmacists, as depicted in Illustration 3-13, can perform foot screens to help identify early-onset foot problems, connect affected patients to podiatrists (as seen in Illustration 3-14), and ultimately help to prevent amputations.[116-118] The American Pharmacists Association's certificate training program "The Pharmacist & Patient-Centered Diabetes Care" teaches pharmacists how to conduct foot screening exams, and many schools and colleges of pharmacy teach students this skill, too.[119,120]

Recommended treatment for all people with diabetes incorporates the lifestyle aspects of healthy eating and exercise.[121] People with type 1 diabetes also require insulin therapy, and people with type 2 diabetes usually need oral and/or injectable medications in addition to lifestyle modifications (Table 3-5). Pharmacists, as members of the interprofessional primary care team, have important responsibilities related to both lifestyle coaching and selection and management of diabetes medications.[20,23,30,117,118,122-126] The types of insulins and categories of oral and injectable medications for diabetes have increased greatly over the past 20 years, and therapy should be tailored to each patient's unique needs and characteristics.[112] Medication selection is determined by drug characteristics such as ability to lower blood glucose; risk of hypoglycemia; propensity for weight gain or to assist with weight loss; benefits or detriments related to cardiovascular disease, heart failure, and kidney disease; medication cost; potential side effects; and frequency that a medication must be taken. Pharmacists are well-positioned within interprofessional teams to formulate therapeutic plans that optimize clinical outcomes.[20,23,30,117,118,122-126] This is a complicated task that involves assessing each patient's situation related to medication needs, as well as additional patient characteristics, such as age, cognitive and mechanical abilities, and economic considerations.

Economic considerations impacting medication use are highlighted in "Holistic," where the pharmacist, throughout the course of the patient visit, discovers a lack of adherence to prescribed medications as a result of financial difficulties. The importance of adherence to diabetes medications cannot be overstated, as many of the severe complications described develop as a result of prolonged periods of hyperglycemia. Rationing the use of medication for cost-saving purposes demonstrates this patient's incredibly complicated, precarious, and sensitive situation. Unfortunately, this unacceptable situation is a common problem.[127,128] Fortunately, the trust the pharmacist has developed with this patient allows for open dialogue and problem solving. His knowledge of other health professionals' skills, including social workers' ability to troubleshoot medication access issues, is also critical. Through interprofessional collaboration, the pharmacist and social worker will help the patient acquire the medications she needs to remain healthy. As stated earlier in the chapter, the illustrated case "Unsung Hero" in Chapter 14 Population Health provides more information about the social determinants of health, including economic considerations.

As an integral member of the interprofessional primary care team, the pharmacist's role and ability to provide patient care is fully reliant upon the relationships both with the patient and other health professionals.[129,130] Illustrations 3-17 and 3-18 convey a caring and trusting relationship between the patient and the pharmacist. Such trust is important and is associated with high patient satisfaction and improved diabetes outcomes, including motivation to improve health, nutrition, and exercise.[129,131-133] Illustration 3-14 relates a professional relationship between the podiatrist and the pharmacist, and Illustration 3-18 indicates a collaborative association between the social worker and the pharmacist. To facilitate teamwork among health professionals, the National Diabetes Education Program has created a toolkit for pharmacists, podiatrists, optometrists, and dentists to enhance collaborations among these professions, as well as with community health workers, nurse educators, physician assistants, and primary care providers.[134] Diabetes care requires a holistic approach, and this can only be accomplished through interprofessional teamwork.

DISCUSSION QUESTIONS FOR "HOLISTIC"

1. The illustrated case "Holistic" highlights interprofessional interactions between a pharmacist, podiatrist, and social worker. What other health professionals and/or community members can you think of that might also be incorporated into the support system for the patient featured in this case?

2. Diabetes can affect almost any part of the body the longer a person has the health condition. Considering the short- and long-term complications presented in this essay, how might a person's life be affected by having one or more diabetes complications? Consider effects on their day-to-day living situation, including home life, employment, leisure activities, and relationships.

3. Pharmacists provide patient care services in many outpatient (i.e., non-hospital) venues, including pharmacies and clinics, as well as through technology (e.g., telephone, video). What other physical locations can you envision that might be conducive to such services? What other technologies might be leveraged to advance pharmacist engagement?

4. Medication selection for people with diabetes is a fascinating yet complex process. What aspects do you think are most important to consider when starting, adjusting, or adding medications for management of blood glucose?

5. Illustration 3-18 reveals the personal connection between the pharmacist and the patient. How do you feel about the pharmacist talking to the patient about a sensitive subject like financial struggles, which some may consider intimate and/or private? Why do you feel that way?

CHAPTER SUMMARY

■ Health delivery in the primary care setting focuses on first-contact care, continuous care, comprehensive care, and care coordination.

■ Primary care pharmacists provide direct patient care for a variety of acute and chronic conditions, including anticoagulation, asthma, diabetes, and high blood pressure.

■ Primary care is a rich environment for interprofessional practice in pharmacy.

■ In support of the interprofessional primary care team, common activities of pharmacists include assisting with evidence-based drug selection, monitoring for and troubleshooting medication side effects, and performing interventions to improve medication adherence.

■ When medications are ineffective or causing side effects, primary care pharmacists will often adjust the medication dose or select a different medication to help the patient meet their health goals.

■ Primary care pharmacists implement population health management initiatives and work collaboratively with members of the interprofessional primary care team to ensure health goals are met for all patients seen in the clinic.

■ Pharmacists in all health settings find and use the best available literature to determine evidence-based answers to clinical questions to support providers and optimize medication use for patients.

■ During appointments, pharmacists in primary care settings educate patients on proper use of medications and how to manage their health conditions. Examples described in this chapter include avoiding asthma triggers, using inhalers, developing asthma action plans, adopting healthy lifestyles, and treating hypo- and hyperglycemia.

REFERENCES

1. Finley CR, Chan DS, Garrison S, et al. What are the most common conditions in primary care? Systematic review. *Can Fam Physician.* 2018;64(11):832-840.

2. Oddone EZ, Boulware EL. Primary care: medicine's Gordian knot. *Am J Med Sci.* 2016;351(1):20-25.

3. American Academy of Family Physicians. Primary Care. Available at https://www.aafp.org/about/policies/all/primary-care.html. Accessed January 5, 2020.

4. Mitchell JD, Haag JD, Klavetter E, et al. Development and implementation of a team-based, primary care delivery model: challenges and opportunities. *Mayo Clin Proc.* 2019;94(7):1298-1303.

5. Vimalananda VG, Meterko M, Waring ME, et al. Tools to improve referrals from primary care to specialty care. *Am J Manag Care.* 2019;25(8):E237-E242.

6. Bodenheimer T, Ghorob A, Willard-Grace R, Grumbach K. The 10 building blocks of primary care. *Ann Fam Med.* 2014;12(2):166-171.

7. Schottenfeld L, Petersen D, Peikes D, Ricciardi R, Burak H, Mc Nellis RJG. Creating patient-centered team-based primary care. Available at https://pcmh.ahrq.gov/page/creating-patient-centered-team-based-primary-care. Accessed January 5, 2020.

8. Schroeder A. What is primary care? University of Utah Health. Available at https://healthcare.utah.edu/healthfeed/postings/2017/01/what-is-primary-care.php. Accessed January 5, 2020.

9. Erickson S, Hambleton J. A pharmacy's journey toward the patient-centered medical home. *J Am Pharm Assoc.* 2011;51(2):156-160.

10. Boren LL, Locke AM, Friedman AS, Blackmore CC, Woolf R. Team-based medicine: incorporating a clinical pharmacist into pain and opioid practice management. *PM R.* 2019;11(11):1170-1177.

11. Herbert C, Winkler H. Impact of a clinical pharmacist–managed clinic in primary care mental health integration at a Veterans Affairs health system. *Ment Heal Clin.* 2018;8(3):105-109.

12. Worth T. Satisfied patients, pharmacists patients, pharmacists at Phoenix VA. *Pharm Today.* 2012;18(8):36-38.

13. Scott MA, Heck JE, Wilson CG. The integral role of the clinical pharmacist practitioner in primary care. *N C Med J.* 2017;78(3):181-185.

14. Heilmann RM, Campbell SM, Kroner BA, et al. Evolution, current structure, and role of a primary care clinical pharmacy

service in an integrated managed care organization. *Ann Pharmacother.* 2013;47(1):124-131.

15. MacDonald DA, Chang H, Wei Y, Hager K. Drug therapy problem identification and resolution by clinical pharmacists in a family medicine residency clinic. *Innov Pharm.* 2018;9(2):4.

16. Fennelly JE, Coe AB, Kippes KA, Remington TL, Choe HM. Evaluation of clinical pharmacist services in a transitions of care program provided to patients at highest risk for readmission. *J Pharm Pract.* 2020;33(3):314-320.

17. Sinclair J, Bentley OS, Abubakar A, Rhodes LA, Marciniak MW. Impact of a pharmacist in improving quality measures that affect payments to physicians. *J Am Pharm Assoc.* 2019;59(4):S85-S90.

18. Bhat S, Kroehl ME, Trinkley KE, et al. Evaluation of a clinical pharmacist-led multidisciplinary antidepressant telemonitoring service in the primary care setting. *Popul Health Manag.* 2018;21(5):366-372.

19. Seckel E, Portillo E, Lehman M, Wilcox A, Vega R. Ambulatory care pharmacy practice advancement: diffusing strong practices. *J Pharm Soc Wis.* 2019;22(4):58-61.

20. Roll A, Pattison D, Baumgartner R, Sublett L, Brown B. The design and evaluation of a pilot covisit model: integration of a pharmacist into a primary care team. *J Am Pharm Assoc.* 2019;60(3):419-496.

21. Jain SH. Can pharmacists help reinvent primary care in the United States? Forbes. Available at https://www.forbes.com/sites/sachinjain/2018/10/10/can-pharmacists-help-reinvent-primary-care-in-the-united-states/#342f7c56590b. Accessed May 31, 2020.

22. Groppi JA, Ourth H, Morreale AP, Hirsh JM, Wright S. Advancement of clinical pharmacy practice through intervention capture. *Am J Heal Pharm.* 2018;75(12):886-892.

23. Prudencio J, Cutler T, Roberts S, Marin S, Wilson M. The effect of clinical pharmacist-led comprehensive medication management on chronic disease state goal attainment in a patient-centered medical home. *J Manag Care Spec Pharm.* 2018;24(5):423-429.

24. Gardea J, Papadatos J, Cadle R. Evaluating glycemic control for patient-aligned care team clinical pharmacy specialists at a large veterans affairs medical center. *Pharm Pract.* 2018;16(2):2-6.

25. Sloeserwij VM, Hazen ACM, Zwart DLM, et al. Effects of non-dispensing pharmacists integrated in general practice on medication-related hospitalisations. *Br J Clin Pharmacol.* 2019;(June):2321-2331.

26. American Pharmacists Association. Pharmacists and primary care. Available at https://www.pharmacist.com/article/pharmacists-and-primary-care. Published 2016. Accessed January 7, 2020.

27. Epplen KT. Patient care delivery and integration: stimulating advancement of ambulatory care pharmacy practice in an era of health reform. *Am J Heal Pharm.* 2014;71(16):1357-1365.

28. National Alliance of State Pharmacy Associations. Collaborative practice agreements: resources and more. Available at https://naspa.us/resource/cpa/. Accessed January 9, 2020.

29. Gebhart F. On the road to provider status. *Drug Topics.* 2019;163(6):13-14.

30. Funk KA, Pestka DL, Roth McClurg MT, Carroll JK, Sorensen TD. Primary care providers believe that comprehensive medication management improves their work-life. *J Am Board Fam Med.* 2019;32(4):462-473.

31. Nguyen M, Zare M. Impact of a clinical pharmacist–managed medication refill clinic. *J Prim Care Community Health.* 2015;6(3):187-192.

32. National Association of Community Health Centers. Action steps toward population health management. Available at http://www.nachc.org/wp-content/uploads/2015/12/NACHC_pophealth_factsheet_FINAL.pdf. Accessed January 9, 2020.

33. Kennedy AG, Biddle MA, Flaherty L, Mosier R, Murphy K. *Practical Strategies for Pharmacist Integration with Primary Care: A Workbook.* Burlington, VA; 2014.

34. Haby HE, Alm RA, Corona AR, Hall AC. Population health model for pharmacist assessment and independent prescribing of statins in an ambulatory care setting. *J Am Pharm Assoc.* 2020;60(1):130-137.

35. Frey M, Margolis AR, Wopat M. Pharmacist led team-based care to improve hypertension management among Veterans in primary care. *J Pharm Soc Wis.* 2019;22(5):53-57.

36. McMurray MA, Schermetzler BJ, Goninen MK. Implementation of a system-wide, telephonic, pharmacist-led population health program: metformin dose optimization. *J Pharm Soc Wis.* 2019;22(6):36-41.

37. Sanborn MD. Population health management and the pharmacist's role. *Am J Heal Pharm.* 2017;74(18):1400-1401.

38. Islam MM, Poly TN, Walther BA, et al. Adverse outcomes of long-term use of proton pump inhibitors: a systematic review and meta-analysis. *Eur J Gastroenterol Hepatol.* 2018;30(12):1395-1405.

39. Odenthal DR, Philbrick AM, Harris IM. Successful deprescribing of unnecessary proton pump inhibitors in a primary care clinic. *J Am Pharm Assoc.* 2020;60(1):100-104.

40. Jalal H, Buchanich JM, Roberts MS, Balmert LC, Zhang K, Burke DS. Changing dynamics of the drug overdose epidemic in the United States from 1979 through 2016. *Science.* 2018;361(6408):eaau1184.

41. Ambulatory Care Pharmacy—Board of Pharmacy Specialties. Available at https://www.bpsweb.org/bps-specialties/ambulatory-care/. Accessed January 5, 2020.

42. Sackett D, Rosenberg W, Gray J, Haynes R, Richardson W. Evidence based medicine: what it is and what it isn't. *Br Med J.* 1996;312(7023):71-72.

43. Guerrera F, Renaud S, Tabbò F, Filosso PL. How to design a randomized clinical trial: tips and tricks for conduct a successful study in thoracic disease domain. *J Thorac Dis.* 2017;9(8):2692-2696.

44. Bhide A, Shah PS, Acharya G. A simplified guide to randomized controlled trials. *Acta Obstet Gynecol Scand.* 2018;97(4):380-387.

45. Kendall JM. Designing a research project: randomised controlled trials and their principles. *Emerg Med J.* 2003;20(2):164-168.

46. Murad MH, Montori VM, Ioannidis JPA, et al. How to read a systematic review and meta-analysis and apply the results to patient care: users' guides to the medical literature. *JAMA.* 2014;312(2):171-179.

47. Guedeney P, Giustino G, Sorrentino S, et al. Efficacy and safety of alirocumab and evolocumab: a systematic review and meta-analysis of randomized controlled trials. *Eur Heart J.* 2019:1-9.

48. Ebell MH, Siwek J, Weiss BD, et al. Strength of Recommendation Taxonomy (SORT): a patient-centered approach to grading evidence in the medical literature. *J Am Board Fam Pract.* 2004;17(1):59-67.

49. Murad MH, Asi N, Alsawas M, Alahdab F. New evidence pyramid. *Evid Based Med*. 2016;21(4):125-127.

50. Mann CJ. Observational research methods. Research design II: cohort, cross sectional, and case-control studies. *Emerg Med J*. 2003;20(1):54-60.

51. Cohen H. How to write a patient case report. *Am J Heal Pharm*. 2006;63(19):1888-1892.

52. Gentry CK, Parker RP, Ketel C, et al. Integration of clinical pharmacist services into an underserved primary care clinic utilizing an interprofessional collaborative practice model. *J Health Care Poor Underserved*. 2016;27(1):1-7.

53. Burkiewicz JS, Zgarrick DP. Evidence-based practice by pharmacists: utilization and barriers. *Ann Pharmacother*. 2005;39(7-8):1214-1219.

54. Kier BKL, Goldwire M. Drug information resources and literature retrieval. In: *Science and Practice of Pharmacotherapy (Pharmacotherapy and Self-Assessment Program)*. Lenexa, KS: American College of Clinical Pharmacy; 2018:619-645.

55. Lexicomp Online. Available at https://www.wolterskluwercdi. com/lexicomp-online/. Accessed February 18, 2020.

56. What is IBM Micromedex? Available at https://www.ibm.com/ watson-health/learn/micromedex. Accessed February 18, 2020.

57. Pharmacist's Letter. Available at https://pharmacist.therapeutic research.com/Home/PL. Accessed February 18, 2020.

58. UpToDate. Available at https://www.uptodate.com/home. Accessed February 18, 2020.

59. Johnson C. Evidence-based practice in 5 simple steps. *J Manipulative Physiol Ther*. 2008;31(3):169-170.

60. Dempsey JT, Matta LS, Carter DM, et al. Assessment of drug therapy-related issues in an outpatient heart failure population and the potential impact of pharmacist-driven intervention. *J Pharm Pract*. 2017;30(3):318-323.

61. Trinkley KE, Weed HG, Beatty SJ, Porter K, Nahata MC. Identification and characterization of adverse drug events in primary care. *Am J Med Qual*. 2017;32(5):518-525.

62. Fedak KM, Bernal A, Capshaw ZA, Gross S. Applying the Bradford Hill criteria in the 21st century: how data integration has changed causal inference in molecular epidemiology. *Emerg Themes Epidemiol*. 2015;12(1):1-9.

63. Hill BA. The environment and disease: association or causation? *Proc R Soc Med*. 1965;58(5):295-300.

64. Gallagher RM, Kirkham JJ, Mason JR, et al. Development and inter-rater reliability of the Liverpool adverse drug reaction causality assessment tool. *PLoS One*. 2011;6(12):e28096.

65. Goldman JL, Chung WH, Lee BR, et al. Adverse drug reaction causality assessment tools for drug-induced Stevens-Johnson syndrome and toxic epidermal necrolysis: room for improvement. *Eur J Clin Pharmacol*. 2019;75(8):1135-1141.

66. Naranjo CA, Busto U, Sellers EM, et al. A method for estimating the probability of adverse drug reactions. *Clin Pharmacol Ther*. 1981;30(2):239-245.

67. Yanto TA, Huang I, Kosasih FN, Lugito NPH. Nightmare and abnormal dreams: rare side effects of metformin? *Case Rep Endocrinol*. 2018;2018:1-3.

68. Bowers RD, Valanejad SM, Holombo AA. Mirtazapine-induced pancreatitis—a case report. *J Pharm Pract*. 2019;32(5):586-588.

69. Bello-Hernández Y, Espinoza-Hernández J, Moreno-Coutiño G. Acneiform rash caused by an unlikely drug: topiramate. *Ski Appendage Disord*. 2018;4(1):25-28.

70. Rudd KM, Panneerselvam N, Patel A. Rash associated with rivaroxaban use. *Am J Heal Pharm*. 2018;75(6):347-349.

71. Sasson E, James M, Russell M, Todorov D, Cohen H. Probable rivaroxaban-induced full body rash: a case report. *J Pharm Pract*. 2018;31(5):503-506.

72. World Health Organisation (WHO). Transitions of care: technical series on safer primary care. 2016:1-26. Available at https://apps.who.int/iris/bitstream/handle/10665/252272/97892-41511599-eng.pdf;jsessionid=F02F4E67BC0581E4B21DE72B23 FC0994?sequence=1. Accessed May 31, 2020.

73. Barrett ML, Wier LM, Jiang J, Steiner CA. All-cause readmissions by payer and age, 2009–2013. Statistical Brief #199. Agency for Healthcare Research and Quality. 2015;166:1-14.

74. Baldwin SM, Zook S, Sanford J. Implementing posthospital interprofessional care team visits to improve care transitions and decrease hospital readmission rates. *Prof Case Manag*. 2018;23(5):264-271.

75. Stranges PM, Marshall VD, Walker PC, Hall KE, Griffith DK, Remington T. A multidisciplinary intervention for reducing readmissions among older adults in a patient-centered medical home. *Am J Manag Care*. 2015;21(2):1-7.

76. White B, Carney PA, Flynn J, Marino M, Fields S. Reducing hospital readmissions through primary care practice transformation. *J Fam Pract*. 2014;63(2):67-74.

77. Elixhauser A, Steiner C. Readmissions to U.S. hospitals by diagnosis, 2010. Statistical Brief #153. Agency for Healthcare Research and Quality. 2013:1-19.

78. Centers for Disease Control and Prevention. Asthma. Available at http://www.cdc.gov/asthma/most_recent_national_asthma_ data.htm. Accessed May 31, 2020.

79. Nunes C, Pereira AM, Morais-Almeida M. Asthma costs and social impact. *Asthma Res Pract*. 2017;3(1):1-11.

80. Centers for Disease Control and Prevention. Asthma-related missed school days among children aged 5–17 years. Available at https://www.cdc.gov/asthma/asthma_stats/AstStatChild_ Missed_School_Days.pdf. Accessed May 31, 2020.

81. Barnett SBL, Nurmagambetov TA. Costs of asthma in the United States: 2002-2007. *J Allergy Clin Immunol*. 2011;127(1):145-152.

82. Global Initiative for Asthma. Pocket guide for asthma management and prevention. Available at https://ginasthma.org/ wp-content/uploads/2019/04/GINA-2019-main-Pocket-Guide-wms.pdf. Accessed November 1, 2020.

83. National Heart, Lung, and Blood Institute. National Asthma Education and Prevention Program Expert Panel Report 3: Guidelines for the Diagnosis and Management of Asthma Full Report 2007. *J Allergy Clin Immunol*. 2007 Nov;120(5 suppl):S94-S138.

84. Allergy Foundation of America. Ethnic disparities in the burden and treatment of asthma. Available at https://www.aafa.org/ media/1633/ethnic-disparities-burden-treatment-asthma-report. pdf. Accessed May 31, 2020.

85. Edwards E. Vaping illnesses may lead to repeat hospitalizations. *NBC News*. Available at https://www.nbcnews.com/health/ vaping/vaping-illnesses-may-lead-repeat-hospitalizations-n1065021. Accessed March 10, 2020.

86. O'Donnell J. I think my kid is vaping: what parents should know about electronic cigarettes, lung injury. *USA Today*. Available at https://www.usatoday.com/story/news/health/2019/10/01/tips-parents-stop-teens-vaping-illness-thc/2429184001/. Accessed March 10, 2020.

87. Balingit M. More than 150 teens have fallen ill from vaping. Is it enough to make their peers stop? *The Washington Post.* Accessed March 10, 2020.

88. Howard J. New vaping study links e-liquids to some lung inflammation. *CNN Health.* Available at https://www.cnn.com/2019/10/16/health/vaping-e-liquids-lung-inflammation-study/index.html. Accessed March 10, 2020.

89. Centers for Disease Control and Prevention. Quick facts on the risks of e-cigarettes for kids, teens, and young adults. Available at https://www.cdc.gov/tobacco/basic_information/e-cigarettes/Quick-Facts-on-the-Risks-of-E-cigarettes-for-Kids-Teens-and-Young-Adults.html#what-are-e-cigarettes. Accessed March 10, 2020.

90. Berry KM, Fetterman JL, Benjamin EJ, et al. Association of electronic cigarette use with subsequent initiation of tobacco cigarettes in US youths. *JAMA Netw open.* 2019;2(2):e187794.

91. Bayly JE, Bernat D, Porter L, Choi K. Secondhand exposure to aerosols from electronic nicotine delivery systems and asthma exacerbations among youth with asthma. *Chest.* 2019;155(1):88-93.

92. American Thoracic Society. ATS health alert—vaping-associated pulmonary illness Available at https://www.atsjournals.org/doi/abs/10.1164/rccm.2007P15. Accessed May 31, 2020.

93. Nathan RA, Sorkness CA, Kosinski M, et al. Development of the asthma control test: a survey for assessing asthma control. *J Allergy Clin Immunol.* 2004;113(1):59-65.

94. Schatz M, Sorkness CA, Li JT, et al. Asthma control test: reliability, validity, and responsiveness in patients not previously followed by asthma specialists. *J Allergy Clin Immunol.* 2006;117(3):549-556.

95. GSK. Childhood asthma control test for children 4 to 11 years. Available at https://www.asthma.com/content/dam/NA_Pharma/Country/US/Unbranded/Consumer/Common/Images/MPY/documents/816205R0_childhoodasthmacontroltest_printable.pdf. Accessed March 10, 2020.

96. Juniper EF, O'Byrne PM, Guyatt GH, Ferrie PJ, King DR. Development and validation of a questionnaire to measure asthma control. *Eur Respir J.* 1999;14(4):902-907.

97. Juniper EF, Bousquet J, Abetz L, Bateman ED. Identifying "well-controlled" and "not well-controlled" asthma using the Asthma Control Questionnaire. *Respir Med.* 2006;100(4):616-621.

98. Grohskopf LA, Alyanak E, Broder KR, Blanton LH, Fry AM, Jernigan DB, Armar RI. Prevention and control of seasonal influenza with vaccines: recommendations of the Advisory Committee on Immunization Practices—United States, 2020–2021 influenza season. *MMWR Recomm Rep.* 2020;69(8):1-24.

99. Centers for Disease Control and Prevention. Candida infections of the mouth, throat, and esophagus. Available at https://www.cdc.gov/fungal/diseases/candidiasis/thrush/index.html. Accessed March 10, 2020.

100. Mayo Clinic. Oral thrush. Available at https://www.mayoclinic.org/diseases-conditions/oral-thrush/symptoms. Accessed March 10, 2020.

101. American Diabetes Association. Available at www.diabetes.org/. Accessed March 10, 2020.

102. American Diabetes Association. The history of a wonderful thing we call insulin. Available at https://www.diabetes.org/blog/history-wonderful-thing-we-call-insulin. Accessed March 10, 2020.

103. Centers for Disease Control and Prevention. National Diabetes Statistics Report, 2020. Available at https://www.cdc.gov/diabetes/data/statistics-report/index.html. Accessed November 1, 2020.

104. Yang W, Dall TM, Beronjia K, et al. Economic costs of diabetes in the U.S. in 2017. *Diabetes Care.* 2018;41(5):917-928.

105. American Diabetes Association. 6. Glycemic targets: standards of medical care in diabetes—2020. *Diabetes Care.* 2020;43(suppl 1):S66-S76.

106. American Diabetes Association. Hyperglycemia (high blood glucose). Available at https://www.diabetes.org/diabetes/medication-management/blood-glucose-testing-and-control/hyperglycemia. Accessed January 9, 2020.

107. American Diabetes Association. Stroke. Available at https://www.diabetes.org/diabetes/complications/stroke. Accessed February 12, 2020.

108. American Heart Association. Cardiovascular disease and diabetes. Available at https://www.heart.org/en/health-topics/diabetes/why-diabetes-matters/cardiovascular-disease-diabetes. Accessed January 9, 2020.

109. American Diabetes Association. Eye complications. Available at https://www.diabetes.org/diabetes/complications/eye-complications. Accessed March 10, 2020.

110. Mark AM. Diabetes and oral health. *J Am Dent Assoc.* 2016;147(10):852.

111. American Diabetes Association. 11. Microvascular complications and foot care: standards of medical care in diabetes—2020. *Diabetes Care.* 2020;43(suppl 1):S135-S151.

112. American Diabetes Association. 9. Pharmacologic approaches to glycemic treatment: standards of medical care in diabetes—2020. *Diabetes Care.* 2020;43(suppl 1):S98-S110.

113. American Diabetes Association. Autonomic neuropathy. Available at https://www.diabetes.org/diabetes/complications/neuropathy/autonomic-neuropathy. Accessed February 14, 2020.

114. American Diabetes Association. Foot complications. Available at https://www.diabetes.org/diabetes/complications/foot-complications. Accessed February 14, 2020.

115. Alexiadou K, Doupis J. Management of diabetic foot ulcers. *Diabetes Ther.* 2012;3(1):1-15.

116. Kiel PJ, McCord AD. Pharmacist impact on clinical outcome in a diabetes disease management program via collaborative practice. *Ann Pharmacother.* 2005;39(11):1828-1832.

117. Pinto SL, Bechtol RA, Partha G. Evaluation of outcomes of a medication therapy management program for patients with diabetes. *J Am Pharm Assoc.* 2012;52(4):519-523.

118. Bluml BM, Watson LL, Skelton JB, Manolakis PG, Brock KA. Improving outcomes for diverse populations disproportionately affected by diabetes: final results of Project IMPACT: diabetes. *J Am Pharm Assoc.* 2014;54(5):477-485.

119. American Pharmacists Association. The pharmacist & patient-centered diabetes care. Available at https://www.pharmacist.com/education/pharmacist-patient-centered-diabetes-care. Accessed March 10, 2020.

120. Waghel RC, Wilson JA, Salem D. Patient assessment skills currently taught in pharmacy curricula. *Curr Pharm Teach Learn.* 2016;8(4):485-491.

121. American Diabetes Association. 5. Facilitating behavior change and well-being to improve health outcomes: standards of medical care in diabetes—2020. *Diabetes Care.* 2020;43(suppl 1):S48-S65.

122. Wubben DP, Vivian EM. Effects of pharmacist outpatient interventions on adults with diabetes mellitus: a systematic review. *Pharmacotherapy.* 2008;28(4):421-436.

123. Fazel MT, Bagalagel A, Lee JK, Martin JR, Slack MK. Impact of diabetes care by pharmacists as part of health care team in ambulatory settings: a systematic review and meta-analysis. *Ann Pharmacother.* 2017;51(10):890-907.

124. van Eikenhorst L, Taxis K, van Dijk L, de Gier H. Pharmacist-led self-management interventions to improve diabetes outcomes. A systematic literature review and meta-analysis. *Front Pharmacol.* 2017;8(December):1-14.

125. Jeong S, Lee M, Ji E. Effect of pharmaceutical care interventions on glycemic control in patients with diabetes: a systematic review and meta-analysis. *Ther Clin Risk Manag.* 2018;14:1813-1829.

126. Ourth HL, Hur K, Morreale AP, Cunningham F, Thakkar B, Aspinall S. Comparison of clinical pharmacy specialists and usual care in outpatient management of hyperglycemia in Veterans Affairs medical centers. *Am J Heal Pharm.* 2019;76(1):26-33.

127. Cohen RA, Cha AE. Strategies used by adults with diagnosed diabetes to reduce their prescription drug costs, 2017–2018. *NCHS Data Brief.* 2019;(349):1-8.

128. Capoccia K, Odegard PS, Letassy N. Medication adherence with diabetes medication: a systematic review of the literature. *Diabetes Educ.* 2016;42(1):34-71.

129. Frazier KR, McKeirnan KC, Kherghehpoush S, Woodard LJ. Rural patient perceptions of pharmacist-provided chronic condition management in a state with provider status. *J Am Pharm Assoc.* 2019;59(2):210-216.

130. Watson LL, Bluml BM. Integrating pharmacists into diverse diabetes care teams: implementation tactics from Project IMPACT: diabetes. *J Am Pharm Assoc.* 2014;54(5):538-541.

131. Hawes EM, Lambert E, Reid A, Tong G, Gwynne M. Implementation and evaluation of a pharmacist-led electronic visit program for diabetes and anticoagulation care in a patient-centered medical home. *Am J Heal Pharm.* 2018;75(12):901-910.

132. Scott DM, Boyd ST, Stephan M, Augustine SC, Reardon TP. Outcomes of pharmacist-managed diabetes care services in a community health center. *Am J Heal Pharm.* 2006;63(21):2116-2122.

133. Schuessler TJ, Ruisinger JF, Hare SE, Prohaska ES, Melton BL. Patient satisfaction with pharmacist-led chronic disease state management programs. *J Pharm Pract.* 2016;29(5):484-489.

134. National Diabetes Education Program. Working together to manage diabetes: a toolkit for pharmacy, podiatry, optometry, and dentistry (PPOD). Centers for Disease Control and Prevention. Available at https://www.cdc.gov/diabetes/ndep/toolkits/ppod.html. Accessed March 10, 2020.

CHAPTER 4

Prevention & Wellness

Featuring the Illustrated Case Studies "Screen,"
"Change Talk," & "Mobilized"

Authors

Beth A. Martin, Eva M. Vivian, Mary S. Hayney, & Joseph A. Zorek

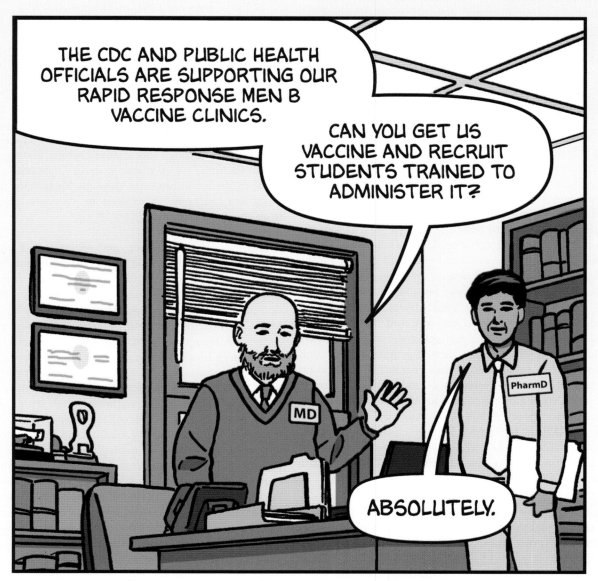

Illustration by George Folz, © 2019 Board of Regents of the University of Wisconsin System

BACKGROUND

Prevention and wellness efforts are frequently associated with public health initiatives. As a concept, public health has been defined as "what we as a society do to assure the conditions in which people can be healthy."[1] Pharmacists, like other health professionals, regularly contribute their skills and expertise to keep people healthy and to prevent diseases; examples include providing education to patients, policy makers, and communities. Oftentimes, the community pharmacy is a patient's first access point within the healthcare system, and it is frequently here where prevention and wellness efforts are initiated.

The American Public Health Association has outlined the role of the pharmacist in public health in an updated policy that identifies several areas where the pharmacist is uniquely positioned to promote prevention and wellness.[2] The policy highlights the value pharmacists have as an accessible source of health and medication information due to their physical location in the community and high degree of clinical training. Pharmacists can serve as educators for other health professionals, patients, and the community. Pharmacists are in an ideal position to promote prevention and wellness initiatives such as health screenings and immunizations, as well as lifestyle modifications linked to diet and the use of alcohol, tobacco, and other substances.[2]

Public health initiatives that pharmacists engage in emphasize three levels of prevention: primary, secondary, and tertiary.[3] Primary prevention focuses on reducing the incidence of disease and injury through direct interventions. Well-known examples of pharmacists contributing to primary prevention efforts include vaccination administration programs and assistance with health behavior change, such as tobacco cessation and improving nutritional status via healthier eating habits.[4] Secondary prevention focuses on decreasing the progression and severity of disease by screening to identify diseases before the symptoms become severe; examples include assessing patients for heart disease and conducting screenings for high blood pressure and blood glucose. Tertiary prevention involves managing disease and injury after diagnosis in order to slow or stop progression through interventions like rehabilitation and promoting medication adherence.[4] Readers interested in a more in-depth discussion of medication adherence are encouraged to explore the illustrated cases "Breathe" and "Opportunities" in Chapter 2 Community Pharmacy and Chapter 15 Administration, respectively. Those who would like more information on rehabilitation efforts should read the illustrated case "Educator" in Chapter 5 Cardiology.

One of the challenges identified within the profession as it relates to pharmacists providing public health-focused services, however, is that pharmacists are often not compensated for their prevention and wellness activities. This limits how often pharmacists can provide these services in lieu of reimbursable activities, such as dispensing medications.[5] New opportunities that can promote pharmacist-delivered wellness services include a shift toward rewarding quality care and increasing use of technology-supported services.[5] The World Health Organization defines quality care as "the extent to which health care services provided to individuals and patient populations improve desired health outcomes. In order to achieve this, health care must be safe, effective, timely, efficient, equitable and people-centred."[6] Examples of quality care outcomes associated with pharmacy services include increases in medication adherence, vaccination rates, and health screening participation, and decreases in blood pressure, blood glucose, tobacco use, and hospital readmissions.[7] Importantly, pharmacists are increasingly leveraging technology to engage patients in rural parts of the country who may otherwise have limited access to healthcare. Electronic prescribing and prescription drug monitoring programs provide two examples.[8]

Healthcare cost management can also be supported by pharmacists impacting prevention and wellness outcomes through the provision of macro-level public health services. In this role, pharmacists design and implement policies and services that can impact primary and secondary prevention outcomes; for example, by establishing policies at government agencies or within hospital and healthcare systems. Pharmacists working in this capacity have reduced hospital readmissions through medication therapy management services.[9] Pharmacists have also promoted safe medication disposal in their communities through Medication Take Back initiatives that remove expired or unwanted medications from the general public.[10]

Another area of prevention and wellness that pharmacists can contribute to is public health planning and emergency preparedness.[2] Disasters such as hurricanes, tornados, and infectious disease outbreaks pose challenges for medication access and distribution. In the aftermath of Hurricane Maria in Puerto Rico, for example, community pharmacists were recognized and applauded for their immediate engagement to maintain patients' access to needed medications.[11] Pharmacists were also critical partners in response to COVID-19. Their work included participating in developing plans early in the outbreak when little was known about effective treatments, collecting specimens for patient diagnosis, and maintaining readiness to immunize.[12] Due to pharmacists' societal role managing the acquisition, storage, security, and distribution of medications, pharmacists are critical and valued members of emergency response teams.[13] Furthermore, drug shortages of lifesaving medications, often due to manufacturing issues or high demand, require pharmacists' expertise within the health team to identify alternative drug therapies and/or administration mechanisms in order to ensure all those who need medications are able to access them.[14,15]

PHARMACISTS IN ACTION

Reducing Fall Risk in Older Adults

Falls are the leading cause of death and injuries in older adults, defined as individuals 65 years of age or older.[16] The US Centers for Disease Control and Prevention (CDC) have developed guidelines to mitigate this problem: Stopping Elderly Accidents, Deaths, and Injuries (STEADI). The STEADI guidelines are intended to help health professionals, including pharmacists, implement fall prevention initiatives.[17] As part of an interprofessional team, pharmacists can use the tools and resources to identify at-risk older adults, review medication use, including vitamin D and calcium, and intervene on the patient's behalf to minimize their fall risk. Medications that affect the central nervous system, like those for sleep, anxiety, and pain, can have side effects like dizziness and drowsiness that are associated with falling.[18] By screening for these medications, pharmacists are able to work with patients' providers to modify dosages, discontinue dangerous medications, or facilitate transition to nondrug therapies. One pharmacist-led service in a community pharmacy setting decreased fall risk by reducing use of dangerous medications and educating patients, who valued the pharmacist's expertise and individualized approach to care.[19]

Healthier Hearts in Iowa

A community pharmacy team in rural Iowa provided a cardiovascular risk reduction program to adults at their work site.[20] When pharmacists visited the workplace, they met one-on-one with participants for an average of seven visits. During visits, they provided education about cardiovascular disease, emphasized the importance of monitoring blood pressure, pulse, and weight, and evaluated medication regimens to identify potential medication-related problems. The pharmacists communicated with participants' prescribers as needed, including recommendations to improve medication use. Importantly, this intervention resulted in improved blood pressure control and cholesterol levels, two markers that significantly impact cardiovascular risk.

Drug Take Back Days

Pharmacists play a significant role in promoting the safe disposal of prescription and nonprescription drugs. The US Drug Enforcement Administration (DEA) enacted National Prescription Drug Take Back Days in 2014, which occur biannually in April and October. Many consumers dispose of unwanted, unused, or expired medications by flushing them down the toilet or throwing them away, which can harm the environment. It is also common for unused medications to remain in medicine cabinets or drawers for extended periods, which increases the risk of accidental exposure/ingestion by children or pets. Unused, unsecured pain medications are also at risk of diversion by those seeking opioid medications. Pharmacies can be authorized collection sites for Take Back Days and provide education to the public on the importance of properly disposing of unused medications, including safe opioid disposal.[21] The DEA reports results of each collection event; on average, each Take Back Day involves over 6000 sites nationally that collectively amass over 450 tons of unused medications.[22] Readers interested in learning more about pharmacists' contributions to the management of accidental ingestions and opioid medications are encouraged to explore the illustrated cases "Accidental" and "Gasping" in Chapter 6 Pediatrics and Chapter 12 Mental Health, respectively.

BECOMING A PHARMACIST WITH PREVENTION & WELLNESS EXPERTISE

It is important to note that all pharmacists, regardless of practice setting, have a role to play in prevention and wellness efforts. Graduates of Doctor of Pharmacy (PharmD) programs accredited by the Accreditation Council for Pharmacy Education (ACPE) achieve learning outcomes that emphasize the pharmacist's role in public health. These outcomes include "exploration of population health management strategies, national and community-based public health programs, and implementation of activities that advance public health and wellness, as well as provide an avenue through which students earn certificates in immunization delivery and other public health-focused skills."[23]

Some pharmacy schools offer dual degrees, combining a Master of Public Health (MPH) degree with a PharmD degree. This pathway establishes a more formal route to contribute to prevention and wellness efforts via the acquisition of knowledge and skills in the public health profession that augment what is acquired while becoming a pharmacist. This generally takes one additional year to complete, and may involve a thesis project/paper. Pharmacists who obtain an MPH are appealing to federal health agencies and healthcare systems, particularly those that focus on population health (see Chapter 14 Population Health for more information on this topic). Additionally, many state and national associations offer advanced training and certification programs to supplement pharmacists' skills and provide resources for implementing prevention and wellness services. Such programs emphasize a wide range of topics, from diabetes, asthma, and high blood pressure to travel health, health coaching, and functional medicine. Importantly, they also often require participants to complete a number of additional patient-directed service hours to become fully certified, as well as a fee to maintain certification.

SCREEN: An Illustrated Case Study

Story by Eva M. Vivian & Joseph A. Zorek
Illustrations by George Folz, © 2019 Board of Regents of the University of Wisconsin System

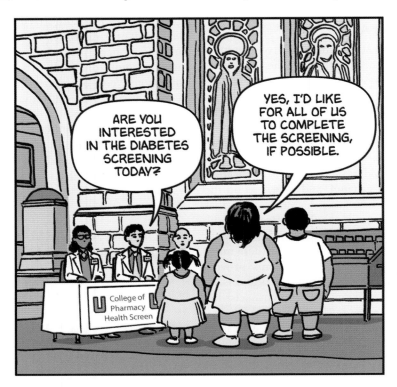

Illustration 4-1

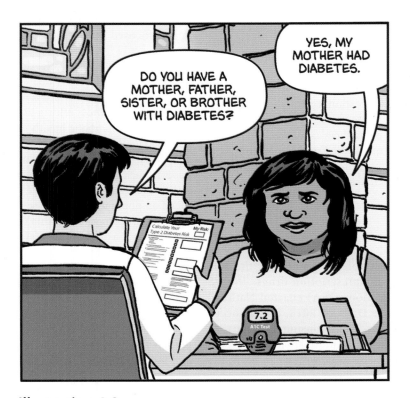

Illustration 4-2

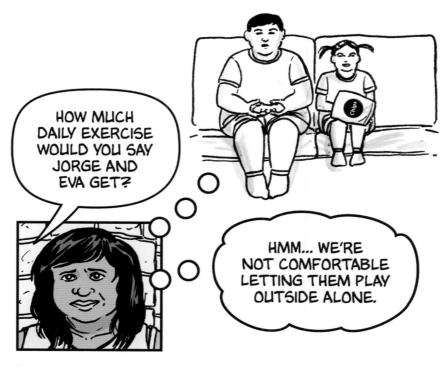

Illustration 4-3

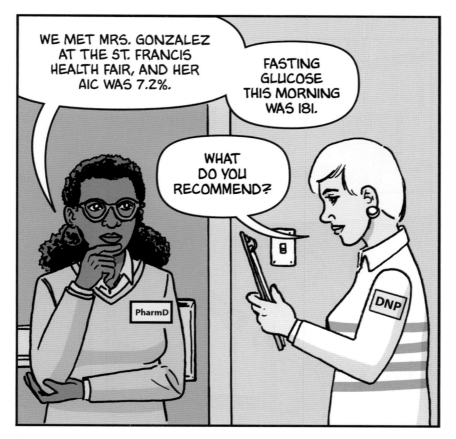

Illustration 4-4

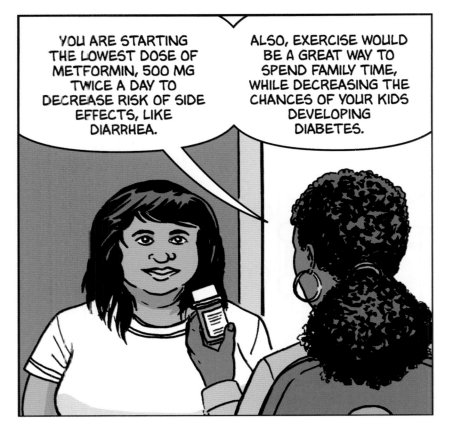

Illustration 4-5

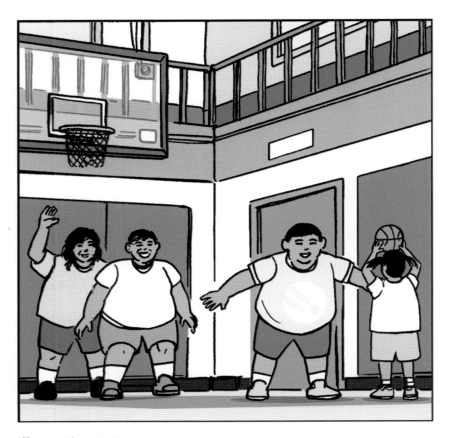

Illustration 4-6

Thoughts on "Screen"

Diabetes mellitus refers to a group of diseases that affect how the body uses glucose (i.e., sugar) that is present in the blood.[24] Glucose is vital to health because it is an important source of energy for the cells that make up muscles and tissues throughout the body. It also serves as the brain's main source of fuel. The underlying cause of diabetes varies according to specific condition. That said, no matter what type of diabetes a person has, it can lead to excess glucose in the blood and serious health problems. Chronic diabetes conditions include type 1 diabetes and type 2 diabetes. Potentially reversible diabetes conditions include prediabetes, when blood glucose levels are higher than normal but not high enough to be classified as diabetes, and gestational diabetes, which occurs during pregnancy but may resolve after the baby is delivered.[25]

The exact cause of type 1 diabetes is unknown.[24] What is known is that the immune system, which normally fights harmful bacteria or viruses, attacks and destroys the insulin-producing cells in the pancreas. This leaves the person with little or no insulin, which is problematic because insulin is required to transport glucose into cells; without insulin, glucose builds up in the bloodstream. Type 1 diabetes is thought to be caused by a combination of genetic and environmental factors, though exactly what those factors are is still unclear. Weight is not believed to be a factor; however, known risks include family history, environmental factors (e.g., exposure to a viral illness), and issues with immune system cells, like autoantibodies.[26] Readers interested in learning more about this topic are encouraged to explore the illustrated case "Type 1" in Chapter 11 Critical Care.

In prediabetes, which can lead to type 2 diabetes, and in type 2 diabetes, cells throughout the body become resistant to the action of insulin. As a result, the pancreas is unable to make enough insulin to overcome this resistance and transport of glucose into cells becomes less effective, causing glucose to build up in the bloodstream.[24,25] Exactly why this happens is uncertain, although it is believed that genetic and environmental factors play a role in the development of type 2 diabetes, too. Being overweight is strongly linked to the development of type 2 diabetes, but not everyone with type 2 diabetes is overweight. Researchers do not fully understand why some people develop prediabetes and type 2 diabetes while others do not. However, it is clear that certain risk factors increase a person's odds; for example, excessive weight, inactivity, increasing age, gestational diabetes, and family history.[26]

The high prevalence of diabetes and prediabetes in the United States presents a major public health problem. According to the CDC, 9.4% of the US population has diabetes, or 30.3 million Americans.[27] Of those affected, it is estimated that only 21 million were formally diagnosed with diabetes; thus, approximately 8 million Americans have diabetes but are unaware of it. Another 84.1 million Americans are estimated to have

Table 4-1. Key Biomarkers Used in the Screening, Diagnosis, and Management of Diabetes		
Name of Test	**Results**	**Interpretation**
Hemoglobin A1c (A1c[*])	<5.7%	Normal
	5.7–6.4%	Prediabetes
	>6.4%	Diabetes
Fasting plasma glucose (FPG[**])	<100 mg/dL	Normal
	100–125 mg/dL	Prediabetes
	>125 mg/dL	Diabetes
Random plasma glucose (RPG[***])	>200 mg/dL plus classic symptoms[****]	Diabetes

[*] A1c is a rough estimate of a patient's average glucose level over the course of approximately 3 months.

[**] FPG is the amount of glucose currently in a patient's blood who has fasted (i.e., not eaten or drank anything but water for at least 8 hours).

[***] RPG is the amount of glucose currently in a patient's blood who has not fasted.

[****] Classic symptoms of hyperglycemia or hyperglycemic crisis include increased thirst, urination, and hunger.

prediabetes, a condition that, as stated, often leads to type 2 diabetes within 5 years.[27] Groups within the United States at higher risk for prediabetes include individuals over 45 years of age, racial and ethnic minorities, women who have had gestational diabetes but do not receive adequate follow-up testing postpartum, and those without access to medical care, such as the uninsured.[26] The number of Americans with diabetes has almost tripled since 1990; therefore, health professionals must engage in outreach efforts to identify those at risk and get them connected to care.[27]

There is strong support for early diagnosis and intervention to minimize the progression of diabetes and the development of associated complications.[28,29] For more information on complications associated with diabetes, see the illustrated cases "Holistic" in Chapter 3 Primary Care and "Type 1" in Chapter 11 Critical Care. Tests commonly used by patients and health professionals to measure blood glucose levels are shown in Table 4-1, along with how results are interpreted. Unless there is a clear clinical diagnosis, two abnormal test results from the same sample or in two separate test samples are required for diagnosis. If using two separate test samples, it is recommended that the second test, which may either be a repeat of the initial test or a different test, be performed without delay.[25]

Many diabetes stakeholder groups and organizations, especially at the local level, advocate for community-based screening (CBS) in venues such as health fairs or diabetes awareness events, as shown in Illustration 4-1. Thousands of individuals throughout the United States have been screened at such events in the hope that those who are undiagnosed will be discovered and connected to care.[28,29] Concerns have been raised that CBS may result in poor identification of those most at risk, and that those at low risk may be inappropriately tested. As a result, it is recommended that CBS take place in communities where the risk of diabetes, or the prevalence of undiagnosed diabetes, is known to be high.[26] As shown in Illustrations 4-1 and 4-2 of the illustrated case "Screen," many CBS events are incorporated into health fairs at community centers and churches located in underserved communities.[28]

While not presented in "Screen," it is important that CBS organizers make every effort to ensure that the individuals who are screened understand what their results mean and the implications of the results for their health. They need to understand that a single elevated blood glucose reading does not meet the criteria for diagnosis of prediabetes or diabetes and no such implication should be expressed or implied. Written materials explaining prediabetes and diabetes, risk factors for these conditions, the tests used for screening, and the meaning of test results, must be provided to all individuals screened. To ensure comprehension, verbal explanation in the language spoken by the individual, a key tenant of culturally competent care, should also be provided.[29,30] For another example of such care, see the illustrated case "Barriers" in Chapter 12 Mental Health.

Because pharmacists are the most accessible health professionals, they are key players in the lifelong management of diabetes and other chronic diseases.[31] Pharmacists receive a comprehensive education that covers disease state etiology, risk factors, prevention, management, and treatment, which gives them a strong foundation for providing lifestyle management counseling.[31] Pharmacists also have the foundational knowledge and skills to perform basic physical assessments and point-of-care testing necessary to identify and counsel persons with prediabetes and those who are overweight or obese.[31-34] For additional examples of point-of-care testing and the important role these tests play in pharmacy, see the illustrated case "Empowerment" in Chapter 5 Cardiology.

The American Diabetes Association (ADA) recommends a non-invasive web- or paper-based questionnaire as the first step of screening. The ADA Type 2 Diabetes Risk Test is commonly used to identify those at high risk for prediabetes or diabetes, as depicted in Illustration 4-2.[25] This test measures risk based on age, sex, family history, body weight, history of gestational diabetes, and a diagnosis of high blood pressure. Illustration 4-2 shows Mrs. Gonzalez completing this test with the help of a pharmacy student, and informing him that her mother had diabetes. This family history, coupled with Mrs. Gonzalez's weight and ethnicity, place her at high risk of developing diabetes on the ADA Risk Test. As a result, a point-of-care testing device that measures hemoglobin A1c is administered. With an A1c reading of 7.2%, Mrs. Gonzalez was referred to a primary care clinic for follow-up testing and diagnosis, as shown in Illustrations 4-4 and 4-5.

Physical inactivity and obesity are important contributors to diabetes. When asked how active her children were in Illustration 4-3, Mrs. Gonzalez reflects on how they spend their time and her fear of letting them play outside unsupervised. Families who live in disadvantaged neighborhoods, where grocery stores and parks may be scarce, sidewalks may not be well maintained, or rates of crime may be high, often gain weight or develop obesity due to lower physical activity levels and poorer nutrition.[35,36] These families are also faced with greater exposure to the marketing of low-nutrition foods and less recreational opportunities.[37] Broadly speaking, factors such as these are referred to as social determinants of health. For more information on this topic, see Chapter 14 Population Health and the illustrated case "Unsung Hero," in particular.

For those who are diagnosed with diabetes or prediabetes, pharmacists are able to provide guidance and advice on how to monitor glucose levels and what to do when levels are out of range. This includes working with patients to develop action plans when glucose levels go too low (i.e., hypoglycemia), which can lead to serious health consequences. For example, a common action plan might include teaching patients how to treat hypoglycemia by consuming fast-acting carbohydrates, foods that are easily converted to glucose in the body, such as glucose tablets or gel, fruit juice, regular soft drinks (not diet), and sugary candy such as licorice. Pharmacist can also encourage patients to eat balanced meals that include carbohydrates and protein. More importantly, pharmacists can recommend alterations in a medication regimen to decrease the likelihood of a patient experiencing hypoglycemia.[31,32]

Medications to treat diabetes are complex, and pharmacists play a critical role collaborating with other members of the interprofessional team, like physicians, physician assistants, nurse practitioners, and social workers, to obtain medications and maximize the impact of medication therapy.[34,38,39] This is demonstrated in Illustration 4-4, which shows the pharmacist who was supervising students earlier in the case collaborating with a nurse practitioner on a treatment plan for Mrs. Gonzalez. The screening event was a success insofar as Mrs. Gonzalez's elevated risk was identified and she was connected to a primary care practice for further workup and diagnosis.

The number of medication options to treat diabetes has increased in recent years, and pharmacists are well positioned to help patients and their prescribers understand the fundamentals and intricacies of using newer, as well as older, medications. Management of adverse drug reactions (ADRs) is a core pharmacist role on interprofessional teams regardless of disease (see the illustrated case "Support" in Chapter 3 Primary Care for more detail on identification and management of ADRs). This is especially important for patients with diabetes given the frequency of ADRs and the need for fast action to prevent serious consequences, particularly from hypoglycemia. Beyond managing ADRs, pharmacists assist patients on proper administration of medications and address common questions and concerns. For patients requiring insulin, this is critically important.[28-31] The diabetes-related illustrated case "Holistic" in Chapter 3 Primary Care provides more detailed information on the medications used to treat diabetes, including how they work.

The pharmacist recommended metformin as an initial treatment for Mrs. Gonzalez, as shown in Illustrations 4-4 and 4-5. Metformin should be started at the time type 2 diabetes is diagnosed unless there are contraindications; for most patients, this will be monotherapy (i.e., no other medications will be used) in combination with lifestyle modifications. Metformin is effective and safe, is inexpensive, and may reduce risk of cardiovascular events and death.[40] Metformin is available in an immediate-release form for twice daily dosing or as an extended-release form that can be given once daily. Compared with sulfonylureas, another oral medication used to lower blood glucose, metformin as first-line therapy has beneficial effects on A1c (refer to Table 4-1), weight, and cardiovascular mortality.[40] The principal side effects of metformin are gastrointestinal intolerance due to bloating, abdominal discomfort, and diarrhea. This drug is cleared by the kidneys, and very high circulating levels (e.g., as a result of overdose or acute kidney failure) have been associated with a serious ADR called lactic acidosis. However, the occurrence of this complication is now known to be very rare, and metformin may be safely administered in patients even if they have moderate impairment in kidney function.[41]

Illustration 4-5 shows the pharmacist recommending a fun physical activity for the entire family, which they follow through on in Illustration 4-6. The health benefits of physical activity for anyone in general cannot be underestimated. Regular physical activity is one of the most important tools to support diabetes management and reduce the risk of complications for people with type 2 diabetes.[42] It is also a proven way to help reduce the risk of diabetes in the first place. The research support for this is impressive, including the finding that regular physical activity in conjunction with healthy eating and weight control can reduce diabetes incidence by 60%.[43] Physical activity can, in some cases, be as effective as a glucose-lowering medication for maintaining diabetes management targets.[42,43] Exercise can reduce, or sometimes even eliminate, the need for medications. Many people with diabetes can literally see their blood pressure going down in front of their eyes during treadmill or other physical activity health tests. In conjunction with healthy eating, regular physical activity can make a huge difference in helping individuals with diabetes reach and maintain their healthy weight and blood glucose targets.[44,45]

Type 2 diabetes most often develops in people over age 45, but more and more children, teens, and young adults are also developing it.[25] As implied in Illustration 4-1, Mrs. Gonzalez would like her children to participate in the diabetes screening because she is concerned about their health. Parents play a big role in shaping children's eating and physical activity habits.[46] First, they are the custodians of daily schedules and can therefore guide issues such as the amount of time spent playing video games (see Illustration 4-3) or engaged in other forms of idle leisure like screen time on devices (tablets, phones, etc.) and television. Second, parental support of physical activity, their own level of physical activity, and their enjoyment of physical activity predict the extent to which their children will engage in physical activity.[47] As shown in Illustration 4-6, when parents engage in physical activity with their children, the impact on physical activity levels in children is impressive, regardless of whether the children are of normal weight or overweight.[47]

DISCUSSION QUESTIONS FOR "SCREEN"

1. In Illustration 4-3, Mrs. Gonzalez does not tell the pharmacy student the reason her children are not as active as they might be; rather, her thoughts reveal concerns for their safety. Why might she have kept this information to herself?

2. Social and environmental factors appear to be influencing the current lifestyle behaviors of the Gonzalez family. Beyond a general recommendation to "be more active," what specific recommendations would you make to encourage a healthier lifestyle? What other health professionals might you consult for guidance?

3. The pharmacist is shown collaborating with a nurse practitioner in Illustration 4-4. What are the similarities and differences between nurse practitioners and pharmacists?

4. The case does not address whether Mrs. Gonzalez has health coverage. What steps should be taken in the event that Mrs. Gonzalez indicates that she does not have health insurance?

5. If a patient does not have health insurance and cannot afford their medications, how are they to obtain and take a prescribed medication like metformin? Can you think of another health professional whose background and training might help in a situation like this?

CHANGE TALK: An Illustrated Case Study

Story by Beth A. Martin & Joseph A. Zorek
Illustrations by George Folz, © 2019 Board of Regents of the University of Wisconsin System

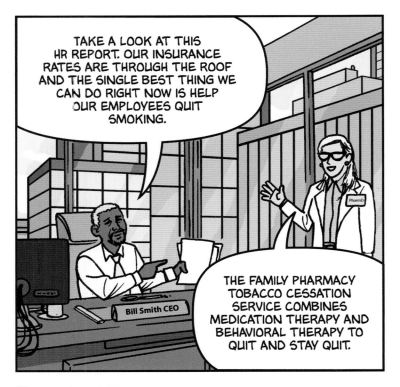

Illustration 4-7

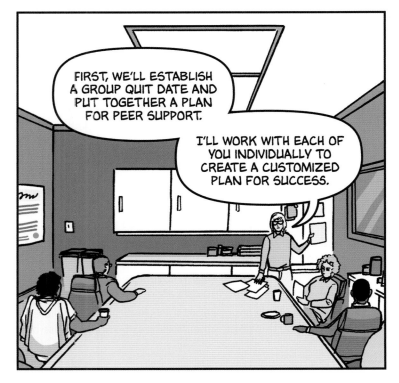

Illustration 4-8

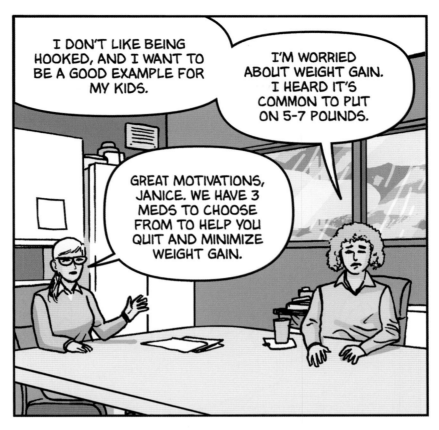

Illustration 4-9

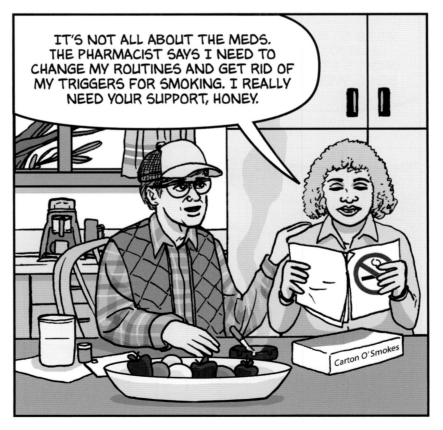

Illustration 4-10

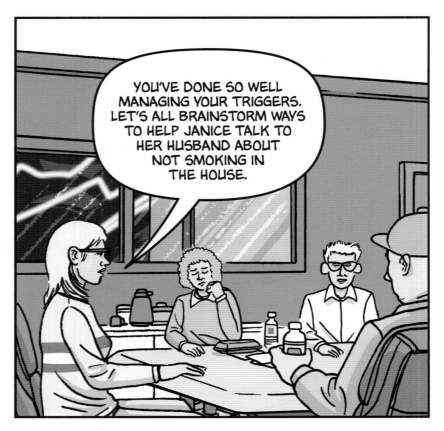

Illustration 4-11

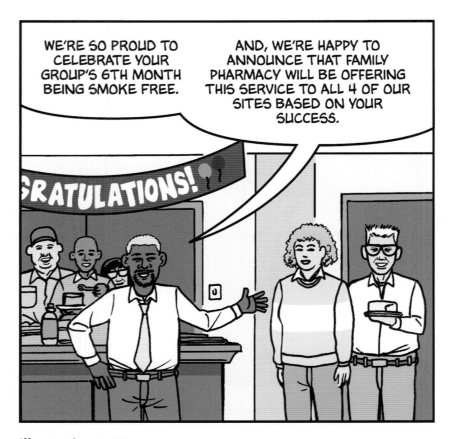

Illustration 4-12

Thoughts on "Change Talk"

Cigarette smoking is the leading known cause of preventable death worldwide, and it is responsible for an estimated 480,000 deaths each year in the United States.[48] In the United States, the annual cost attributable to smoking has been estimated at a staggering $300 billion, which includes smoking-related health expenditures and lost productivity at work.[48] Sustained efforts to reduce cigarette smoking in the United States over the last several decades have resulted in demonstrable change; for example, approximately 20.8% of US adults reported regularly smoking cigarettes in 2006, down from 24.7% in 1997.[49] The downward trend in US adult smoking has been slow and steady, and it is currently estimated that roughly 14% of the US population smokes either every day or some days.[50] The magnitude of this overall change is impressive, especially in light of the physiologically addictive nature of cigarette smoking. It is well known that medication therapies exist to assist with attempts to quit smoking, and combining behavioral interventions, such as counseling or support groups, can facilitate this positive change.[51] The illustrated case "Change Talk" attempts to highlight the importance of combining such interventions with direct medication support via an entrepreneurial pharmacist with expertise in both.

While nicotine is the addictive component in cigarettes and other products, the negative effects of smoking are due to the tobacco and other additives in these highly engineered products. The negative effects impact nearly the entire body and have been shown to cause numerous health issues, including cardiovascular diseases (e.g., hypertension), respiratory diseases (e.g., chronic obstructive pulmonary disease, or COPD), and many forms of cancer.[49] Readers interested in learning more about the role of pharmacists in the interprofessional care of patients with hypertension, COPD, and cancer are encouraged to read the illustrated cases "Underlying Cause" in Chapter 5 Cardiology, "Breathe" in Chapter 2 Community Pharmacy, and "Compromising" and "Compassion" in Chapter 9 Oncology, respectively.

When all nicotine-containing products (NCPs) are taken into account, including combustible (e.g., cigarettes), noncombustible (e.g., dips, chews), and electronic products (e.g., vaping devices), the number of US adults exposed to related health risks jumps from the 14% reported above to 19.3%, or roughly 47.4 million adults.[50] Among those, nearly 20% (9 million) regularly used two or more NCPs.[50] This trend has alarmed health professionals, who worry that the positive public health progress made with reduced cigarette smoking is now in jeopardy.[52] As it can take years for researchers to systematically study health behaviors, make sense of data acquired, and publish results, most of the supporting evidence shared in this essay does not account for electronic NCPs (i.e., vaping devices) or the recent surge in their use; the trend is simply too new. What is clear is that nicotine, the primary ingredient in both traditional and newer products, is highly addictive and that health professionals, like the pharmacist featured in the illustrated case "Change Talk," will continue to play an integral

role assisting patients in their attempts to quit NCPs regardless of whether they are smoked, chewed, or vaped.

It has been well documented that the prevalence of tobacco use varies in accordance with socioeconomic factors (e.g., race/ethnicity, age, education level). Rates of cigarette smoking, for example, are highest among non-Hispanic American Indians/Alaska Natives (24%) and lowest among non-Hispanic Asians (7.1%).[50] Smoking is more common among people ages 45 to 64 years (16.5%) and those living below the federal poverty level (21.4%). It is also more prevalent for those whose highest level of education is a high school diploma, especially individuals who completed the General Educational Development (GED) test (36.8%).[50] Thirty-six percent of patients with mental health conditions smoke cigarettes, the highest prevalence among patients with chronic medical conditions. This group is also responsible for approximately one-third of all cigarettes sold in the United States.

While public health efforts have helped reduce rates of cigarette smoking, vaping is on the rise. Vaping devices have a reservoir of flavored solution that contains nicotine in various concentrations. Powered by a battery, these devices vaporize the solution, creating a mist that can be inhaled (i.e., vaped). Researchers categorize individuals as frequent users if they vape more than 20 days per month. Interestingly, the prevalence of high school students categorized as frequent vapers increased from 20% in 2017 to 27.7% in 2018.[53] Another study found that rates of teenagers who reported vaping in the past month had more than doubled in a 2-year period.[54] Among eighth graders, the numbers nearly tripled between 2017 and 2019.[54] The biggest concern is that adolescents believe vaping is mostly harmless.[55] The CDC and others are encouraging increased restrictions on vaping products based on investigations of illnesses associated with vaping.[56,57] Furthermore, data have shown that youth and young adults who had vaped in the past 30-day period were nearly twice as likely to have an intention to smoke conventional cigarettes compared with those who had never smoked or vaped before.[58] Readers interested in health issues associated with, and exacerbated by, vaping are encouraged to read the illustrated case "Swish" in Chapter 3 Primary Care.

Nicotine dependence is considered a chronic condition and often requires multiple attempts to quit long term.[51] Nicotine dependence is characterized by the difficulty to reduce or refrain from smoking or vaping for extended periods of time, continued use despite knowledge of harm, and, for most daily users, nicotine withdrawal symptoms when abruptly stopped or withheld. Withdrawal symptoms can vary by type and severity, and even from one person to another; typically, they include strong cravings, irritability, anxiety, difficulty concentrating, restlessness, hunger and sleep disturbances. They usually manifest within the first 1 to 2 days of cessation and gradually resolve over 2 to 4 weeks. Importantly, cravings can continue for months to years after quitting and may contribute to relapse episodes.[59,60]

Because nicotine use is a complex, addictive behavior, helping patients quit and preventing relapse are best achieved by combining appropriate medication therapy with behavioral counseling.[51] For any patient who uses NCPs, the primary goal is to achieve complete, long-term abstinence. The benefits of quitting smoking, for example, are substantial and although it is best to quit earlier in life, benefits can occur at any age.[61]

Nearly 7 in 10 US adult smokers report that they want to quit; therefore, it is important to have multiple access points to receive cessation services.[52] Pharmacists are in a unique position to provide these services because of their extensive medication expertise and, importantly, their status as one of the most accessible health professionals in the United States. Over 90% of US residents, for example, live within 5 miles of a pharmacy.[63] Importantly, pharmacists also receive education and training associated with facilitating behavioral changes to improve health.[23] Coupling medication expertise, know-how related to behavior change, and ease of accessibility makes pharmacists ideal health professionals to help patients tackle addiction to NCPs.

Cessation services focused on tobacco-containing products (e.g., cigarettes, chews) have been best studied. These services include individualized counseling, medication prescribing and management, and the ability to assist patients throughout their quit attempt. Pharmacists and other health professionals can engage in these services in multiple settings, including hospitals, emergency departments, primary care offices, and community pharmacies. Pharmacists have been shown to impact quit rates for patients equal to or better than usual care.[64] They make recommendations for medication therapy, provide behavioral counseling, and refer patients to established cessation programs and/or the national telephone quitline: 1-800-QUIT-NOW (1-800-784-8669).[51] The "5As" counseling process is promoted nationally:

1) Ask patients about tobacco use;
2) Advise all smokers to quit tobacco use;
3) Assess their readiness to quit tobacco;
4) Assist smokers in the quit process, including medication therapy and behavioral strategies; and
5) Arrange for follow-up to monitor their success and prevent relapse.[51]

Even brief advice is associated with increased odds of quitting. That said, more intensive approaches have been shown to result in increased quit rates; these typically include longer and more frequent counseling sessions and use of medication therapy.[51] Although time is often a barrier to any health professional offering tobacco cessation services, pharmacists who use the Ask-Advise-Refer (AAR) method to support patients have been successful at increasing referrals to quitlines and providing quitline materials to interested patients.[65,66] In addition, student pharmacists have been shown to help pharmacy staff deliver tobacco cessation interventions by increasing their utilization of the AAR method.[67]

Workplace wellness programs, like tobacco cessation programs, are often offered by employers to promote positive health habits. Illustration 4-7 depicts an entrepreneurial pharmacist from an independently owned pharmacy working with Bill Smith, the Chief Executive Officer (i.e., CEO) of a local company, to secure a contract for a tobacco cessation program. Such programs have been shown to improve employee health, productivity, and job satisfaction. Importantly, from the CEO's perspective, they have also been associated with reduced healthcare costs associated with heart disease and other smoking-related conditions.[68] Group counseling services can be provided on site and during work hours to make it easier for workers who lack the time or transportation options to access the service outside of their workplace. Sometimes incentives are offered which help to offset costs associated with acquiring medications that may be recommended to assist with individuals' quit attempts.[68,69] A review of workplace-based interventions for smoking cessation found that programs targeting group behavior therapy, use of individual counseling, medications to treat nicotine addiction, or a combination thereof, helped increase the likelihood of success.[70] Illustration 4-12 shows the CEO spearheading a celebration to reward employees who have remained smoke-free for 6 months. Based on this success, he has decided to expand this workplace wellness program to other worksites so more employees can reap the benefits.

First-line medication therapy options include both prescription and over-the-counter, or OTC, medications. Table 4-2 lists medications approved by the FDA for use in the United States. These medications can be used as monotherapy (i.e., alone) or in certain combinations. Examples of combination therapies include use of a nicotine patch plus a gum or lozenge product, or use of a nicotine patch plus bupropion SR. Specific combinations are tailored to fit individual characteristics for best quit results. National guidelines suggest that medications should be used with caution in certain patient populations either due to health conditions or lack of evidence; these patient populations include those who have serious heart disease, adolescents, smokeless tobacco users, light smokers, and pregnant or breast-feeding women.[51]

Group-based counseling is one approach to help people quit smoking. Participants meet regularly with a facilitator or coach trained in smoking cessation counseling. In Illustration 4-8, participants establish a group quit date and plan for regular meetings at their workplace. Participants not only have the benefit of the pharmacist's expertise, but also peer support and encouragement. Group-based programs have been shown to increase participants' chance of quitting by 50% to 130% compared to self-help programs. Interestingly, such programs have shown equal effectiveness to individual face-to-face counseling.[71]

If an individual is ready to quit in the next month, it is ideal to have them select a quit date that is within the next 2 weeks, allowing time to create a personal action plan. This involves identifying triggers and strategies for managing them,

Table 4-2. Categories and Examples of Medications Commonly Used to Help Patients Quit Nicotine-Containing Products

Category	Medication Examples[*]	Physiologic Effect
Nicotine replacement therapy	<ul><li>nicotine gum (Nicorette)[**]</li><li>nicotine inhaler (Nicotrol)</li><li>nicotine lozenge (Nicorette)[**]</li><li>nicotine nasal spray (Nicotrol NS)</li><li>nicotine patch (NicoDerm CQ)[**]</li></ul>	Replaces some nicotine to help reduce physical withdrawal symptoms associated with quitting, allowing the patient to focus on behavior changes
Antidepressant	<ul><li>bupropion SR (Zyban)</li></ul>	Inhibits dopamine reuptake, which attenuates nicotine withdrawal symptoms
Nicotinic receptor partial agonist	<ul><li>varenicline (Chantix)</li></ul>	Blocks nicotinic receptors in the brain, reducing the pleasurable sensations experienced with using nicotine-containing products

[*] Medication examples presented in alphabetical order as "generic name (Brand Name)."

[**] Available over the counter (i.e., without a prescription).

preparing the environment (i.e., removing tobacco products, ashtrays, etc.), and discussing their desire to quit with family and friends to build social support. Once a quit date is determined, medication options can be discussed. Bupropion SR and varenicline are prescription medications, and both need to be started 1 to 2 weeks prior to the established quit date to ensure they are tolerated and working by the time the individual stops smoking. Time to schedule a visit with a prescriber to obtain the prescription must be accounted for in the planning process.

Preferences for medication therapy should be identified, including previous experience with cessation medications and ability to adhere to the regimen. In Illustration 4-9, the featured participant, Janice, expresses concern about weight gain that may occur when she quits. Three medication options in Table 4-2 have been shown to delay weight gain; including the 4 mg nicotine products (gum and lozenge) and bupropion SR. Although e-cigarettes were initially considered as a possible alternative to approved tobacco cessation medications, the data remain insufficient to support their safety and efficacy in reducing or eliminating smoking and the nicotine concentrations can vary from device to device.[72]

Illustration 4-9 also demonstrates how the pharmacist identifies the participant's motivations for quitting. Reviewing participants' desire, ability, reasons, and/or need for quitting tobacco helps lay the foundation for behavior change.[73] Behavioral counseling, including motivational interviewing communication skills, can be provided in a variety of ways, including established appointment-based programs, group classes, internet-based programs, or referral to the aforementioned national quitline. Motivational interviewing is a client-centered counseling style that helps smokers explore and resolve ambivalence about making changes in their nicotine use behavior. The counselor evokes the individual's own motivations for change and how they would approach making changes, then assists in developing an individual quit plan.[73] During behavioral counseling, it is most helpful

to review cognitive and behavioral strategies (see Table 4-3) that patients can employ on their quit date to help refrain from smoking, manage stress and cravings, and remain a nonsmoker.

Illustration 4-10 draws attention to the complexities that may arise when one person in a partnership decides to quit while the other does not. Janice is shown speaking with her partner in preparation for her quit date. It is revealed that, working with the pharmacist, she has decided to incorporate medication and behavioral strategies to strengthen her chances of quitting. Janice mentions her desire to modify daily routines and avoid triggers she has identified that frequently lead her to reach for a cigarette. While not explicitly stated, the routine of morning coffee at the kitchen table is implied. Further, both Janice and her husband likely enjoy this routine; this time spent together before heading off to work. A necessary change Janice sees as a positive step in the right direction for her may be seen by her partner as problematic, something that may challenge their relationship.

In Illustration 4-11, Janice appears dejected, and the storm in the background captures her inner thoughts. The potential issue foreshadowed in Illustration 4-10 has come to fruition, and it appears Janice is struggling to engage her partner as a supportive element in her quit attempt. The valuable role of peer support is demonstrated, as well, and the group is shown brainstorming ways to help Janice convince her husband to stop smoking in the house and around her. Peer group support has been shown to benefit those with chronic conditions; it helps to improve self-efficacy (i.e., a person's belief in their own abilities) and medication adherence, as well as to sustain behavior change.[74] The celebration depicted in Illustration 4-12 indicates that support from her peers helped Janice weather the storm.

What is not shown between Illustrations 4-10, 4-11, and 4-12 are the different ways the pharmacist provided follow-up support both individually and within the group regarding

Table 4-3. Examples of Non-Medication Interventions for Nicotine Dependence

Intervention	Description	Examples
Cognitive	Focus on retraining how individuals think about nicotine use.	▪ Commitment to quit (e.g., "I am a nonsmoker") ▪ Distractive thinking to refocus on other things ▪ Positive self-talk (e.g., "I can do this!") ▪ Relaxation through imagery and positive thoughts ▪ Mental rehearsal and visualization
Behavioral	Applied based on specific triggers, routines, or situations individuals have associated with nicotine use. Avoiding triggers, finding alternatives, or using healthy substitutes is encouraged. Extrinsic motivators to reward progress may also be considered (e.g., monetary incentives, workplace rewards).	▪ Alleviate stress (e.g., deep breaths, step away from the situation) ▪ Avoid or minimize alcohol use during early phase of quit attempt ▪ Avoid situations where others are using NCPs* ▪ Use oral gratification (e.g., chew gum/toothpicks, drink water) ▪ Change automatic smoking routines ▪ Manage post-cessation weight gain (e.g., choose healthy snacks, walk) ▪ Manage cravings for nicotine (e.g., use mindfulness, use cessation medications)

*NCPs = nicotine-containing products.

medication use. Pharmacists regularly assess whether participants are experiencing medication side effects, and whether medication therapies are helping to manage withdrawal symptoms. Participants using nicotine replacement therapies should be slowly reducing the use and dose of these products in order to be completely free from nicotine within 3 or more months. When someone has quit smoking for at least 6 months, they are considered a former smoker. It is beneficial to seek opportunities to congratulate them on their success and also anticipate if there is any likelihood they would return to smoking. Relapse risk occurs most frequently within the first month of quitting; however, relapse can still occur even after a year of abstinence.[75] Participants' self-efficacy to remain quit is also a strong independent predictor of long-term cessation success.[76]

Health professionals continue their efforts to make nicotine product assessment and cessation services a routine component of all healthcare visits, whether in a community pharmacy, hospital room, dentist office, clinic, or workplace wellness program. Trained health professionals, including pharmacists, can have a meaningful impact on the individual and national burden that nicotine dependence causes. Behavior change is critical to prevention and wellness efforts. In the illustrated case "Change Talk," the power of combining medication expertise with knowledge of cognitive and behavioral interventions is revealed. Pharmacists throughout the United States apply this unique combination of knowledge and skills to not only reduce nicotine dependence, but also to advance other prevention- and wellness-focused initiatives such as nutritious eating and increased exercise to improve the health of patients with chronic conditions such as heart disease or diabetes.

DISCUSSION QUESTIONS FOR "CHANGE TALK"

1. In Illustration 4-9, Janice shares some of her motivations or reasons for wanting to quit smoking. Think of someone you know who may smoke or vape. Beyond the motivations Janice shared, what might be some additional reasons someone might want to quit smoking or vaping?

2. In conversation with her partner, Janice reveals that she is considering behavioral strategies for reducing her smoking triggers. Certain routines have been associated with triggers; for example, first thing in the morning, after meals, with coffee, while driving, and while talking on the phone. What advice and/or recommendations would you provide someone preparing for their quit date related to these triggers?

3. In Illustration 4-11, Janice's peer group is asked to brainstorm ways to help her talk to her husband about not smoking in the house. If you were part of this peer group, what suggestions would you have to help?

4. What barriers do you think exist for health professionals to provide smoking or vaping cessation services to patients? What are some differences that might exist between providing such services for individuals who use tobacco versus vaping products?

5. In "Change Talk," the pharmacist is shown providing tobacco cessation services in the workplace. What advantages can you think of to this approach versus a similar program delivered in a healthcare setting?

MOBILIZED: An Illustrated Case Study

Story by Mary S. Hayney & Joseph A. Zorek
Illustrations by George Folz, © 2019 Board of Regents of the University of Wisconsin System

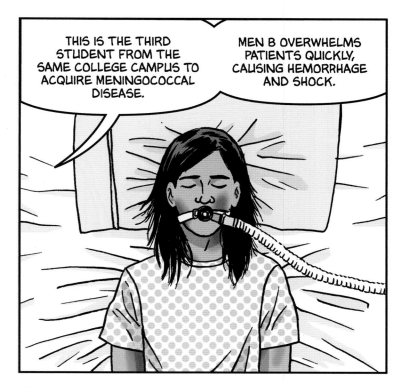

Illustration 4-13

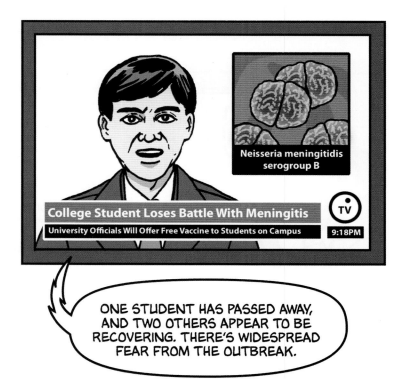

Illustration 4-14

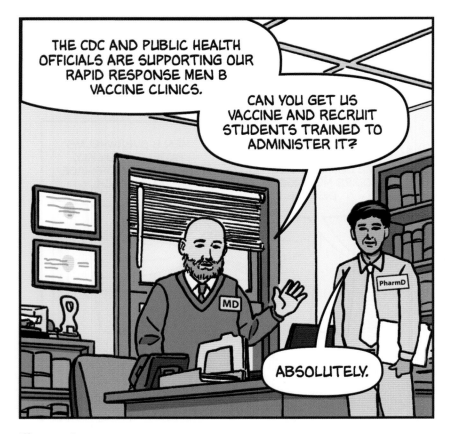

Illustration 4-15

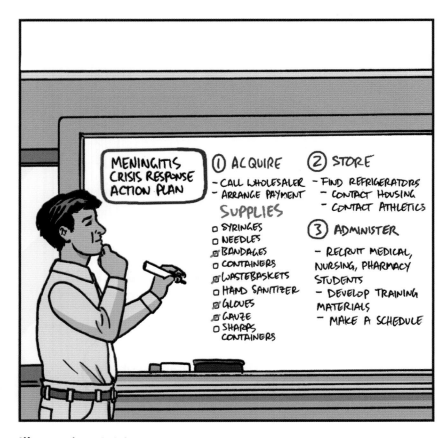

Illustration 4-16

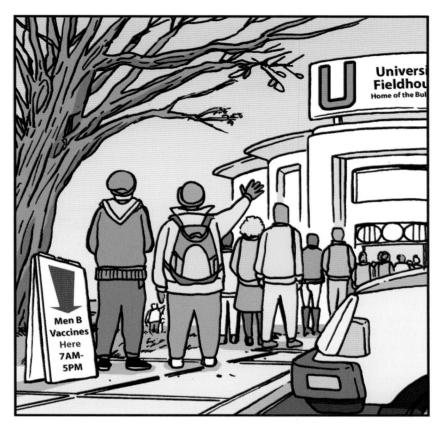

Illustration 4-17

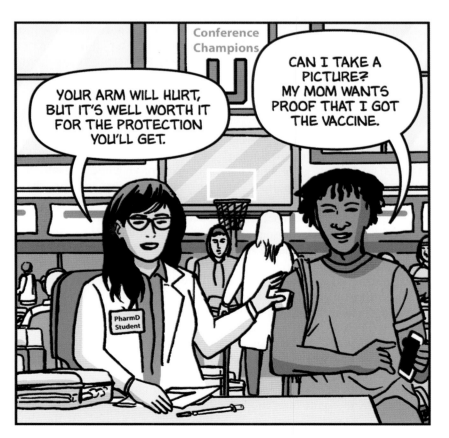

Illustration 4-18

Thoughts on "Mobilized"

Infectious diseases are the third leading cause of death in the United States and the second leading cause worldwide.[77,78] These diseases are caused by microorganisms, such as bacteria, fungi, or viruses, that bypass natural human defenses and cause harm, becoming pathogenic. The most dangerous pathogens, at least from a societal viewpoint, are ones that are able to spread easily from one person to another. When infections spread to more people in an area than is expected, the official term applied is *epidemic*, also often called an *outbreak*. Outbreaks that spread throughout the world are called *pandemics*. For a more in-depth discussion of microorganisms and infections, including the role of antibiotics to treat infections, readers are encouraged to explore the illustrated cases "Wounded" and "Superinfection" in Chapter 8 Infectious Diseases.

History is replete with scary examples of outbreaks that led to pandemics. Perhaps the best-known historical example is the bubonic plague, also called the Black Death, which occurred in the mid-1300s and killed up to half of the population of Europe between 1347 and 1353.[79] This was caused by the bacterial pathogen *Yersina pestis*, which was spread by rodents. The Spanish Flu of 1918, caused by an influenza virus of avian origin, provides a more recent example of a catastrophic pandemic.[80] It is estimated that 500 million people contracted the infection, about one-third of the world's population at that time, and that over 50 million people died. Even more recent is the human immunodeficiency virus (HIV) pandemic, which has infected 75 million people globally since it was first identified in 1981.[81] Thirty-eight million people have HIV currently. HIV attacks the immune system; however, unlike most viruses, the body is unable to mount an effective immune response and the infection lasts for life. HIV is transmitted through sexual activity, sharing needles for drug injection, or from mother to baby during pregnancy, birth, or breastfeeding.[82]

The first pandemic of the 21st century was caused by severe acute respiratory syndrome (SARS) coronavirus. Beginning with an outbreak in China in 2003, SARS spread to 29 countries worldwide with 8000 cases and 775 deaths reported.[83] In 2009, a novel influenza virus (subtype H1N1) caused an outbreak that turned into a pandemic. Interestingly, in contrast to seasonal influenza infections which mainly cause hospitalizations and death in the elderly, the 2009 H1N1 influenza virus was more dangerous for those ages 24 years and younger.[84] The Zika virus provides another example. Zika caused sporadic outbreaks since its discovery in 1947. An outbreak that began in Brazil in 2015 was associated with cases of Guillain-Barré, a paralytic syndrome followed by recovery that can happen within weeks, but may also last several years.[85] It was observed during the latest Zika outbreak that infection during pregnancy is associated with microcephaly (i.e., head circumference smaller than normal) and other abnormalities present at birth. The Zika virus is transmitted by mosquito bites and has spread to 86 countries.

Compared to SARS and Zika, the Ebola virus outbreak in West Africa in 2014, and then in the Democratic Republic of the Congo, while contained geographically to a single region of the world, was much more devastating, with nearly 30,000 cases.[86] Ebola virus infection is transmitted from an animal, often a bat, porcupine, or nonhuman primate, and is fatal about 50% of the time. The virus is transmitted from person to person through contact with blood or body fluids. An Ebola virus vaccine is now licensed, and it is expected to be used to immunize individuals who were in contact with Ebola-infected individuals to prevent its spread.[87]

In late 2019, an outbreak of severe acute respiratory syndrome coronavirus 2 (SARS-CoV-2) was observed in China, which caused an illness that came to be known as coronavirus disease (COVID-19). By early 2020, in response to mounting cases in other countries, the World Health Organization declared COVID-19 a global pandemic.[88] Efforts to control the spread of this virus caused widespread social disruption, including business and school closures, travel restrictions, and self-quarantine.[89,90] Social distancing to avoid contact with potentially infected individuals and the donning of face masks became the norm for months on end; those who could work from home did, and schools around the world shifted to online and/or asynchronous instruction. The economic impact in the United States and globally was substantial. Unemployment rates hit near-historic levels as only businesses deemed essential were allowed to maintain operations.[91] At the time of the writing of this book, the COVID-19 pandemic was active, with nearly 28 million cases and 900,000 deaths documented worldwide.[92] With no end currently in sight, an all-out effort to control the pandemic is underway, and scientists from around the world are racing to develop vaccines capable of inducing an immune response to this novel and menacing virus.[93]

Many infectious microorganisms persist in human populations even after outbreaks and pandemics come under control. When this occurs, the official term applied is *endemic*. Examples of endemic diseases in the United States include pertussis, influenza, and varicella. Many readers will recognize these names from childhood visits to physician offices or pharmacies, as they are kept under control through the widespread use of targeted vaccines (see Table 4-4). Even though new measles outbreaks have occurred over the past few years, measles has not been endemic in the United States since 2000. These new outbreaks were initiated by someone who traveled abroad, returned with the infection, then exposed others who were unimmunized, incompletely immunized, or too young to be immunized. Fortunately, immunization rates were sufficiently high so as to prevent widespread transmission and persistance.[94]

An English physician named Edward Jenner is considered the father of modern vaccinology based on his work developing the smallpox vaccine.[95] At the time, little was known about the immune system. In fact, this took place long before Louis Pasteur's experiments solidified the germ theory of disease. Since the time of Jenner's and Pasteur's discoveries, scientists and health professionals have been in constant pursuit of vaccines to prevent the debilitating and deadly effects of infectious diseases. Vaccines work with an individual's immune system to prevent infection, essentially by educating the immune system to be able to recognize an infectious microorganism and attack it upon future exposure.

Receiving a vaccine is called vaccination. Once the body mounts the desired immune response, the person is considered immunized. Immunization is a routine and critical intervention for both children and adults. Thanks to vaccines, diseases like rubella, tetanus, and diphtheria are almost unheard of nowadays. Smallpox has been eradicated, and polio is on the verge of global eradication, as well.[96] Before being licensed by the US Food and Drug Administration (FDA), vaccines are tested in thousands of individuals for their ability to protect against the target infection and for safety. Actually, both effectiveness and safety continue to be monitored after a vaccine is licensed and used in the general population.[97] Table 4-4 lists common vaccines and a description of the infectious disease each is intended to prevent. For detailed information on vaccine schedules (i.e., recommended ages for administration), readers are encouraged to consult the CDC website.[98]

Vaccines have had an incredibly positive impact on human societies worldwide. It is estimated that 6 million lives are saved each year because of vaccines.[99] In low-income countries, infectious diseases cause a disproportionate death rate. Immunizations can economically decrease this inequity. In the United States, the annual number of paralytic polio cases prior to vaccine licensure peaked at 58,000; in 2000, it was zero. An estimated 580 annual cases of tetanus, with muscle spasms and contractions strong enough to break the spines of those infected, occurred in the 1900s; in 2016, just 33.[100]

A growing skepticism in the United States around the value of vaccines has been described in recent years. Many scientists and health professionals attribute this to the success of vaccines and vaccination programs;[101] along the lines of the old adage "out of sight, out of mind." What is not well understood within the public, though, is that decreasing participation in vaccine programs, even in what some might describe as small numbers, can create a pathway for outbreaks. This pathway is through the loss of *herd immunity*, a term used to describe the limited ability of an infection to spread throughout a population when a high percentage of individuals are immune, either from past infection or via immunization. Some people within a group cannot be immunized because of underlying medical conditions or allergies, making herd immunity incredibly important for them. In this way, high immunization rates protect all members of a community. If immunization rates slip below a critical threshold, an outbreak can occur.[102]

Vaccine skepticism and hesitancy have posed a risk to herd immunity in recent years, and both increased following the publication of a scientific paper in 1998 in a reputable journal linking the measles, mumps, and rubella (MMR) vaccine with autism. Retracted (i.e., withdrawn and disavowed by the publisher) in 2010, this paper is often cited within the modern "Anti-Vaxxer Movement."[103] Individuals within this movement have taken a true anti-vaccine stance; they are against vaccines and believe that vaccines are neither necessary nor safe. Vaccine-hesitant individuals, on the other hand, are skeptical of vaccines but have not taken a true anti-vaccine stance.[104] Those who are vaccine-hesitant often seek additional information and education, and the accessibility of pharmacists makes them ideal resources to provide this information.[105] A number of strategies have been developed to do so; one such strategy called CASE is highlighted here.[106] CASE is a communication strategy that includes four parts:

1) Corroborate: The pharmacist acknowledges the individual's concerns about the vaccine, attempting to connect with the individual in a way that will allow the conversation to be successful

2) About me: The pharmacist tells the individual about how she/he came to possess expert knowledge of vaccines and recent vaccine developments

3) Science: The pharmacist talks about the risks and benefits of vaccines, attempting to directly address the individual's concerns

4) Explain/advise: The pharmacist ends with a strong recommendation for the vaccine emphasizing their shared desire to have the best health outcome

The involvement of pharmacists in immunization on a widespread and routine basis began in the mid-1990s.[107] Their unique access to the public offers the opportunity to improve immunization rates in populations. Approximately one-third of influenza vaccines administered to US adults are done in a pharmacy.[108] Pharmacy schools offer specific education to prepare their graduates to provide this important public health service to their patients.

The illustrated case "Mobilized" focuses on a pharmacist's role in an outbreak of invasive meningococcal disease (MenB), which is rare but very serious.[109] Sporadic cases of MenB are much more common compared to outbreaks, such as the one depicted in this illustrated case. MenB is caused by *Neisseria meningitidis* serogroup B, a bacteria that can colonize the nose and throat of healthy individuals. However, sometimes it causes infection of the blood (i.e., sepsis) or the protective covering of the brain and spinal cord called the meninges (i.e., meningitis).[110,111] The infection quickly causes fever, rash, low blood pressure, bleeding, and organ failure, which can be fatal in about 10% to 15% of cases. The college student shown in Illustration 4-13, with bruising throughout her body and requiring mechanical ventilation to breathe, has been infected

Table 4-4. Commonly Used Vaccines and the Infectious Diseases They Prevent

Vaccine	Causative Microorganism and Description of Disease
Bacterial targets	
Diphtheria	Toxin produced during infection with *Corynebacterium diphtheriae* bacteria results in coating and blocking the airway; can also affect the heart.
Haemophilus influenzae type b	Infection with *Haemophilus influenzae* bacteria that causes a range of manifestations from colonization of the nose and throat to meningitis[*]; most common in infants.
Neisseria meningitidis	Infection with a type of *Neisseria meningitidis* called serogroup A, B, C, W, or Y that causes a range of manifestations from colonization of the nose and throat to meningitis[*].
Pertussis	Commonly referred to as whooping cough. The bacteria *Bordetella pertussis* causes serious coughing spells; most dangerous for infants who may require hospitalization or die from infection.
Pneumococcal disease	Infection caused by the bacteria *Streptococcus pneumoniae* causes pneumonia[*], sepsis[*], or meningitis[*].
Tetanus	Toxin produced during infection with *Clostridium tetani* bacteria results in spasms and contractions in all muscles; infected individuals may not be able to open mouth (lockjaw) or breathe.
Viral targets	
Hepatitis A	Infection of the liver caused by the hepatitis A virus, typically transmitted through fecal-oral route and more serious in adults; causes muscle aches, fever, loss of appetite, and yellowing of the skin (i.e., jaundice).
Hepatitis B	Infection of the liver caused by the hepatitis B virus, typically transmitted through blood and body fluids; causes muscle aches, fever, loss of appetite and jaundice, and can lead to chronic infection and irreversible liver damage (i.e., cirrhosis).
Herpes zoster	Reactivation of varicella zoster virus, which is the virus that causes chickenpox and is commonly called shingles[*]; risk of reactivation increases with age or if an individual's immune system is compromised.
Human papillomavirus	Human papillomavirus (HPV) leads to warts on the skin and mucous membranes at the site of infection; most HPV infections are asymptomatic, but some can cause cervical, anogenital, or oropharyngeal cancer.
Influenza	Respiratory illness caused by different strains of influenza A virus and/or influenza B virus that leads to abrupt onset of fever, chills, muscles aches, sore throat, dry cough, and fatigue; can cause severe illness requiring hospitalization, most commonly in older adults.
Measles	Highly contagious illness caused by the measles virus that leads to rash, fever, and watery eyes; complications include diarrhea, pneumonia,[*] seizures, brain damage, or death.
Mumps	Illness caused by the paramyxovirus that leads to swelling of parotid glands; may cause meningitis[*], encephalitis[*], or hearing loss.
Polio	Illness caused by poliovirus that is transmitted fecal-orally and can lead to meningitis[*]; may cause paralysis in its serious form.
Rotavirus	Illness caused by rotavirus that causes fever, vomiting, abdominal pain, and watery diarrhea; may lead to severe dehydration requiring hospitalization, particularly dangerous in infants.
Rubella	Illness caused by the rubella virus that causes rash and fever; can cause blindness, deafness, brain abnormalities, or heart defects in a fetus if the mother is infected.
Varicella	Illness also referred to as chickenpox caused by the varicella-zoster virus that leads to itchy rash and fever; complications may include bacterial infection on top of rash, pneumonia[*], encephalitis[*], or death.

[*] Types of infection defined by their location in the body, presented in alphabetical order as "name of infection (location in body)": encephalitis (brain), hepatitis (liver), meningitis (meninges, i.e., lining of brain and spinal cord); pneumonia (lungs), sepsis (blood), shingles (nerves).

with MenB. Unfortunately, Illustration 4-14 reveals that she did not survive this infection.

Illustration 4-14 shows a local news anchor educating the public about MenB and not only one, but three cases. He also reports about the widespread fear that often accompanies outbreaks such as these. The two survivors reported are not described in detail; however, survivors of MenB may experience hearing loss, brain or kidney damage, or loss of a limb. Infants, adolescents, young adults, and people with compromised immune systems are much more likely to develop MenB compared to otherwise healthy individuals.

Invasive meningococcal disease can be prevented with immunization. Two different types of vaccines are currently available. The quadrivalent meningococcal conjugate vaccine (MenACWY) is routinely recommended as a two-dose series for all adolescents; dose one at age 11 to 12 years, and dose two administered at age 16 years. Two meningococcal serogroup B (MenB) vaccines have recently been licensed and may be used in adolescents aged 16 to 18 years.[110,111] These require either two or three doses based on the product and situation. The appropriate MenB vaccine may also be used in the event of a meningococcal outbreak as described in "Mobilized."[112,113] In consultation with public health experts, Illustration 4-15 shows the medical director of the student health department and a pharmacist at this university working together in an excellent example of interprofessional practice to offer MenB vaccine to their students in an effort to end the outbreak on campus (Illustrations 4-16 and 4-17). Readers are encouraged to explore the illustrated case "Organized Chaos" in Chapter 2 Community Pharmacy for an example of how community pharmacists work such vaccines into their daily workflow.

Emergency preparedness and response is the process by which government agencies, businesses, organizations, and individuals prepare for large-scale emergencies that threaten the health or safety of a population.[83] Preparation involves a continuous cycle of planning, practicing, and evaluating emergency plans. These plans involve many interprofessional partnerships, including among public health officials and a variety of different health professionals (e.g., physicians, nurses, pharmacists). Law enforcement, communications professionals, and lay volunteers may also be involved. Lay volunteers contribute in a variety of ways, such as setting up rooms, delivering and moving supplies, and managing schedules. Communications professionals take responsibility for disseminating information about the situation, including the status of the emergency and where the public can go for help. Law enforcement officials typically take responsibility for security and, depending on the nature of the event, may need to investigate a crime. Importantly, as depicted in "Mobilized" (Illustration 4-18), students in various health professions programs who have completed the requisite training can also contribute to the effort.

Vaccines have become an indispensable tool to advance public health. They have reduced the burden of disease across communities and have provided vital protection against once-devastating infectious diseases like smallpox and polio. Vaccines have prevented more deaths than any other modern medical innovation.[114] Importantly, vaccines have also increased life expectancy for entire populations.[99] For maximal impact, vaccine programs require public trust and participation. Unfortunately, some of this has eroded in recent decades, as evidenced by the rise of anti-vaccination movements. Health professionals, like the pharmacist and physician featured in "Mobilized," will have to educate not only their students, but also the population at large, if tragic scenarios like the one depicted in this illustrated case are to be prevented.

DISCUSSION QUESTIONS FOR "MOBILIZED"

1. In the past two decades, multiple types of coronavirus have caused severe respiratory diseases. Zika virus also spread to several countries. What social factors do you think contribute to the spread of these diseases?

2. What are some of the factors you think may have contributed to the meningococcal serogroup B (i.e., MenB) outbreak shown in this illustrated case?

3. From your perspective, why do you think some people have come to question the necessity and safety of vaccines?

4. The American Pharmacists Association has coined the term "immunization neighborhood." What do you think this means? And who might belong to this neighborhood?

5. Consider the effort and financial investment necessary for emergency preparedness and responses, such as the one depicted in this case. Some argue that greater investment in prevention efforts, such as research, development, and distribution of more vaccines, might be a better approach. What do you think about this?

CHAPTER SUMMARY

- Considering their physical location in the community and high degree of clinical training, pharmacists are uniquely positioned to promote prevention and wellness initiatives.

- Pharmacists serve as educators for other health professionals, patients, and community members, and they provide services such as health screenings and immunizations, as well as lifestyle modifications linked to diet and the use of alcohol, tobacco, and other substances.

- Well-known prevention and wellness activities of pharmacists include diabetes screenings, tobacco cessation services, and vaccination programs, all highlighted by the illustrated cases "Screen," "Change Talk," and "Mobilized" in this chapter.

- Medications to treat diabetes are complex, and pharmacists play a critical role in preventing disease progression and the development of health complications by collaborating with other members of the interprofessional team, and helping patients obtain medications and maximize the impact of medication therapy.

- Pharmacists provide guidance and advice on how to monitor glucose levels, treat hypoglycemia, eat balanced meals, and incorporate physical activity into routines to advance prevention and wellness for patients with diabetes, and they do this for patients with a host of other chronic conditions, as well, such as high blood pressure, high cholesterol, and depression.

- The negative effects of tobacco use and smoking impact nearly the entire body and have been shown to cause numerous health issues, including cardiovascular diseases, respiratory diseases, and many forms of cancer.

■ Pharmacists and other health professionals can help patients quit nicotine-containing products and prevent relapse by combining appropriate medication therapy with behavioral counseling.

■ Vaccines have become an indispensable tool to advance public health, reducing the burden of disease and preventing more deaths than any other modern medical innovation.

■ Pharmacists have improved immunization rates due to their accessibility to the public; for example, approximately one-third of influenza vaccines administered to US adults are done in a pharmacy.

■ All pharmacists receive education and training to contribute to prevention and wellness initiatives throughout healthcare, regardless of practice setting.

REFERENCES

1. Committee for the Study of the Future of Public Health. *The Future of Public Health*. Washington, DC: National Academies Press; 1998:1.

2. American Public Health Association. The role of the pharmacist in public health. Available at https://www.apha.org/policies-and-advocacy/public-health-policy-statements/policy-database/2014/07/07/13/05/the-role-of-the-pharmacist-in-public-health. Accessed May 31, 2020.

3. Ali A, Katz DL. Disease prevention and health promotion: how integrative medicine fits. *Am J Prev Med.* 2015;49 (5 suppl 3):S230-S240.

4. Centers for Disease Control and Prevention. Prevention. Available at https://www.cdc.gov/pictureofamerica/pdfs/picture_of_america_prevention.pdf. Accessed February 17, 2020.

5. Sorensen T. Wellness services in community pharmacies—what will drive success? Available at https://www.pharmacytimes.com/publications/directions-in-pharmacy/2015/october2015/wellness-services-in-community-pharmacieswhat-will-drive-success. Accessed February 18, 2020.

6. World Health Organization. What is quality of care and why is it important? Available at https://www.who.int/maternal_child_adolescent/topics/quality-of-care/definition/en/. Accessed March 7, 2020.

7. American Pharmacists Association. Patient care. Available at https://www.pharmacist.com/resources/patient-care?is_sso_called=1. Accessed February 18, 2020.

8. Delcher C, Wagenaar AC, Goldberger BA, Cook RL, Maldonado-Molina MM. Abrupt decline in oxycodone-caused mortality after implementation of Florida's Prescription Drug Monitoring Program. *Drug Alcohol Depend.* 2015;150:63-68.

9. Woodard LJ, Kahaleh AA, Nash JD, Truong H, Goginenie H, Barbosa-Leikertf C. Healthy People 2020: assessment of pharmacists' priorities. *Public Health.* 2018;155:69-80.

10. U.S. Food and Drug Administration. Drug disposal: drug take back locations. Available at https://www.fda.gov/drugs/disposal-unused-medicines-what-you-should-know/drug-disposal-drug-take-back-locations. Accessed February 18, 2020.

11. Melin K, Conte N. Community pharmacists as first responders in Puerto Rico after hurricane Maria. *J Am Pharm Assoc.* 2018;58(2):149.

12. American Pharmacists Association. Executive summary: pharmacists as front-line responders for COVID-19 patient care. Available at https://www.pharmacist.com/sites/default/files/files/APHA%20Meeting%20Update/PHARMACISTS_COVID19-Final-3-20-20.pdf. Accessed March 28, 2020.

13. Landesman LY. *Public Health Management and Disasters: The Practice Guide.* 3rd ed. Washington, DC: American Public Health Association; 2012.

14. Lenox ER, Tyler LS. Managing drug shortages: seven years' experience at one health system. *Am J Health Syst Pharm.* 2003;60:245-253.

15. Clark SL, Levasseur-Franklin K, Pajoumand M, et al. Collaborative management strategies for drug shortages in neurocritical care. *Neurocrit Care.* 2020;32(1):226-237.

16. Bergen G, Stevens MR, Burns ER. Falls and fall injuries among adults aged ≥65 years—United States, 2014. *MMWR Morb Mortal Wkly Rep.* 2016;65:993-998

17. Stevens JA, Phelan EA. Development of STEADI: a fall prevention resource for health care providers. *Health Promot Pract.* 2013;14(5):706-714.

18. 2019 American Geriatrics Society Beers Criteria Update Expert Panel. American Geriatrics Society 2019 updated AGS Beers Criteria for Potentially Inappropriate Medication Use in older adults. *J Am Geriatr Soc.* 2019;67(4):674-694.

19. Mott DA, Martin B, Breslow R, Michaels B, Kirchner J, Mahoney J, et al. Impact of a medication therapy management intervention targeting medications associated with falling: results of a pilot study. *J Am Pharm Assoc.* 2016;56(1):22-28.

20. John EJ, Vavra T, Farris K, et al. Workplace-based cardiovascular risk management by community pharmacists: impact on blood pressure, lipid levels, and weight. *Pharmacotherapy.* 2006;26(10):1511-1517.

21. Bonner L. Drug Take Back Day: help patients properly dispose of medication. Available at https://www.pharmacytoday.org/article/S1042-0991(19)31150-8/fulltext. Accessed March 7, 2020.

22. Drug Enforcement Administration. Take Back Day. Available at https://takebackday.dea.gov/. Accessed March 7, 2020.

23. Accreditation Council for Pharmacy Education. Available at https://www.acpe-accredit.org/about/. Accessed January 11, 2020.

24. American Diabetes Association. Diabetes. Available at https://www.diabetes.org/diabetes. Accessed May 31, 2020.

25. American Diabetes Association. Classification and diagnosis of diabetes: standards of medical care in diabetes—2019. *Diabetes Care.* 2019;42(suppl 1):S13-S28.

26. American Diabetes Association. Diabetes risk. Available at https://www.diabetes.org/diabetes-risk. Accessed May 31, 2020.

27. Centers for Disease Control and Prevention. *National Diabetes Statistics Report, 2017.* Atlanta, GA: Centers for Disease Control and Prevention, US Department of Health and Human Services; 2017.

28. American Diabetes Association. Improving care and promoting health in populations: standards of medical care in diabetes—2019. *Diabetes Care.* 2019;42(suppl 1):S7-S12.

29. Beck J, Greenwood DA, Blanton L, et al. National standards for diabetes self-management education and support. *Diabetes Educ.* 2017;43(5):449-464.

30. American Diabetes Association. Lifestyle management: standards of medical care in diabetes—2019. *Diabetes Care.* 2019;42(suppl 1):S46-S60.

31. Smith M. Pharmacists' role in improving diabetes medication management. *J Diabetes Sci Technol.* 2009;3:175-179.

32. Ragucci KR, Fermo JD, Wessell AM, Chumney EC. Effectiveness of pharmacist-administered diabetes mellitus education and management services. *Pharmacotherapy.* 2005;25:1809-1816.

33. Kiel PJ, McCord AD. Pharmacist impact on clinical outcomes in a diabetes disease management program via collaborative practice. *Ann Pharmacother.* 2005;39:1828-1832.

34. McCord AD. Clinical impact of a pharmacist-managed diabetes mellitus drug therapy management service. *Pharmacotherapy.* 2006;26:248-253.

35. Lopez R. Neighborhood risk factors for obesity. *Obesity.* 2007;15:2111-2119.

36. Black J, Macinko J. Neighborhoods and obesity. *Nutr Rev.* 2008;66:2-20.

37. Morland K, Wing S, Diez Roux A, et al. Neighborhood characteristics associated with the location of food stores and food service places. *Am J Prev Med.* 2002;22(1):23-29.

38. Fera T, Bluml BM, Ellis WM, et al. The Diabetes Ten City Challenge: interim clinical and humanistic outcomes of a multisite community pharmacy diabetes care program. *J Am Pharm Assoc.* 2008;48:181-190.

39. Cranor CW, Christensen DB. The Asheville Project: factors associated with outcomes of a community pharmacy diabetes care program. *J Am Pharm Assoc.* 2003;43:160-172.

40. American Diabetes Association. Pharmacologic approaches to glycemic treatment: standards of medical care in diabetes—2019. *Diabetes Care.* 2019;42(suppl 1):S90-S102.

41. Diabetes Prevention Program Research Group. Long-term safety, tolerability, and weight loss associated with metformin in the Diabetes Prevention Program Outcomes Study. *Diabetes Care.* 2012;35:731-737.

42. Church TS, Blair SN, Cocreham S, et al. Effects of aerobic and resistance training on hemoglobin A1c levels in patients with type 2 diabetes: a randomized controlled trial. *JAMA.* 2010;304:2253-2262.

43. Balk EM, Earley A, Raman G, Avendano EA, Pittas AG, Remington PL. Combined diet and physical activity promotion programs to prevent type 2 diabetes among persons at increased risk: a systematic review for the community preventive services task force. *Ann Intern Med.* 2015;163:437-451.

44. Rejeski WJ, Ip EH, Bertoni AG, et al. Lifestyle change and mobility in obese adults with type 2 diabetes. *N Engl J Med.* 2012;366:1209-1217.

45. American Diabetes Association. Obesity management for the treatment of type 2 diabetes: standards of medical care in diabetes—2019. *Diabetes Care.* 2019;42(suppl 1):S81-S89.

46. Savage JS, Orlet Fisher J, Birch LL. Parental influence on eating behavior. *J Law Med Ethics.* 2007;35(1):22-34.

47. Barr-Anderson DJ, Adams-Wynn AW, DiSantis KI, Kumanyika S. Family-focused physical activity, diet and obesity interventions in African-American girls: a systematic review. *Obes Rev.* 2013;14(1):29-51.

48. GBD 2015 Tobacco Collaborators. Smoking prevalence and attributable disease burden in 195 countries and territories, 1990–2015: a systematic analysis from the Global Burden of Disease Study 2015. *Lancet.* 2017;389:1885-1906.

49. U.S. Department of Health and Human Services. The health consequences of smoking—50 years of progress: a report of the surgeon general. Atlanta, GA: U.S. Department of Health and Human Services, Centers for Disease Control and Prevention; 2014.

50. Wang TW, Asman K, Gentzke AS, et al. Tobacco product use among adults—United States, 2017. *MMWR Morb Mortal Wkly Rep.* 2018;67:1225-1232.

51. Fiore MC, Jaen CR, Baker TB, et al. *Treating Tobacco Use and Dependence: Quick Reference Guide of Clinicians—2008 Update.* Rockville, MD: U.S. Department of Health and Human Services, Public Health Service; 2009.

52. Newman, K. Vaping and e-cigarettes: the new public health problem. *U.S. News & World Report.* Available at https://www.usnews.com/news/healthiest-communities/articles/2019-09-30/vaping-and-e-cigarettes-a-new-public-health-problem. Accessed February 2, 2020.

53. Gentzke AS, Creamer M, Cullen KA, et al. Vital signs: tobacco product use among middle and high school students—United States, 2011–2018. *MMWR Morb Mortal Wkly Rep.* 2019;68:157-164.

54. National Institute on Drug Abuse. Monitoring the future 2019 survey results: vaping. Available at https://www.drugabuse.gov/related-topics/trends-statistics/infographics/monitoring-future-2019-survey-results-vaping. Accessed February 2, 2020.

55. Miech R, Johnston L, O'Malley PM, Bachman JG, Patrick ME. Trends in adolescent vaping 2017–2019. *N Engl J Med.* 2019;381:1490-1491.

56. U.S. Food and Drug Administration. Trump administration combating epidemic of youth e-cigarette use with plan to clear market of unauthorized, non-tobacco-flavored e-cigarette products. Available at https://www.fda.gov/news-events/press-announcements/trump-administration-combating-epidemic-youth-e-cigarette-use-plan-clear-market-unauthorized-non. Accessed May 31, 2020.

57. Raven K. Teen vaping linked to more health risks. Available at https://www.yalemedicine.org/stories/teen-vaping/. Accessed May 31, 2020.

58. US Department of Health and Human Services. E-cigarette use among youth and young adults. a report of the surgeon general. Atlanta, GA: U.S. Department of Health and Human Services, CDC; 2016. Available at https://www.cdc.gov/tobacco/data_statistics/sgr/e-cigarettes/pdfs/2016_sgr_entire_report_508.pdf. Accessed May 31, 2020.

59. American Psychiatric Association. *Diagnostic and Statistical Manual of Mental Disorders.* 5th ed. Washington, DC: American Psychiatric Association; 2013.

60. Hughes JR. Effects of abstinence from tobacco: valid symptoms and time course. *Nicotine Tob Res.* 2007;9(3):315-327.

61. U.S. Department of Health and Human Services. How tobacco smoke causes disease: the biology and behavioral basis for smoking-attributable disease: a report of the surgeon general. Atlanta, GA: U.S. Department of Health and Human Services, Centers for Disease Control and Prevention, National Center for Chronic Disease Prevention and Health Promotion, Office on Smoking and Health; 2010.

62. Babb S, Malarcher A, Schauer G, Asman K, Jamal A. Quitting smoking among adults—United States, 2000–2015. *MMWR Morb Mortal Wkly Rep.* 2017:65(52):1457-1464.

63. National Association of Chain Drug Stores. Face-to-face with community pharmacies. Available at http://www.nacds.org/pdfs/about/rximpact-leavebehind.pdf. Accessed May 31, 2020.

64. Chen T, Kazerooni R, Vannort EM, et al. Comparison of an intensive pharmacist-managed telephone clinic with standard of care for tobacco cessation in a veteran population. *Health Promot Pract*. 2014;15(4):512-520.

65. Patwardhan PD, Chewning BA. Effectiveness of intervention to implement tobacco cessation counseling in community chain pharmacies. *J Am Pharm Assoc*. 2012;52(4):507-514.

66. Hudmon KS, Corelli RL, de Moore C, et al. Outcomes of a randomized trial evaluating two approaches for promoting pharmacy-based referrals to the tobacco quitline. *J Am Pharm Assoc*. 2018;58(4):387-394.

67. Wahl KR, Woolf BL, Hoch MA, et al. Promoting pharmacy-based referrals to the tobacco quitline: a pilot study of academic detailing administered by pharmacy students. *J Pharm Pract*. 2015;28(2):162-165.

68. Matson Koffman DM, Lanza A, Phillips Campbell K. A purchaser's guide to clinical preventive services: a tool to improve health care coverage for prevention. *Prev Chronic Dis*. 2008;5(2):A59.

69. Cahill K, Perera R. Quit and win contests for smoking cessation. *Cochrane Database Syst Rev*. 2008;4:CD004986.

70. Cahill K, Lancaster T. Workplace interventions for smoking cessation. *Cochrane Database Syst Rev*. 2014;2:CD003440.

71. Stead LF, Carroll AJ, Lancaster T. Group behaviour therapy programmes for smoking cessation. *Cochrane Database Syst Rev*. 2017;3:CD001007.

72. Cobb NK, Abrams DB. E-cigarette or drug-delivery device? Regulating novel nicotine products. *N Engl J Med*. 2011;365(3):193-195.

73. Miller W, Rollnick S. *Motivational Interviewing: Helping People Change*. 3rd ed. New York, NY: Guilford Press; 2013.

74. University of North Carolina Gillings School of Global Public Health. Peers for progress. Science behind peer support. Available at http://peersforprogress.org/learn-about-peer-support/science-behind-peer-support/. Accessed May 31, 2020.

75. Herd N, Borland R, Hyland A. Predictors of smoking relapse by duration of abstinence: findings from the International Tobacco Control (ITC) Four Country Survey. *Addiction*. 2009;104:2088-2099.

76. Gwaltney CJ, Metrik J, Kahler CW, et al. Self-efficacy and smoking cessation: a meta-analysis. *Psychol Addict Behav*. 2009;23:56-66.

77. Centers for Disease Control and Prevention. Leading causes of death. Available at https://www.cdc.gov/nchs/fastats/leading-causes-of-death.htm. Accessed February 21, 2020.

78. World Health Organization. The top 10 causes of death. Available at https://www.who.int/news-room/fact-sheets/detail/the-top-10-causes-of-death. Accessed February 21, 2020.

79. Spyrou Maria A, Tukhbatova Rezeda I, Feldman M, et al. Historical *Y. pestis* genomes reveal the European black death as the source of ancient and modern plague pandemics. *Cell Host Microbe*. 2016;19:874-881.

80. Centers for Disease Control and Prevention. 1918 Pandemic (H1N1 virus). Available at https://www.cdc.gov/flu/pandemic-resources/1918-pandemic-h1n1.html. Accessed February 21, 2020.

81. World Health Organization. Global Health Observatory (GHO) data. HIV/AIDS. Available at https://www.who.int/gho/hiv/en/. Accessed February 21, 2020.

82. Centers for Disease Control and Prevention. About HIV/AIDS. Available at https://www.cdc.gov/hiv/basics/whatishiv.html. Accessed February 21, 2020.

83. World Health Organization. Update 74. Global decline in cases and deaths continues. WHO emergency preparedness response—disease outbreak news. June 5, 2003. Available at https://www.who.int/csr/don/2003_06_05/en/. Accessed February 21, 2020.

84. Centers for Disease Control and Prevention. Use of influenza A (H1N1) 2009 monovalent vaccine. Recommendations of the Advisory Committee on Immunization Practices (ACIP), 2009. *MMWR Morb Mortal Wkly Rep*. 2009;58:1-8.

85. World Health Organization. Zika virus. Available at https://www.who.int/news-room/fact-sheets/detail/zika-virus. Accessed February 21, 2020.

86. World Health Organization. Ebola virus disease. Available at https://www.who.int/news-room/fact-sheets/detail/ebola-virus-disease. Accessed February 21, 2020.

87. Henao-Restrepo AM, Camacho A, Longini IM, et al. Efficacy and effectiveness of an rVSV-vectored vaccine in preventing Ebola virus disease: final results from the Guinea ring vaccination, open-label, cluster-randomised trial (Ebola). *Lancet*. 2017;389:505-518.

88. World Health Organization. WHO director-general's opening remarks at the media briefing on COVID-19, 11 March 2020. Available at https://www.who.int/dg/speeches/detail/who-director-general-s-opening-remarks-at-the-media-briefing-on-covid-19---11-march-2020

89. Brenan M. Most U.S. adults expect long-term COVID-19 disruption. Available at https://news.gallup.com/poll/304493/adults-expect-long-term-covid-disruption.aspx. Accessed March 28, 2020.

90. Griffiths J, Woodyatt A. 780 million people in China are living under travel restrictions due to the coronavirus outbreak. Available at https://edition.cnn.com/2020/02/16/asia/coronavirus-covid-19-death-toll-update-intl-hnk/index.html. Accessed February 21, 2020.

91. Schwartz ND, Casselman B, Koeze E. How bad is unemployment? "Literally off the charts." Available at https://www.nytimes.com/interactive/2020/05/08/business/economy/april-jobs-report.html. Accessed May 16, 2020.

92. Johns Hopkins University & Medicine. Coronavirus Resource Center. Available at https://www.coronavirus.jhu.edu/map.html. Accessed September 10, 2020.

93. Callaway E. The race for coronavirus vaccines: a graphical guide. *Nature*. 2020;580(7805):576-577.

94. Hecht H, Hayney MS. Understanding the role of vaccination exemption in the recent measles outbreaks. *J Am Pharm Assoc*. 2019;59:753-755.

95. Immunization Action Coalition. Vaccine timeline. Historic dates and events related to vaccination. Available at https://www.immunize.org/timeline/. Accessed February 21, 2020.

96. Kroger A, Duchin J, Vazquez M. General best practice guidelines for immunization. Best practices guidance of the Advisory Committee on Immunization Practices (ACIP). Available at www.cdc.gov/vaccines/hcp/acip-recs/general-recs/downloads/general-recspdf. Accessed February 21, 2020.

97. Centers for Disease Control and Prevention. In: Hamborsky J, Kroger A, Wolfe S, eds. *Epidemiology and Prevention of Vaccine-Preventable Diseases*. 13th ed. Washington, DC: Public Health Foundation; 2015.

98. Recommended immunization schedules for persons aged 0 through 18 years—United States, 2020. 2020. Available at

https://www.cdc.gov/vaccines/schedules/downloads/child/0-18yrs-child-combined-schedule.pdf. Accessed February 21, 2020.

99. Andre F, Booy R, Bock HL, et al. Vaccination greatly reduces disease, disability, death and inequity worldwide. *Bull World Health Organ.* 2008;86:140-146.

100. Centers for Disease Control and Prevention. Reported cases and deaths from vaccine-preventable diseases, United States. 2017. Available at https://www.cdc.gov/vaccines/pubs/pinkbook/downloads/appendices/e/reported-cases.pdf. Accessed February 21, 2020.

101. Chen RT, Shimabukuro TT, Martin DB, Zuber PLF, Weibel DM, Sturkenboom M. Enhancing vaccine safety capacity globally: a lifecycle perspective. *Am J Prev Med.* 2015;49:S364-S376.

102. Friedlander NJ, Hayney MS. The strength of the community: herd protection. *J Am Pharm Assoc.* 2019;59:905-907.

103. Shelby A, Ernst K. Story and science: how providers and parents can utilize storytelling to combat anti-vaccine misinformation. *Hum Vaccin Immunother.* 2013;9:1795-1801.

104. MacDonald NE. Vaccine hesitancy: definition, scope and determinants. *Vaccine.* 2015;33:4161-4164.

105. Sharpe AR, Hayney MS. Strategies for responding to vaccine hesitancy and vaccine deniers. *J Am Pharm Assoc.* 2019;59:291-292.

106. Singer A. Making the CASE for vaccines: a new model for talking to parents about vaccines. 2010. Available at http://www.vicnetwork.org/wp-content/uploads/VICNetworkWebinarSept-23SlidesFinal1.pdf. Accessed February 21, 2020.

107. Hogue M, Grabenstein JD, Foster SL, Rothholz M. Pharmacist involvement with immunizations: a decade of professional advancement. *J Am Pharm Assoc.* 2006;46:168-182.

108. Centers for Disease Control and Prevention. Flu vaccination coverage, United States, 2018–19 influenza season. Available at https://www.cdc.gov/flu/fluvaxview/coverage-1819estimates.htm. Accessed February 21, 2020.

109. Heidi MS, Lucy AM, Amy EB, et al. University-based outbreaks of meningococcal disease caused by serogroup B, United States, 2013–2018. *Emerg Infect Dis.* 2019;25:434.

110. Centers for Disease Control and Prevention. Prevention and control of meningococcal disease. *MMWR Morb Mortal Wkly Rep.* 2013;62:1-32.

111. Centers for Disease Control and Prevention. Use of serogroup B meningococcal vaccines in persons aged >10 years at increased risk for serogroup B meningococcal disease: recommendation of the Advisory Committee on Immunization Practices, 2015. *MMWR Morb Mortal Wkly Rep.* 2015;62:608-612.

112. Ritscher AM, Ranum N, Malak JD, et al. Meningococcal serogroup B outbreak response University of Wisconsin-Madison. *J Am Coll Health.* 2019;67:191-196.

113. Soeters HM, McNamara LA, Blain AE, et al. University-based outbreaks of meningococcal disease caused by serogroup B, United States, 2013–2018. *Emerg Infect Dis.* 2019;25:434-440.

114. The Jordan Report: Accelerated development of vaccines, 1996. Division of Microbiology and Infectious Disease, National Institute of Allergy and Infectious Disease, National Institutes of Health.

CHAPTER 5

Cardiology
Featuring the Illustrated Case Studies "Underlying Cause," "Educator," & "Empowerment"

Authors

Karen J. Kopacek, Andrea L. Porter, John M. Dopp, & Joseph A. Zorek

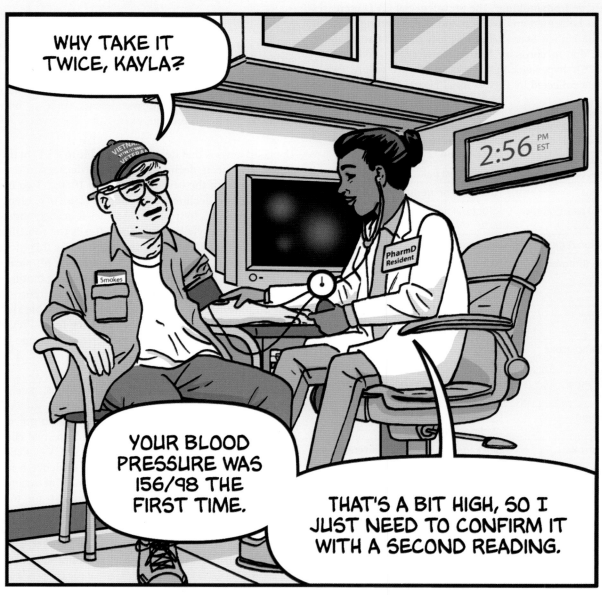

Illustration by George Folz, © 2019 Board of Regents of the University of Wisconsin System

BACKGROUND

Cardiology, a term derived from the Greek "cardia" (heart) and "logy" (study of), is a branch of medicine that specializes in the treatment of cardiovascular diseases (CVD).[1] Health conditions that involve the heart or circulatory system are categorized under CVD. Common examples of CVD include high blood pressure (i.e., hypertension), high cholesterol (i.e., dyslipidemia), and deep vein thrombosis. Heart disease, in contrast, refers to disorders of only the heart and is a subset of CVD. Common examples of heart disease are angina pectoris, arrhythmias, coronary heart disease, and heart failure. Table 5-1 includes a list of other CVDs and conditions related to the heart that readers may have heard of previously.[2,3]

Roughly 122 million Americans 20 years of age and older, or 48% of the adult population in the United States, had one or more form of CVD in 2016.[4] Furthermore, approximately 47% of all Americans have at least one of three key risk factors for developing CVD: elevated blood pressure, abnormal cholesterol levels, and/or smoking.[5] The prevalence of CVD increases with age in both men and women and is the leading cause of death in the United States.[2] The majority of CVD-attributable deaths are due to coronary heart disease (43%), followed by stroke (17%), hypertension (11%), and heart failure (9%).[2] Annual data collected by the National Heart, Lung, and Blood Institute demonstrate that CVD contributes to more deaths in the United States than all forms of cancer.[6] Unfortunately, many Americans are not aware of this important fact. For example, a survey conducted by the American Heart Association (AHA) found that only 56% of women were aware that heart disease was the leading cause of death among females.[7] Globally, CVD is also the leading cause of death.[8] Worldwide projections estimate that CVD will account for more than 22 million deaths annually by 2030.

There are serious, potentially life-threatening events associated with CVD. For example, stroke, hypertension, and heart disease are leading causes of disability in the United States, leaving many people with significant physical limitations that impact their ability to perform everyday tasks.[9] Cardiovascular diseases like hypertension and dyslipidemia, combined with risk factors like advancing age, diabetes, obesity, smoking, and family history put patients at significant risk for experiencing a myocardial infarction (i.e., heart attack).[10] It is estimated that one American will have a heart attack every 40 seconds.[2] Patients with coronary heart disease and heart failure are also at increased risk for experiencing sudden cardiac arrest (SCA), a condition in which the heart suddenly, and without warning, stops beating.[11] Only 10% of victims who experience SCA outside of a hospital survive.[12] Those who do survive typically experience multiple medical problems, including cognitive deficits such as diminished ability to think and remember.[2]

The good news is that deaths attributable to CVD in the United States have been declining in recent decades, after steadily increasing from the early 1900s to the 1980s.[2] Two important reasons for this decline are the increased use of evidence-based medical therapies to treat disease once it occurs, and adoption of healthier lifestyle habits.[10] The latter is the most important way to prevent heart disease throughout life; this includes not smoking, eating a healthy diet, engaging in physical activity, maintaining a healthy weight, and controlling blood pressure, blood glucose, and cholesterol levels.[13] For more information on pharmacists' efforts to impact modifiable risk factors for CVD and other conditions, see Chapter 4 Prevention & Wellness and the illustrated cases "Screen," "Change Talk," and "Mobilized."

Guidelines from professional organizations, such as the American College of Cardiology (ACC) and the AHA, recommend aggressive reduction in risk factors to prevent future cardiovascular events.[13] Medications and lifestyle changes are critical for the treatment and prevention of CVD. Patients with CVD are often under-prescribed critical, evidence-based therapies.[14] Those who are non-adherent to guideline-recommended medication regimens, meanwhile, are at risk for medication errors due to multiple chronic medications. These patients may experience adverse drug events leading to serious side effects, like bleeding or falling.[14] As medication experts, pharmacists who specialize in cardiology play an important role assisting

Table 5-1. Common Cardiovascular Diseases

Disease*	Description
Angina pectoris	Stable chest pain
Arrhythmias	Fast, slow, or irregular heart rhythms
Congenital heart disease	Structural heart defects present at birth
Coronary heart disease	Blockage in arteries of the heart
Deep vein thrombosis	Blood clots in deep veins
Dyslipidemia	Consistently abnormal cholesterol levels over time
Heart failure	Impairment of the heart to fill or pump blood
Hemorrhagic stroke	Bleeding in or around the brain from a ruptured blood vessel.
Hyperlipidemia	Consistently high cholesterol levels over time
Hypertension	Consistently high blood pressure readings over time
Ischemic stroke	Blockage of one or more arteries leading to or in the brain
Myocardial infarction	Heart attack
Peripheral artery disease	Blockage in one or more arteries of the legs and/or arms
Valvular heart disease	Damaged or defective heart valves

* Diseases listed in alphabetical order.

patients and prescribers to mitigate such risks as they contribute to the management of complex drug regimens. In addition, cardiology pharmacists provide critically important education about medications and CVD, which has been shown to improve adherence to drug therapies and pharmacotherapeutic outcomes.[14,15]

Members of the Interprofessional Cardiovascular Team

Many health professionals contribute to interprofessional cardiovascular teams, each sharing a unique perspective based on specialized education and training. Pharmacists who specialize in cardiology work on interprofessional teams located in coronary care units, surgical intensive care units, cardiovascular intensive care units, and emergency departments within hospitals.[16] They also collaborate with other health professionals outside of hospital settings, including outpatient clinics focused on treating patients with a variety of cardiovascular conditions ranging from hypertension and dyslipidemia to heart failure, arrhythmias, blood clots, and cardiac transplant.

The types of health professionals that cardiology pharmacists interact with vary depending upon the setting in which care is provided. Comprehensive interprofessional cardiovascular teams are found within hospitals certified as comprehensive cardiac centers.[17] Team members other than pharmacists include cardiologists and other prescribers, such as nurse practitioners and physician assistants, as well as case managers, dietitians/nutritionists, exercise specialists, nurses, physical therapists, respiratory therapists, and social workers.[17-19] Cardiology pharmacists engage with many additional specialty cardiac physicians in their pursuit of maximizing the safe and effective use of medications.[19-21] Robust interprofessional teamwork for patients with CVD is a hallmark of many practice settings outside of hospitals, as well, as indicated in the illustrated cases in this chapter.

Role of Pharmacists within the Interprofessional Cardiovascular Team

Pharmacists play a pivotal role in the interprofessional cardiovascular team by maintaining accurate medication lists, which has been shown to minimizing medication-related mistakes when patients transition from one care setting to another.[22] Cardiology pharmacists also focus on disease and drug therapy monitoring, medication dosing and management, drug interaction screening, and clinician and patient education.[14,22] The latter is important to increase the likelihood that patients will take their medications as prescribed, which is also referred to as medication adherence. Such activities have led to impressive outcomes; examples include reduced length of hospital stay, medication errors, adverse drug reactions, and costs, as well as increased patient survival. The illustrated cases "Underlying Cause," "Educator," and "Empowerment" thoroughly address the role of pharmacists in outpatient (i.e., clinic) settings; that

said, the remainder of this Background section will focus on the roles and impact of cardiology pharmacists embedded within hospitals.

Unfortunately, medication errors are common, and they have been associated with patient harm.[23] Given the complexity of medication regimens, patients with CVD are susceptible to medication errors related to inaccurate medication histories when their care is transitioned between different settings and providers.[22] Examples of such transitions include admission to hospitals for acute issues (e.g., heart attack, worsening heart failure symptoms), as well as upon discharge from hospitals when acute issues have been resolved. Medication reconciliation, a process whereby a health professional develops a comprehensive and accurate list of medications used by the patient, has been proven to reduce errors and drug-related incidents.[24,25]

Upon each care transition, cardiology pharmacists provide patient education on new medications, as well as dosing and/or administration changes. Unfortunately, medication adherence following care transitions is challenging. It is not uncommon, for example, for patients to be discharged with six to nine prescription medications to manage their condition.[26] Adherence to daily medications for heart failure, for example, has been estimated at approximately 50%.[27] Medication counseling and disease education by cardiology pharmacists can uncover adherence issues to drug therapy and resolve misunderstandings that patients may have about their condition. For an example of a poor outcome linked to a failed transition of care, readers are encouraged to explore the illustrated case "Breakdown" in Chapter 1 Interprofessional Practice in Pharmacy.

Cardiology pharmacists minimize medication errors by monitoring the daily administration patterns of medications and intervening when necessary. Such interventions frequently come in the form of recommendations to other members of the interprofessional team. Combined with knowledge of treatment guidelines for various cardiovascular conditions, such as those published by ACC and AHA, close monitoring like this leads to safer and more effective use of medications. Pertinent treatment guidelines include those related to hypertension, dyslipidemia, coronary heart disease (e.g., angina pectoris and myocardial infarction), atrial fibrillation, venous thromboembolism, heart failure, and ventricular arrhythmias.[28]

Cardiology pharmacists also monitor disease status and response to drug therapy with the goal of determining optimal treatment options.[16] To do this, they must develop a familiarity with common diagnostic tests, like electrocardiograms (ECG, measures the heart's electrical activity) and echocardiograms (ECHO, ultrasound test that examines the heart's structure and function). Combining expert knowledge of cardiovascular medications with a good working knowledge of such tests positions cardiology pharmacists for positive impact.

Pharmacists must also understand and be able to interpret laboratory values and therapeutic drug concentrations from blood tests, which allows for direct interventions to address issues before harm is caused. One example includes the close monitoring of low blood pressure readings (i.e., hypotension) so dosing can be adjusted to avoid a major adverse drug event, such as an injury caused by dizziness and a fall. Such activities have been shown to decrease medication errors and adverse drug events.[22]

A direct application of treatment guidelines within hospital settings involves cardiopulmonary resuscitation (CPR) and Advanced Cardiovascular Life Support (ACLS).[29,30] The participation of pharmacists in CPR/ACLS is associated with fewer adverse drug reactions and medication errors, and reductions in mortality.[31] Members of emergency cardiopulmonary response teams, including pharmacists, are certified in both CPR and ACLS. Pharmacists have many different roles during these situations; for example, they provide drug therapy recommendations and drug information, calculate drug dosages, determine when medications should be given, and prepare drugs for administration. Pharmacists trained in ACLS drug treatments not only reduce mortality, they increase the correct drug being given during codes by 35%, and their participation in ACLS teams improves overall adherence to ACLS guidelines by nearly 30%.[31] Pharmacists are also trained to set up infusion pumps, directly administer drugs, and perform chest compressions. As the drug information expert, pharmacists on these teams also scrutinize patients' chronic medications to identify potential causes for the cardiac arrest.

CARDIOLOGY PHARMACISTS IN ACTION

Every Second Counts!

Ischemic stroke occurs when blood supply to the brain is suddenly obstructed by a clot.[32] Rapid intervention is necessary to save stroke victims' lives and minimize long-term disability. Guidelines from the AHA and American Stroke Association (ASA) recommend early treatment for eligible patients, which involves administration of alteplase, a "clot busting" medication, within 60 minutes of hospital arrival.[33] Timely administration of alteplase is challenging as patients must be appropriately screened. Additionally, patients' blood pressures must be reduced to a certain level to ensure its safe use. Administration of alteplase to patients outside of certain parameters can cause serious and fatal bleeding. One university medical center incorporated pharmacists into their stroke team in an effort to decrease the time required to determine eligibility, achieve adequate blood pressure, and administer treatment.[34] Pharmacists completed medication histories, screened for risk factors, and made interventions to speed patient eligibility. They also calculated appropriate alteplase doses and answered questions from patients, family members, and health professionals on the team. Pharmacists prepared alteplase at bedside and jointly administered it with a nurse. During and after administration, pharmacists closely monitored patients for potential side effects and any signs of major bleeding. Incorporating pharmacists in this manner reduced the time it took to administer lifesaving medications to patients by 23.5 minutes and increased the percentage of patients meeting the AHA/ASA goal time of 60 minutes by 49%.[34] For another example of pharmacist involvement in the care of a patient experiencing stroke, see the illustrated case "One Day" in Chapter 10 Emergency Medicine.

Survival at 30,000 Feet

Sudden cardiac arrest is the abrupt loss of heart function.[11] If witnesses do not immediately begin CPR, the vast majority of those who experience SCA will die.[12] Patients with heart disease, particularly those experiencing an acute heart attack, are at high risk for SCA. A common heart arrhythmia associated with SCA is ventricular fibrillation, during which the lower chambers of the heart (i.e., ventricles) suddenly beat chaotically, causing them to lose the ability to pump blood out of the heart. This leads to unconsciousness and death if CPR is not started immediately. On an international flight, a man developed chest pain due to a heart attack and went into SCA.[35] Three passengers sprung into action and immediately began CPR: a physician, a police officer, and a pharmacist. The police officer performed chest compressions and the physician provided rescue breaths using a face mask. Once the automatic external defibrillator (AED) arrived, which identified ventricular fibrillation as the cause of the victim's SCA, the pharmacist used the AED to deliver a shock. After two shocks, the victim began to spontaneously move and his pulse returned. The pharmacist then took responsibility for monitoring the patient's blood pressure and pulse. Unfortunately, the victim went back into ventricular fibrillation and CPR resumed. The physician was able to place an intravenous line in the victim's arm and the pharmacist took over administration of medications. Due to the limited amount of supplies and the projected flight time remaining, the pharmacist prepared an infusion bag of epinephrine and gave small bolus doses every 5 minutes to ration supplies. The airplane was diverted to the closest metropolitan city, and the patient was transported to a cardiac hospital. Thankfully, the quick actions of this impromptu interprofessional team saved the victim's life. For another example of pharmacist involvement in the care of a patient experiencing SCA, see the illustrated case "Life & Death" in Chapter 10 Emergency Medicine.

BECOMING A CARDIOLOGY PHARMACIST

Upon completing a Doctor of Pharmacy (PharmD) degree and passing licensure exams, all pharmacists are able to provide medication recommendations and education to patients with CVD, regardless of the healthcare setting. However, pharmacists who wish to practice on interprofessional teams within specialized cardiac units in a hospital, or those who would like to work in outpatient cardiology-focused clinics, require postgraduate training.[14] Most pharmacists interested in this career path choose to pursue advanced training through residencies and/or fellowships. A general postgraduate year 1 (PGY-1) pharmacy residency prepares the individual to be competent in patient-centered care and pharmacy operational services applicable to multiple practice settings. Pharmacists who desire specialization in cardiology typically complete a postgraduate year 2 (PGY-2) cardiology-focused residency, through which they receive training in the care of patients with CVD, clinical research, teaching and educational activities, leadership, and practice management.[14,36] A research fellowship is a highly individualized postgraduate program intended to train pharmacists to conduct scientific research.

Beyond residency and/or fellowship training, pharmacists can obtain recognition for their specialized cardiology knowledge and skills through the Board of Pharmacy Specialties, which offers a nationally recognized credential called the Board Certified Cardiology Pharmacist (BCCP).[37] The BCCP credential validates that the pharmacist has met the eligibility criteria to deliver direct patient care as a member of an interprofessional cardiovascular team, working to ensure safe and effective use of medications in patients with CVD. Pharmacists may also choose to obtain more broad-based certifications available to health professionals regardless of specific profession; examples include various areas associated with CVD, such as anticoagulation (i.e., using medications to prevent blood clots and reduce the risk of ischemic stroke), diabetes, and dyslipidemia.[14] Readers interested in more information about BCCP are encouraged to visit the Board of Pharmacy Specialties website.[37]

UNDERLYING CAUSE: An Illustrated Case Study

Story by John M. Dopp & Joseph A. Zorek
Illustrations by George Folz, © 2019 Board of Regents of the University of Wisconsin System

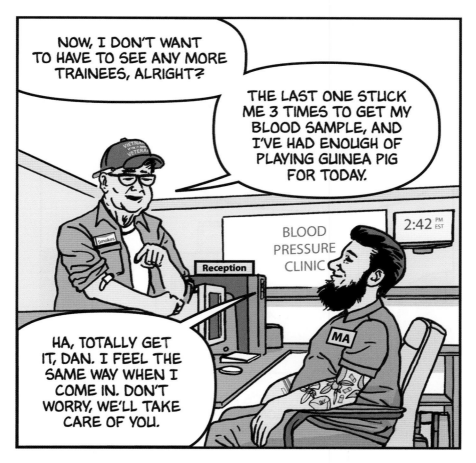

Illustration 5-1

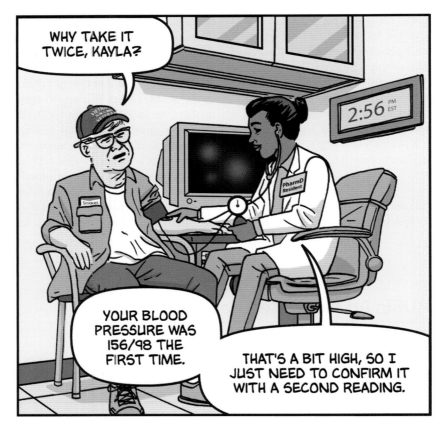

Illustration 5-2

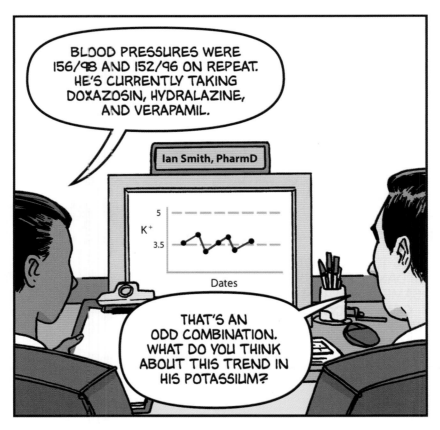

Illustration 5-3

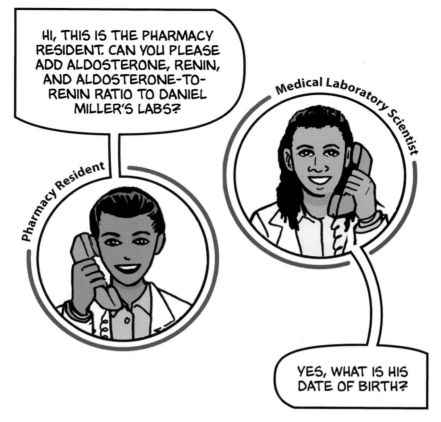

Illustration 5-4

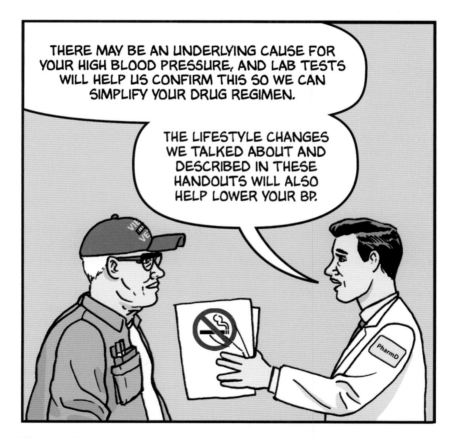

Illustration 5-5

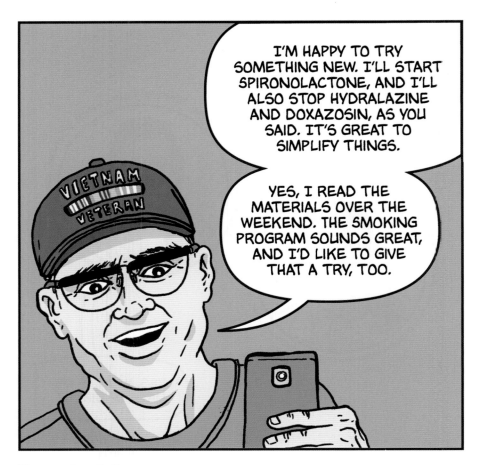

Illustration 5-6

Thoughts on "Underlying Cause"

The illustrated case "Underlying Cause" begins with a Vietnam veteran named Daniel Miller arriving for his first pharmacy appointment at a Veterans Affairs (VA) clinic in his new hometown. Prior to Mr. Miller's recent move, he had only sporadically visited the doctor. One of his favorite mantras, "if it ain't broke, don't fix it," had been, until engaging with the VA, the driving force behind his approach to healthcare. Mr. Miller was content to remain on the blood pressure (BP) medications that were started years ago, as he thought they were working just fine.

Illustration 5-2 depicts the work of a pharmacy resident, Dr. Kayla Johnson, assessing Mr. Miller's current BP status. While not explicitly stated, Kayla also learns via completion of Mr. Miller's medication history that he experienced significant side effects in the past while taking a diuretic, considered a first-line medication. This experience made him resistant to changing his BP medications, and it reinforced his favorite mantra. As a result, Mr. Miller has been taking the same three-drug BP regimen for years.

Kayla and Dr. Ian Smith, her pharmacist supervisor, recognize that this particular combination of medications is not ideal.

Importantly, they also recognize that Mr. Miller's BP should still be better controlled than what Kayla measured in Illustration 5-2. Together, Kayla and Ian explore laboratory results to further investigate potential explanations for this problem (Illustrations 5-3 and 5-4). After identifying an underlying cause, Kayla and Ian simplify Mr. Miller's medication regimen (Illustrations 5-5 and 5-6). Effective interprofessional practice between these pharmacists, a medical assistant (Illustrations 5-1), and a medical laboratory scientist (Illustration 5-4) is highlighted throughout.

High BP (i.e., hypertension) is one of the most common medical conditions in the United States. Prior to 2018, approximately 30% of American adults met criteria for a hypertension diagnosis.[38] With the publication of new criteria for diagnosing and classifying hypertension in 2018 (Table 5-2), nearly 50% of US adults are now classified as having this condition.[39] Unfortunately, only about half of patients with a hypertension diagnosis bring this health issue under control, and the consequences are devastating.[40,41] For example, hypertension is linked to the development of kidney disease, heart disease, and other heart complications such as myocardial infarction (i.e., heart attack), stroke, and heart failure. Reducing BP reduces the risk of heart and kidney problems, so it is essential to lower patients' BP to help minimize the potential for long-term complications.[42]

Table 5-2. Categorization System for Hypertension

Category	Systolic Blood Pressure		Diastolic Blood Pressure
Normal	<120 mm Hg	AND	<80 mm Hg
Elevated	120–129 mm Hg	AND	<80 mm Hg
Hypertension			
Stage 1	130–139 mm Hg	OR	80–89 mm Hg
Stage 2	≥140 mm Hg	OR	≥90 mm Hg

The reasons for lack of BP control are numerous, including imperfect adherence to medications and lack of patient understanding of the condition and its treatment.[43] Additional reasons include suboptimal coordination between health professionals about who is managing BP, and barriers within the healthcare system, such as shortages of available appointments with providers.[39] To learn more about medication adherence, readers are encouraged to explore the illustrated case "Opportunities" in Chapter 15 Administration.

One of the most important factors associated with lack of hypertension control is that patients cannot feel that their BP is high; in other words, there are no symptoms. For this reason, leading health organizations such as the AHA frequently refer to hypertension as a "silent killer."[44] Unlike other health conditions, where symptoms (e.g., pain, seasonal allergies) may reinforce healthy behaviors, like taking medications, the absence of symptoms from hypertension can sometimes lead to it being ignored. As a result, there is a need for changes in how care is delivered for hypertension to help patients control BP and improve their health. One such approach is to maximize use of the knowledge and skills possessed by every health professional who can meaningfully contribute. In the current hypertension treatment guidelines, there is a clear recommendation to leverage team-based care to improve outcomes; this includes contributions from, and collaborations among, cardiologists, community health workers, dietitians/nutritionists, nurses, pharmacists, physician assistants, primary care physicians, and social workers.[29]

Research has shown that pharmacists can play an important role in helping patients improve their BP control.[45–49] Pharmacists are medication experts who provide detailed and personalized information about hypertension medications prescribed by cardiologists, nurse practitioners, physician assistants, and primary care physicians. Examples of this personalized approach include monitoring for side effects and drug interactions, as well as intervening on behalf of patients to optimize dosing and following up to ensure patients are getting to their BP goal. The roles of cardiology pharmacists working in direct patient care, like Kayla and Ian, have expanded in the last several decades. In many health systems, pharmacists work as direct providers of care with other members of the interprofessional health team to help select medications, determine optimal dosing and monitoring, and perform patient assessments to evaluate the efficacy of therapies chosen.[50] Pharmacists are increasingly able to order laboratory tests and prescribe medications in certain health systems.[51,52] Direct patient care activities are completed in-person, as shown in "Underlying Cause," over the phone, or using telehealth video technologies.[53] For more information on incorporation of technologies to advance interprofessional practice in pharmacy, see the illustrated cases "Leverage," "Integrated," and "Innovator" in Chapter 13 Technology. Those seeking an example of a telehealth video appointment are encouraged to read the illustrated case "Wounded" in Chapter 8 Infectious Diseases.

Hypertension is an ideal health condition for pharmacists to manage. First, unlike pain or other symptoms, BP can be measured objectively. Decisions about therapy are based directly on BP readings, such as medication initiation, modification, and/or lifestyle changes. Illustration 5-2 depicts Kayla utilizing correct BP measurement technique to obtain Mr. Miller's latest reading. His feet are flat on the floor, he is sitting upright in his chair, and his cuffed arm is resting at or near the level of his heart. The other potential issues are whether Mr. Miller refrained from smoking or consuming caffeine in the 30 minutes prior to his visit, if he emptied his bladder, and if he was allowed to rest quietly for a minimum of 5 minutes prior to the initial reading.[39] Kayla makes a wise decision to recheck Mr. Miller's BP reading as the first one was elevated. This also provided her an important opportunity to teach Mr. Miller about proper technique to ensure his home BP readings, which will also be used to optimize his therapy, are accurate.

The complexity of hypertension medications provides another compelling reason for pharmacists to manage patients with hypertension. It is revealed in Illustration 5-3 that Mr. Miller takes three BP medications, which creates numerous opportunities for adverse drug events. For example, BP medications may have interactions with each other and may need to be used cautiously in patients who have additional health conditions. Some BP medications have additive side effects, raising the risk of dizziness and falls from low BP. Other hypertension medications may work opposite each other and cancel out potential problems. BP medications can also change body concentrations of electrolytes like potassium, as depicted in Illustration 5-3. This requires routine laboratory monitoring, as abnormal blood levels of potassium have been associated with serious consequences, such as heart arrhythmias, cardiac arrest, and death.[54] Third, regular patient contact is essential when starting and modifying medications and lifestyle changes. Pharmacists in hypertension clinics generally have greater availability than other providers, such as physicians, which allows for more frequent visits to conduct patient monitoring and follow-up.[55]

Adequate BP is normal and necessary to provide blood flow, oxygen, and nutrients to organs and other tissues. Blood pressure is measured in blood vessels (arteries) at two times: systolic

BP is measured during contraction (systole) of the heart, and diastolic BP is measured during relaxation (diastole). The BP reading is most commonly written as systolic/diastolic, and it is expressed in millimeters of mercury (mm Hg). Mr. Miller's first BP reading in Illustration 5-2 (158/98), therefore, tells us that his systolic BP is 158, and that his diastolic BP is 98. This is a troublesome reading, particularly if it is consistently this high. If it were to hold upon repeat measurement, he would fit the category of stage 2 hypertension (Table 5-2).[39] The current hypertension treatment guidelines recommend lifestyle modifications for all patients, but especially for those with elevated, stage 1, or stage 2 hypertension. Illustrations 5-5 and 5-6 highlight that lifestyle modifications, including quitting smoking, are key elements in BP management. For more information on behavior modifications with an emphasis on stopping use of nicotine-containing products (e.g., cigarettes, vaping devices), see the illustrated case "Change Talk" in Chapter 4 Prevention & Wellness.

Blood pressure increases naturally with aging. In certain individuals, BP becomes elevated on a daily basis.[56] Systolic BP increases about 7 mm Hg for each decade of life for people over the age of 40 in Western societies.[41] In contrast, diastolic BP increases until around age 50, then plateaus and may even decrease thereafter.[57] The increase in systolic BP over time is a result of hardening of the large arteries that regulate BP; this is, in fact, the most common cause of hypertension. While less frequent, secondary factors may also cause hypertension. Examples of secondary factors include sleep breathing disorders (e.g., sleep apnea), as well as hormonal, physiologic, and anatomic abnormalities such as narrowing of blood vessels in the kidney or damage to the kidney.[58] Approximately 5% to 10% of hypertension diagnoses stem from secondary causes, and the risk of secondary hypertension increases with age.[59]

In general, patients at highest suspicion of secondary hypertension fall within one of the following categories:[58,59]

1. Diagnosed before age of 30 years;
2. Resistant hypertension (i.e., uncontrolled despite three BP medications at optimal doses, one of which is a diuretic);
3. Severe hypertension (i.e., BP >180/110 mm Hg)
4. Sudden increases in BP; and
5. Damage to organs from high BP.

In most patients with secondary hypertension, identification of the specific cause and targeted therapy will help achieve BP goals.[58,59] Thus, identification of a possible secondary cause is important to help find the right treatments for each patient. In order to do so, health professionals need to order the correct laboratory tests, perform the appropriate patient assessments, and use other appropriate diagnostic methods as necessary. Once the contributing secondary cause of hypertension is identified, targeted treatment can be planned and implemented. As depicted in Illustration 5-3, Ian is beginning to zero in on low potassium (i.e., K^+) as a clue that might help him and Kayla pinpoint the secondary cause responsible for Mr. Miller's difficult-to-control hypertension.

For healthy patients who are low risk, BP medications should be initiated when readings reach 140/90 mm Hg or higher.[39] For patients at higher risk, however, or for those with certain health conditions like chronic kidney disease or diabetes, medications should be started when BP readings rise above 130/80 mm Hg. Once treated with medications, the target BP is less than 130/80 mm Hg. In "Underlying Cause," Mr. Miller is taking three BP medications: doxazosin (Cardura), hydralazine (Apresoline), and verapamil (Calan). For more information about these medications, as well as others used to treat hypertension, see Table 5-3.[60]

Revisiting Illustration 5-3, Kayla and Ian notice that Mr. Miller's potassium levels, as evidenced by the graph, consistently remain low. Together, unexplained low potassium and difficult-to-control hypertension are suggestive of a condition called primary hyperaldosteronism, which is a frequent cause of secondary hypertension.[58] Hyperaldosteronism is estimated to be present in approximately 10% of patients with hypertension.[61] In this condition, excess amounts of aldosterone are released from the adrenal gland. Within the kidney, this excess aldosterone causes sodium and water to be retained, which leads to increased BP. When the body reabsorbs sodium, potassium is exchanged and is excreted into the urine, causing low potassium levels in the blood. In addition, a hallmark of hyperaldosteronism is elevated aldosterone concentrations in the blood.

In Illustration 5-4, Kayla is shown talking to a medical laboratory scientist. Kayla requests that aldosterone, renin, and aldosterone-to-renin ratio be added to Mr. Miller's most recent laboratory test, which we know from Illustration 5-1 occurred earlier that day. Under normal conditions, the hormone renin regulates the amount of aldosterone secreted from the adrenal gland.[62] Measuring renin and the ratio between aldosterone and renin is necessary, as hyperaldosteronism can be diagnosed when aldosterone is elevated with accompanying low renin activity. It is important to note that most BP medications will influence either aldosterone and/or renin, and subsequently, the aldosterone-to-renin ratio.[58] In order to get a definitive and correct diagnosis of hyperaldosteronism, all BP medications that influence these laboratory parameters would need to be switched to non-interfering medications.

When hyperaldosteronism is diagnosed, the preferred and targeted therapy is spironolactone (Aldactone) (see Table 5-3). Spironolactone is a medication that blocks aldosterone and lowers BP. In most cases, use of targeted therapy in secondary hypertension will lower BP to goal. Patients less than 40 years old with secondary hypertension are more likely than older

Table 5-3. Categories and Examples of Medications Commonly Used to Treat Hypertension

Category	Medication Examples*	Physiologic Effect
Alpha-blockers	▪ doxazosin (Cardura) ▪ prazosin (Minipress) ▪ terazosin (Hytrin)	Block alpha-1 receptors, which relaxes blood vessels and causes reductions in blood pressure
Angiotensin-converting enzyme (ACE) inhibitors	▪ benazepril (Lotensin) ▪ captopril (Capoten) ▪ enalapril (Vasotec) ▪ lisinopril (Prinivil, Zestril) ▪ quinapril (Accupril) ▪ ramipril (Altace)	Prevent formation of angiotensin II, a hormone that constricts blood vessels and increases body fluid volume through its impact on the kidney; blocking angiotensin II stops these effects, which reduces blood pressure
Angiotensin receptor blockers	▪ candesartan (Atacand) ▪ irbesartan (Avapro) ▪ losartan (Cozaar) ▪ olmesartan (Benicar) ▪ telmisartan (Micardis) ▪ valsartan (Diovan)	Block angiotensin II receptors, preventing the angiotensin II hormone from exerting its negative effects on blood pressure as stated above for ACE inhibitors
Beta-blockers	▪ atenolol (Tenormin) ▪ bisoprolol (Zebeta) ▪ carvedilol (Coreg) ▪ metoprolol (Lopressor, Toprol) ▪ nebivolol (Bystolic) ▪ propranolol (Inderal)	Block beta-receptors in the heart, which decreases the number of heart beats per minute, causing reduced blood pressure; also block beta-receptors in the kidney, which decreases renin, a hormone that leads to formation of angiotensin II
Calcium channel blockers	▪ amlodipine (Norvasc) ▪ diltiazem (Cardizem) ▪ felodipine (Plendil) ▪ nifedipine (Adalat CC, Procardia XL) ▪ verapamil (Calan, Verelan)	Block the movement of calcium into blood vessel and heart cells, causing them to relax, which results in reduced blood pressure and heart rate
Central alpha-2 agonists	▪ clonidine (Catapres) ▪ guanfacine (Intuniv, Tenex) ▪ methyldopa (Aldomet)	Bind to receptors in the brain and spinal cord that reduce heart rate and relax blood vessels, leading to decreased blood pressure
Mineralocorticoid antagonists	▪ eplerenone (Inspra) ▪ spironolactone (Aldactone)	Block the hormone aldosterone, which reduces blood pressure by decreasing sodium and fluid retention in the kidneys
Thiazide diuretics	▪ chlorthalidone (Hygroton) ▪ hydrochlorothiazide (Hydrodiuril) ▪ indapamide (Lozol)	Block reabsorption of sodium and fluid in the kidney, reducing body fluid and relaxing blood vessels which results in decreased blood pressure
Vasodilators	▪ hydralazine (Apresoline) ▪ minoxidil (Loniten)	Cause relaxation of blood vessels, which leads to a decrease in blood pressure

* Medication examples presented in alphabetical order as "generic name (Brand Name)."

patients to reach goal BP with specific treatments but even two-thirds of older patients reach BP goals.[59] In some cases, doses of other medications that do not specifically target aldosterone can be reduced, or the medication may be discontinued altogether, if satisfactory BP reduction is achieved with spironolactone at adequate doses.[63]

In Illustration 5-6, Ian is on the phone with Mr. Miller, who is ecstatic to learn that he is going to see a decrease in the number of medications he has to take; doxazosin and hydralazine will be replaced by a single medication, spironolactone. Through this process, Kayla and Ian were able to use their knowledge and skills to build a trusting relationship with Mr. Miller. This is evidenced not only by his positive reaction toward the end, but also in Mr. Miller's willingness to enter the smoking cessation program. Careful patient assessment, coupled with curiosity and a willingness to investigate, allowed these cardiology pharmacists to identify and correctly treat the underlying cause of Mr. Miller's hypertension. By identifying hyperaldosteronism and using a targeted therapy, Kayla and Ian have increased Mr. Miller's odds of reaching his BP goal of less than 130/80 mm Hg, ultimately reducing the likelihood that this "silent killer" will claim another victim.

DISCUSSION QUESTIONS FOR "UNDERLYING CAUSE"

1. The illustrated case "Underlying Cause" opens with Mr. Miller expressing frustration with his blood draw, which he jokingly attributes to an inexperienced trainee. Have you or a loved one ever received care from a health professional-in-training, such as a student or resident? What is your reaction to Mr. Miller describing himself as a guinea pig? How does this compare to your experience?

2. Illustration 5-2 shows the pharmacy resident Kayla taking Mr. Miller's blood pressure a second time because the first reading was elevated. There are two clues hidden in Illustrations 5-1 and 5-2 that might explain this elevated reading. Kayla will need to consider these clues before she can confidently attribute Mr. Miller's elevated blood pressure to inadequate medication therapy. Can you identify these? What other factors should be taken into consideration?

3. Kayla and Ian were able to work with the medical laboratory scientist in Illustration 5-4 to use Mr. Miller's earlier blood sample to run additional tests. What are the benefits of this approach to Mr. Miller and to the health system? Can you think of other health professionals Kayla and Ian might collaborate with on a regular basis as they work to improve blood pressure control for their patients?

4. Illustration 5-6 depicts Mr. Miller as ecstatic after Ian shares with him results of the laboratory tests and associated medication-related changes. What are some reasons that might explain Mr. Miller's joyous response?

5. Unlike other health conditions, hypertension is largely asymptomatic; meaning, patients do not feel sick. How might this impact medication adherence? What are some ways you can think of to motivate patients to take their hypertension medications?

EDUCATOR: An Illustrated Case Study

Story by Karen J. Kopacek & Joseph A. Zorek
Illustrations by George Folz, © 2019 Board of Regents of the University of Wisconsin System

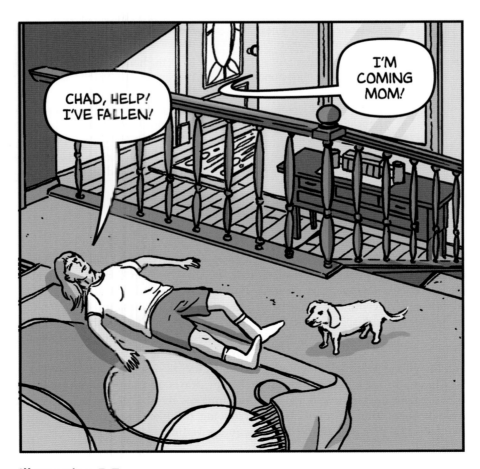

Illustration 5-7

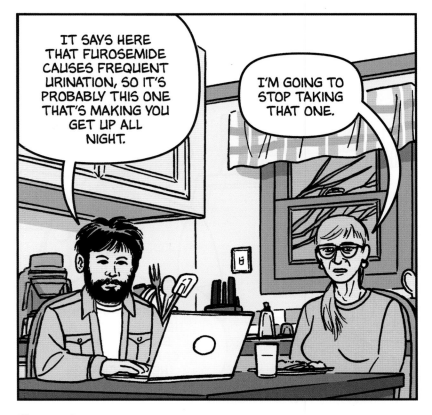

Illustration 5-8

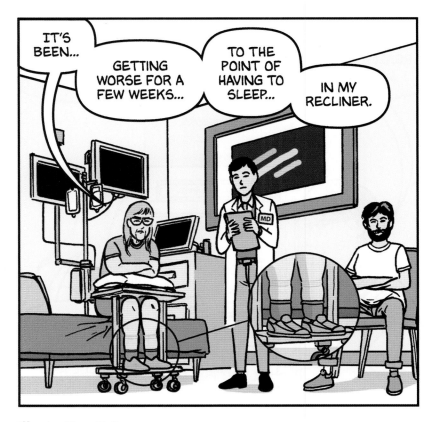

Illustration 5-9

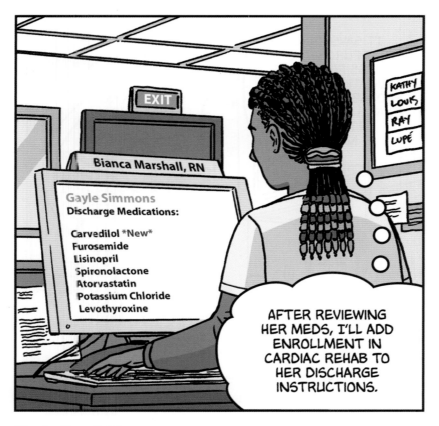

Illustration 5-10

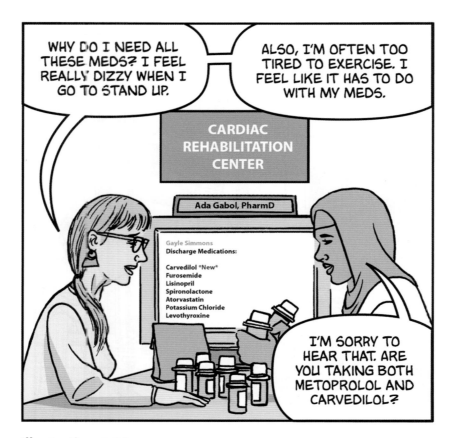

Illustration 5-11

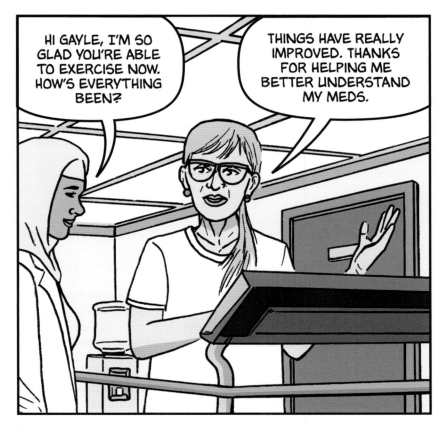

Illustration 5-12

Thoughts on "Educator"

The illustrated case "Educator," told through the lens of a recently widowed, older adult named Gayle Simmons, highlights the difficulties of living with heart failure (HF). One such difficulty is the challenge patients and their families experience as they attempt to manage complex medication regimens. Illustrations 5-7, 5-8, and 5-9 reveal a troubling series of adverse drug events. The story opens with Mrs. Simmons lying flat on her back, having tripped and fallen in the middle of the night. While not explicitly stated, it is implied that frequent nighttime trips to the bathroom associated with furosemide (Lasix), a critically important medication to treat HF, are to blame. A misinformed decision by Mrs. Simmons to withhold furosemide, which is understandable from the perspective of someone terrified of falling and injuring herself, leads to the rapid deterioration of Mrs. Simmons' condition that results in her hospitalization. What is abundantly clear by the end of the story is that education was missing from Mrs. Simmons' previous treatment regimen. Fortunately, a cardiology pharmacist named Dr. Ada Gabol is as good at teaching her patients as she is knowledgeable about their medications, and the story ends on a promising note.

The heart is a complex organ, approximately the size of a clenched first, that is responsible for circulating blood throughout the body.[64] It is divided into two sides, the left and right, and is comprised of two upper chambers called atria and two lower chambers called ventricles. The right atrium (RA) sits on top of the right ventricle (RV) and the left atrium (LA) sits on top of the left ventricle (LV). The walls of the heart consist of muscles that contract to pump blood out of each chamber with every heartbeat. The right side of the heart (RA and RV) is responsible for pumping oxygen-poor blood to the lungs to exchange carbon dioxide for oxygen. The newly oxygenated blood returns to the left side of the heart (LA and LV), where it is pumped out to the rest of the body. Cells throughout the body remove oxygen from the blood and the cycle continues with the return of oxygen-poor blood to the RA.

Heart failure is a complex syndrome that results from any structural or functional impairment of the ventricles to fill with or eject blood.[65,66] Patients with HF are classified into two groups based on the ability of the LV to pump or eject blood. A measurement called ejection fraction (EF) is used to help health professionals understand the severity of a patient's condition. Ejection fraction is the percentage of blood pumped out of the LV with each heartbeat. There are two types of HF, one in which EF is preserved and remains normal, and another in which EF is reduced to abnormal levels.

When the LV contracts poorly and the ejection of blood declines, delivery of oxygen and nutrients to other organs is reduced. This reduction in blood flow triggers several compensatory systems in the body to increase blood volume. The kidneys, for example, are stimulated by the reduction of blood flow to trigger production and release of two hormones, angiotensin II and aldosterone, to compensate for reduced blood volume.

Simultaneously, norepinephrine is released, leading to increases in the number of times the heart beats, as well as the strength of heart muscle contraction. Unfortunately, both angiotensin II and norepinephrine increase blood pressure by constricting the blood vessels that transport blood throughout the body, which ultimately makes it harder for the LV to pump blood out of the heart. This increase in blood volume and workload on the heart worsens the function of the already-failing LV. Left ventricular failure frequently leads to fluid accumulation in certain parts of the body called edema, most commonly the lungs, abdomen, and lower extremities (e.g., ankles and feet).

Illustration 5-9 portrays Mrs. Simmons in the midst of a HF exacerbation, with her condition acutely worsening. The fluid buildup in her lungs is causing several common symptoms associated with this condition; for example, dyspnea (shortness of breath), orthopnea (difficulty breathing while lying flat), and cough. The pop-out in Illustration 5-9 also highlights fluid buildup in Mrs. Simmons' lower extremities, called peripheral edema. Mrs. Simmons has rolled her socks down in order to show the physician the indentations in her skin. This is called pitting edema, where fluid retention is so great that an indentation (i.e., a pit) remains even when the pressure that caused it is removed. Other common signs and symptoms of HF include reduced exercise capacity, fatigue, confusion, loss of appetite, and frequent urination. Many of these signs and symptoms occur at the same time, which has negative consequences on patients' quality of life.[66]

It is estimated that 6.2 million adults in the United States had HF in 2016; this number is projected to increase to more than 8 million adults by 2030.[2] The prevalence of HF progressively increases with age, starting after the age of 50 years.[65] In the last decade, the average age of patients with HF has increased to 77 years, and many of these patients have at least four other medical conditions (i.e., comorbidities) that may negatively impact the management of their HF.[67–69] Examples of such comorbidities include chronic obstructive pulmonary disease (COPD), chronic kidney disease, diabetes, glaucoma, and osteoarthritis.[65–69] For a patient with HF, the risk of adverse drug interactions increases as the number of daily medications increases.[70] Unfortunately, medications used to manage other chronic medical conditions can negatively affect the beneficial effects of HF meds.[70] An older adult who takes an over-the-counter medication like ibuprofen or naproxen for arthritis pain exemplifies this issue. These pain medications, also called nonsteroidal anti-inflammatory agents, cause sodium and water retention by the kidneys, which leads to additional fluid retention and worsening of HF symptoms.

Common risk factors for developing HF include heart disease, high blood pressure (i.e., hypertension), diabetes, obesity, and use of nicotine-containing products (cigarettes, vaping devices).[2] Risk factors vary around the world, but hypertension is the risk factor most strongly associated with HF in all regions of the world. An important goal in managing HF is treating the patient's other medical conditions through medications and lifestyle changes, like adopting a heart-healthy diet, increasing aerobic exercise, and stopping the use of nicotine-containing

products. Even when stable, these other conditions can increase a patient's risk for polypharmacy and medication side effects, as well as competing for a patient's attention and financial resources.[68] Those interested in a more in-depth review of hypertension are encouraged to read the illustrated case "Underlying Cause" in this chapter. For information on, and an example of, pharmacist assistance quitting nicotine-containing products, see the illustrated case "Change Talk" in Chapter 4 Prevention & Wellness. The illustrated cases "Holistic" and "Screen" in Chapter 3 Primary Care and Chapter 4 Prevention & Wellness, respectively, provide more details on the treatment of diabetes. Finally, the illustrated case "Burden" in Chapter 7 Geriatrics describes a pharmacist's efforts to reduce polypharmacy.

While HF affects both men and women, women are more likely to die from it compared to men.[2,65] Death due to HF is declining, primarily due to management of risk factors, use of evidence-based medications, high-tech surgically implanted devices, and medical procedures that improve blood flow in the coronary arteries (i.e., coronary revascularization).[2] While HF-associated mortality has declined, the costs associated with treating HF are rising dramatically. The total cost for diagnosing and treating HF in the United States was estimated to be $30.7 billion in 2012; by 2030, it is projected to be $69.8 billion.[2] Two-thirds of the total cost to treat HF is due to direct medical expenditures, particularly from hospital readmissions. Heart failure is the primary diagnosis of approximately 800,000 hospitalizations annually and continues to be a frequent cause of 30-day readmissions for Medicare patients.[2,66]

Hospital admission and readmissions have serious consequences for patients with HF. As the heart weakens over time, patients require frequent hospitalizations when they accumulate too much fluid and struggle to breath, like Mrs. Simmons in "Educator." These hospitalizations tend to result in increasing intensity of drug therapies to control symptoms, as well as a corresponding decrease in the patient's overall quality of life. Therefore, it is important that health professionals ensure that patients (1) are on evidence-based medications as early as possible, (2) receive appropriate education on their medications, and (3) receive a care plan that includes how to monitor their condition and what to do if symptoms return (i.e., self-care) to avoid readmissions.[67,71] The consequences of a lack of such knowledge are highlighted by Mrs. Simmons' experience in this illustrated case.

Appropriate drug therapies depend on the type of HF with which the patient has been diagnosed; either preserved or reduced EF. While not explicitly stated, Mrs. Simmons suffers from the latter, also called HF with reduced ejection fraction, or HFrEF for short. Evidence-based medication therapies for patients with HFrEF,[66,70,72] described in detail in Table 5-4, include the following combination:

(1) An angiotensin-converting enzyme inhibitor (ACEI), an angiotensin receptor blocker (ARB), or an angiotensin receptor-neprilysin inhibitor (ARNI) with

(2) A beta-blocker (BB);

(3) A mineralocorticoid receptor antagonist (MRA); and

(4) A loop diuretic.

Table 5-4. Categories and Examples of Medications Commonly Used to Treat Heart Failure

Category	Medication Examples*	Physiologic Effect
Angiotensin-converting enzyme inhibitors	■ enalapril (Vasotec) ■ lisinopril (Prinivil, Zestril) ■ ramipril (Altace)	Decrease blood pressure and protect kidney function
Angiotensin receptor blockers	■ candesartan (Atacand) ■ losartan (Cozaar) ■ valsartan (Diovan)	
Angiotensin receptor blocker combined with a neprilysin inhibitors	■ sacubitril/valsartan (Entresto)	In addition to blood pressure lowering and kidney protective effects of valsartan, inhibits neprilysin, the enzyme that breaks down natriuretic peptides, leading to increased sodium and water excretion
Beta-blockers	■ bisoprolol (Zebeta) ■ carvedilol (Coreg) ■ metoprolol (Lopressor, Toprol XL)	Decrease heart rate and blood pressure
Loop diuretics	■ bumetanide (Bumex) ■ furosemide (Lasix) ■ torsemide (Demadex)	Promote sodium and water excretion by the kidneys, decreasing blood pressure
Mineralocorticoid receptor antagonists	■ eplerenone (Inspra) ■ spironolactone (Aldactone)	Promote sodium and water excretion by the kidneys, decreasing blood pressure, and prevent formation of scar tissue in the heart

* Medication examples presented in alphabetical order as "generic name (Brand Name)."

Illustration 5-10 depicts Mrs. Simmons' nurse, Bianca Marshall, preparing to discharge Mrs. Simmons from the hospital. One of the critical steps at this phase of a HF patient's hospitalization is ensuring accuracy of the home medication list, as well as the patient's understanding of any medication changes that have been made. The computer screen in Illustration 5-10 shows that Mrs. Simmons is being discharged on the appropriate combination of HF medications (carvedilol [BB], lisinopril [ACEI], spironolactone [MRA], and furosemide [loop diuretic]), as well as medications to control cholesterol (atorvastatin) and hypothyroidism (levothyroxine). The intense diuresis (intentional water loss) that takes place during a hospitalization for a HF exacerbation can impact electrolyte concentrations in the blood, notably potassium. Mrs. Simmons' discharge medication list includes a potassium supplement, which is appropriate and commonly seen in this setting.

Unfortunately, medication adherence is challenging as patients can be discharged with six to nine prescription medications to manage HF symptoms and associated conditions (e.g., hypertension, diabetes) or treat common side effects associated with these drugs.[73] Adherence to daily medications has been estimated at approximately 50% in patients with HF.[27] There are many factors that can explain medication non-adherence in this patient population, such as pill burden (i.e., the number of tablets or capsules taken per day), the complexity of the drug therapies (i.e., number of times per day each medication must be taken), side effects or intolerances, and cost.[70,73]

Side effects from evidence-based medication therapies, like the regimen Mrs. Simmons is being discharged on, contribute to adherence issues.[70,74] As Table 5-4 depicts, these HF medications decrease strain on the heart by decreasing blood pressure. As a result, patients frequently experience hypotension (i.e., low blood pressure). In Illustration 5-11, Mrs. Simmons reports to Ada that she feels dizzy when standing up. This complaint is referred to as orthostatic hypotension, which is caused by a sudden decrease in blood pressure when patients change their body positions (i.e., laying to sitting, sitting to standing). This change in position results in decreased blood flow to the brain, which causes dizziness and increases the risk of injuries from falls. For a patient like Mrs. Simmons, who has a history of abandoning medication therapy after falls, this is a serious risk factor for another HF exacerbation, hospitalization, and worsening of her overall health.

Fortunately, the cardiology pharmacist Ada requested that Mrs. Simmons bring all of her medications to her first cardiac rehabilitation appointment. While not visible, Ada is holding in her hands two beta-blockers: metoprolol, which Mrs. Simmons was taking before her hospitalization, and carvedilol, which was prescribed upon discharge. While the nurse instructed Mrs. Simmons to discard her metoprolol during discharge counseling, she was tired, stressed, feeling overwhelmed, and simply missed this critical point. As a result, she had been taking both metoprolol and carvedilol, which Ada rightfully identified as the cause of Mrs. Simmons' hypotension, dizziness, and fatigue.

Adherence to drug therapy improves when patients become more engaged in their medical care through positive interactions with health professionals. Patients who receive medication education, like the kind provided by Ada, make fewer medication errors and experience fewer adverse drug events.[27] When patients have questions about the purpose or efficacy of their treatments and are not involved in making decisions related to their HF care with their healthcare providers, they are more likely to turn to family members or the Internet to help with managing their medications, which is exactly what precipitated Mrs. Simmons' recent hospitalization.[75,76]

Cardiac rehabilitation is an important component of care in patients diagnosed with various cardiovascular diseases. ACC and AHA strongly recommend that patients with HFrEF, like Mrs. Simmons, participate in cardiac rehab to reduce hospital readmissions, prevent future cardiovascular events (e.g., heart attack, stroke), decrease the risk of death, and improve exercise capacity, as shown in Illustration 5-12.[72,77,78] Cardiac rehabilitation combines exercise therapy with targeted programming to address heart disease risk factors like high cholesterol and tobacco cessation with education on disease management, medications, and nutrition, as well as social and emotional support to improve well-being.[72,77-79]

Cardiac rehabilitation starts while patients are hospitalized and continues after hospital discharge in an outpatient clinic for 12 weeks.[68] Patients typically attend group sessions 3 to 5 days per week, exercising at 50% to 80% of their maximal exercise capacity.[79] The workout routine consists of a brief warmup, followed by supervised aerobic exercise lasting 20 to 60 minutes, and a brief cool down. Exercise training has been shown to lower blood pressure, improve blood glucose control, relieve anxiety and stress, and lead to weight loss, which greatly benefits the management of HF.

Multiple health professionals collaborate to advance improved patient outcomes in this program, making it an excellent model of interprofessional practice; some examples include cardiologists, dietitians/nutritionists, nurses, pharmacists, physical therapists, and psychologists. Pharmacists like Ada serve as educators to both patients and other health professionals.[14,15] An important role of the pharmacist is to review all medications that the patient is taking, screening for potential drug interactions, duplications in therapy, and medication-related side effects.[15,27] They also review the patient's self-care plan, evaluating home blood pressure, heart rate, and weight measurements to optimize medication therapies.[80] Patients receive education on each medication, which includes indication for use, instructions on how to take, potential side effects, and how to monitor effectiveness. Pharmacists create individualized medication schedules and offer concrete steps patients can take to ensure adherence. Importantly, they also help patients recognize the early symptoms of HF exacerbations, which can allow for interventions that might stave off hospitalizations like Mrs. Simmons'.

Heart failure is a complex condition associated with substantial burden on patients and health systems. Management of HF includes evidence-based medication therapy, which can be difficult to manage for patients and caregivers. Engagement with a cardiology pharmacist in cardiac rehabilitation has many positive benefits, including reductions in medication errors, improvements in medication adherence, decreased hospitalizations, and improvements in quality of life.[73,80,81] Patients with HF report that the information received from cardiology pharmacists positively influences their beliefs about medications and improves their adherence to critically important medications.[75] Additionally, medication adherence improves when patients have a good relationship with their pharmacist, as seen in this illustrated case.

DISCUSSION QUESTIONS FOR "EDUCATOR"

1. Medical and medication misinformation is common online, with real consequences, as depicted in the illustrated case "Educator." What can pharmacists and other health professionals do to guard against this?

2. In Illustration 5-9, Mrs. Simmons tells the physician that she has had to sleep in her recliner. Based on your understanding of heart failure, what might be an appropriate physiological explanation for this?

3. Mrs. Simmons stopped taking furosemide because she attributed a recent fall to this medication. After her hospitalization, she was re-prescribed this medication, along with other medications associated with dizziness and falls. Presumably, this would cause anxiety and stress, something no one seems to have directly addressed. What would you tell this patient to help alleviate her concerns?

4. Significant health benefits are gained by enrollment in cardiac rehabilitation, yet only 20% to 30% of eligible patients with cardiovascular disease participate. What are potential reasons for this trend?

5. Cardiac rehabilitation involves group exercise sessions where patients can share with each other their own experiences and challenges with HF. What are possible benefits of patients sharing information and advice with each other? What are potential negative consequences?

EMPOWERMENT: An Illustrated Case Study

Story by Andrea L. Porter & Joseph A. Zorek
Illustrations by George Folz, © 2019 Board of Regents of the University of Wisconsin System

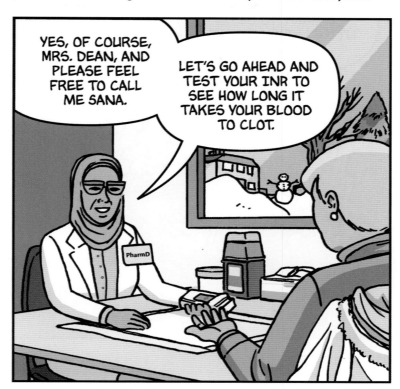

Illustration 5-13

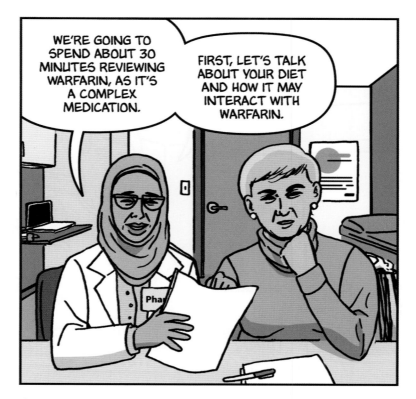

Illustration 5-14

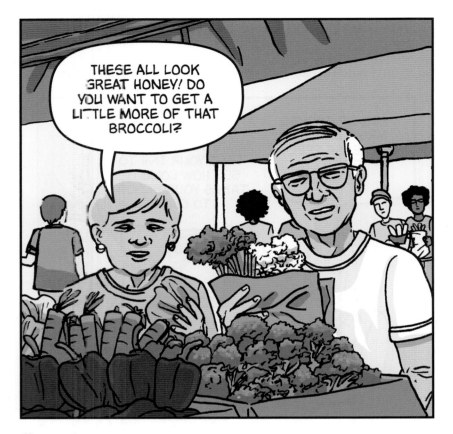

Illustration 5-15

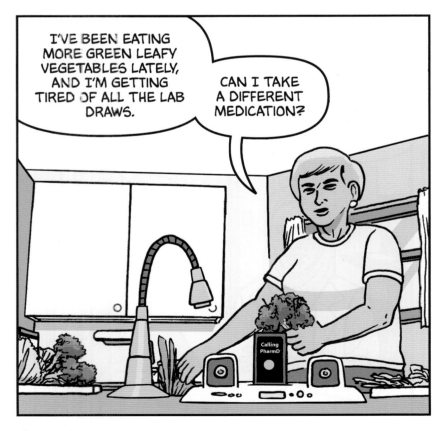

Illustration 5-16

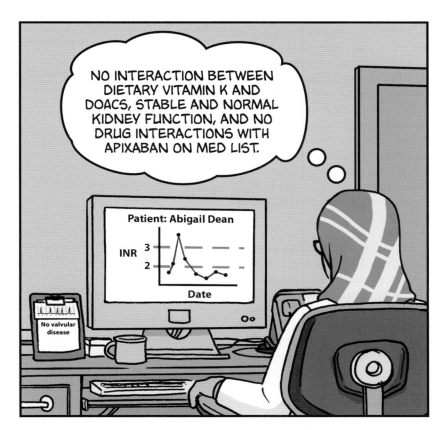

Illustration 5-17

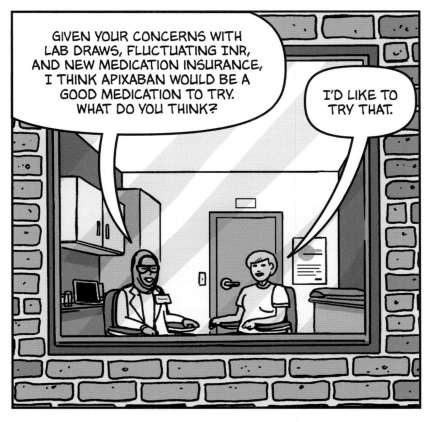

Illustration 5-18

Thoughts on "Empowerment"

The main character in the illustrated case "Empowerment" is an older adult named Abigail Dean, who was recently diagnosed with a common heart rhythm disorder called atrial fibrillation (AFib).[81,82] The heart has four chambers: two atria located in the top of the heart and two ventricles located in the bottom. The coordinated contraction and relaxation of these chambers produces the heartbeat. In a healthy heart, this cycle of contraction and relaxation leads to a smooth and predictable flow of blood through each chamber (i.e., inside the heart). This ultimately allows for blood to get pumped out of the heart and into the arteries, where it delivers oxygen to tissues and vital organs, such as the brain, liver, and kidneys.

Atrial fibrillation occurs when the atria beat irregularly and faster than normal, something Mrs. Dean felt that prompted her to visit her physician.[82] When this happens, the blood does not flow normally through the chambers of the heart. Typically, this results in a slowing down of blood flow. This is dangerous because blood that does not move normally is at risk of clotting through a process called coagulation, where blood-clotting proteins come together with platelets to form a blood clot. This is the same process that allows a cut to stop bleeding, ultimately forming a scab that allows a wound to heal. The consequences of this happening inside the chambers of the heart can be catastrophic. If a clot forms there, a heartbeat can cause the clot to move out of the heart and into the brain. A blood clot in the brain can be devastating as it blocks the flow of blood from reaching that part of the brain, depriving it of oxygen. The end result is an ischemic stroke (i.e., stroke caused by restricted blood flow) or mini-stroke, also known as a transient ischemic attack, or TIA.[83]

Common symptoms of a stroke include weakness, numbness, or facial drooping on one side of the body, as well as difficulty speaking.[83] If a patient is experiencing these symptoms, they should call 9-1-1 and seek medical attention immediately, as the window of time available to break up the clot and restore blood flow and oxygen to the brain is small before permanent damage is caused. Oxygen deprivation to the brain can lead to the affected brain tissue essentially dying, and all bodily functions controlled or impacted by that part of the brain will be affected. This might take the form of permanent loss of speech, or the inability to walk, for example. Sadly, the primary cause of serious long-term disability in the United States is stroke, occurring in approximately 3% of males and 2% of females with a disability.[2] Patients with AFib are at a five times greater risk for stroke compared to patients with a regular and normal heart rhythm.[81] That said, the critical importance of cardiology pharmacists, like the one depicted in "Empowerment," to maximize the safe and effective use of medications to prevent blood clots and stroke, cannot be overstated. To learn more about pharmacists' contributions to the treatment of ischemic stroke, see the illustrated case "One Day" in Chapter 10 Emergency Medicine.

Based on recent studies, the risk of developing AFib is between one in three to one in four individuals.[2] By 2030, it is estimated that 12.1 million people will have AFib in the United States.[2] There is a strong correlation between increasing age and the incidence of AFib.[81] Other risk factors include high blood pressure, heart disease, alcohol consumption, family history, and other chronic conditions such as diabetes, asthma, and hyperthyroidism.[84]

The most common symptom of AFib is fatigue or tiredness.[81,82] Patients may also experience palpitations or a noticeable heartbeat, shortness of breath, low blood pressure, heart failure, or a loss of consciousness or syncope. Some patients experience no symptoms at all.

There are two main treatment strategies with AFib.[82] The first is to regulate the heartbeat (i.e., heart rate, heart rhythm), and the other is to prevent blood clots from forming inside the heart (Table 5-5).[85-89] The good news is that blood clots and stroke can be largely prevented by taking a medication called an anticoagulant.[82] Anticoagulants prevent blood from clotting by blocking the action of proteins that help form blood clots.[90] There are two main categories of anticoagulants: vitamin K antagonists and direct oral anticoagulants (DOACs).

In the 1930s, a team of chemists led by Dr. Karl Paul Link at the University of Wisconsin–Madison set out to identify the chemical compound responsible for sweet clover disease.[91,92] It was known at the time that spoiled, moldy sweet clover hay induced an anticoagulated state in animals who ate it. Many cattle, for example, experienced significant bleeding and died. After many years, Link and his team isolated the causative chemical compound. Further research led to a more potent version, which was used initially to kill rodents by causing internal bleeding. The resulting medication for humans was named warfarin after the Wisconsin Alumni Research Foundation, or WARF. Warfarin began to be used to prevent blood clots in humans beginning in the 1950s.[81,92]

The history of contemporary pharmacy practice is rooted in warfarin therapy. Anticoagulation clinics were established in the United States shortly after warfarin use gained in popularity, and it was not long until pharmacists became directly involved.[93,94] One of the earliest published examples involved pharmacists at the Medical College of Virginia in 1979 directly managing patients taking warfarin, including adjusting doses, and ordering labs to monitor safety and effectiveness. This pioneering work has since become standard practice throughout the United States, where pharmacist-run anticoagulation clinics have been shown to reduce bleeding and clotting events, as well as healthcare utilization, including hospitalizations, emergency department visits, and healthcare costs.[95-100] Those interested in a more in-depth exploration of pharmacists contributing to interprofessional care in emergency departments are encouraged to read Chapter 10 Emergency Medicine and the illustrated cases "Life & Death" and "One Day."

Illustration 5-13 depicts an exchange between Dr. Sana Nazir, a cardiology pharmacist who specializes in anticoagulation, and

Table 5-5. Categories and Examples of Medications Commonly Used to Treat Atrial Fibrillation		
Category	**Medication Examples***	**Physiologic Effect**
Medications to prevent blood clots		
Vitamin K antagonists	▪ warfarin (Coumadin)	Prevent the formation of blood clots by blocking the action of proteins that lead to their formation
Direct oral anticoagulants	▪ apixaban (Eliquis) ▪ dabigatran (Pradaxa) ▪ edoxaban (Savaysa) ▪ rivaroxaban (Xarelto)	
Medications to control heart rate		
Beta-blockers	▪ atenolol (Tenormin) ▪ bisoprolol (Zebeta) ▪ carvedilol (Coreg) ▪ metoprolol (Lopressor, Toprol) ▪ propranolol (Inderal)	Control and reduce the rate of the heartbeat to improve symptoms of atrial fibrillation
Digitalis glycosides	▪ digoxin (Lanoxin)	
Non-dihydropyridine calcium channel blockers	▪ diltiazem (Cardizem) ▪ verapamil (Calan, Verelan)	
Medications to control heart rhythm		
Antiarrhythmics	▪ amiodarone** (Cordarone) ▪ dofetilide (Tikosyn) ▪ dronedarone (Multaq) ▪ flecainide (Tambocor) ▪ propafenone (Rhythmol) ▪ sotalol (Betapace)	Restore and maintain a normal heartbeat rhythm to improve symptoms of atrial fibrillation

* Medication examples presented in alphabetical order as "generic name (Brand Name)."

** Amiodarone can also be used to control heart rate.

Mrs. Dean. After diagnosis, Mrs. Dean's cardiologist started her on warfarin with a referral to Sana. The cardiologist performed a risk-benefit analysis, balancing results from a variety of laboratory and diagnostic tests with Mrs. Dean's preferences, to determine if anticoagulation therapy would be appropriate.[81,101] For some patients, even though they have AFib, their risk for stroke may not be high enough to warrant starting an anticoagulant. For others, their risk of experiencing a serious adverse drug event, such as severe bleeding, may be too high to initiate anticoagulation.

Sana runs an anticoagulation clinic, which she operates through a collaborative practice agreement with the cardiologist who diagnosed Mrs. Dean's AFib.[102] Based on this agreement, Sana will work with Mrs. Dean the same way she works with hundreds of other patients; that is, directly managing her anticoagulation therapy with a laser-sharp focus on preventing blood clots and the serious adverse drug events that have been associated with anticoagulants. These clinics monitor blood levels, educate patients, reverse over-anticoagulation, and manage anticoagulants around the time of surgical or invasive procedures. Most of these clinics are associated with hospitals or health systems and care is provided by pharmacists, nurses, and physician assistants.[103]

Wearing protective gloves and holding a point-of-care testing machine in Illustration 5-13, Sana is poised to prick Mrs. Dean's finger with a sharp device called a lancet to draw a drop of blood. She will transfer a sample of blood to a test strip, which will then be inserted into the machine to produce a reading called the International Normalized Ratio, or INR. The INR is a number that helps health professionals assess the amount of time it takes a warfarin patient's blood to clot compared to patients who are not taking warfarin.[94] The higher the INR, the more anticoagulated the patient's blood. For patients not on warfarin, a normal INR is around 1.0. For patients with AFib, the desired INR goal is between 2.0 and 3.0.[85] If the INR is too high, it increases the risk of bleeding, and if it is too low, there is an increased risk of clotting. Because INRs can vary based on many factors, it is critical for patients to maintain close contact with the health professionals managing their care. This is especially true at the start of warfarin therapy, as depicted in Illustration 5-13, when the daily dose is modified regularly until a stable, safe regimen is identified. Initially, the INR is monitored every 3 to 5 days, then every 1 week, 2 weeks, 4 weeks, and finally every 6 to 12 weeks if the patient is stable.

While the benefits of anticoagulation therapy in preventing stroke are clear, the associated risk of excessive bleeding is a serious concern.[81] Patients taking anticoagulants may notice increased bruising, gum bleeding when brushing their teeth, nosebleeds, or that minor cuts take longer to stop bleeding. More serious bleeding events such as gastrointestinal bleeding, bleeding inside the head, or severe bleeding elsewhere that does not stop can also occur. Because of these significant risks, healthcare organizations have additional precautions and processes in place for the safe use of all anticoagulants.[104]

Concerns about anticoagulation, for health professionals and patients alike, are warranted. An analysis of US emergency department visits related to adverse drug events identified the top 15 drugs implicated.[105] Highlighting the seriousness of their risk, and the importance of anticoagulation pharmacists like Sana, over 25% (4/15) of these were anticoagulants: warfarin, rivaroxaban, dabigatran, and an injectable anticoagulant not commonly used in AFib called enoxaparin (listed in order of most emergency department visits per medication). Medications that can cause significant harm to patients when not used correctly are called high-alert medications. The Institute for Safe Medication Practices has created lists of high-alert medications for a variety of healthcare settings, and anticoagulants appear on all of these lists due to their significant risks.[106-108]

Once anticoagulation is determined to be appropriate for the patient and a medication is selected, one of the next steps in the process is to empower the patient through education. Illustration 5-14 provides a snapshot of Sana providing this critically important service with regard to warfarin. Patient education tools, such as the handout Sana is using, can be helpful for patients to remember information covered during the education session.[109] Several key education points for all patients on anticoagulation therapy include signs and symptoms of bleeding and clotting, how to take the medication correctly, laboratory monitoring required, potential drug interactions, and what to do around the time of surgery or other procedures.

Illustration 5-14 emphasizes Sana's efforts to teach Mrs. Dean about drug-drug and drug-food interactions that are unique to warfarin. Warfarin has a significant number of drug interactions.[85] Some of these interactions increase the anticoagulant effect of warfarin while others decrease its effectiveness. As a result of warfarin's long history, the magnitude of interactions and the dose adjustments necessary are known for most medications, but not all. Alcohol interacts with warfarin and excess alcohol can increases its effectiveness, which can also increase the risk of bleeding.

Warfarin is also affected by the amount of vitamin K patients eat, as vitamin K prevents warfarin from working in the body.[90] An increase in vitamin K intake, in other words, will decrease the effectiveness of warfarin. If intake of vitamin K-rich food fluctuates, the patient's INR will fluctuate accordingly. Pharmacists like Sana work with patients taking warfarin to ensure they understand this connection, especially the heightened bleeding and clotting risks associated with an inconsistent vitamin K diet. The key is consistency; patients who enjoy eating vitamin K-rich foods can do so, as long as their intake remains stable from one week to the next. Examples of foods that are high in vitamin K include green leafy vegetables such as spinach, kale, and asparagus. Additional examples include broccoli, brussel sprouts, cabbage, collard greens, coleslaw, lettuce, and green tea.

The change of seasons between Illustrations 5-13 and 5-16 implies that several months have elapsed since initiation of Mrs. Dean's warfarin therapy. Set in a farmer's market replete with vitamin K-rich vegetables, Illustration 5-15 foreshadows a looming internal struggle for Mrs. Dean, which she shares via a telehealth appointment with Sana in Illustration 5-16. Due to her increased intake of vitamin K-containing vegetables, as well as her growing frustration with the amount of INR blood tests and frequent changes to her warfarin regimen, Mrs. Dean expresses an interest in switching to a different anticoagulant therapy, a DOAC, that requires less monitoring and is covered by her new medication insurance.

There are many patient characteristics and other considerations that play a role in determining optimal anticoagulant therapy. Since warfarin has been on the market since 1954, it has a broad range of indications (i.e., conditions approved for treatment by the US Food and Drug Administration).[85] The DOACs are a newer category of medications, having first come to market in the United States in 2010. That said, they are still being studied in some indications, and they have been found to be less effective than warfarin for patients with other conditions, such as those with AFib who also have certain types of valvular heart disease.[86-89,101,110] A reference to this valvular heart disease exclusion can be found on Sana's desk in Illustration 5-17, where she is shown deliberating if a DOAC can be used to address Mrs. Dean's preference to try something other than warfarin. The DOACs are more expensive than warfarin, and this can also play a role in medication selection.[81]

The most recent AFib treatment guidelines from the AHA recommend DOACs over warfarin, except for situations in which patients are unable to take a DOAC.[101] The illustrated case "Empowerment" draws attention to several comparative benefits of DOACs over warfarin, at least from the patient's perspective; namely, not needing to monitor vitamin K-containing food intake, and reducing the number of blood tests. Additionally, while there are important drug interactions with DOACs, the number of these is smaller in comparison to warfarin.[86-89] Perhaps the most important reasons for Sana to facilitate a change of therapy is that Mrs. Dean prefers one and her insurance now covers the cost of the medication. Empowering patients through shared decision making is a hallmark of the patient-centered, high-quality care that pharmacists provide in such settings.[111]

Management of anticoagulation is a common and vitally important role for pharmacists due to the severity of complications from bleeding and clotting if medications are used inappropriately. For many decades, pharmacists have improved the care and health outcomes of patients with atrial fibrillation through the careful and judicious management of warfarin. This level of high-quality care has continued with the newest category of anticoagulants, DOACs.[112] The illustrated case "Empowerment" shows the impact of a knowledgeable, engaging pharmacist who, through trusting relationships with her patients and physician partners, maximizes the safe and effective use of lifesaving medications.

DISCUSSION QUESTIONS FOR "EMPOWERMENT"

1. In the illustrated case "Empowerment," the pharmacist Sana manages Mrs. Dean's anticoagulation through a collaborative practice agreement with her cardiologist. What other health professionals might be involved in the care of patients like Mrs. Dean? How do you think Sana collaborates with them, coordinating her efforts with theirs?

2. Shared decision making is an important component of patient-centered care, as demonstrated in Illustration 5-18. Drawing upon your personal experiences receiving care from different health professionals, what do you think are the most effective ways to get patients engaged in their own care? How can health professionals activate, or empower, patients?

3. In Illustrations 5-15 and 5-16, we see that Mrs. Dean enjoys going to the farmer's market and that her diet is impacting the effectiveness of her medication. Have you ever had to make changes to your diet, or do you know someone who has (e.g., allergies, gluten intolerance, drug interactions)? Based on this experience/knowledge, what do you think the most pressing challenges are when it comes to behavior changes like these?

4. In Illustration 5-17, Mrs. Dean is shown discussing her health concerns with Sana over the phone. Have you ever received care or advice from a health professional over the phone or via computer? How did that differ from an in-person interaction? Which do you prefer, and why?

5. Warfarin requires frequent blood draws, which can become a nuisance as depicted in this illustrated case. However, confirming on a regular basis that the risks of stroke and bleeding have been minimized can be comforting to some patients. For most medications, patients do not typically have access to this real-time information. Which would you prefer, enduring frequent tests to obtain knowledge of efficacy and safety, or simply trusting that the medication you are taking is doing what it was designed to do?

CHAPTER SUMMARY

- Cardiovascular disease (CVD) is the most common medical condition in the United States and is the leading cause of death worldwide.

- Cardiology pharmacists engage with patients and other health professionals in hospitals, outpatient clinics, and through cardiac rehabilitation programs, where they contribute to medication selection and monitoring, as well as provide education to help patients safely manage medications and nondrug therapies to control their CVD.

- The participation of pharmacists on interprofessional cardiovascular teams improves health outcomes and decreases medication errors and adverse drug events.

- Hypertension is the most common CVD in the world—uncontrolled, it puts patients at risk of developing heart failure and/or experiencing a heart attack or stroke.

- Pharmacists are well-trained and -positioned within healthcare to help patients reach their blood pressure goals by educating them on their medications and lifestyle changes, as well as appropriate blood pressure measurement techniques.

- Medication management by pharmacists improves patient adherence to evidence-based therapies for heart failure and engagement in self-care, which decreases the risk of hospitalizations due to heart failure exacerbations.

- Cardiac rehabilitation is an important component of care for patients with CVD to prevent hospitalizations, reduce the risk for future cardiovascular events, and improve exercise capacity.

- Pharmacist-run anticoagulation clinics have been shown to reduce bleeding and clotting events in patients who have atrial fibrillation and other conditions, which minimizes hospitalizations, emergency department visits, and healthcare costs.

REFERENCES

1. Brazier Y. What is cardiology? Available at http://www.medicalnewstoday.com/ articles/248935.phpMedicalnewstoday.com. Accessed April 13, 2020.

2. Benjamin EJ, Munter P, Alonso A, et al. Heart disease and stroke statistics—2019 update: a report from the American Heart Association. *Circulation.* 2019;139:e56-e528.

3. Cardiology Today. What is cardiology? Available at http://www.healio.com/cardiology/news/online /%7B5d853196-9296-42f2-8b94-340a34f3d605%7D/what-is-cardiology. Accessed April 13, 2020.

4. National Center for Health Statistics. National Health and Nutrition Examination Survey (NHANES) public use data files. Available at http://www.cdc.gov/nchs/nhanes/. Accessed April 1, 2020.

5. Fryar CD, Chen TC, Li X. Prevalence of uncontrolled risk factors for cardiovascular disease: United States, 1999–2010. *NCHS Data Brief.* 2012;103:1-8.

6. National Center for Health Statistics. National Vital Statistics System: public use data file documentation: mortality multiple cause-of-death microdata files. Available at http://www.cdc.gov/nchs/data/nvsr/nvsr68/ nvsr68_06-508.pdf. Accessed April 15, 2020.

7. Mosca L, Hammond G, Mochari-Greenberger H, Towfighi A, Albert MA. Fifteen-year trends in awareness of heart disease in women: results of a 2012 American Heart Association national survey. *Circulation.* 2013;127:1254-1263.

8. Global Status Report on Noncommunicable Diseases 2014. Geneva, Switzerland: World Health Organization; 2014. Available at http://apps.who.int/iris/bitstream/10665/148114/1/9789241564854_eng.pdf. Accessed April 25, 2020.

9. Centers for Disease Control and Prevention. Prevalence and most common causes of disability among adults: United States, 2005. *MMWR Morb Mortal Wkly Rep.* 2009;58:421-426.

10. Yang Q, Cogswell ME, Flanders WD, et al. Trends in cardiovascular health metrics and associations with all-cause and CVD mortality among US adults. *JAMA*. 2014;307:1273-1283.

11. American Heart Association. Heart attack or sudden cardiac arrest: how are they different? Available at http://www.heart.org/en/health-topics/heart-attack/about-heart-attacks/heart-attack-or-sudden-cardiac-arrest-how-are-they-different. Accessed April 14, 2020.

12. American Heart Association. About cardiac arrest. Available at http://www.heart.org/en/health-topics/cardiac-arrest/about-cardiac-arrest. Accessed April 25, 2020.

13. Arnett DK, Blumenthal RS, Albert MA, et al. 2019 ACC/AHA guidelines on the primary prevention of cardiovascular disease. *J Am Coll Cardiol*. 2019;74:e177-e232.

14. Dunn SP, Birtcher KK, Beavers CJ, et al. The role of the clinical pharmacist in the care of patients with cardiovascular disease. *J Am Coll Cardiol*. 2015;66:2129-2139.

15. Omboni S, Caserini M. Effectiveness of pharmacist's intervention in the management of cardiovascular disease. *Open Heart*. 2018;5:e000687.

16. Ng TM, DiDomenico RJ, Ripley TL, et al. An opinion paper of the cardiology practice and research network of the American College of Clinical Pharmacy: recommendations for training of cardiovascular pharmacy specialists in postgraduate year 2 residency programs. *J Am Coll Clin Pharm*. 2020;3:95-108.

17. The Joint Commission. Comprehensive Cardiac Center Certification Review Process Guide. Available at http://www.jointcommission.org/en/accreditation-and-certification/certification/certifications-by-setting/hospital-certifications/cardiac-certification/advanced-cardiac/comprehensive-cardiac-center-certification/. Accessed April 15, 2020.

18. CardioSmart. Your health care team. Available at http://www.cardiosmart.org/Heart-Basics/Your-Health-Care-Team. Accessed April 13, 2020.

19. American Heart Association. Your heart failure healthcare team. Available at http://www.heart.org/en/health-topics/heart-failure/living-with-heart-failure-and-managing-advanced-hf/your-heart-failure-healthcare-team. Accessed April 13, 2020.

20. CardioSmart. What is a cardiologist? Available at http://www.cardiosmart.org/Heart-Basics/What-is-a-Cardiologist. Accessed April 13, 2020.

21. Bello D, Shah NB, Edep ME, Tateo IM, Massie BM. Self-reported differences between cardiologists and heart failure specialists in the management of chronic heart failure. *J Am Coll Cardiol*. 1999;138:100-107.

22. Milfred-LaForest SK, Chow SL, DiDomenicao RJ, et al. Clinical pharmacy services in heart failure: An opinion paper from the Heart Failure Society of America and American College of Clinical Pharmacy Cardiology Practice and Research Network. *Pharmacotherapy*. 2013;33:529-548.

23. Magalhaes GF, Santos GN, Rosa ME, Nobalat Lde A. Medication reconciliation in patients hospitalized in a cardiology unit. *PLoS One*. 2014;9(12):e115491.

24. The Joint Commission. National patient safety goals effective July 2020 for the hospital program. Available at http://www.jointcommission.org/-/media/tjc/documents/standards/national-patient-safety-goals/2020/npsg_chapter_hap_jul2020.pdf. Accessed April 16, 2020.

25. Rogers G, Alper E, Brunelle D, et al. Reconciling medications at admission: safe practice recommendations and implementation strategies. *Jt Comm Qual Patient Saf*. 2006;32:37-50.

26. Anderson SL, Marrs JC. A review of the role of the pharmacist in heart failure transition of care. *Adv Ther*. 2018;35:311-323.

27. Ferdinand KC, Yadav K, Nasser SA, et al. Disparities in hypertension and cardiovascular disease in blacks: the critical role of medication adherence. *J Clin Hypertens*. 2017;19:1015-1024.

28. American College of Cardiology. Clinical topics. Available at https://www.acc.org/clinical-topics. Accessed April 26, 2020.

29. Soar J, Connino MW, Maconochie I, et al. 2018 international consensus on cardiopulmonary resuscitation and emergency cardiovascular care science with treatment recommendations summary. *Circulation*. 2018;138:e714-e730.

30. Link MS, Berkow LC, Kudenchuk PJ. Part 7: adult advanced cardiovascular life support: 2015 American Heart Association guidelines update for adult cardiopulmonary resuscitation and emergency cardiovascular care. *Circulation*. 2015;132 (18 suppl 2):s444-s464.

31. Lipshutz AKM, Morloc LL, Shore AD, et al. Medication errors associated with code situation in U.S. hospitals: direct and collateral damage. *Jt Comm J Qual Patient Saf*. 2008;34:46-56.

32. American Stroke Association. About stroke. Available at http://www.stroke.org/en/about-stroke. Accessed April 25, 2020.

33. Powers WJ, Rabins AA, Ackerson T, et al. 2018 guidelines for the early management of patients with acute ischemic stroke: a guideline for healthcare professionals from the American Heart Association/American Stroke Association. *Stroke*. 2018;49:e46-e99.

34. Rech MA, Bennett S, Donahey E. Pharmacist participation in acute ischemic stroke decreases door-to-needle time to recombinant tissue plasminogen activator. *Ann Pharmacother*. 2017;51:1084-1089.

35. Monks DT, Springer M, Goomber R, Li PC. Did you hear the one about the policeman, the doctor, and the pharmacist at 30,000 feet? *BMJ Case Rep*. 2014;2014:bcr2014206485.

36. American Society of Health-System Pharmacists. Residency information. Available at https://www.ashp.org/Professional-Development/Residency-Information?loginreturnUrl=SSOCheckOnly. Accessed May 31, 2020.

37. Board of Pharmacy Specialties. Cardiology pharmacy. Available at http://www.bpsweb.org/bps-specialties/cardiology-pharmacy/#1517761118361-6c02bae3-f5a01517780015777. Accessed April 15, 2020.

38. National Center for Health Statistics NCHS Fact Sheet, 2017. National Health and Nutrition Examination Survey. Available at http://www.cdc.gov/nchs/data/factsheets/factsheet_nhanes.pdf. Accessed January 13, 2020.

39. Whelton PK, Carey RM, Aronow WS, et al. 2017 ACC/AHA/AAPA/ABC/ACPM/AGS/APhA/ASH/ASPC/NMA/PCNA guideline for the prevention, detection, evaluation, and management of high blood pressure in adults: a report of the American College of Cardiology/American Heart Association task force on clinical practice guidelines. *Hypertension*. 2018;71(6):e13-e115.

40. Flint AC, Conell C, Ren X, et al. Effect of systolic and diastolic BP on cardiovascular outcomes. *N Engl J Med*. 2019;381:243-251.

41. Centers for Disease Control and Prevention. Health, United States, 2011: Table 51. End-stage renal disease patients, by selected characteristics: United States, selected years 1980–2010. Available at www.cdc.gov/nchs/data/hus/2011/051.pdf. Accessed May 31, 2020.

42. Ettehad D, Emdin CA, Kiran A, et al. BP lowering for prevention of cardiovascular disease and death: a systematic review and meta-analysis. *Lancet.* 2015;387:957-967.

43. Clement D. Poor BP control. What can we do? *J Hypertens.* 2017;35:1368-1370.

44. American Heart Association. Available at https://www.heart.org/en/health-topics/high-blood-pressure/why-high-blood-pressure-is-a-silent-killer. Accessed April 20, 2020.

45. Margolis KL, Asche SE, Dehmer SP, et al. Long-term outcomes of the effects of home BP telemonitoring and pharmacist management on BP among adults with uncontrolled hypertension: follow-up of a cluster randomized clinical trial. *JAMA Netw Open.* 2018;1:e181617.

46. Anderegg MD, Gums TH, Uribe L, et al. Pharmacist interventions for BP control in patients with diabetes and/or chronic kidney disease. *Pharmacotherapy.* 2018;38:309-318.

47. Okada H, Onda M, Shoji M, et al. Effects of lifestyle advice provided by pharmacists on BP: The COMmunity Pharmacists ASSist for BP (COMPASS-BP) randomized trial. *Biosci Trends.* 2018;11:632-639.

48. Asche SE, O'Connor PJ, Dehmer SP, et al. Patient characteristics associated with greater BP control in a randomized trial of home BP telemonitoring and pharmacist management. *J Am Soc Hypertens.* 2016;10:873-880.

49. Carter BL, Rogers M, Daly J, Zheng S, James PA. The potency of team-based care interventions for hypertension. *Arch Intern Med.* 2009;169:1748-1755.

50. Manolakis PG, Skelton JB. Pharmacists' contribution to primary care in the United States collaborating to address unmet patient care needs: the emerging role for pharmacists to address the shortage of primary care providers. *Am J Pharm Educ.* 2010;74:S7.

51. Irons BK, Meyerrose G, Laguardia S, Hazel K, Seifert CF. A collaborative cardiologist-pharmacist care model to improve hypertension management in patients with or at high risk for cardiovascular disease. *Pharm Pract.* 2012;10:25-32.

52. Hirsch JD, Steers N, Adler DS, et al. A randomized pragmatic trial of primary care based pharmacist-physician collaborative medication therapy management for hypertension. *Clin Ther.* 2014;36:1244-1254.

53. Heisler M, Hofer TP, Schmittdiel JA, et al. Improving BP control through a clinical pharmacist outreach program in patients with diabetes mellitus in 2 high-performing health systems. *Circulation.* 2012;125:2863-2872.

54. Hunter RW, Bailey MA. Hyperkalemia: pathophysiology, risk factors, and consequences. *Nephrol Dial Transplant.* 2019;34(suppl 3):iii2-iii11.

55. Tsuyuki RT, Beahm NP, Okada H, Al Hamarneh YN. Pharmacists as accessible primary health care providers: review of the evidence. *Can Pharm J.* 2018;151:4-5.

56. Sun Z. Aging, arterial stiffness and hypertension. *Hypertension.* 2015;65:252-256.

57. Franklin SS, Gustin W4th, Wong ND, et al. Hemodynamic patterns of age-related changes in BP. The Framingham Heart Study. *Circulation.* 1997;96:308-315.

58. Rimoldi SF, Scherrer U, Messerli FH. Secondary arterial hypertension: when, who, and how to screen? *Eur Heart J.* 2014;35:1245-1254.

59. Streeten DH, Anderson GHJr, Wagner S. Effect of age on response of secondary hypertension to specific treatment. *Am J Hypertens.* 1990;3:360-365.

60. Sinha AD, Agarwal R. Clinical pharmacology of antihypertensive therapy for the treatment of hypertension in CKD. *Clin J Am Soc Nephrol.* 2019;14:757-764.

61. Rossi GP, Bernini G, Caliumi C, et al. A prospective study of the prevalence of primary aldosteronism in 1,125 hypertensive patients. *J Am Coll Cardiol.* 2006;48:2293-2300.

62. Byrd JB, Turcu AF, Auchus RJ. Primary aldosteronism. Practical approach to diagnosis and management. *Circulation.* 2018;138:823-835.

63. Holaj R, Rosa J, Zelinka T, et al. Long-term effect of specific treatment of primary aldosteronism on carotid intima-media thickness. *J Hypertens.* 2015;33:874-882.

64. CardioSmart. How the heart works. Available at https://www.cardiosmart.org/Heart-Basics/How-the-Heart-Works. Accessed on April 9, 2020.

65. Mosterd A, Hoes AW. Clinical epidemiology of heart failure. *Heart.* 2007;93:1137-1146.

66. Yancy CW, Jessup M, Bozkurt B, et al. 2013 ACCF/AHA guideline for the management of heart failure: a report of the American College of Cardiology Foundation/American Heart Association Task Force on practice guidelines. *Circulation.* 2013;128:e240-e319.

67. Hill L, Carson MA, Vitale C. Care plans for the older heart failure patient. *Eur Heart J Suppl.* 2019;21(suppl L):L32-L35.

68. Flint KM, Pastva AM, Reeves GR. Cardiac rehabilitation in older adults with heart failure: fitting a square peg in a round hole. *Clin Geriatr Med.* 2019;35:517-526.

69. Page RL, O'Bryant CL, Dheng D, et al. Drugs that may cause or exacerbate heart failure. *Circulation.* 2016;134(6):e32-e69.

70. Goyal P, Gorodeski EZ, Marcum ZA, Forman DE. Cardiac rehabilitation to optimize medication regimens in heart failure. *Clin Geriatr Med.* 2019;35:549-560.

71. Clark AM, Davidson P, Currie K, et al. Understanding and promoting effective self-care during heart failure. *Curr Treat Options Cardiovasc Med.* 2010;12:1-9.

72. Yancy CW, Jessup M, Bozkurt B, et al. 2017 ACC/AHA/HFSA focused update of the 2013 ACCF/AHA guideline for the management of heart failure: a report of the American College of Cardiology/American Heart Association task force on clinical practice guidelines and the Heart Failure Society of America. *J Am Coll Cardiol.* 2017;70:776-803.

73. Anderson SL, Marrs JC. A review of the role of the pharmacist in heart failure transition of care. *Adv Ther.* 2018;35:311-323.

74. Goldgrab D, Balakumaran K, Kim MJ, Tabtabai SR. Updates in heart failure 30-day readmission prevention. *Heart Fail Rev.* 2019;24:177-187.

75. Mondesir FL, Levitan EB, Malla G, et al. Patient perspectives on factors influencing medication adherence among people with coronary heart disease (CHD) and CHD risk factors. *Patient Pref Adherence.* 2019;13:2017-2027.

76. Samsky MD, Lin L, Greene SJ, et al. Patient perceptions and familiarity with medical therapy for heart failure. *JAMA Cardiol.* 2019;5(3). [Epub ahead of print].

77. Kumar KR, Pina IL. Cardiac rehabilitation in older adults: new options. *Clin Cardiol.* 2020;43(2):163-170.

78. Thomas RJ, Huang HH. Cardiac rehabilitation for secondary prevention of cardiovascular disease: 2019 update. *Curr Treatment Options Cardiovasc Med.* 2019;21(10):56.

79. McMahon SR, Ades PA, Thompson PD. The role of cardiac rehabilitation in patients with heart disease. *Trends Cardiovasc Med*. 2017;27(6):420-425.

80. Pape ZA, Hale G, Joseph T, Moreau C, Wolowich WR. Impact of pharmacist-led heart failure tool kits on patient-reported self-care behaviors in a primary care-based accountable care organization. *J Am Pharm Assoc*. 2019;59:891-895.

81. January CT, Wann LS, Alpert JS, et al. 2014 AHA/ACC/HRS guideline for the management of patients with atrial fibrillation: a report of the American College of Cardiology/American Heart Association Task Force on Practice Guidelines and the Heart Rhythm Society. *J Am Coll Cardiol*. 2014;64:e1-e76.

82. Parmet S, Lynm C, Glass RM. JAMA patient page. Atrial fibrillation. *JAMA*. 2007;298:2820.

83. Jin J. JAMA patient page. Warning signs of a stroke. *JAMA*. 2014;311:1704.

84. American Heart Association. Who is at risk for atrial fibrillation (AF or AFib)? Available at http://www.heart.org/en/health-topics/atrial-fibrillation/who-is-at-risk-for-atrial-fibrillation-af-or-afib. Accessed May 30, 2020.

85. Coumadin Package Insert. Bristol-Myers Squibb Company. July 2017. Available at https://packageinserts.bms.com/pi/pi_coumadin.pdf. Accessed May 31, 2020.

86. Eliquis Package Insert. Bristol-Myers Squibb Company. November 2019. Available at http://packageinserts.bms.com/pi/pi_eliquis.pdf. Accessed May 31, 2020.

87. Xarelto Package Insert. Janssen Pharmaceuticals, Inc. November 2019. Available at http://www.janssenlabels.com/package-insert/product-monograph/prescribing-information/XARELTO-pi.pdf. Accessed May 31, 2020.

88. Savaysa Package Insert. Daiichi Sankyo, Inc. August 2019. Available at https://dsi.com/prescribing-information-portlet/getPIContent?productName=Savaysa&inline=true. Accessed May 31, 2020.

89. Pradaxa Package Insert. Boehringer Ingelheim Pharmaceuticals, Inc. November 2019. Available at https://docs.boehringer-ingelheim.com/Prescribing%20Information/PIs/Pradaxa/Pradaxa.pdf. Accessed May 31, 2020.

90. Sugerman DT. JAMA patient page. Blood thinners. *JAMA*. 2013;310:2579.

91. Wardrop D, Keeling D. The story of the discovery of heparin and warfarin. *Br J Haematol*. 2008;141:757-763.

92. Copeland CE, Six CK. A tale of two anticoagulants: warfarin and heparin. *J Surg Educ*. 2009;66:176-181.

93. Nutescu EA. The future of anticoagulation clinics. *J Thromb Thrombolysis*. 2003;16(1-2):61-63.

94. Reinders TP, Steinke WE. Pharmacist management of anticoagulant therapy in ambulant patients. *Am J Hosp Pharm*. 1979;36:645-648.

95. Scrivens JJ, Magalian P, Crozier GA. Cost-effective clinical pharmacy services in a veterans administration drop-in clinic. *Am J Hosp Pharm*. 1983;40:1952-1953.

96. Manzoor BS, Cheng WH, Lee JC, Uppuluri EM, Nutescu EA. Quality of pharmacist-managed anticoagulation therapy in long-term ambulatory settings: a systematic review. *Ann Pharmacother*. 2017;51:1122-1137.

97. Downing A, Mortimer M, Hiers J. Impact of a pharmacist-driven warfarin management protocol on achieving therapeutic International Normalized Ratios. *Am J Health Syst Pharm*. 2016;73(5 suppl 1):S69-S73.

98. Rudd KM, Dier JG. Comparison of two different models of anticoagulation management services with usual medical care. *Pharmacotherapy*. 2010;30:330-338.

99. Zhou S, Sheng XY, Xiang Q, Wang ZN, Zhou Y, Cui YM. Comparing the effectiveness of pharmacist-managed warfarin anticoagulation with other models: a systematic review and meta-analysis. *J Clin Pharm Ther*. 2016;41:602-611.

100. Witt DM, Clark NP, Kaatz S, Schnurr T, Ansell JE. Guidance for the practical management of warfarin therapy in the treatment of venous thromboembolism. *J Thromb Thrombolysis*. 2016;41:187-205.

101. January CT, Wann LS, Calkins H, et al. 2019 AHA/ACC/HRS focused update of the 2014 AHA/ACC/HRS guideline for the management of patients with atrial fibrillation: a report of the American College of Cardiology/American Heart Association task force on clinical practice guidelines and the Heart Rhythm Society in collaboration with the Society of Thoracic Surgeons. *Circulation*. 2019;140:e125-e151.

102. Centers for Disease Control and Prevention. Collaborative practice agreements and pharmacists' patient care services: a resource for pharmacists. Atlanta, GA: US Department of Health and Human Services, Centers for Disease Control and Prevention; 2013. Available at http://www.cdc.gov/dhdsp/pubs/docs/ Translational_Tools_Pharmacists.pdf. Accessed April 17, 2020.

103. Nutescu EA. Anticoagulation management services: entering a new era. *Pharmacotherapy*. 2010;30:327-329.

104. The Joint Commission. National patient safety goals effective January 2020: hospital accreditation program. Available at https://www.jointcommission.org/assets/1/6/NPSG_Chapter_HAP_Jan2020.pdf. Accessed May 31, 2020.

105. Shehab N, Lovegrove MC, Geller AI, Rose KO, Weidle NJ, Budnitz DS. US emergency department visits for outpatient adverse drug events, 2013-2014. *JAMA*. 2016;316:2115-2125.

106. Institute for Safe Medication Practices. High-alert medications in community/ambulatory settings. Available at http://www.ismp.org/recommendations/high-alert-medications-community-ambulatory-list. Accessed May 31, 2020.

107. Institute for Safe Medication Practices. High-alert medications in acute care settings. Available at http://www.ismp.org/recommendations/high-alert-medications-acute-list. Accessed May 31, 2020.

108. Institute for Safe Medication Practices. High-alert medications in long-term care (LTC) settings. Available at http://www.ismp.org/recommendations/high-alert-medications-long-term-care-list. Accessed May 31, 2020.

109. U.S. National Library of Medicine: Medline Plus. Choosing effective patient education materials. Available at http://medlineplus.gov/ency/patientinstructions/000455.htm. Accessed May 31, 2020.

110. Pengo V, Denas G, Zoppellaro G, et al. Rivaroxaban vs warfarin in high-risk patients with antiphospholipid syndrome. *Blood*. 2018;132:1365-1371.

111. Zeballos-Palacios CL, Hargraves IG, Noseworthy PA, et al. Developing a conversation aid to support shared decision making: reflections on designing anticoagulation choice. *Mayo Clin Proc*. 2019;94:686-696.

112. Barnes GD, Nallamothu BK, Sales AE, Froehlich JB. Reimagining anticoagulation clinics in the era of direct oral anticoagulants. *Circ Cardiovasc Qual Outcomes*. 2016;9:182-185.

CHAPTER 6

Pediatrics

Featuring the Illustrated Case Studies "Accidental" & "All In"

Authors

Sarah E. Kubes, Monica C. Bogenschutz, Jessica M. Bergsbaken, & Joseph A. Zorek

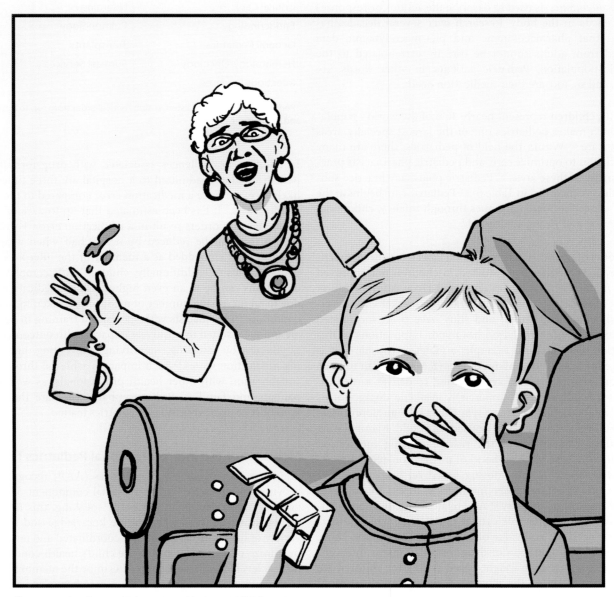

Illustration by George Folz, © 2020 McGraw-Hill Education

BACKGROUND

Pediatrics is a field devoted to the health and well-being of infants, children, and adolescents up to the age of 18 years.[1] A common framework for categorizing pediatric patients by age is presented in Table 6-1.[1,2] A holistic approach to caring for the physical, mental, social, and psychological needs of children is required for them to achieve their full potential.[3] Growth and development during this phase of life is characterized by ongoing and often rapid change, which presents challenges that make caring for this population unique. Medications may act differently when administered to a child compared to an adult.[1] For example, the amount of drug absorbed through the gastrointestinal tract into the bloodstream, how efficiently the drug is then broken down by the liver, and how quickly it gets eliminated from the body through the kidneys can differ within the pediatric population.[4] The movement of drugs, how they get into and out of the body, is called *pharmacokinetics*. A similar term, *pharmacodynamics*, is used to describe the actions or responses a drug elicits in the body. Research over several decades has revealed that pharmacokinetic and pharmacodynamic data obtained from adults cannot be directly extrapolated to the pediatric population. Pediatric patients, in other words, are unique, and so, too, are their medication needs.

Currently, children represent nearly 30% of the world's population, which makes pediatrics one of the largest specialty areas in healthcare.[2,5] Within the field of pediatrics, there are many subspecialties to optimize care, and pediatric pharmacists practice in many of these areas.[6,7] Pediatric pharmacy practice subspecialties are included in Table 6-2.[7] Pediatric care begins at the time of conception and continues through infancy, childhood, adolescence, and young adulthood.[1]

Nearly 50% of medications are used off label in children; meaning, they have neither been studied in children nor approved for use in children by the US Food and Drug Administration (FDA).[8] Most medications available on the market were developed with adults in mind, and thus have been formulated accordingly. Drug formulation has major implications in this population. Consider, for example, a tablet or capsule that is too large for a child to swallow, or a device, such as an inhaler, that requires sophisticated coordination to deliver a medication. As a result, many commercially available dosage forms require manipulation to transform them into an appropriate formulation that can be taken or used by a child. Manipulating medications can introduce the risk of causing medication errors and increase the likelihood of medication-related problems. Medication use and dosing based on body weight in children often require closer monitoring to ensure safe and effective medication delivery.[1,8] As it relates to medications, children represent a vulnerable patient population, which underscores the need for, and value of, pediatric pharmacists. Those interested in manipulation of drug formulations or interventions to ensure accurate weight-based dosing for children are encouraged to explore the illustrated cases "Transformation" and "Organized Chaos," respectively, in Chapter 2 Community Pharmacy.

Table 6-1. Categorization Scheme for Pediatric Patients by Age

Age Group	Age Range
Premature neonate	Any age prior to 37 weeks' gestation
Neonate	Birth–1 month
Infant	1 month–2 years
Child	2–11 years
Early adolescence	12–14 years
Middle adolescence	15–17 years
Late adolescence	18–21 years

Table 6-2. Subspecialties* in Pediatric Pharmacy Practice

Antimicrobial Stewardship	Neonatology
Cardiology	Nephrology
Critical Care	Neurology
Endocrinology	Pulmonology
General Pediatrics	Transplant
Hematology/Oncology	Surgical Services
Infectious Diseases	

* Pediatric subspecialties listed in alphabetical order from top to bottom and left to right.

In addition to challenges associated with drug formulations, pediatric patients admitted to a hospital are three times more likely to experience a medication error compared to their adult counterparts.[9] It has been estimated that up to 27% of pediatric medication orders result in a medication error. Fortunately, such errors can be reduced by nearly half when a pediatric pharmacist is embedded as a member of the interprofessional pediatrics team.[9] Additionally, children with complex health conditions can be at an even higher risk of medication errors due to an increasing number of medications taken to treat each condition.[10] Pharmacists with specialized training in pediatrics are uniquely suited to positively impact health outcomes in this population by assessing, identifying, preventing, and resolving medication issues.[11] Such impact is achieved through close collaboration with other health professionals, as well as with patients and families. Pediatric pharmacists are thus valued members of interprofessional pediatrics teams.

Members of the Interprofessional Pediatrics Team

The American Academy of Pediatrics (AAP) recognizes that providing team-based care is a crucial component of a child's growth and development.[12] Broadly speaking, this is a model of healthcare delivery whereby the knowledge and skills of a variety of health professionals are coordinated and leveraged to maximize patient outcomes.[12] The child's health condition and his/her level of acuity will often determine the members and size of the interprofessional team. Team members also vary by setting or a child's specific needs; that said, frequent team members include, in alphabetical order, child life personnel (trained to improve the experience of pediatric patients with illness), dentists, dietitians/nutritionists, nurse practitioners, nurses, occupational therapists, pharmacists, physical therapists, physician assistants, physicians, respiratory therapists, social workers, and speech-language pathologists.[13,14] Within the profession of medicine, there are many pediatric specialties, and these specialists play a crucial role in the health and well-being of children.[15]

Role of Pharmacists within the Interprofessional Pediatrics Team

The American Society of Health-System Pharmacists (ASHP) and the Pediatric Pharmacy Association (PPA) collaborated to develop recommendations to guide the provision of pediatric pharmacy services in hospitals and health systems.[11] This guidance clarifies, for stakeholders inside and outside of pharmacy, the professional activities and contributions that can be expected of pediatric pharmacists to address numerous medication-related challenges in the provision of care to children.[11] Additionally, the AAP recommends that prescribers and other health professionals utilize pediatric pharmacists whenever available.[12] Given the array of pediatric subspecialties, as described, pharmacists can establish a practice site in nearly any setting. For example, a pediatric pharmacist with an interest in chronic conditions may work in a clinic setting. Alternatively, those interested in acute care may thrive in a hospital setting. Areas within hospitals where pediatric pharmacists have become well established include neonatal intensive care units (NICUs), pediatric intensive care unit (PICUs), medical or surgical general care units, hematology/oncology care units, and pediatric emergency departments. The roles of pediatric pharmacists vary widely depending on practice setting.

Within the hospital setting, many pharmacy-related activities take place in a large pharmacy located in a centralized part of the hospital.[16] Centralized pharmacists oversee the production of sterile products, such as liquid medications to be administered intravenously (IV); meaning, directly into patients' bloodstreams through a vein. They also ensure that all medication orders throughout the entire hospital are safe and optimized through a process called verification, while also managing processes involved in the distribution of medications. Other pharmacy-related activities, termed decentralized, take place within NICUs, PICUs, or other care units.[14,16] Pediatric pharmacists working in a decentralized manner may take responsibility for medication distribution within a specific unit, while also providing additional clinical services to pediatric patients. Table 6-3 highlights services provided by pediatric pharmacists embedded within interprofessional teams.[17,18] In addition to each of these professional activities, pediatric pharmacists may also lend their expertise to advance hospital-wide initiatives related to medication use, serve on committees, and participate in other administrative capacities.

Decentralized pediatric pharmacists working in general care units with less acutely ill patients must have a broad knowledge base given the wide variety of health conditions treated. Common conditions treated range from appendicitis, asthma,

Table 6-3. Common Professional Activities of Pediatric Pharmacists on Interprofessional Teams

Professional Activity	Description
Collaborate with other health professionals	Optimize medication use and patient care through teamwork and coordination with other health professionals
Optimize drug selection	Recommend preferred drug therapy based on expert-developed guidelines, clinical trial data, and/or hospital formularies, while incorporating patient-specific factors
Optimize drug dosing	Recommend changes to drug dosages based on best available evidence from published literature, as well as patient-specific factors such as kidney and liver function
Verification of medication orders and prescriptions	Review pediatric medication orders and prescriptions for indication (i.e., approved usage and age), safety, and accuracy, and work with prescribers to correct identified issues
Vaccine advocacy	Recommend vaccines for preventable diseases based on current guidelines, previous vaccination history, medical conditions, and age
Educate patients, families, caregivers, and health professionals	Provide medication counseling regarding side effects and how to take and measure doses of medications, answer drug information questions, and provide education for other health professionals
Monitor patient response to medications for efficacy and safety	Recommend dose adjustments or different medications based on changes in kidney and liver function, laboratory data, and/or patient-reported side effects or adverse drug events (diarrhea, vomiting, confusion, agitation, etc.)
Ensure access to medications	Address insurance and cost barriers, utilize medication assistance programs, direct families to a specialty outpatient pharmacy, and navigate drug shortages

and dehydration to diabetes and epilepsy.[19] Expertise in transplant medications and medications used for end-of-life or palliative care is also required. Pediatric pharmacists work in close collaboration with patients, parents, caregivers, and members of the interprofessional team to maximize medication outcomes for such conditions. Once stabilized and ready for hospital discharge, pediatric pharmacists often identify ways to make difficult-to-take medications palatable for children.[11,16,20] They also perform the vitally important task of educating patients and caregivers about medications, including potential side effects and how to respond should one occur, as well as the necessity of medication adherence (i.e., taking medications as prescribed) to improve health. Readers are encouraged to explore the illustrated case "Type 1" in Chapter 11 Critical Care for an example of this.

Critically ill neonates, including those born prematurely, are cared for in the NICU. Premature neonatal patients may weigh less than 500 grams, approximately 1.1 pounds, while full-term neonates may weigh up to 5 kilograms, approximately 11 pounds.[21] This represents a 10-fold difference in weight, which has incredibly important implications for medication selection and dosing.[22] Patients in this setting can also be at high risk for infections, and NICU pharmacists must be knowledgeable about their prevention and treatment. Infections can arise from invasive procedures like mechanical ventilation or the insertion of tubes intended to stay in place for extended periods of time, such as a feeding tube or an IV line. Many antibiotics require specialized dosing based on body weight, gestational age, and/or postnatal age. Gestational age is defined as the age from the time of conception to birth, while postnatal age is defined as the age in days of life after birth.[1] Differences in these values can drastically change how antibiotics are dosed.

NICU pharmacists play many additional important roles on the team. One example is working in collaboration with dietitians and nutritionists to optimize nutrients administered to neonates through an IV line to ensure appropriate growth and bone mineralization, which is called parenteral nutrition.[23] Another important role NICU pharmacists play is decreasing the severity of withdrawal for neonates exposed in utero to substances or medications, such as opioids, that can lead to physiological dependency.[24] NICU pharmacists also contribute to a host of other health conditions, including low blood glucose (i.e., sugar), bleeding complications, and respiratory distress syndrome.[25]

The NICU and PICU populations differ greatly. Key differences include not only age, but also common disease states and the medications used to treat them. Health conditions commonly managed in the PICU include a life-threatening complication from type 1 diabetes, called diabetic ketoacidosis, and uncontrolled seizures, called status epilepticus.[26] PICU pharmacists must also become familiar with postoperative management of repaired congenital heart defects, as well as medication management associated with trauma.[26,27] PICU pharmacists are an integral part of the team and have a significant impact not only on patient outcomes, but also on the costs associated with hospitalized pediatric patients.[28] Some of the most complicated and sickest patients will be treated in the PICU, which lends opportunities to maximize care while simultaneously containing costs. Critically ill pediatric patients often require multiple medications to support their recovery, such as sedation and pain medications to prevent them from fighting against breathing tubes.

Critically ill patients with sepsis and infection require close monitoring of organ function and may require medication dosage adjustments to accommodate ongoing changes in both kidney and liver function. Patients with multiorgan dysfunction or failure may require life support therapies, which require medication adjustments due to alterations in pharmacokinetics. Finally, PICU pharmacists also participate in pediatric advanced life support, where they prepare weight-specific medications that are administered to patients during resuscitation efforts, or when a patient is

"coding." Incorporation of pediatric pharmacists into emergency response teams has a positive impact on patient-specific outcome measures, timely medication administration, optimization of therapy, medication safety, and cost avoidance.[29]

PEDIATRIC PHARMACY IN ACTION

Taste Is a Big Deal

Medication adherence rates in children have been found to vary widely, with the bottom end of the range reported to be as low as 11%; meaning, up to 89% of children do not take their medications as prescribed.[30] This is a major problem that pediatric pharmacists are well-positioned to address. Common reasons reported for medication non-adherence include formulation and issues with palatability. Palatability concerns stem from the taste of the active pharmaceutical ingredients, which may be very bitter. This is problematic for many children, as their taste perception differs from adults, leading to a preference for sweet tastes and a heightened distain for bitter flavors.[31] Poor medication taste results in poor medication adherence and treatment failure, highlighting the seriousness of this issue.[30] Some children with complex health conditions, like epilepsy, may require multiple medication doses per day to control their symptoms. One pharmacist, the grandfather of a child with epilepsy, identified several strategies to optimize palatability as he searched for a way to improve her medication-taking behavior, and therefore, her health.[32] This search led to the development of a medication flavoring company that continues to provide pharmacists in community and hospital settings with the tools they need to effectively flavor medications.

Pediatric Pharmacist–Led Medication Weans Work

In NICUs and PICUs, use of powerful medications that can lead to physiological dependency is often necessary; examples include opioids to control pain and benzodiazepines to reduce anxiety as an adjunct to sedation during mechanical ventilation. After as little as 5 days of use, roughly half of pediatric patients will experience withdrawal symptoms if these medications are stopped. After 10 days of opioid use, all pediatric patients will experience withdrawal if medications are abruptly discontinued.[33] Methadone has been used to prevent withdrawal symptoms in pediatric patients since the 1990s.[34] Methadone is ideal for weaning pediatric patients off opioids because of its many desirable characteristics, including high oral absorption of around 85%, accessibility at retail pharmacies, and long history of use. Additionally, methadone tapers may be completed at home which can decrease hospital length of stay in some cases. Recently, the role of pediatric pharmacists managing protocols and dosing tapers to facilitate safely weaning pediatric patients off of these powerful medications was evaluated.[35] The pharmacist-managed taper for methadone weaning resulted in positive outcomes; for example, reduced withdrawal symptoms and decreases in the amount of time needed to complete the taper. The use of standardized pediatric pharmacist–led protocols also decreased practice variability, which has been shown to improve overall patient outcomes.[24,34,35]

BECOMING A PEDIATRIC PHARMACIST

Pediatric pharmacists practice in hospital and clinic settings. After graduating from a Doctor of Pharmacy (PharmD) program accredited by the Accreditation Council for Pharmacy Education, most pharmacists interested in pediatrics pursue additional training in the form of a general postgraduate year 1 (PGY-1) residency.[36,37] First-year residency training can be completed either in a facility that offers both adult and pediatric training experiences or solely at a pediatric facility. PGY-1 residents interested in a career in pediatric care may also complete a postgraduate year 2 (PGY-2) residency dedicated exclusively to pediatric care.[37] This additional 1-year residency provides intense training under the guidance of experienced pediatric pharmacists. PGY-2 pediatric pharmacy residencies are designed to build upon knowledge and skills gained during PGY-1 training with a specific focus on the pediatric population.

Several national organizations successfully advocated for pediatric pharmacy practice to be recognized as specialty, including the American College of Clinical Pharmacy, PPA, ASHP, and the American Pharmacists Association.[11] In 2015, the Board of Pharmacy Specialties granted this specialty recognition in the form of a national credential; namely, the Board Certified Pediatric Pharmacotherapy Specialist (BCPPS). The acquisition of BCPPS status, via a written examination, demonstrates advanced knowledge and expertise in the care of pediatric patients.[18] To sit for the BCPPS exam, pharmacists must first qualify by meeting one of the following three criteria: 4 years of post-licensure practice with at least 50% of time spent in pediatrics, completion of a PGY-1 residency in pediatric pharmacy and at least 2 additional years of post-licensure practice with 50% of practice time focused in pediatrics, or completion of a PGY-2 residency in pediatric pharmacy. BCPPS certification is valid for 7 years, after which point the pediatric pharmacist must either earn 100 hours of approved continuing education credit or achieve a passing score on a recertification examination.

ACCIDENTAL: An Illustrated Case Study

Story by Jessica M. Bergsbaken & Joseph A. Zorek
Illustrations by George Folz, © 2020 McGraw-Hill Education

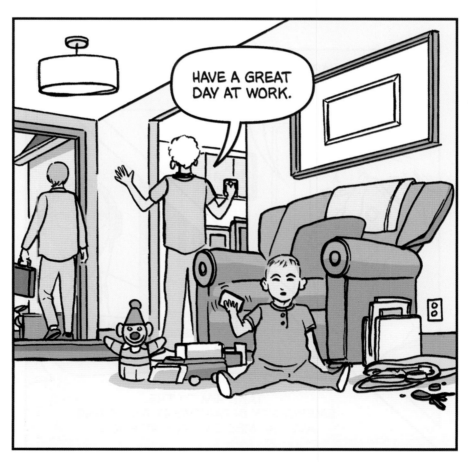

Illustration 6-1

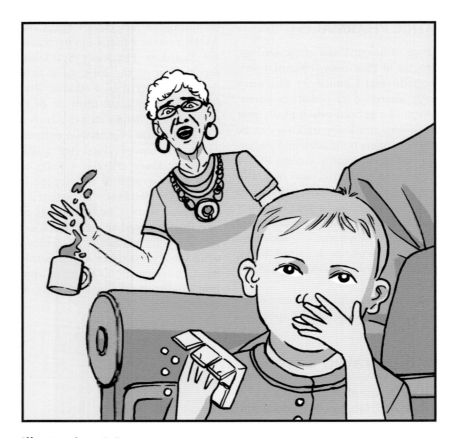

Illustration 6-2

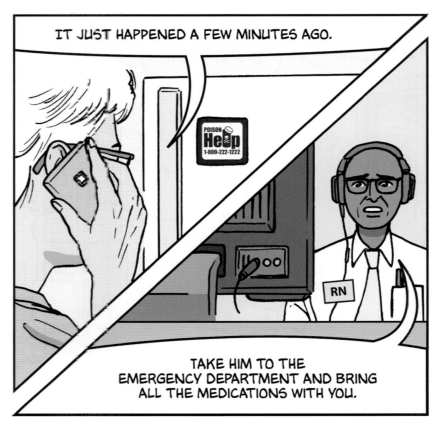

Illustration 6-3

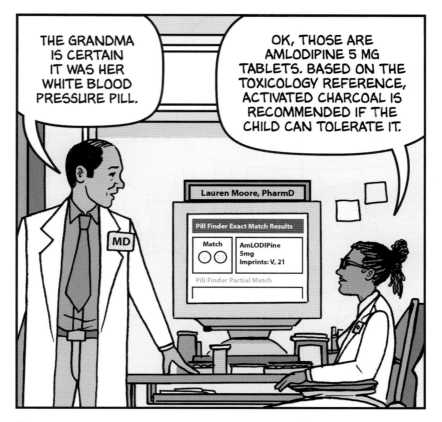

Illustration 6-4

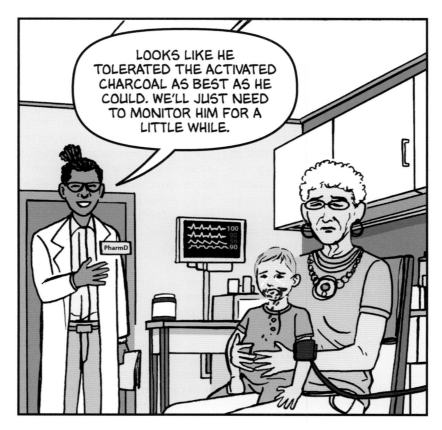

Illustration 6-5

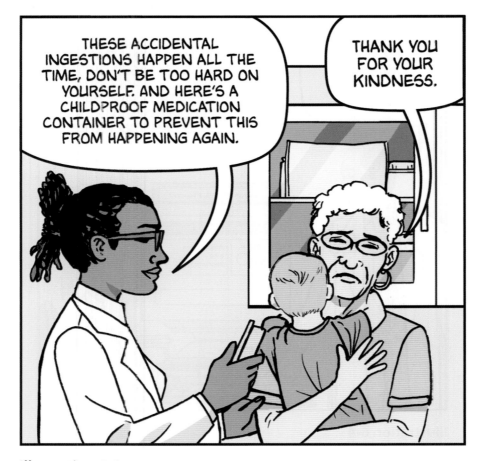

Illustration 6-6

Thoughts on "Accidental"

As depicted in the illustrated case "Accidental," toxic exposures involving medications are terrifying and, unfortunately, a relatively common occurrence. According to the American Association of Poison Control Centers, nearly half of the reported 2.5 million toxic exposures reported in 2018 occurred in children less than 6 years old at a home residence.[38] Each year, these exposures result in approximately 450,000 calls to poison control centers and 60,000 visits to the emergency department.[38,39] The top types of chemical exposures vary slightly depending on age; that said, the most commonly reported over the last 10 years were analgesics (i.e., pain medications), household cleaning substances, cosmetics/personal care products, psychotropics (e.g., sedatives/hypnotics, antipsychotics, antidepressants), and cardiovascular drugs.[38]

Causes of toxic exposures in the pediatric population vary across the age spectrum. Infants less than 1 year of age represent only 5% of all exposures and are considered a low-risk group because they are not yet ambulatory. It is important to point out that while this age group is considered low risk, when exposures do occur, health professionals should consider child abuse as a top cause for the intoxication. Unintentional medication dosing errors are also common in this age group on account of many factors, including breakdowns in coordination between multiple caregivers, confusion resulting from multiple medication types (e.g., infant, child, and adult strengths of the same medication), and the lack of appropriate measuring devices in households. Toddlers up to 6 years of age account for nearly half of all poisoning exposures due to their curious nature and need to explore. Children aged 6 to 12 years and teens account for about 13% of all cases of ingestion, with the most frequent reasons being misuse, abuse, or suicide attempt.[40]

Significant harm and death can result from ingestion of toxic substances in children, and not all children are as lucky as Sam, the child featured in the illustrated case "Accidental. There were over 3000 fatalities in 2018 as a result of toxic exposures, and 51 of these deaths involved children less than 6 years of age.[38] Of these, 57% were related to unintentional exposures. Analgesics, antihistamines, and cardiovascular drugs were the top medications most frequently involved in deaths of children less than 6 years old, whiles fumes/gases/vapors, batteries, and household cleaners accounted for the top non-medication-related substances.

Accidental ingestions in children can occur within any family. Even a previous director of a poison control center experienced this, when her 1-year-old child found a loose pill and attempted to ingest it.[41] The pill, identified as the pain medication tramadol, had fallen out of the pocket of a friend who had visited. Certain medications can be very harmful or deadly if accidentally ingested by a child. In some cases, ingestion of a single pill may lead to the death of a child.[42] In this illustrated case, Sam ingested the blood pressure-lowering medication amlodipine, which can cause serious harm in a child of his size and age.

There are several contributing factors associated with accidental ingestions in young children. Medications placed on countertops, tables, low shelves, or in pocketbooks are easily accessible.[43] Supervision by grandparents and the use of medication containers other than original prescription bottles are also associated with pediatric ingestions.[44] Adults often forget that children are natural explorers, curious about their environment, and unable to discriminate safe from unsafe products due to their age.[45] Several of these factors contributed to the accidental ingestion by Sam, captured in Illustrations 6-1 and 6-2, including his grandmother's use of a non-childproof container and the storage of this container in her purse, which was left on the floor and within Sam's reach.

Poison control centers throughout the United States are available to assist with management of accidental ingestions, like Sam's, and other exposures to toxic substances. The general public and health professionals may call the toll-free poison control helpline (1-800-222-1222) 24 hours a day, 365 days a year, to receive assistance with poisoning emergencies. All calls are answered by specially trained poison experts, including nurses, pharmacists, physicians, and other health professionals with specific training in toxicology.[46–48] In Illustration 6-3, Sam's grandmother appropriately called the poison control center phone number, thankfully present on the family's refrigerator as a magnet, to receive guidance on what to do following his accidental ingestion. Contacting the poison control center can be beneficial, as many times ingestions can be managed over the phone rather than calling 9-1-1 or going to the emergency department.[48] In Illustration 6-3, the nurse who received this call advised Sam's grandmother to take him to the emergency department immediately, with the pill box.

Childhood poisonings were identified as a significant problem as far back as the 1930s, but the full magnitude of this problem was not captured until an epidemiological study was completed in the 1950s.[47,49] Investigation of pediatric accidental ingestions in the United States was prompted after a report in the British literature exposed the frequency of accidental poisonings occurring in young children. In the United States from 1940 to 1950, deaths from accidental poisoning occurred in approximately 4000 children less than 6 years of age. The rate of accidental poisoning was identified

to be four times higher than the British rate, likely due to easy access to poisonous substances. One-third of deaths were caused by medications with petroleum products and materials for external use such as lead, lye, and arsenic accounting for the remainder of deaths. Aspirin, salicylates, and barbiturates were the most common medications associated with these deaths, which are still sources of pediatric ingestions today.

Prior to this study, during World War II, Louis Gdalman, a pharmacist from Chicago, began to develop a toxicological information system to catalog substances, which eventually included over 9000 commercial and consumer products.[50] Gdalman and a physician colleague, Edward Press, established the first formal poison control center using this information system in 1953. Over the next decade, the number of poison control centers rapidly increased and spread across the country. Some of today's poison control center operations originated from the interprofessional teamwork of Gdalman and Press. The 24-hour services provided by today's poison control centers stemmed from Gdalman's history of personally taking phone calls at all hours of the day and night. Additionally, Gdalman and Press recognized that utilizing phone triage allowed for treatment of some exposures at home and prevented unnecessary hospital or emergency department visits.

In 1970, undoubtedly inspired by the work of Gdalman and Press, the US Congress passed the Poison Prevention Packaging Act (PPPA), which required child-resistant packaging for over-the-counter and prescription medications, as well as hazardous household products.[51] PPPA requires that packaging must be designed to be significantly difficult for children under 5 years of age to open within a reasonable time, but not difficult for normal adults to use properly. For the sake of the elderly and those with disabilities who might have difficulty opening such containers, the PPPA states that a regulated product available for purchase on store shelves may be packaged in one non-complying size provided it carries a warning that it is not recommended for use in households with children, and provided that the product is also supplied in complying popular size packages. Upon assessment of this impact in 1982, it was estimated that the PPPA had resulted in the prevention of nearly 200,000 accidental ingestions since 1973 and that it contributed significantly to a decreased poison-related death rate, from 2 per 100,000 to 0.5 per 100,000 children under the age of 5 years.[52]

As more than 90% of exposures documented by poison control calls occur in the home, safe storage of medications and hazardous substances is one way to minimize accidental ingestions.[53] Pharmacists play an important role in educating and counseling the general public on how to properly store medications and other household products. Medications, both prescription and over-the-counter, should be stored out of sight and reach of children and pets, as should cleaning and laundry products, which are top substances for toxic exposures in young children. Medications should also be kept in their original containers with childproof caps.[53,54] For additional security, medication lock boxes may also be purchased for storage of medications to prevent unintentional and intentional ingestions from children, adolescents, or adults.

Equally important to proper medication storage is proper medication disposal to minimize accidental and intentional exposures. The best and safest way to dispose of expired, unwanted, or unused medications is through community take-back days.[55] The US Drug Enforcement Agency (DEA) sponsors two national take-back events each year where temporary drug collection sites are set up to collect medications dropped off by individuals in the community for proper disposal.[55,56] Outside of drug take-back days, there are authorized permanent collection sites for medication disposal in retail, hospital, or clinic pharmacies, or at police stations or other law enforcement locations.[56] If unable to dispose of medications at temporary or permanent collection sites, there are other methods to dispose of medications at home. Medications, left whole and intact, may be mixed with kitty litter or used coffee grounds, placed in a sealed container, such a plastic bag or used food container, and thrown into the trash.[55] Certain medications that may be harmful if accidentally ingested can be flushed down the sink or toilet only if unable to be disposed at a medication take-back collection site. A list of medications recommended to be flushed is listed on the FDA website.[56]

Children with acute ingestions are assessed starting with the ABCD method; namely, airway, breathing, circulation, and diagnosis of poisoning.[57] Since most ingestions do not have a specific antidote, supportive care is often employed as the main treatment modality. The patient should be assessed to ensure they are hemodynamically stable while notifying a poison control center and obtaining their assistance. Next, the team should decide if the patient would benefit from gastric decontamination, or removal of the ingested substance from the stomach to decrease absorption. The ingested substance, time of the ingestion, tolerability, and stability of the patient are some factors that determine if gastric decontamination is appropriate. Illustration 6-4 depicts the emergency department physician conferring with Dr. Lauren Moore, a pharmacist with specialty training in pediatrics. Lauren utilized a drug information resource to identify the name and dose of the medication Sam ingested, as well as the recommended treatment strategy; that is, gastric decontamination using activated charcoal.

Gastric decontamination exists in many forms and is indicated for use in several situations.[57] Single-dose activated charcoal should be considered in asymptotic patients who present for care within an hour of ingestion.[58] Activated charcoal works by absorbing toxins in the stomach, which decreases the amount of the toxin available to be absorbed into the bloodstream. Activated charcoal comes as black powder that is mixed with liquid and given to the patient to drink. It has maximal efficacy when given within 1 hour of ingestion, so prompt arrival to an emergency department is crucial.[59] Unfortunately, this modality is not effective for all types of ingestions; for example, it does not absorb iron, lithium, or alcohol. Its use has also decreased over the last several decades in response to reports of adverse events, such as lack of tolerability and aspiration (i.e., when vomit and/ or saliva are breathed into the airway). Less serious, but still problematic, adverse effects of activated charcoal include vomiting and constipation.[60] Multi-dose activated charcoal may be considered in cases where the toxin ingested undergoes extensive metabolism by the liver.

Whole bowel irrigation is another method to mitigate complications from ingestions of known long-acting substances that are not well absorbed by activated charcoal.[61] Whole bowel irrigation works by rinsing the intestines with a concentrated medication called polyethylene glycol, which causes diarrhea. Readers may recognize this medication due to its use by patients required to complete "bowel prep" ahead of a colonoscopy. The rate of administration for this decontamination is much faster than a normal bowel cleanout in preparation for colonoscopy. Whole bowel irrigation should not be used in a patient with no bowel sounds (indicating that their bowels have stopped working), as use may cause gastrointestinal discomfort and perforation of the colon.[61]

Gastric lavage, which removes ingested toxins by flushing the stomach with saline and removing stomach contents via a tube inserted into the stomach through the nose or mouth, is a high-risk procedure that may be considered in patients who present to the emergency department or hospital within 2 hours of ingesting a substance with no effective antidote that may result in significant toxicity.[62] Patients often need to be intubated to protect their airway and breathe for the patient during the procedure. Due to the lack of supporting efficacy and the invasive requirements of the procedure, however, this is not often attempted. It is important to note that gastric lavage will not remove large pills or objects, carries the risk of injury to the esophagus and trachea, and can lead to hypoxia and significant electrolyte disturbances.[62]

In Illustration 6-5, Lauren checks on Sam and his grandmother to see how well he tolerated the activated charcoal treatment. Lauren informs Sam's grandmother that the emergency medicine team will need to continue to monitor his blood pressure and heart rate, which is an important step. If a patient's condition deteriorates despite an initial decontamination attempt, other measures, including use of antidotes, may be necessary. Table 6-4 provides a select list of antidotes prescribed and dosed with pharmacist recommendations.[63]

In addition to providing recommendations for acute treatment of ingestions, pharmacists like Lauren are often

Table 6-4. Select Antidotes for Treatment of Poisoning/Toxicity in Children

Substance	Intended Use	Antidote(s) in Poisoning/Toxicity Situations
Acetaminophen	Over-the-counter pain medication	▪ Acetylcysteine
Benzodiazepines	Psychoactive medications	▪ Flumazenil
Beta-blockers, calcium channel blockers	Blood pressure medications	▪ Calcium ▪ Glucagon
Iron	Iron-containing medications (e.g., vitamins)	▪ Deferoxamine
Lead	Lead-based paint, soil, water, toys, jewelry, cosmetics	▪ Calcium disodium EDTA
Methotrexate	Chemotherapy, anti-rheumatic medication	▪ Glucarpidase
Opioids	Narcotic pain medications	▪ Naloxone
Organophosphates	Pesticides, insecticides	▪ Atropine ▪ Pralidoxime
Sulfonylureas	Type 2 diabetes medications	▪ Octreotide
Valproic acid	Seizure medication	▪ Levocarnitine
Warfarin	Anticoagulant medication	▪ Phytonadione (vitamin K)

involved in identification of unknown pills, as depicted in Illustration 6-4. To identify a medication, the pharmacist will enter the description of the pill, such as the shape, color, and imprints on the pill, into a drug identification resource. The drug identification resource will query the database to determine matches based on the inputted data. Pharmacists may also use drug reference resources such as LexiComp or Micromedex, which include drug identification resources, as well as websites like Drugs.com.[64-66] In addition to online databases, pill identification applications have been developed and can be downloaded for use on smartphones.[67]

Pediatric pharmacists use creativity to develop strategies for helping to get children to take unpleasant medications, like the activated charcoal shown in this illustrated case. Pharmacists recommend specific administration instructions to improve palatability and increase tolerability of medications. Activated charcoal and oral acetylcysteine are two examples of medications commonly used for accidental ingestions that have a very unpleasant taste. The taste of activated charcoal can be improved by mixing with

milk, cola, or fruit juice rather than water.[68] Acetylcysteine has a strong sulfur odor, similar to the smell of rotten eggs, which can be masked by putting the dose on ice, in a cup with a cover, and drinking through a straw.[69] There are many other strategies that can be used with pediatric patients to improve tolerance of all types of medications. Flavoring can be added directly to the medication by the pharmacist, and tablets may be crushed or capsules may be opened and mixed with soft foods, such as yogurt, pudding, or applesauce. Giving a cold treat such as a popsicle immediately before and after giving a medication can numb taste buds and minimize aftertaste.[31,70]

Beyond medication-related activities in cases of accidental ingestion, pharmacists are uniquely positioned in pediatric care settings to connect with patients, parents, or caregivers by showing compassion and kindness. As demonstrated in Illustration 6-6, there is still work to be done even after the acute health risks associated with Sam's accidental ingestion have been mitigated. Lauren's emotional intelligence is on display as she recognizes the guilt and anguish Sam's grandmother is experiencing. While providing empathetic and heartfelt words, and a childproof medication container to prevent future accidental ingestions, Lauren's deft touch proves invaluable not only for Sam, but for his grandmother, too.

DISCUSSION QUESTIONS FOR "ACCIDENTAL"

1. Has anyone in your life ever experienced a medication-related poisoning, either accidental or intentional? After reading Thoughts on "Accidental," what recommendations can you make to minimize future risks for family or friends?

2. Activated charcoal can be very hard to tolerate, as seen in Illustration 6-5. What are some ways pharmacists and other health professionals can improve this experience?

3. Many acute ingestions are unidentified initially, but a family member reports certain attributes of a medication lying near the patient, like in Illustration 6-4. What resources can you utilize to assist in identifying the unknown substance?

4. In Illustration 6-3, Sam's grandmother frantically calls the poison control center. Imagine you are the health professional answering the call. What can you do to decrease her anxiety and help her during this scary time?

5. Upon discharge from the emergency department or hospital, many families are nervous, hesitant, and often feel guilt when they are going home after an acute ingestion. What resources can you recommend for the family and what can you do to put them at ease?

ALL IN: An Illustrated Case Study

Story by Monica C. Bogenschutz & Joseph A. Zorek
Illustrations by George Folz, © 2019 Board of Regents of the University of Wisconsin System

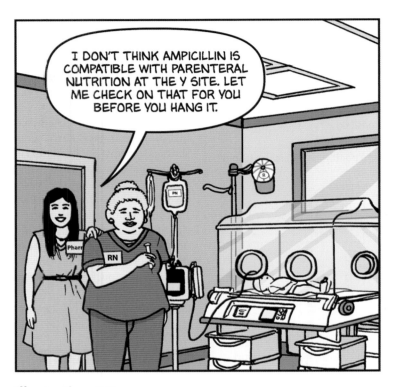

Illustration 6-7

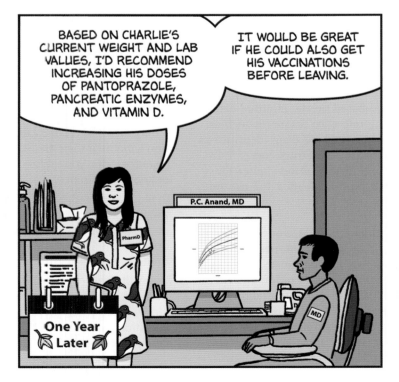

Illustration 6-8

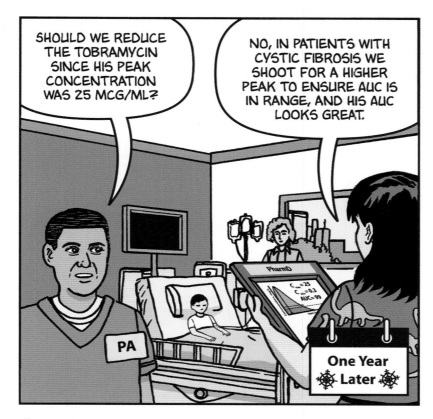

Illustration 6-9

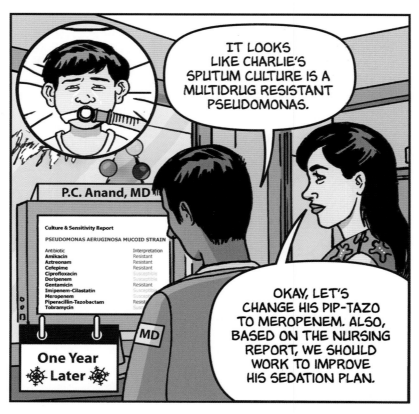

Illustration 6-10

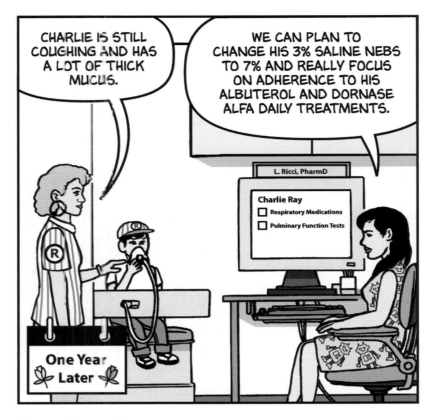

Illustration 6-11

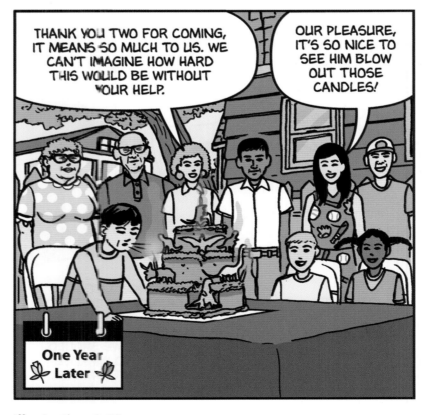

Illustration 6-12

Thoughts on "All In"

The illustrated case "All In" tells the story of Charlie Ray, a child born with cystic fibrosis (CF). Each illustration provides an annual update on Charlie's health and his interactions with the healthcare system over the first 5 years of his life. Charlie's journey features the work of an interprofessional pediatrics team, with an emphasis on the role and contributions of Dr. Liana Ricci, a pediatric pharmacist.

Charlie's story begins in the NICU, where as a premature newborn he is being treated for neonatal sepsis, a condition that results from a bloodstream infection. Illustration 6-7 depicts an intervention by Liana to prevent a medication error. One critically important role of pediatric pharmacists is to ensure that the route of medication administration is safe for patients. As it relates to the IV route, physical properties of coadministered drugs must be considered, as inactivation of medications may occur if they are incompatible. Charlie's nurse is preparing to administer ampicillin, an antibiotic to treat his infection, through the same IV line being used for his source of nutrition (called parenteral nutrition [PN]). Coadministration of medications through the same IV line is common; however, some medications are known to react negatively inside the IV line, and these reactions can jeopardize their effectiveness. Fortunately, Liana recognizes this problem before it occurs, and she works in a collaborative manner with Charlie's nurse to address it.

Charlie's interprofessional pediatrics team is on high alert this particular morning, as his newborn screening results came back abnormal for CF, a genetic disease caused by a mutation of a gene called cystic fibrosis transmembrane conductance regulator, or CFTR for short.[71] There are over 1700 reported CFTR mutations grouped into one of five reported classes.[72] The CFTR gene produces a protein that is located on various cell surfaces throughout the body, which collectively help to transport water and electrolytes into and out of cells.[71] A CFTR mutation may lead to a protein that does not work well, is not produced in sufficient quantities, or is not produced at all. As a result, patients with CF have abnormally thick and sticky secretions. Because this protein is found throughout the body, disease symptoms may manifest in several organ systems, most commonly in the lungs and gastrointestinal tract.[73] Common clinical manifestations of CF are described in Table 6-5.[73,74]

CF is the most common genetic disease in the Caucasian population, and recent estimates suggest that there are about 80,000 CF cases worldwide.[75] In the United States, there are roughly 30,000 people living with CF. It is estimated that 1 in every 3500 infants worldwide is born with this disease. Currently, there is no cure for CF and the life expectancy of people living with this disease is about 46 years. As recent as 25 years ago, the life expectancy was 34 years. Much of this extended life expectancy is attributable to medication and respiratory therapies, and additional progress is portended for the future. For example, new data suggest that the median predicted survival age of babies born in 2018 with CF will be 47 years or older.[76]

Universal newborn screening is performed in the United States in the first days of a baby's life, testing for several genetic diseases that are known to impede normal development.[74,77,78] While screening for specific disorders varies by state, the recommended panel includes screening for conditions such as phenylketonuria, CF, sickle cell disease, critical congenital heart disease, and hearing loss.[79,80] A positive screen does not confirm diagnosis of CF, as it could be a false positive.[81-83] Additional testing called a sweat chloride test is the gold standard for diagnosis. Recall that the CFTR mutation leads to deficiencies in the transport of water and electrolytes into and out of cells. Chloride is one of the most prevalent electrolytes in the human body, and the sweat chloride test quantifies the amount of it excreted though sweat. Healthy individuals have a sweat chloride test result of less than 29 mmol/L. A chloride level greater than 60 mmol/L on a sweat test confirms CFTR protein dysfunction and a diagnosis of CF. Babies born with CF may be born prematurely or have a low birth weight. Additionally, they often require hospitalization in a NICU for respiratory distress and/or meconium ileus.[81-83]

In Illustration 6-7, in addition to receiving antibiotics and PN, Charlie is also undergoing a medical workup for the diagnosis of CF based on results of his newborn screen. A team of pediatric pulmonary experts were contacted and they recommended conducting a sweat chloride test when Charlie is about 2 weeks old to confirm diagnosis.[84] While Charlie remains in the NICU, the team decides to increase his nutritional intake by the IV route through PN and to slowly integrate some breast milk by mouth.

Adequate nutrition is critical to support normal growth and development. Many children with CF have nutritional deficiencies as a result of CFTR protein dysfunction, as this affects the absorption and digestion of food and essential nutrients in the gastrointestinal tract.[71,73,85,86] It is imperative to optimize nutrition in children with CF as normal weight and stature for age is associated with improved lung function and survival.[85-87] Certain CFTR protein mutations may completely inhibit the release of digestive enzymes from the pancreas, while other mutations may lead to impaired pancreatic function. If left untreated, such chronic impairment can lead to complete insufficiency over time. To ensure maintenance of proper nutrition, individuals with pancreatic insufficiency should consume a high-calorie diet, up to 200% of the energy intake of that of a healthy individual, with 40% coming from fat calories.[85,88]

The pancreas is considered a glandular organ that is part of the digestive tract, and it serves a critical function of secreting digestive enzymes into the small intestine. These digestive enzymes include lipase, amylase, and protease, all of which help to break down fats, carbohydrates, and proteins present in food. Without these necessary enzymes to aid in digestion, the nutrients in food will not be absorbed, and patients will have poor growth and development as a result. Additionally, the inability to effectively digest foods can lead to vitamin and mineral deficiencies. To mitigate these problems, patients with CF take medications to replace pancreatic enzymes. This group

Table 6-5. Clinical Manifestations of Cystic Fibrosis by Organ System

Organ System	Clinical Manifestation	Description
Pulmonary system	Asthma	A condition that causes airways to narrow, swell, and produce extra mucus, all of which can make breathing difficult
	Bronchiectasis	A condition that causes cough, sputum production, and recurrent respiratory infections
	Chronic cough	A cough that lasts greater than 4 weeks in a pediatric patient
	Digital clubbing	A deformity of the finger or toe nails associated with diseases of the heart and lungs
	Recurrent respiratory infections	Repeated infections that occur in the lungs
	Sinusitis	Infections and swelling in the cavities surrounding the nasal passages
	Nasal polyps	Soft, painless, noncancerous growths on the lining of nasal passages or sinuses
	Hemoptysis	Coughing up of blood or blood-stained mucus from the lungs
Gastrointestinal system	Distal intestinal obstruction syndrome (DIOS)	Blockage or obstruction of the small intestines causing constipation
	Hepatobiliary disease	A disease affecting the bile ducts, gallbladder, and other structures involved in the production and transportation of bile
	Meconium ileus	A bowel blockage that occurs when the meconium (first bowel movement in a newborn) in the intestine is thicker and stickier in the intestines
	Pancreatic insufficiency	Inflammation of the pancreas, which causes issues with secreting important enzymes needed to digest food
	Vitamin deficiencies	Lack of vitamins absorbed in the body which result in feelings of weakness and bone loss or fractures
	Steatorrhea	Presence of excess fat in the stool
Endocrine, renal, reproductive systems	Cystic fibrosis–related diabetes	Type of diabetes that is common in people with cystic fibrosis, resulting in elevated blood glucose levels
	Electrolyte imbalances	Electrolyte levels in the body are either too high or too low
	Hyponatremic dehydration	Sodium level in the blood is too low, usually as a result of diarrhea
	Male infertility	A health issue that makes it hard to conceive a child
	Osteoporosis	Porous bone structure which may result in fractures
	Nephrolithiasis	Small deposits that build up in the kidneys; also called kidney stones

of medications come in capsule form and are dosed based on the patient's weight, clinical symptoms, and the amount of fat present in his/her stool.[89,90] For patients who are unable to swallow whole capsules, the capsules may be opened, and the contents mixed with a small amount of acidic food, such as applesauce, and then consumed. In addition to continually titrating the dose of enzyme therapy, adjustments to vitamin and mineral supplementation are made on a regular basis according to routine laboratory monitoring.

As children with CF grow, medication regimens must be continually assessed to ensure that they, too, "grow" with the child. Unlike most medications in adult patients, pediatric medications are dosed by patient weight until they reach an adult age or size. In Illustration 6-8, Liana works collaboratively with Charlie's pulmonologist (i.e., physician who specializes in respiratory conditions) to evaluate Charlie's growth, making the recommendation to increase his medication doses based on his continued increase in weight. Weight-based dose adjustments

are vital in CF patients, as dose adjustments ensure optimal outcomes from these drugs. In addition to optimizing medication dosing, Liana also recommends administering Charlie's scheduled childhood vaccinations. Staying current with childhood vaccines is essential for CF patients as they are at high risk for negative outcomes from vaccine preventable diseases.[91,92] Not only should CF patients receive recommended vaccinations on time, it is imperative that caregivers and/or household contacts also remain up-to-date, including the annual influenza vaccination, to prevent exposure and disease transmission. Pharmacists can administer vaccines to both adults and children; however, regulations for certification, type of vaccines, and age of administration varies by state.[93]

Given the severity of this disease and immediate onset, patients with CF are likely to begin medications very early in life. Variations in CFTR genetic mutations make medication selection and dosing incredibly complex. Because of these differences, variability in medication regimens prescribed to patients with CF is common. Patients with CF are prescribed an average of about 10 medications at any given time, which poses a challenge when it comes to adherence.[94] Furthermore, it has been documented that adherence rates decrease as patients with CF age.[94] Such complexities underscore the importance of pediatric pharmacists in the care of patients with CF. Table 6-6 highlights examples of common medications prescribed to patients with CF.[95-99]

Inhaled medication therapies along with airway clearance are performed multiple times daily to promote expectoration of mucus from the lungs.[98] Many devices such as postural percussion therapy or chest physiotherapy are utilized in combination with medications like inhaled hypertonic saline, dornase alfa, and albuterol to prevent excessive pulmonary irritation.[100] With progression of disease, inhaled anti-infectives may be integrated into daily therapies to decrease the colonization and growth of

Table 6-6. Categories and Examples of Medications Commonly Used to Treat Cystic Fibrosis

Category	Medication Examples*	Physiologic Effect
Anti-infectives	▪ amoxicillin (Amoxil) ▪ amoxicillin/clavulanate (Augmentin) ▪ aztreonam for inhalation (Cayston) ▪ cefepime (Maxipime) ▪ cephalexin (Keflex) ▪ ciprofloxacin (Cipro) ▪ colistimethate (Colistin) ▪ levofloxacin (Levaquin) ▪ linezolid (Zyvox) ▪ meropenem (Merrem) ▪ piperacillin-tazobactam (Zosyn) ▪ sulfamethoxazole-trimethoprim (Bactrim) ▪ tobramycin (Tobi) ▪ vancomycin (Vancocin)	Prevent and treat infections in the airway
Anti-inflammatories	▪ azithromycin (Zithromax)** ▪ ibuprofen (Advil, Motrin)	Decrease inflammation, improve lung function, and reduce exacerbations
Acid suppressing medications	▪ famotidine (Pepcid) ▪ omeprazole (Prilosec) ▪ pantoprazole (Protonix)	Decrease pain associated with gastric reflux and increase gastric pH
Bronchodilators	▪ albuterol (Ventolin, ProAir)	Make it easier to breathe by relaxing the airway
CFTR modulators	▪ elexacaftor/tezacaftor/ivacaftor and ivacaftor (Trikafta) ▪ ivacaftor (Kalydeco) ▪ lumacaftor/ivacaftor (Orkambi) ▪ tezacaftor/ivacaftor (Symdeko)	Correct problems with the CFTR protein that causes disease symptoms
Inhaled corticosteroids	▪ beclomethasone (Qvar) ▪ budesonide (Pulmicort) ▪ fluticasone (Flovent)	Reduce swelling in the airway for people who also have asthma
Inhaled corticosteroids with long-acting bronchodilators	▪ budesonide/formoterol (Symbicort) ▪ fluticasone/salmeterol (Advair) ▪ mometasone/formoterol (Dulera)	Reduce swelling in the airway and help to make it easier to breathe by relaxing the airway
Laxatives	▪ lactulose (Enulose) ▪ polyethylene glycol (Miralax)	Prevent constipation
Mucolytics	▪ dornase alpha (Pulmozyme) ▪ hypertonic saline 3% and 7% (HyperSal)	Break down thick, sticky mucus within the lungs
Pancreatic enzyme replacement therapy	▪ lipase/amylase/protease (Creon, Pancreaze, Pertzye, Viokace, Zenpep)	Aid in digestion when pancreas is not releasing enzymes
Vitamins	▪ cholecalciferol (Vitamin D) ▪ iron (Fer-in-Sol) ▪ multivitamin with additional fat-soluble vitamins (AquADEK, MVW Complete Formulation, Vitamax) ▪ phytonadione (Mephyton, Vitamin K)	Prevent nutritional deficiencies

* Medication examples presented in alphabetical order as "generic name (Brand Name)."

** Azithromycin is an antibiotic that is also used for anti-inflammatory purposes.

dangerous bacterial organisms, such as *Pseudomonas aeruginosa*, also called *P. aeruginosa*. These anti-infectives decrease bacterial burden, improve lung function, and decrease the risk of systemic side effects which may occur with IV antibiotic formulations. The addition of azithromycin is recommended when a patient is chronically colonized with *P. aeruginosa*, as it may improve lung function, reduce lung inflammation, and thus reduce respiratory exacerbations.[101] For CF patients with an acute exacerbation requiring hospitalization, IV anti-infectives are utilized to treat significant bacterial infections.[97–99,102]

Histamine-2 receptor antagonists and proton pump inhibitors are often utilized to decrease acid in the stomach and improve absorption of pancreatic enzymes.[103] Constipation and distal intestinal obstructive syndrome (DIOS) are complications seen in the CF population, which may require chronic use of oral laxatives and stool softeners, such as polyethylene glycol, to prevent or to acutely treat these conditions.[95,96]

Historically, CF therapy was aimed at treating the manifestations and complications of the disease; however, recent advancements in research have targeted the CFTR genetic mutation, working to restore and optimize the function of the affected CFTR gene. These new medications are known as CFTR modulators.[71] The CFTR modulators are reported to be well tolerated and to improve quality of life, lung function, and results of sweat chloride tests. A combination therapy of elexacaftor/tezacaftor/ivacaftor and ivacaftor (Trikafta) was approved by the FDA in 2019. Studies have shown this drug combination to be effective with minimal safety concerns for patients with CF 12 years of age or older with a specific CFTR mutation.[104] While the new therapies are proving to be life changing, they are also very costly and, even with insurance, may be difficult for some to afford.[105]

Patients with CF are at a much higher risk of infections due to bacteria that can hide in the thick mucus that can build up in the lungs. Common bacterial species that cause respiratory infections, and subsequent hospitalization, in patients with CF include *P. aeruginosa*, *Stenotrophomonas maltophilia*, *Burkholderia cepacia*, *Haemophilus influenzae*, and methicillin-resistant *Staphylococcus aureus*, also known as MRSA.[106] As depicted in Illustrations 6-9 and 6-10, Charlie is admitted to the hospital on two different occasions for an acute exacerbation of CF, one of which required mechanical ventilation due to respiratory failure (Illustration 6-10).

Illustration 6-10 highlights Liana's valuable contribution to selection of anti-infective therapy via collaboration with Dr. P.C. Anand, Charlie's physician. Culture and sensitivity data reveal that the strain of *P. aeruginosa* causing Charlie's respiratory failure is resistant to multiple medications. It is important to note that cultures and sensitivities take time to develop, and patients experiencing a CF exacerbation are therefore started on empiric therapy, which is essentially an informed, educated guess as to what treatment is most likely to be effective. In Charlie's case, piperacillin-tazobactam and tobramycin were chosen as empiric therapy, and unfortunately the culture and sensitivities

revealed that it may not be effective. Liana, therefore, recommends changing piperacillin-tazobactam to a different antibiotic called meropenem.[107]

Pediatric pharmacists work collaboratively with other health professionals to ensure appropriate selection, dosing, and optimization of antibiotics for patients with CF. Knowledge of common pathogenic bacteria is equally important as anti-infective therapy must be tailored accordingly. The stakes are high in this regard, as inappropriate antibiotic use has been associated with the development of antibiotic resistance, including multidrug-resistant bacterial organisms that pose an incredible threat to the health and lives of patients with CF, like MRSA.[108] Cultures grown from sputum or mucus allow medical laboratory scientists to identify causative organisms. These cultures are then sensitivity tested by applying a variety of antibiotics, which allows laboratory professionals to report out which antibiotics will be effective for treatment.

When a patient is admitted to the hospital for a CF exacerbation, cultures and sensitivities of bacterial organisms are performed. Based on this information, anti-infective therapies are selected to best match the bacteria likely causing the exacerbation. Too high of a dose or too broad of an anti-infective agent can lead to toxicity or spur the development of antimicrobial resistance, while too low of a dose or narrow of a selected agent can lead to treatment failure. Treatment of infections in CF must be finely tuned, and the route of administration, duration of therapy, and anti-infective selection are key.[107,108] In Illustration 6-9, Liana provides reassurance to the physician assistant that the dose of tobramycin, an antibiotic, is appropriate for Charlie's infection. Specifically, Liana uses her expert knowledge of pharmacokinetics to explain that patients with CF, for a variety of reasons, tend to require larger doses than non-CF patients to reach the desired body exposure, also called the area under the curve, or AUC.[102,109] For more information on infectious diseases, anti-infective use, and antimicrobial resistance, readers are encouraged to explore Chapter 8 Infectious Diseases and the illustrated cases "Wounded" and "Superinfection."

As depicted in Illustration 6-11, pediatric pharmacists can improve both adherence to medications and the overall health of patients with CF. Key activities performed include reviewing medications at different transitions of care, addressing barriers to medication access (e.g., insurance or other financial concerns), conducting patient interviews and establishing a relationship with the family, reviewing and addressing potential drug interactions, providing education on new and chronic medications, and working with other health professionals to improve medication use.[110] Adherence to airway clearance therapies can be a significant challenge in children due to the time required for therapy administration and the overall tolerability. Based on Charlie's pulmonary function tests, cough, and thick mucus, Liana recommends stepping up his respiratory medication regimen to help with airway clearance in Illustration 6-11.[100,111] Additionally, Liana emphasizes the need to focus on adherence to his daily treatments. While this case addresses adherence during childhood, it is important to continue to reinforce medication adherence into the adolescent and young adulthood age group.[112]

Adherence to medication therapies in childhood is crucial not only to prevent CF-related hospitalizations, but also to decrease healthcare-related costs.[113] Establishing an effective medication schedule during early childhood is crucial for patients and their caregivers. Poor adherence to medications may lead to a significant decline in lung function and overall health, which may require hospitalization and administration of oral, aerosolized, and/or IV antibiotics.[113] Pharmacists can play a critical role in optimizing therapy by helping with adherence and providing education and support needed to help families integrate therapy into their lifestyle.

The illustrated case "All In" ends with a celebration of another year and another birthday, with Charlie's good health on display via his ability to blow out his birthday candles (Illustration 6-12). The presence of Charlie's physician and pharmacist at this celebration is clearly meaningful to Charlie and his family. Charlie and his family will continue to interact with his interprofessional team for the entirety of his life. Throughout the 5 years depicted in this illustrated case, from Charlie's time in the NICU to his fifth birthday party, it is clear that Charlie and his family have bonded with his interprofessional team. Such bonds are important, and the benefits cut both ways; that is, while they undoubtedly lead to improvements in patient care, health professionals involved also derive a great amount of career satisfaction.

DISCUSSION QUESTIONS FOR "ALL IN"

1. What barriers to care do you think might exist for pediatric and adolescent patients compared to adult patients related to medication management?

2. Medication adherence is vital for improved lung function and overall quality of life for patients with CF. What are some ways you can think of that might help increase adherence to medications?

3. There are many chronic diseases in the pediatric population and many pediatric patients take multiple medications. What are some ways pharmacists and other health professionals can ensure that correct medications are selected and administered to pediatric patients?

4. Patients experiencing a CF pulmonary exacerbation are often admitted to the hospital for two weeks or more to receive appropriate therapy. What are some strategies the team might employ to improve the patient's quality of life during these extended hospital stays?

5. Vaccinations are critically important for patients with and without CF. What controversies related to vaccine administration have you heard of? What are some reasons for these controversies?

CHAPTER SUMMARY

- Pediatrics is a field devoted to the health and well-being of infants, children, and adolescents up to the age of 18 years.

- Pediatric pharmacists practice in both hospital and clinic settings and work collaboratively with other health professionals to optimize drug and dose selection; educate patients, families, and other health professionals; and ensure the safe and effective use of medications.

- Pediatric pharmacist participation in patient care improves health outcomes, decreases medication errors and adverse drug events, and reduces healthcare costs.

- Accidental ingestions in children less than 6 years old are common, yet preventable.

- Pediatric pharmacists play multiple roles in accidental ingestions, from recommending decontamination strategies to increasing the palatability of antidotes.

- Cystic fibrosis is a genetic disorder that affects many body systems, including the lungs and the gastrointestinal tract, and pediatric pharmacists play an important role managing and monitoring medication therapies to ensure safety and efficacy.

- Pediatric pharmacists regularly counsel patients and families regarding the importance of medication adherence.

- Pediatric pharmacists play a critical role in optimizing medication therapy across many chronic health conditions, much of which involves building strong, supportive relationships with patients and their families.

REFERENCES

1. Lu H, Rosenbaum S. Developmental pharmacokinetics in pediatric populations. *J Pediatr Pharmacol Ther.* 2014;19(4):262-276.

2. Hardin AP, Hackell JM, Committee On Practice and Ambulatory Medicine. Age limit of pediatrics. *Pediatrics.* 2017;140(3):e20172151.

3. Kemper KJ. Holistic pediatrics = good medicine. *Pediatrics.* 2000;105(1 pt 3):214-218.

4. Fernandez E, Perez R, Hernandez A, Tejada P, Arteta M, Ramos JT. Factors and mechanisms for pharmacokinetic differences between pediatric population and adults. *Pharmaceutics.* 2011;3(1):53-72.

5. Gapminder. The world has reached peak number of children! Available at https://www.gapminder.org/news/world-peak-number-of-children-is-now/. Accessed May 17, 2020.

6. Council of Pediatric Subspecialties. Pediatric subspecialties. Available at https://www.pedsubs.org/about-cops/subspecialty-descriptions/. Accessed May 24, 2020.

7. Teskey SMA. Pediatric pharmacy practice. In: Austin Z, ed. *Encyclopedia of Pharmacy Practice and Clinical Pharmacy.* Vol. 1. 1st ed. Ontario, Canada: Elsevier Inc; 2019:360-370.

8. Verbanas P. Off-label medication orders on the rise for children: office-based doctors are ordering medication off-label to children at increasing rates, particularly for unapproved

conditions. Available at https://www.sciencedaily.com/releases/2019/09/190916081423.htm. Accessed May 13, 2020.

9. Rinke ML, Bundy DG, Velasquez CA, et al. Interventions to reduce pediatric medication errors: a systematic review. *Pediatrics*. 2014;134(2):338-360.

10. Neuspiel DR, Taylor MM. Reducing the risk of harm from medication errors in children. *Health Serv Insights*. 2013;6:47-59.

11. Eiland LS, Benner K, Gumpper KF, et al. ASHP-PPAG guidelines for providing pediatric pharmacy services in hospitals and health systems. *J Pediatr Pharmacol Ther*. 2018;23(3):177-191.

12. Council on Children with Disabilities and Medical Home Implementation Project Advisory Committee. Patient- and family-centered care coordination: a framework for integrating care for children and youth across multiple systems. *Pediatrics*. 2014;133(5):e1451-e1460.

13. Association of Child Life Professionals. What is a certified child life specialist? Available at https://www.childlife.org/the-child-life-profession. Accessed May 24, 2020.

14. Are decentralized pharmacy services the preferred model of pharmacy service delivery within a hospital? *Can J Hosp Pharm*. 2015;68(2):168-171.

15. Mayer ML, Skinner AC. Too many, too few, too concentrated? A review of the pediatric subspecialty workforce literature. *Arch Pediatr Adolesc Med*. 2004;158(12):1158-1165.

16. Webster S, Kane C, Brown C, Warhurst H, Sedgley S, Slaughter W. Pediatric pharmacy services: current models and justification for expansion. *J Pediatr Pharmacol Ther*. 2019;24(5):438-444.

17. Pediatric Pharmacy Association. What is a pediatric pharmacist? Available at https://www.ppag.org/index.cfm?pg=profession. Accessed May 13, 2020.

18. Board of Pharmacy Specialties. Pediatric pharmacy fact sheet. Available at https://www.bpsweb.org/media/pediatric-pharmacy-fact-sheet/. Accessed May 13, 2020.

19. Ernst KD, Committee on Hospital Care. Resources recommended for the care of pediatric patients in hospitals. *Pediatrics*. 2020;145(4):e20200204.

20. Bonner L. Pharmacists work to make medications safer for pediatric patients. Available at https://www.pharmacytoday.org/article/S1042-0991(17)30393-6/pdf. Accessed May 11, 2020.

21. Murthy K, Dykes FD, Padula MA, et al. The Children's Hospitals Neonatal Database: an overview of patient complexity, outcomes and variation in care. *J Perinatol*. 2014;34(8):582-586.

22. O'Hara K, Wright IM, Schneider JJ, Jones AL, Martin JH. Pharmacokinetics in neonatal prescribing: evidence base, paradigms and the future. *Br J Clin Pharmacol*. 2015;80(6):1281-1288.

23. Krzyzaniak N, Bajorek B. A global perspective of the roles of the pharmacist in the NICU. *Int J Pharm Pract*. 2017;25(2):107-120.

24. Johnson MR, Nash DR, Laird MR, Kiley RC, Martinez MA. Development and implementation of a pharmacist-managed, neonatal and pediatric, opioid-weaning protocol. *J Pediatr Pharmacol Ther*. 2014;19(3):165-173.

25. Hashim MJ, Guillet R. Common issues in the care of sick neonates. *Am Fam Physician*. 2002;66(9):1685-1692.

26. Ibiebele I, Algert CS, Bowen JR, Roberts CL. Pediatric admissions that include intensive care: a population-based study. *BMC Health Serv Res*. 2018;18(1):264.

27. PedsCCM.org. Pediatric critical care. Available at http://www.pedsccm.org/clinical-resources.php. Accessed May 12, 2020.

28. Tripathi S, Crabtree HM, Fryer KR, Graner KK, Arteaga GM. Impact of clinical pharmacist on the pediatric intensive care practice: an 11-year tertiary center experience. *J Pediatr Pharmacol Ther*. 2015;20(4):290-298.

29. Farmer BM, Hayes BD, Rao R, Farrell N, Nelson L. The role of clinical pharmacists in the emergency department. *J Med Toxicol*. 2018;14(1):114-116.

30. Walsh J, Cram A, Woertz K, et al. Playing hide and seek with poorly tasting paediatric medicines: do not forget the excipients. *Adv Drug Deliv Rev*. 2014;73:14-33.

31. Mennella JA, Spector AC, Reed DR, Coldwell SE. The bad taste of medicines: overview of basic research on bitter taste. *Clin Ther*. 2013;35(8):1225-1246.

32. FLAVORx. What's FLAVORx all about? Available at https://www.flavorx.com/about-us/. Accessed May 11, 2020.

33. Roth A. Methadone weaning: the role of the pharmacist. Available at https://pediatricsnationwide.org/2015/10/23/methadone-weaning-the-role-of-the-pharmacist/. Accessed May 11, 2020.

34. Steineck KJ, Skoglund AK, Carlson MK, Gupta S. Evaluation of a pharmacist-managed methadone taper. *Pediatr Crit Care Med*. 2014;15(3):206-210.

35. Tobias JD. Methadone: who tapers, when, where, and how? *Pediatr Crit Care Med*. 2014;15(3):268-270.

36. Accreditation Council for Pharmacy Education. PharmD program accreditation. Available at https://www.acpe-accredit.org/pharmd-program-accreditation/. Accessed May 11, 2020.

37. American Society of Health System Pharmacists. Residency information. Available at https://www.ashp.org/Professional-Development/Residency-Information. Accessed May 11, 2020.

38. Gummin DD, Mowry JB, Spyker DA, et al. 2018 Annual Report of the American Association of Poison Control Centers' National Poison Data System (NPDS): 36th annual report. *Clin Toxicol (Phila)*. 2019;57(12):1220-1413.

39. Lovegrove MC, Weidle NJ, Budnitz DS. Trends in emergency department visits for unsupervised pediatric medication exposures, 2004–2013. *Pediatrics*. 2015;136(4):e821-e829.

40. Matteucci MJ. One pill can kill: assessing the potential for fatal poisonings in children. *Pediatr Ann*. 2005;34(12):964-968.

41. Long D. 7 drugs that can kill kids in a single pill. Available at https://abcnews.go.com/Health/Wellness/accidental-ingestion-common-pills-kill-toddlers/story?id=10130146. Accessed May 19, 2020.

42. Abbruzzi G, Stork CM. Pediatric toxicologic concerns. *Emerg Med Clin North Am*. 2002;20(1):223-247.

43. Salzman M, Cruz L, Nairn S, Bechmann S, Karmakar R, Baumann BM. The prevalence of modifiable parental behaviors associated with inadvertent pediatric medication ingestions. *West J Emerg Med*. 2019;20(2):269-277.

44. Agarwal M, Lovegrove MC, Geller RJ, et al. Circumstances involved in unsupervised solid dose medication exposures among young children. *J Pediatr*. 2020;219:188-195.e6.

45. Peden M. World report on child injury prevention calls for evidence-based interventions. *Int J Inj Contr Saf Promot*. 2009;16(1):57-58.

46. American Association of Poison Control Centers. About poison control centers. Available at https://aapcc.org/about-centers. Accessed May 19, 2020.

47. Institute of Medicine (US) Committee on Poison Prevention and Control. *Forging a Poison Prevention and Control System*.

Washington, DC: National Academies Press; 2004. Available at https://www.ncbi.nlm.nih.gov/books/NBK215795/. doi:10.17226/10971.

48. Health Resources & Services Administration. Poison centers. Available at https://poisonhelp.hrsa.gov/poison-centers. Accessed May 19, 2020.

49. Bain K. Death due to accidental poisoning in young children. *J Pediatr*. 1954;44(6):616-623.

50. Botticelli JT, Pierpaoli PG. Louis Gdalman, pioneer in hospital pharmacy poison information services. *Am J Hosp Pharm*. 1992;49(6):1445-1450.

51. U.S. Consumer Product Safety Commission. Poison Prevention Packaging Act. Available at https://www.cpsc.gov/Regulations-Laws--Standards/Statutes/Poison-Prevention-Packaging-Act. Accessed May 23, 2020.

52. Walton WW. An evaluation of the Poison Prevention Packaging Act. *Pediatrics*. 1982;69(3):363-370.

53. American Association of Poison Control Centers. In the home. Available at https://aapcc.org/prevention/home. Accessed May 19, 2020.

54. American Academy of Pediatrics. Poison prevention & treatment tips. Available at https://www.healthychildren.org/English/safety-prevention/all-around/Pages/Poison-Prevention.aspx. Accessed May 19, 2020.

55. American Association of Poison Control Centers. Safe medication disposal. Available at https://aapcc.org/prevention/medication-safety. Accessed May 19, 2020.

56. U.S. Food and Drug Administration. Disposal of unused medicines: what you should know. Available at https://www.fda.gov/drugs/safe-disposal-medicines/disposal-unused-medicines-what-you-should-know#MEDICINES. Accessed May 19, 2020.

57. Mangus CW, Canares TL. Toxic ingestions: initial management. *Pediatr Rev*. 2018;39(4):219-221.

58. Chyka PA, Seger D, Krenzelok EP, et al. Position paper: single-dose activated charcoal. *Clin Toxicol (Phila)*. 2005;43(2):61-87.

59. Lapus RM. Activated charcoal for pediatric poisonings: the universal antidote? *Curr Opin Pediatr*. 2007;19(2):216-222.

60. Position statement and practice guidelines on the use of multi-dose activated charcoal in the treatment of acute poisoning. American Academy of Clinical Toxicology; European Association of Poisons Centres and Clinical Toxicologists. *J Toxicol Clin Toxicol*. 1999;37(6):731-751.

61. Thanacoody R, Caravati EM, Troutman B, et al. Position paper update: whole bowel irrigation for gastrointestinal decontamination of overdose patients. *Clin Toxicol (Phila)*. 2015;53(1):5-12.

62. Benson BE, Hoppu K, Troutman WG, et al. Position paper update: gastric lavage for gastrointestinal decontamination. *Clin Toxicol (Phila)*. 2013;51(3):140-146.

63. Marraffa JM, Cohen V, Howland MA. Antidotes for toxicological emergencies: a practical review. *Am J Health Syst Pharm*. 2012;69(3):199-212.

64. Drug I.D. 2020. Available at http://online.lexi.com. Accessed May 19, 2020.

65. Drug Identification. Truven Health Analytics; 2020. Available at http://micromedex.com. Accessed May 19, 2020.

66. U.S. National Library of Medicine. Identify or search for a pill. Available at https://pillbox.nlm.nih.gov. Accessed May 23, 2020.

67. Aungst T. Upgrading the way we identify pills with new technology. *Pharmacy Times*. 2015.

68. Activated Charcoal. Wolters Kluwer Health, Inc; 2020. Available at http://online.lexi.com. Accessed May 19, 2020.

69. Acetylcysteine. Wolters Kluwer Health, Inc; 2020. Available at http://online.lexi.com. Accessed May 19, 2020.

70. Cabaleiro J. Flavoring meds for children and adults so it goes down easy! *Home Healthc Nurse*. 2003;21(5):295-298.

71. Egan ME. Cystic fibrosis transmembrane conductance receptor modulator therapy in cystic fibrosis, an update. *Curr Opin Pediatr*. 2020;32(3):384-388.

72. Cystic Fibrosis Foundation. Types of CFTR mutations. Available at https://www.cff.org/What-is-CF/Genetics/Types-of-CFTR-Mutations/. Accessed May 14, 2020.

73. Goetz D, Ren CL. Review of cystic fibrosis. *Pediatr Ann*. 2019;48(4):e154-e161.

74. Rosenfeld M, Sontag MK, Ren CL. Cystic fibrosis diagnosis and newborn screening. *Pediatr Clin North Am*. 2016;63(4):599-615.

75. Cystic Fibrosis Foundation. 2018 Patient Registry Annual Data Report. Available at https://www.cff.org/Research/Researcher-Resources/Patient-Registry/2018-Patient-Registry-Annual-Data-Report.pdf. Accessed May 14, 2020.

76. Cystic Fibrosis Foundation. Understanding changes in life expectancy. Available at https://www.cff.org/Research/Researcher-Resources/Patient-Registry/Understanding-Changes-in-Life-Expectancy/. Accessed May 14, 2020.

77. Grosse SD, Boyle CA, Botkin JR, et al. Newborn screening for cystic fibrosis: evaluation of benefits and risks and recommendations for state newborn screening programs. *MMWR Recomm Rep*. 2004;53(RR-13):1-36.

78. U.S. National Library of Medicine. What is newborn screening? Available at https://ghr.nlm.nih.gov/primer/newbornscreening/nbs. Accessed May 14, 2020.

79. Farrell PM, White TB, Ren CL, et al. Diagnosis of cystic fibrosis: consensus guidelines from the Cystic Fibrosis Foundation. *J Pediatr*. 2017;181S:S4-S15.e1.

80. U.S. National Library of Medicine. What disorders are included in newborn screening? Available at https://ghr.nlm.nih.gov/primer/newbornscreening/nbsdisorders. Accessed May 16, 2020.

81. Schluter DK, Griffiths R, Adam A, et al. Impact of cystic fibrosis on birthweight: a population based study of children in Denmark and Wales. *Thorax*. 2019;74(5):447-454.

82. Sosnay PR, White TB, Farrell PM, et al. Diagnosis of cystic fibrosis in nonscreened populations. *J Pediatr*. 2017;181S:S52-S57.e2.

83. Farrell PM, White TB, Howenstine MS, et al. Diagnosis of cystic fibrosis in screened populations. *J Pediatr*. 2017;181S:S33-S44.e2.

84. Cystic Fibrosis Foundation. Sweat test. Available at https://www.cff.org/What-is-CF/Testing/Sweat-Test/. Accessed May 31, 2020.

85. Stallings VA, Stark LJ, Robinson KA, et al. Evidence-based practice recommendations for nutrition-related management of children and adults with cystic fibrosis and pancreatic insufficiency: results of a systematic review. *J Am Diet Assoc*. 2008;108(5):832-839.

86. Yen EH, Quinton H, Borowitz D. Better nutritional status in early childhood is associated with improved clinical outcomes and survival in patients with cystic fibrosis. *J Pediatr*. 2013;162(3):530-535.e1.

87. Borowitz D, Baker RD, Stallings V. Consensus report on nutrition for pediatric patients with cystic fibrosis. *J Pediatr Gastroenterol Nutr.* 2002;35(3):246-259.

88. Matel JL. Nutritional management of cystic fibrosis. *JPEN J Parenter Enteral Nutr.* 2012;36(1 suppl):60S-67S.

89. Sinaasappel M, Stern M, Littlewood J, et al. Nutrition in patients with cystic fibrosis: a European consensus. *J Cyst Fibros.* 2002;1(2):51-75.

90. Pancrelipase. Wolters Kluwer Clinical Drug Information, Inc.; 2020. Available at http://online.lexi.com. Accessed May 9, 2020.

91. Lahiri T, Hempstead SE, Brady C, et al. Clinical practice guidelines from the Cystic Fibrosis Foundation for preschoolers with cystic fibrosis. *Pediatrics.* 2016;137(4):e20151784.

92. Centers for Disease Control and Prevention. Recommended child and adolescent immunization schedule for ages 18 years or younger, United States, 2020. Available at https://www.cdc.gov/vaccines/schedules/hcp/imz/child-adolescent.html. Accessed May 17, 2020.

93. Xavioer SaG, J. Authority and scope of vaccination: how states differ. *Pharmacy Times.* 2017. Available at https://www.pharmacytimes.com/about-us. Accessed May 17, 2020.

94. Quittner AL, Zhang J, Marynchenko M, et al. Pulmonary medication adherence and health-care use in cystic fibrosis. *Chest.* 2014;146(1):142-151.

95. Haller W, Ledder O, Lewindon PJ, Couper R, Gaskin KJ, Oliver M. Cystic fibrosis: an update for clinicians. Part 1: nutrition and gastrointestinal complications. *J Gastroenterol Hepatol.* 2014;29(7):1344-1355.

96. Ledder O, Haller W, Couper RT, Lewindon P, Oliver M. Cystic fibrosis: an update for clinicians. Part 2: hepatobiliary and pancreatic manifestations. *J Gastroenterol Hepatol.* 2014;29(12):1954-1962.

97. Rafeeq MM, Murad HAS. Cystic fibrosis: current therapeutic targets and future approaches. *J Transl Med.* 2017;15(1):84.

98. Mogayzel PJ Jr, Naureckas ET, Robinson KA, et al. Cystic fibrosis pulmonary guidelines. Chronic medications for maintenance of lung health. *Am J Respir Crit Care Med.* 2013;187(7):680-689.

99. Flume PA, Mogayzel PJ Jr, Robinson KA, et al. Cystic fibrosis pulmonary guidelines: treatment of pulmonary exacerbations. *Am J Respir Crit Care Med.* 2009;180(9):802-808.

100. Nenna R, Midulla F, Lambiase C, et al. Effects of inhaled hypertonic (7%) saline on lung function test in preschool children with cystic fibrosis: results of a crossover, randomized clinical trial. *Ital J Pediatr.* 2017;43(1):60.

101. Nichols DP, Durmowicz AG, Field A, Flume PA, VanDevanter DR, Mayer-Hamblett N. Developing inhaled antibiotics in cystic fibrosis: current challenges and opportunities. *Ann Am Thorac Soc.* 2019;16(5):534-539.

102. Zobell JT, Young DC, Waters CD, et al. Optimization of anti-pseudomonal antibiotics for cystic fibrosis pulmonary exacerbations: VI. Executive summary. *Pediatr Pulmonol.* 2013;48(6):525-537.

103. Ng SM, Jones AP. Drug therapies for reducing gastric acidity in people with cystic fibrosis. *Cochrane Database Syst Rev.* 2003;(2):CD003424.

104. Middleton PG, Mall MA, Drevinek P, et al. Elexacaftor-tezacaftor-ivacaftor for cystic fibrosis with a single Phe508del allele. *N Engl J Med.* 2019;381(19):1809-1819.

105. Starner C. How much is too much? Available at https://www.primetherapeutics.com/en/news/prime-insights/2019-insights/Story_Cystic_Fibrosis_Treatments.html. Accessed May 21, 2020.

106. Coutinho HD, Falcao-Silva VS, Goncalves GF. Pulmonary bacterial pathogens in cystic fibrosis patients and antibiotic therapy: a tool for the health workers. *Int Arch Med.* 2008;1(1):24.

107. Barlam TF, Cosgrove SE, Abbo LM, et al. Implementing an Antibiotic Stewardship Program: guidelines by the Infectious Diseases Society of America and the Society for Healthcare Epidemiology of America. *Clin Infect Dis.* 2016;62(10):e51-e77.

108. Waters VJ, Ratjen FA. Is there a role for antimicrobial stewardship in cystic fibrosis? *Ann Am Thorac Soc.* 2014;11(7):1116-1119.

109. Safi KH, Damiani JM, Sturza J, Naer SZ. Extended-interval aminoglycoside use in cystic fibrosis exacerbation in children and young adults: a prospective quality improvement project. *Glob Pediatr Health.* 2016;3:2333794X16635464.

110. Zobell JT, Schwab E, Collingridge DS, Ball C, Nohavec R, Asfour F. Impact of pharmacy services on cystic fibrosis medication adherence. *Pediatr Pulmonol.* 2017 52(8):1006-1012.

111. Rosenfeld M, Ratjen F, Brumback L, et al. Inhaled hypertonic saline in infants and children younger than 6 years with cystic fibrosis: the ISIS randomized controlled trial. *JAMA.* 2012;307(21):2269-2277.

112. Bishay LC, Sawicki GS. Strategies to optimize treatment adherence in adolescent patients with cystic fibrosis. *Adolesc Health Med Ther.* 2016;7:117-124.

113. Eakin MN, Riekert KA. The impact of medication adherence on lung health outcomes in cystic fibrosis. *Curr Opin Pulm Med.* 2013;19(6):687-691.

CHAPTER 7

Geriatrics
Featuring the Illustrated Case Studies "Burden" & "Sleuth"

Authors

Robert M. Breslow, Mara A. Kieser, & Joseph A. Zorek

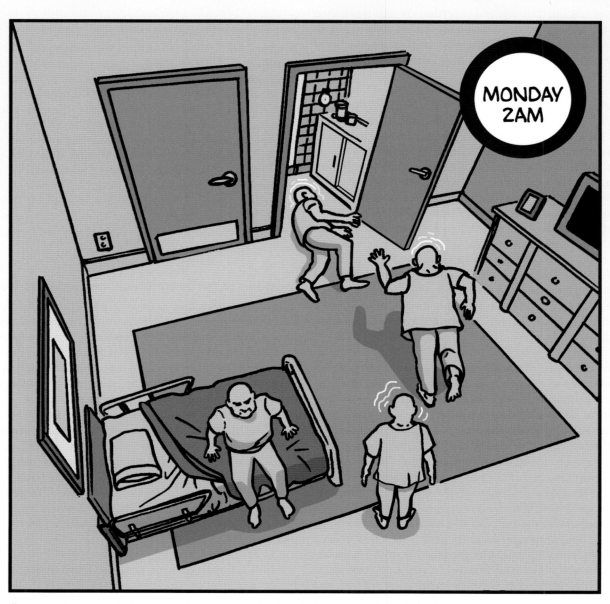

Illustration by George Folz, © 2019 Board of Regents of the University of Wisconsin System

BACKGROUND

Within the next 40 years, one in four Americans will be older than age 65.[1] It is common for older adults to have at least one chronic health condition (e.g., diabetes, depression, heart failure, urinary incontinence), and many older adults have more than one. The greater the number of chronic health conditions, the greater the number of medications prescribed to manage them. Thirty to 40% of older adults take 5 or more medications and 10% take more than 10.[2-5] While medications can do a lot of good, they can also produce significant drug-related harm in older adults. For example, risks associated with drug interactions are high in this population. Complicating this situation, older adults are more prone to the adverse effects of medications because of age-related changes in the way medications get into and out of the body (i.e., pharmacokinetics) and changes in the body's response to medications (i.e., pharmacodynamics).[6] Geriatric pharmacists, by virtue of their education, training, and expertise, are well positioned to manage, either directly or as a contributing member of an interprofessional team, implications for medication use based on pharmacokinetic and pharmacodynamic changes associated with aging.

Consider, as an example, a class of medications called benzodiazepines used to treat anxiety and sleep problems in older adults.[7] The changes that occur in pharmacokinetics and pharmacodynamics with aging can result in adverse drug events if not accounted for when they are prescribed. Metabolism of benzodiazepines can be slowed with aging, prolonging the time these drugs remain in the body. Furthermore, as we age, our brains become more sensitive to the effects of benzodiazepines, which can exacerbate side effects and lead to troubling adverse drug events. Consequences of benzodiazepine use in older adults include an increased risk for falls and motor vehicle accidents, as well as impairments in cognition (i.e., thinking and memory) and development of dependency with withdrawal-like effects if suddenly discontinued.[7-10] As a result, this class of medications is considered inappropriate for older adults.[11]

Nationwide recognition of the value of geriatric pharmacists dates back over 45 years.[12] Given the inherent risks associated with medication use in this special population, the federal government passed legislation in the mid-1970s mandating that pharmacists perform monthly drug regimen reviews (DRRs), also referred to as medication regimen reviews, for persons residing in skilled nursing facilities. These settings are also referred to as nursing homes, or long-term-care facilities. Monthly DRRs generally entail a review of all medications the long-term care resident is prescribed at the time of the review, with the purpose of identifying ineffective or potentially inappropriate drug therapy, side effects, drug interactions, and duplicate drug therapy.[13] If any of these circumstances are noted, the geriatric pharmacist intervenes with recommendations to optimize medication therapy and minimize risks of harm. Findings and recommendations are reported to the interprofessional team of health professionals responsible for the patient's care, including nursing staff and providers such as nurse practitioners, physician assistants, and physicians.[14]

Geriatric pharmacists outside of long-term-care settings employ a similar technique to systematically review medication regimens of older adults called a comprehensive medication review, or CMR.[15] Interventions by geriatric pharmacists through DRRs and CMRs result in positive outcomes.[16-20] Some important examples include the following:

- Decreased use of inappropriate medications;
- Reduced number of adverse drug events;
- Reduced health expenditures;
- Achievement of desired therapeutic endpoints; and
- Improved health-related quality of life.

Founded in 1969, the American Society of Consultant Pharmacists (ASCP) has long served as a primary professional home for pharmacists who provide care to older adults, also called senior care pharmacy.[21] ASCP supports high-quality patient care by geriatric pharmacists through education, resources, and opportunities for innovation. One of ASCP's signature contributions is development of the professional credential Certified Geriatric Pharmacist, which solidified this practice area in 1997 as a specialty within the profession.[21,22] In 2018, this credential transitioned to the Board Certified Geriatric Pharmacist (BCGP).[23] Stakeholders throughout healthcare acknowledge that effectively caring for older adults requires the meaningful contributions of geriatric pharmacists with specialized knowledge and skills.

Members of the Interprofessional Geriatrics Team

As a distinct branch of healthcare, geriatrics has a long tradition of interprofessional practice, and pharmacists have been valued team members.[24,25] Historically, key non-pharmacist members of interprofessional geriatrics teams have been physicians of all specialty areas, but especially geriatricians, as well as gerontological nurse practitioners and a variety of nursing professionals ranging from registered nurses (RNs) and licensed practical nurses (LPNs) to certified nurse's assistants (CNAs). Other health professionals who make important contributions to high-quality care of older adults include dentists, dietitians/nutritionists, occupational therapists, physical therapists, psychologists, physician assistants, recreational therapists, social workers, and speech therapists.[25] More recently, animal-assisted therapists, art therapists, and music therapists have been leveraged to improve the health and well-being of older adults.[26-28]

Interprofessional care in geriatrics has been shown to improve the management of complex health conditions.[24] The benefits of team-based care include improvements in physical and mental function, as well as improved sense of well-being. For example, improved physical function can help the older adult perform daily activities such as dressing and bathing and can reduce the risk of injury due to falling by increasing lower extremity strength and improving balance and gait. Improvements in mental function are generally associated with a decrease in the severity of depressive symptoms and anxiety. The overall effect of interprofessional geriatrics teams on healthcare utilization and costs has been more difficult to demonstrate because older adults have multiple health problems that complicate this assessment.[29] However, case reports of this positive effect abound; for example, the efforts of an interprofessional team composed of a geriatric pharmacist, nurse case manager, nurse practitioner, and social worker demonstrated reductions in hospital readmission rates and healthcare consumption.[30] In recent years, interprofessional teams with actively engaged geriatric pharmacists have had a meaningful impact on preventive care efforts, with documented positive outcomes related to medication-related problems (MRPs), vaccination rates, and patient and provider satisfaction, to name a few.[31–33] For more information on pharmacists' contributions to reducing hospital readmission rates, see the illustrated case "Support" in Chapter 3 Primary Care. Those interested in preventive care services are encouraged to explore the illustrated cases "Screen," "Change Talk," and "Mobilized" in Chapter 4 Prevention & Wellness.

Role of Pharmacists within the Interprofessional Geriatrics Team

Geriatric pharmacists play an important role in the care of older adults individually and as members of interprofessional teams. Ultimately, the goal is to optimize care and minimize unwanted outcomes. Geriatric pharmacists contribute to this goal by ensuring the safe and effective use of medications in a variety of practice settings. While opportunities for interprofessional collaboration may differ based on setting, the overarching responsibility to protect patients from medication-related harm remains consistent.

Geriatric pharmacists play an important role in the management of chronic health conditions, such as heart failure, diabetes, chronic obstructive pulmonary disease, and others.[20] In this role, these pharmacists recommend appropriate medications for older adults and minimize chances of adverse drug events by identifying potentially inappropriate medications, or potentially inappropriate medication doses. Recommendations are developed through a variety of mechanisms; some examples include patient/caregiver interviews, medication reconciliation activities, and CMRs.[34]

There is evidence that patients who adhere to their appropriately prescribed medication regimens will receive the intended benefits of those medications.[35] One important role of geriatric pharmacists is to counsel and educate patients and caregivers about their medications, ensuring they understand the importance of adherence, as well as how to respond if side effects are experienced. Geriatric pharmacists also provide special medication packaging for patients and caregivers to streamline the medication-taking process.[36,37] Patients with severe arthritis, for example, may struggle to open pill bottles and some patients may also struggle to remember how or when to take their medications. Geriatric pharmacists help them troubleshoot through use of reminder systems or technologies designed to overcome barriers to medication adherence.[38]

Pharmacists' knowledge about, and ability to use, medication risk assessments and tools to evaluate the appropriateness of medications in older adults makes them an invaluable member of the interprofessional geriatrics team. By assisting in identifying higher-risk drugs, the geriatric pharmacist can help prevent unnecessary healthcare costs such as emergency department visits and hospitalizations. For older adults, approximately 10% of hospital admissions are the result of medications.[39–41] Twenty-five percent of older adults who are hospitalized will experience an adverse drug event, and a quarter to one-half of these could have been prevented.[42]

Interprofessional teams caring for older adults can be found in a variety of practice settings. Contributing to the care of older adults is not necessarily dependent on the care team itself specializing in geriatrics. Patients 65 years and older are hospitalized at a rate nearly twice as often as the adult population under age 65, but they comprise less than 15% of the US population.[43] In addition, adults over age 65 frequent physician offices more than twice as often as adults under the age of 65.[44] In short, a pharmacist with expertise and training in geriatrics can be an invaluable resource as a formal or informal member of many care teams to improve a wide range of outcomes.

Care provided by geriatric pharmacists is associated with positive effects on medication use, safety, and adherence, as well as hospitalization rates.[45] In addition to these positive outcomes, the integration of pharmacists into interprofessional geriatrics teams is a fiscally smart decision.[46] Medication management by geriatric pharmacists is an effective solution to caring for older adults with high-risk, high-cost health conditions. Geriatric pharmacists should be considered an essential member of interprofessional care teams based on their demonstrated ability to improve the overall care of older adults.

GERIATRIC PHARMACISTS IN ACTION

Making House Calls

As patients age, increasingly in their own homes, or in the homes of their children, traveling to medical appointments can become burdensome. This extends to visiting community pharmacies. For older adults of advanced age, or those who may be frail, a trip to the pharmacy for advice about medications can be impractical due to physical limitations. A geriatric pharmacist developed a solution to this problem; namely, making house calls.[47] One such visit involved a family's efforts to help their 90-year-old mother, who was experiencing oral health issues including dry mouth, sores, and cavities. Having read a story in the local newspaper about the geriatric pharmacist, the daughter of this older adult arranged a visit. To her surprise, the visit began with conversation about her mother's well-being rather than rushing to discuss medications. After obtaining her mother's health history, the pharmacist then assessed home safety (e.g., loose carpeting or rugs that might serve as trip hazards) and asked questions about quality of life. Having taken the time to establish rapport with the family, the geriatric pharmacist then gathered additional information about medications. A complete assessment of the patient's medication list, including screening for drug interactions and side effects, was developed in real time. A full report was mailed to the family, who shared this with the mother's primary care provider at her next visit. This resulted in medication adjustments and the discontinuation of one medication associated with dry mouth, which resolved many of the oral health issues experienced and led to much-appreciated improvements in the mother's quality of life.

Precision Medicine to Improve the Care of Older Adults

It has been shown that genetic differences contribute to variable responses to medications.[48] Identifying these variations through pharmacogenomic testing can have important implications for drug therapy. For example, knowledge of genetic variations linked to how drugs are metabolized can lead to safer and more effective drug selection, drug dosing, and avoidance of drug interactions. One group studied the feasibility of a centralized pharmacy model for performing pharmacogenomic testing with associated recommendations to improve medication use.[49] This group partnered with a company that manages the pharmacy needs of patients who participate in the Program of All-Inclusive Care for the Elderly (PACE), a long-term-care model for qualifying community-dwelling adults that has been adopted across many states.[50] PACE programs serve individuals who are 55 years of age or older who have been certified by their state to need long-term care, but who are able to live safely in

the community. PACE programs provide the entire range of services for older adults with chronic care needs with the goal of keeping them in their homes for as long as possible. Pharmacogenomic testing was completed for PACE participants, and results were reviewed by pharmacists for potential interventions to improve drug therapy. Pharmacists recommended improvements to medication regimens to the patients' healthcare providers; 89% of which were accepted. Given the economics of caring for older adults, the use of pharmacogenomic testing to optimize medication use in this manner has the potential to lower healthcare costs by improving outcomes and preventing additional expenditures associated with adverse drug events.

BECOMING A GERIATRIC PHARMACIST

While all Doctor of Pharmacy (PharmD) students are exposed to medication management in the older adult population, the depth and breadth of that education can vary widely. By and large, most of the training to be a geriatric pharmacist occurs after completion of the PharmD degree. It is possible to develop expertise in geriatric pharmacy through a combination of continuing professional development and practice experience, but this can take years. The more direct path is to complete a general postgraduate year 1 residency followed by a postgraduate year 2 specialty residency focused on geriatrics.[51] A specialty residency in geriatrics provides an intensive training experience with robust patient care opportunities and exposure to geriatric pharmacy in multiple practice settings, such as in clinics, long-term care facilities, and hospitals. There are also geriatric pharmacy-focused fellowships for individuals who would like to receive research training.

The BCGP credential is another avenue to demonstrate expertise in the care of older adults. Pharmacists with the BCGP credential have met specific eligibility criteria that serve to provide evidence of their advanced knowledge about the care of older adults. To obtain BCGP status, pharmacists must graduate from a PharmD program accredited by the Accreditation Council for Pharmacy Education (ACPE), or a qualifying program outside the United States. In addition to achieving a passing score on a written examination, the pharmacist must demonstrate a minimum of 2 years of practice experience following licensure, with at least 50% of time spent in geriatric pharmacy activities. Recertification is required every 7 years and can be obtained by taking a recertification examination or completing approved continuing education.[23]

BURDEN: An Illustrated Case Study

Story by Robert M. Breslow & Joseph A. Zorek
Illustrations by George Folz, © 2019 Board of Regents of the University of Wisconsin System

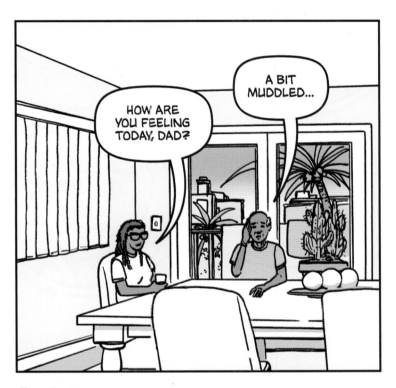

Illustration 7-1

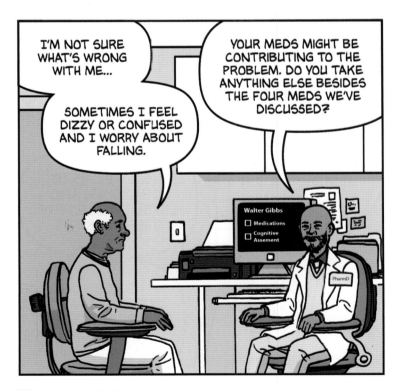

Illustration 7-2

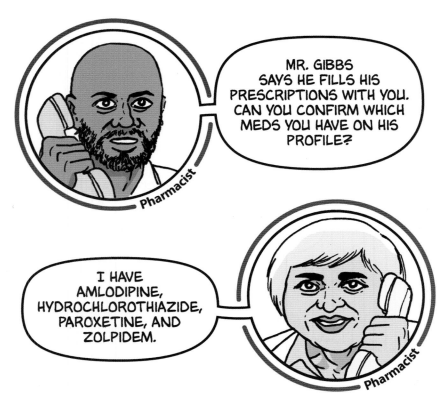

Illustration 7-3

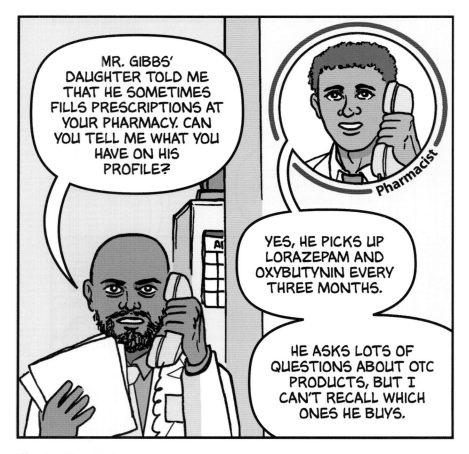

Illustration 7-4

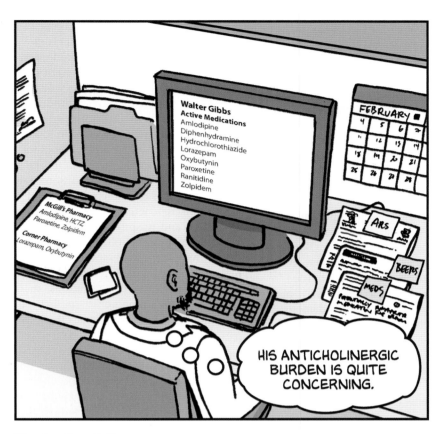

Illustration 7-5

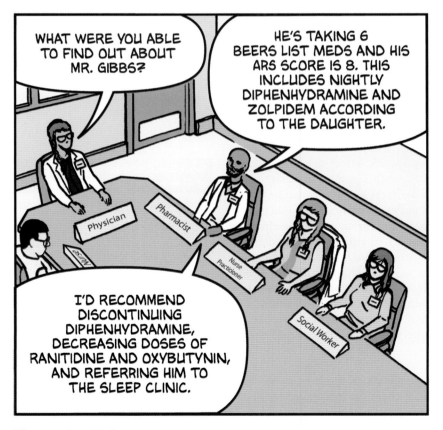

Illustration 7-6

Thoughts on "Burden"

The illustrated case "Burden" highlights the importance of medication reconciliation for the health and well-being of older adults. It also shines a light on a vitally important role of caregivers. The burden caregivers shoulder, especially as dependency increases with advancing age, can be quite large. It can also be highly variable based on a loved one's health condition (e.g., chronic obstructive pulmonary disease, heart failure, dementia). Without his daughter's engagement and encouragement (Illustration 7-1), Mr. Gibbs may not have scheduled the medical visit depicted in Illustration 7-2. Nor would the pharmacist's efforts to reconcile his medication list have succeeded, for it was Mr. Gibbs' daughter who filled in important details, such as the revelation of multiple pharmacies and use of an over-the-counter medication, diphenhydramine (Benadryl), that is likely contributing to his mental state. As patients age, they become more susceptible to another kind of burden frequently discussed in geriatric pharmacy circles; namely, medications with anticholinergic properties. This case demonstrates one pharmacist's efforts, working in concert with other pharmacist colleagues (Illustrations 7-3 and 7-4), to reduce risks associated with these medications via contributions as a valued member of an interprofessional geriatrics team (Illustrations 7-5 and 7-6).

As we age, our organ systems undergo predictable changes.[52,53] Kidneys, for example, become less efficient at filtering blood. The rate at which these changes take place varies from person to person.[52] This is important because organ function plays a critical role determining the concentration of medications in our bodies, and hence the ultimate effect they have on us. In pharmacy terms, this is referred to as pharmacokinetics and pharmacodynamics, respectively, as noted briefly in the Background section above.[53,54]

Pharmacokinetics is the fate of a medication in the body; how it moves, where it accumulates, what concentration it reaches in the blood. Pharmacodynamics describes the effect a drug has on the body once it reaches its intended site of action; in other words, the drug attaches to a specific receptor on a specific organ and produces a specific effect (e.g., slows down heart rate). Most of the time, this results in desired outcomes; however, unwanted effects sometimes occur. While chronological age alone is not necessarily an absolute predictor of organ function or potential for adverse drug effects, it has been associated with increased risk for unwanted effects and MRPs. Examples of MRPs include missing medications (i.e., medications a patient is not taking that they should be taking for a specific health condition), incorrect medication doses, adverse drug reactions, unnecessary medications, and inappropriate medications.[53] Geriatric pharmacists, like the protagonist in "Burden," are trained to identify and correct these MRPs.

Anticholinergic effects of medications result from blockade of a neurotransmitter (i.e., a chemical messenger inside the body) called acetylcholine.[56] Acetylcholine is involved in learning and memory, making its blockade problematic. In addition to the central nervous system (i.e., the brain and spinal cord), where anticholinergic effects have a deleterious effect on learning and memory, acetylcholine receptors can be found throughout the body. As such, medications that block acetylcholine can produce many undesirable effects. The potency of anticholinergic drugs can range from high to low. When medications with high anticholinergic potency are taken by an older adult, the older adult can be said to have high anticholinergic burden. The magnitude of this burden increases with each additional anticholinergic medication taken. This is problematic because anticholinergic effects can result in cognitive decline, delirium, dizziness, confusion, falls, and hospitalizations.[57-59] Other adverse effects associated with anticholinergic medications include blurry vision, constipation, dry mouth, urinary retention, and impairment of thermoregulation causing the older adult to be susceptible to heat-related complications, such as heat stroke. Table 7-1 describes a mnemonic that is used to remind health professionals about the adverse effects that can occur with anticholinergic medications.[60]

Assessment tools have been designed to estimate anticholinergic burden, and geriatric pharmacists leverage these tools to minimize use of such medications. There are many examples of these tools, including the Anticholinergic Activity Scale, Anticholinergic Burden Classification, Anticholinergic Cognitive Burden Scale, Anticholinergic Drug Scale, Anticholinergic Loading Scale, and the Anticholinergic Risk Scale (ARS).[61,62] Each contains a list of medications with anticholinergic properties and some mechanism to assign a score to provide the user with a sense of overall potency of their anticholinergic actions. They provide geriatric pharmacists a framework to help guide clinical decisions to minimize medication risks; that is, to identify problematic medications, reduce their doses, or eliminate them altogether (i.e., de-prescribe them).

Table 7-1. Common Mnemonic Describing Physiologic Effects of Anticholinergic Medications		
Mnemonic	**Medical Terminology**	**Physiologic Effect**
Hot as a hare	Hyperthermia	Increased body temperature
Blind as a bat	Mydriasis	Dilated pupils
Dry as a bone	Xerostomia	Dry mouth
	Keratoconjunctivitis sicca	Dry eyes
	Hypohidrosis	Decreased sweat
Red as a beet	Flushing	Redness of face, neck, other parts of body
Mad as a hatter	Cognitive impairment	Change in mental status, inability to concentrate, delirium

Another key phrase in the geriatric pharmacy literature is "potentially inappropriate medications," or PIMs. This phrase gained in popularity with the publication of what has become a seminal work in this field; namely, the Beers Criteria for Potentially Inappropriate Medication Use in Older Adults.[11] The Beers Criteria is updated regularly by the American Geriatrics Society. It includes PIMs related to anticholinergic burden, as well as a whole host of additional medication-related concerns. Illustration 7-5 reveals that the pharmacist is using both the Beers Criteria and the ARS to establish his recommendations to address Mr. Gibbs' primary concern of mental confusion. Mr. Gibbs' complete medication list includes six Beers Criteria medications and an anticholinergic burden that is quite high, indicated by his ARS score of 8 (Illustration 7-6). Together, these tools are used in a complementary manner to guide clinical decision making within the interprofessional geriatrics team.

Irrespective of Beers Criteria and ARS score, the sheer number of medications Mr. Gibbs is taking (eight total) puts him at risk due to polypharmacy.[63,64] Polypharmacy can be a significant problem for older adults, as it has been shown to be associated with hospitalizations, increased healthcare costs, and MRPs such as adverse drug events, drug interactions, and even death.[63,64] There is no standard definition of polypharmacy. Studies have defined polypharmacy using a wide range of criteria, from as low as 2 medications to more than 11 medications.[64] The majority of studies, however, have defined polypharmacy using five medications as the cutoff; in other words, a patient is experiencing polypharmacy if they take five or more medications. Approximately 40% of adults age 65 and older satisfy these criteria.[2]

Polypharmacy generally has a negative connotation. However, there is rational (i.e., appropriate) polypharmacy and indiscriminate (i.e., inappropriate) polypharmacy.[64] In the case of rational polypharmacy, the use of multiple medications may be appropriate for the number of underlying health conditions. So long as their use is guided by an evidence-based framework to optimize care and improve clinical outcomes, this is not seen as problematic. On the other hand, indiscriminate polypharmacy embodies the use of medications for which there is no clear indication, or in situations where its presence may do more harm than good.

The use of multiple prescribers and multiple pharmacies has also been associated with polypharmacy.[65] The illustrated case "Burden" highlights the challenges of keeping track of medication use, for patients, caregivers, and health professionals, when medications are purchased from multiple community pharmacies. Before the pharmacist can troubleshoot Mr. Gibbs' complaints of feeling dizzy, confused, and afraid of falling (Illustration 7-2), he must first reconcile Mr. Gibbs' medication list. As depicted in Illustrations 7-3 and 7-4, this involves cooperation with two different pharmacists; some important information is derived from dispensing records,

while other details, such as over-the-counter medication use, are provided from memory. The latter highlights the critical role of relationship-building in the community pharmacy setting. For a more in-depth discussion of this practice area, readers are encouraged to explore the illustrated cases "Organized Chaos," "Transformation," and "Breathe" in Chapter 2 Community Pharmacy.

There are times when a medication is prescribed to treat a suspected medical problem when the symptom reported by the patient is actually an adverse effect caused by an existing medication. This is called the prescribing cascade, and geriatric pharmacists must constantly be on the lookout for it.[66] Consider the example, unrelated to the case of Mr. Gibbs, of medications used to treat the symptoms of Alzheimer's dementia. Some of these are associated with urinary incontinence (i.e., loss of bladder control that leads to involuntary urination).[67] Urinary incontinence, completely unrelated to medications, is considered a geriatric syndrome and is experienced by an estimated 40% to 45% of older adults.[68] If a patient taking one of the Alzheimer's medications associated with urinary incontinence meets with a prescriber who is unfamiliar with this adverse drug effect, a new medical diagnosis is likely to be made. This, in turn, can initiate the prescribing cascade with the addition of a new medication to treat urinary incontinence. Mr. Gibbs is actually taking one of these; namely, oxybutynin (Ditropan). Oxybutynin works by decreasing muscle spasms in the bladder; however, it is also highly anticholinergic.[59,69] In formulating his recommendations, one of the puzzles the geriatric pharmacist in "Burden" needs to figure out is whether oxybutynin, which is likely contributing to Mr. Gibbs' complaints, is a necessary medication, or whether it was added as part of a prescribing cascade.

Pharmacists can help to minimize polypharmacy in several ways.[20] Some of the most impactful are listed below:

1. Perform a thorough medication history to generate a complete list of prescription and over-the-counter medications;
2. Identify drug-related problems and work with prescribers to eliminate problematic or unnecessary medications and reduce pill burden/polypharmacy; and
3. Counsel patients on remaining medications to ensure complete understanding of their purpose and importance, including how to take them and what to expect, in order to facilitate medication adherence.

Step 2 involves an important process called de-prescribing, which is intended to reduce polypharmacy by eliminating PIMs.[70,71] A number of tools and algorithms have been developed to help pharmacists and other health professionals identify PIMs and other high-risk medications.[64] The Beers Criteria and several anticholinergic scales have already been addressed. Another important tool is called the STOPP/START Criteria.[72] This tool, like the Beers Criteria, was developed to identify potentially inappropriate prescribing and, in so doing, reduce the risk of harm to the older adult. Another tool is the Medication Appropriateness Index (MAI), which is predicated on a series of questions that leads the health professional to conclude whether a PIM can/should be de-prescribed.[73] Each of the tools has strengths and weaknesses, and it is important for geriatric pharmacists to familiarize themselves with these prior to use.[64,74]

To have the most positive impact, geriatric pharmacists must work interprofessionally with other health professionals and closely with caregivers. According to data from the US Census Bureau, 35% of older adults have some type of disability.[1] This includes difficulties in hearing, vision, cognition, ambulation, self-care, and independent living. Changes in physical and cognitive function associated with aging can result in increasing dependency on caregivers. The percentage of older adults age 85 and over needing help with personal care is more than twice the percentage for older adults ages 75 to 84, and more than six times the percentage for adults ages 65 to 74.[75] These age-related changes have important implications as they relate to managing medications. As pointed out already, the number of medications prescribed generally increases in each of these decades of life.

Informal caregivers, such as Mr. Gibbs' daughter, are indispensable partners in medication management.[76] A caregiver's role in medication management can include ordering and picking up medications at the pharmacy, splitting tablets, setting up pill boxes, teaching how to use medication-related devices (e.g., inhalers, glucose meters, blood pressure machines), and administering medications. Such caregivers frequently take responsibility for communicating with health professionals about their loved one's health status and, in some cases, may also be involved in healthcare decisions.

Monitoring medication adherence (i.e., keeping track of medications to be sure they are taken appropriately) can be a challenging task for an informal caregiver, especially in the case of a dependent older adult who is cognitively impaired. Geriatric pharmacists often provide caregivers with medication adherence support. Such support may include preparing medication lists, calendars, and checklists; setting up and programming electronic reminder devices; and filling pill organizing systems.[55] Adherence approaches must be tailored to individual and family needs. The roles/responsibilities of the caregiver could be limited by their own mental and/or physical limitations. Such situations often involve multiple informal caregivers, and it is incumbent upon the geriatric pharmacist to develop relationships with all involved to ensure the safe and effective use of medications.[76]

The illustrated case "Burden" highlights a number of issues that underscore the challenges of caring for older adults. It is common for informal caregivers, often family, to assist in medication management. Aging can affect how medications act in the body and this can lead to unwanted consequences like falls. This is compounded by the number of medications prescribed for Mr. Gibbs and Mr. Gibbs' use of multiple pharmacies, making it difficult for the pharmacist to obtain a complete medication list. Incomplete information makes it difficult to identify or anticipate drug interactions that would increase Mr. Gibbs' risk for adverse drug effects as is the case for multiple medications with anticholinergic effects. In order to mitigate unwanted consequences, there are a number of assessment tools that are available to pharmacists, as well as other health professionals, to stop or alter the doses of medications that can do more harm than good. Finally, this illustrated case showcases the benefits of team-based care to develop strategies for safer medication use in older adults.

DISCUSSION QUESTIONS FOR "BURDEN"

1. Illustration 7-6 highlights interprofessional practice. When looking around the table at the participants, what knowledge and skills do you think each team member contributes to the care of older adults like Mr. Gibbs?

2. The illustrated case "Burden" demonstrates the complex nature of the care of older adults and is notable for the involvement of family members. Have you been involved in the care of an older family member? Or has anyone you know been in a situation like this? What impact do you think this type of family member engagement has on the quality of care received?

3. The main pharmacist in this illustrated case, originally depicted in Illustration 7-2, found it necessary to contact other pharmacists who might be able to contribute information about Mr. Gibbs' medication regimen, given Mr. Gibbs' medication-related purchasing patterns. Of these pharmacists, who should ultimately bear responsibility for maintaining Mr. Gibbs' complete medication list? Why?

4. The main pharmacist focuses his attention on the medications with anticholinergic effects that can cause unwanted side effects. What other monitoring might the main pharmacist perform to ensure the appropriateness of all of Mr. Gibbs' medications? Think about predictable physiologic changes associated with aging.

5. Illustrations 7-1 and 7-2 highlight that thinking and memory can be affected by medications, but they also suggest that Mr. Gibbs might have an underlying memory problem. Besides not remembering the names of his medications, how else could memory problems affect his medication taking?

SLEUTH: An Illustrated Case Study

Story by Mara A. Kieser & Joseph A. Zorek
Illustrations by George Folz, © 2019 Board of Regents of the University of Wisconsin System

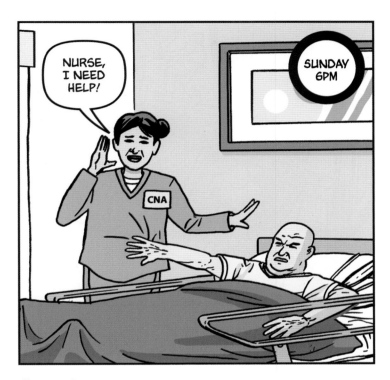

Illustration 7-7

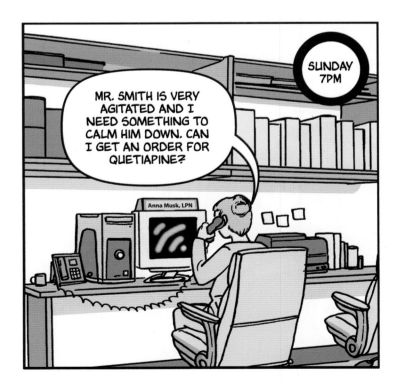

Illustration 7-8

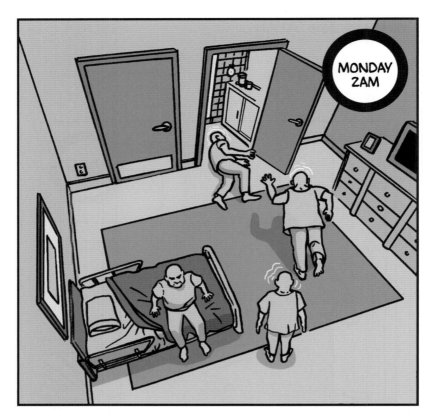

Illustration 7-9

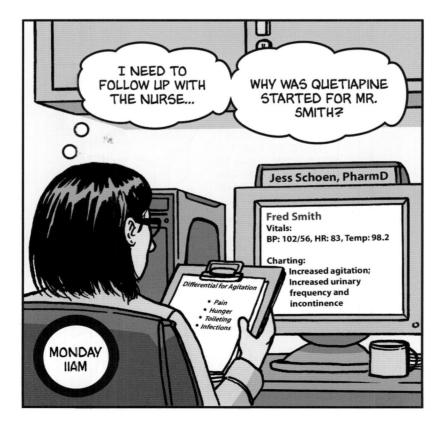

Illustration 7-10

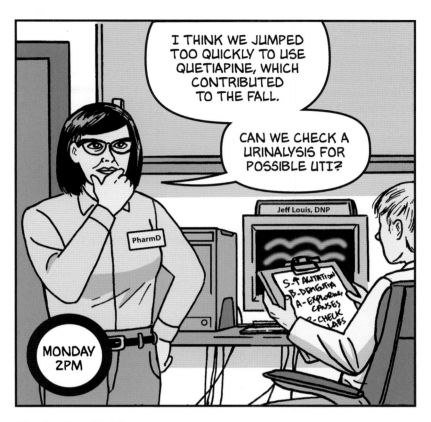

Illustration 7-11

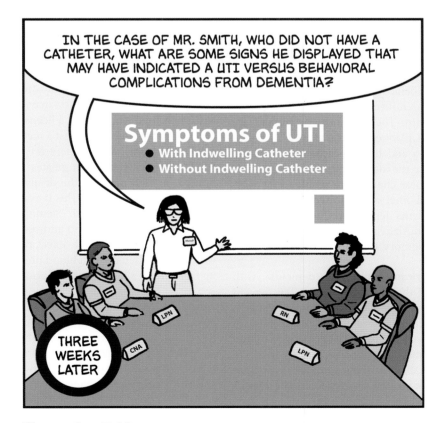

Illustration 7-12

Thoughts on "Sleuth"

The illustrated case "Sleuth" highlights the challenges health professionals face providing care for patients with dementia. The protagonist, Dr. Jess Schoen, serves as a consultant pharmacist to a skilled nursing facility. Another formal name for this practice setting is long-term care facility, while many refer to these settings informally as nursing homes. A patient named Fred Smith is experiencing what appears to be behavioral symptoms associated with dementia (Illustration 7-7), which initiates a string of events that ultimately lead to a serious adverse drug event (Illustrations 7-8 and 7-9). Jess tracks down, or sleuths, the cause of this medication error. She collects facts (Illustration 7-10), works collaboratively with a nurse practitioner (Illustration 7-11), and provides education to team members to avoid similar medication errors in the future (Illustration 7-12).

In simple terms, dementia refers to loss of memory and the symptoms associated with memory loss.[77] There are multiple types of dementia, and each is characterized by abnormal changes within the brain. Different parts of the brain control and correspond with different functions. Examples include interpreting body sensations, processing sight, sound, and smells; thinking, problem solving, and planning; forming and controlling memories; and controlling voluntary movements. Alzheimer's disease is the most common form of dementia, accounting for between 60% to 80% of cases.[78] Other less common forms include vascular, Lewy body, and frontotemporal dementia. While these dementias differ according to brain changes, onset of symptoms, and types of symptoms experienced, they all share memory loss as a main problem.

Mr. Smith suffers from Alzheimer's disease, which was discovered in the early 1900s by Dr. Alois Alzheimer, a practicing psychiatrist in Germany.[79] Dr. Alzheimer identified brain abnormalities in one of his patients after her death and linked these changes to abnormal behaviors associated with dementia. Scientists have since identified abnormal formations of proteins present in the brain. The two most prominent are referred to as beta-amyloid plaques and tangles of a protein called tau.[80,81] These plaques and tangles cause brain cells to die, which ultimately leads to the loss of brain tissue in patients with Alzheimer's disease. These changes are visible using magnetic resonance imaging and other sophisticated technologies.[82] Symptoms exhibited by patients depend on the location of the damaged cells in the brain. In Alzheimer's disease, areas affected typically control learning, memory, thinking, and planning.

More than 5 million Americans suffer from dementia, with Alzheimer's dementia being the most prevalent.[78] Ten percent of Americans over 65 years of age have Alzheimer's, which is the sixth-leading cause of death in the United States. In terms of economic impact, this disease was projected to cost $305 billion in 2020. People age 65 and older live an average of 4 to 8 years after an Alzheimer's diagnosis, but some live as long as 20 years, which highlights the variable progression of the disease.

While dementia is not a normal part of aging, increased age is one risk factor for dementia.[83] Additional risk factors for developing dementia have been identified and are multifactorial. In 2017, the Lancet Commission estimated that a third of dementia cases are caused by potentially modifiable risk factors such as educational attainment, midlife hypertension and obesity, hearing loss, late-life depression, diabetes, physical inactivity, smoking, and social isolation.[84] Identifying modifiable risk factors is extremely important in preventing dementia, as this disease currently has no cure.

Dementia is typically divided into three stages: early, mild-to-moderate, and severe.[81] It is important for health professionals and caregivers to recognize symptoms associated with each stage, as they provide clues as to the speed with which the disease is progressing, as well as the potential efficacy of therapeutic approaches being used (Table 7-2).[81,85]

Beyond modifying risk factors listed above, a mainstay in dementia treatment is the use of medications to slow progression and improve dementia symptoms. Several examples of medications used for these purposes are described in Table 7-3.[77,86]

In addition to cognitive deficits, patients with dementia also suffer from behavioral and psychological symptoms, commonly referred to as BPSD.[87] The nurse assistant in Illustration 7-7 finds herself in a challenging situation, whereby Mr. Smith is agitated and physically striking out at her. These are hallmark features of BPSD that are frequently referred to as "behaviors." Additional common BPSD symptoms include apathy, anxiety, insomnia, depression, delusions, and hallucinations.[88] Ninety percent of people with dementia experience BPSD.[87] The burden associated with BPSD is high; for example, it accounts for one-third of all dementia costs, and it is the leading cause of nursing home placement. Patients with dementia who experience severe BPSD, such as psychotic symptoms, have been shown to demonstrate an accelerated cognitive decline, as well as increased mortality.[87,88]

Mr. Smith's residence in a nursing home and the actions of the nurse assistant and nurse in Illustrations 7-7 and 7-8, respectively, imply that his dementia may be progressing. In response to his behavior, Anna Musk, a licensed practical nurse, contacts the on-call provider to request a medication to treat Mr. Smith's BPSD symptoms. While there are many drugs used to treat BPSD, the evidence as it relates to their efficacy is pretty limited. In fact, many of the drugs used for BPSD may cause more harm than good.[89,90] This is exactly what happens with Mr. Smith in the illustrated case "Sleuth," whereby the antipsychotic medication administered to address his aggression, quetiapine (Seroquel), results in a side effect called postural hypotension, which is a sudden drop in blood pressure when a person stands up from either a lying or seated position.[86]

Table 7-4 contains psychoactive (also called psychotropic) medications commonly used to treat both acute and chronic BPSD. For acute aggression, like that displayed by Mr. Smith, antipsychotic medications are used when there is a threat to the safety of the resident or others. However, it is required to assess and address any underlying causes that may contribute to the acute condition.[91] This step is important to verify the need for a psychotropic drug. Interprofessional teams in long-term care settings need to ensure that the acute condition is not due to underlying medical conditions that may resolve, environmental

Table 7-2. Stages of Dementia

Stage	Approximate Duration*	Symptoms
Mild	2–4 years	• Difficulty concentrating • Decreased memory of recent events • Difficulty managing finances • Difficulty traveling alone to new locations • Difficulty completing complex tasks accurately
Moderate	2–10 years	• Major memory deficiencies • Need for assistance to complete daily living activities (dressing, bathing, preparing meals, etc.) • Prominent memory loss including major relevant aspects of current life • Difficulty remembering details of earlier life • Incontinence (loss of bladder or bowel control) • Ability to speak declines • Personality/emotional changes may occur, such as delusions (believing something to be true that is not), compulsions (repeating a simple behavior, such as cleaning), or anxiety and agitation
Severe	1–1.5 years	• Inability to speak or communicate • Need for assistance with most activities (e.g., using the toilet, eating) • Loss of psychomotor skills (e.g., the ability to walk)

* Approximate duration of stages listed here are estimates. Duration is different for each person and some stages may overlap.

Table 7-3. Categories and Examples of Medications Commonly Used to Treat Dementia

Category	Medication Examples*	Physiologic Effect
Cholinesterase inhibitors	• donepezil (Aricept) • galantamine (Razadyne) • rivastigmine (Exelon)	Increase the levels of acetylcholine in the brain, which is thought to maintain memory
NMDA receptor antagonist	• memantine (Namenda)	Decreases the effects of glutamate in the brain, which is thought to decrease damage to the brain and maintain memory

* Medication examples presented in alphabetical order as "generic name (Brand Name)."

factors that can be addressed, or psychological stressors that may improve. For chronic BPSD, the American Psychiatric Association recommends a combination of medication and non-medication therapies.[92] Examples of non-medication therapies include physical activities and music therapy.[93] Evidence supports these non-medication therapies to improve BPSD.

In Illustration 7-9, Mr. Smith experiences postural hypotension when he stands up to use the bathroom several hours after receiving quetiapine to treat the aggression incident, which causes severe dizziness that ultimately results in a fall. While the outcome of Mr. Smith's fall is unclear, studies suggest that 10% to 25% of falls that take place in nursing homes result in serious injury, such as hip or spinal fractures.[94] The association between psychoactive drugs and falls is well established. One study demonstrated that fall risk increased by 54% for patients using antipsychotic medications, 57% for antidepressants, and

42% for anxiolytics.[95] Another study found that polypharmacy, defined by study authors as taking four or more medications, increased fall risk by 75%.[96] Forty percent of nursing home residents take nine or more medications, which underscores how risky this environment can be as it relates to falls.[97]

The US Centers for Medicare and Medicaid Services (CMS), the largest funder of nursing home care, launched an initiative in 2012 to reduce the use of antipsychotic medications in nursing homes.[98,99] When using psychotropic drugs, CMS requires clear documentation of their necessity, that they be gradually reduced in an effort to discontinue when they are used, and that psychotropic drug use on an as-needed basis is limited to 14 days.[91] This initiative began due to the high use of these drugs in nursing homes without an appropriate diagnosis, usage as chemical restraints, and the increased risk of morbidity and mortality when used in patients with dementia. In 2012, the national average for psychotropic drug use in nursing home patients was 23.9%.[98] By 2018, psychotropic drug use in this setting declined to 14.6%.[100]

The National Partnership to Improve Dementia Care in Nursing Homes was created to improve the quality of care for individuals with dementia living in nursing homes.[101] The National Partnership has a mission to deliver healthcare that is person-centered, comprehensive, and interprofessional with a specific focus on protecting residents from being prescribed antipsychotic medications unless there is a valid clinical indication, as well as a systematic process to evaluate each individual's need. This partnership provides multiple educational tools for nursing home staff and families on appropriate use of psychotropic drugs in patients with dementia.

Geriatric pharmacists like Jess in the illustrated case "Sleuth" play an important role in improving medication therapy for patients in long-term-care facilities. CMS requires that

Table 7-4. Categories and Examples of Medications Commonly Used to Treat Behavioral and Psychological Symptoms of Dementia

Category	Medication Examples[*]	Physiologic Effect
Antidepressants	▪ bupropion (Wellbutrin) ▪ citalopram (Celexa) ▪ fluoxetine (Prozac) ▪ mirtazapine (Remeron) ▪ sertraline (Zoloft) ▪ venlafaxine (Effexor)	Act within the brain to alter neurotransmitters[**], such as serotonin, norepinephrine, and dopamine that have been shown to improve mood, sleep, and appetite
Antipsychotics	▪ aripiprazole (Abilify) ▪ haloperidol (Haldol) ▪ olanzapine (Zyprexa) ▪ quetiapine (Seroquel) ▪ risperidone (Risperdal) ▪ ziprasidone (Geodon)	Alter neurotransmitters in the brain, such as dopamine and serotonin, that effect mood, emotions, and behaviors; these include reductions in delusions, hallucinations, and other symptoms of psychosis
Anxiolytics	▪ alprazolam (Xanax) ▪ diazepam (Valium) ▪ lorazepam (Ativan)	Produce a calming effect through activation of benzodiazepine receptors in the brain and by enhancing effects of the neurotransmitter GABA[***]; also affect muscle relaxation and motor coordination
Sedative-hypnotics	▪ eszopiclone (Lunesta) ▪ ramelteon (Rozerem) ▪ zaleplon (Sonata) ▪ zolpidem (Ambien)	Increase neurotransmitters in the brain, such as GABA and melatonin, to produce drowsiness and to induce and/or maintain sleep

[*] Medication examples presented in alphabetical order as "generic name (Brand Name)."

[**] Neurotransmitters are chemical messengers that transmit signals from one part of the body to another; these signals have a wide-ranging impact on physiology.

[***] GABA is an acronym for a neurotransmitter within the brain called gamma-aminobutyric acid.

pharmacists review medications of all patients in these facilities at least monthly.[102] Pharmacists have the training and expertise to identify and mitigate drug therapy problems, including use of inappropriate medications, doses that are too high or too low, drug interactions, and drug side effects. Most facilities do not employ pharmacists on a full-time basis; rather, they are hired as consultants to provide medication review and use services, including educational services to train staff. Oftentimes, this requires some detective-type work on the part of the consultant pharmacist to retrospectively make sense of drug use patterns or, as in "Sleuth," to identify the cause of medication errors.

Geriatric pharmacists' roles have evolved over the years from being product- to patient-focused, and the services provided have shifted toward a more clinical perspective, including medication reviews and medication management. A recent study identified the impact of geriatric pharmacists ensuring the safe and effective use of medications in long-term-care facilities.[103] Interventions by geriatric pharmacists through medication reviews decreased falls among nursing home residents and improved BPSD through participation in interprofessional behavior teams. Pharmacists in this role assume responsibility for ensuring appropriate medication use for patients on psychotropic medications. In addition, pharmacist-led reviews have reduced the number of medications taken per patient and identified and resolved medication therapy problems.

In the illustrated case "Sleuth," Jess arrives to her long-term-care facility Monday morning, a few hours after Mr. Smith's fall.

Illustration 7-10 shows her in the middle of her monthly review of Mr. Smith's medications, during which she learns of the facility's recent use of quetiapine to address his aggressive behavior. She begins the sleuthing process by first trying to determine why quetiapine was used at all, which will help inform recommendations for its gradual dose reduction and discontinuation in accordance with CMS guidance. After reading that he hit a team member, an out-of-the-ordinary event for Mr. Smith, Jess begins to explore alternative causes for his behavior. She starts by looking for medication-related causes, then moves on to other possibilities when nothing turns up. Clues that his behavior may stem from an infection begin to emerge, as evidenced by nurses' charting of increased urine output and Jess's research that pain, hunger, toileting, and infections can also lead to agitation/aggression (Illustration 7-10).

A casual observer might rule out an infectious source because Mr. Smith's body temperature does not meet the classic threshold of fever; that is, 100.4 degrees Fahrenheit (Illustration 7-10).[104] It is common, however, for elevation in body temperature to go unnoticed in this population because the basal (i.e., baseline) temperature for many older adults can be markedly lower than for younger patients. Furthermore, several infections manifest in older adults with atypical symptoms; this includes urinary tract infections (UTIs).[105] Many older adults do not present with the typical UTI symptoms of urgency or burning on urination; rather, some present with other symptoms such as falls or confusion. To determine if older adults have an infection, an established aid called the McGeer criteria provides health professionals with specific definitions and guidance.[106] This tool was developed to assess for true infections and to avoid unwarranted use of antibiotics. Urinary incontinence and frequency are listed in the McGeer criteria for a UTI. In noting the patient's agitation, increased incontinence and urinary frequency, Jess asks Dr. Jeff Louis, the nurse practitioner who serves as the on-site provider, to consider checking a urinalysis to rule out UTI as a cause for Mr. Smith's agitation and abnormal behavior (Illustration 7-11).

The illustrated case "Sleuth" closes with a depiction of another valuable service consultant pharmacists provide to skilled nursing facilities. In Illustration 7-12, Jess is shown in the middle of an educational in-service to nursing home employees. Attendees include nurses like Anna, who initiated quetiapine use with the on-call physician in Illustration 7-8. The goal of in-services like these is not to ridicule, embarrass, or punish mistakes; rather, it is to share lessons learned from adverse drug events like Mr. Smith's fall to avoid similar problems in the future. In addition to symptoms of UTI, Jess will also teach about the McGeer criteria, atypical presentation of infections, common medications used to treat UTIs, medication side effects, and, importantly, how to avoid unnecessary psychotropic drug use.

DISCUSSION QUESTIONS FOR "SLEUTH"

1. Mr. Smith resides in a long-term-care facility, also called a nursing home. Draw upon your knowledge of and/or experiences with this setting; for example, a prior visit to a relative. What are your overall impressions of people living out the remainder of their lives in this setting?

2. Considering what you learned in the description of the illustrated case "Sleuth," what do you think would be the hardest part about being diagnosed with dementia? How might this differ if you were the caregiver of someone diagnosed with dementia?

3. There is currently no curative treatment for Alzheimer's disease, the most common form of dementia. Available medications are intended to slow its progression, yet the side effects can cause harm, presenting a classic challenge in medication management; namely, balancing benefits against risks. Do you think the benefits outweigh the risks in this situation, or vice versa? Explain your rationale.

4. Illustration 7-7 depicts a certified nurse's assistant being physically struck by Mr. Smith. This initiated the use of a psychotropic medication to control his behavior that ultimately led to Mr. Smith's fall. What was your initial reaction to this violent act? How did reading this illustrated case influence your thoughts on the use of medications in this manner?

5. The illustrated case "Sleuth" highlights interprofessional practice between a pharmacist and nurse practitioner to get to the bottom of a complex problem. What changes to medication ordering and use might this long-term-care facility make to prevent such problems in the future?

CHAPTER SUMMARY

- The population of adults 65 years of age and older in the United States is projected to grow over the next 40 years, with a commensurate increase in the use of medications and other healthcare resources.

- With specialized education and training, geriatric pharmacists are well-positioned to improve care delivered to this population, as well as to reduce costs and resource utilization required to do so.

- Geriatric pharmacists work in healthcare settings ranging from community pharmacies, hospitals, and long-term-care facilities to primary care clinics, rehabilitation facilities, and specialty clinics.

- Pharmacists are recognized as important members of interprofessional geriatrics teams, within which they collaborate with a host of health professionals including animal-assisted therapists, art therapists, dentists, dietitians/nutritionists, music therapists, occupational therapists, physical therapists, psychologists, physician assistants, recreational therapists, social workers, and speech therapists.

- Older adults are prone to adverse drug events due to several age- and medication-related factors, and geriatric pharmacists are uniquely qualified to identify, mitigate, and/or manage these factors.

- Geriatric pharmacists use a variety of resources and tools to ensure the safe and effective use of medications, including compilations of potentially inappropriate medications and guides to reduce the use of risky medications, such as those with high anticholinergic burden.

- A growing trend within geriatric pharmacy is the intentional effort to reduce polypharmacy and the use of potentially inappropriate medications through de-prescribing efforts.

- Geriatric pharmacists have factored prominently in federal efforts to curb inappropriate and unsafe medication practices throughout the United States, perhaps most prominently in nursing homes where monthly drug regimen reviews are mandated by law.

REFERENCES

1. U.S. Department of Health and Human Services Administration on Aging. A profile of older Americans: 2017. Available at https://acl.gov/sites/default/files/Aging%20and%20 Disability%20in%20America/2017OlderAmericansProfile.pdf. Accessed May 31, 2020.

2. Charlesworth CJ, Smit E, Lee DS, Alramadhan F, Odden MC. Polypharmacy among adults aged 65 years and older in the United States: 1988-2010. *J Gerontolog A Biol Sci Med Sci*. 2015; 989-995.

3. Farrell B, Thompson W, Black CD, et al. Health care providers' roles and responsibilities in management of polypharmacy: results of a modified Delphi. *Can Pharm J*. 2018;151:395-407.

4. Gu Q, Dillon CF, Burt V. Prescription drug use continued to increase: US prescription drug data for 2007–2008. CDC/NCHS Data Brief No. 42. 2010:1-2.

5. Kantor ED, Rehm CD, Haas JS, Chan AT, Giovannucci EL. Trends in prescription drug use among adults in the United States from 1999–2012. *JAMA.* 2015;314(17):1818-1831.

6. Hutchison LC. Chapter 3: Biomedical principles of aging. In: Hutchison LC, Sleeper RB, eds. *Fundamentals of Geriatric Pharmacotherapy.* 2nd ed. Bethesda, MD: American Society of Health-System Pharmacists; 2015:57-76.

7. Markota M, Rummans TA, Bostwick M, Lapid M. Benzodiazepine use in older adults: dangers, management, and alternative therapies. *Mayo Clin Proc.* 2016;91(11):1632-1639.

8. Gallagher HC. Addressing the issue of chronic, inappropriate benzodiazepine use: how can pharmacists play a role? *Pharmacy.* 2013;1: 65-93.

9. Maust DT, Lin LA, Blow FC. Benzodiazepine use and misuse among adults in the United States. *Psychiatric Services.* 2019;70(2):97-106.

10. Triscott J, Dobbs B, Carr F, et al. Use and misuse of benzodiazepines in the elderly. Available at http://www.cpsa.ca/use-misuse-benzodiazepines-elderly/. Accessed April 21, 2020.

11. The 2019 American Geriatrics Society Beers Criteria Update Expert Panel. American Geriatrics Society 2019 updated AGS Beers Criteria for potentially inappropriate medication use in older adults. *J Am Geriatr Soc.* 2019;67:674-694.

12. Code of Federal Regulations. 42 CFR §482.25—conditions of participation: pharmaceutical services. Available at https://www.govinfo.gov/app/details/CFR-2011-title42-vol5/CFR-2011-title42-vol5-sec482-25. Accessed May 31, 2020.

13. Harjivan C, Lyles A. Improved medication use in long-term care: building on the consultant pharmacist's drug regimen review. *Am J Manag Care.* 2002;8(4):318-326.

14. Code of Federal Regulations. 42 CFR §483.45—pharmacy services. Available at https://www.law.cornell.edu/cfr/text/42/483.45. Accessed May 31, 2020.

15. Kiel WJ, Phillips SW. Impact of pharmacist-conducted comprehensive medication reviews for older adult patients to reduce medication related problems. *Pharmacy.* 2017;6(1):2.

16. Chisholm-Burns MA, Lee JK, Spivey CA, et al. US pharmacists' effect as team members on patient care: systematic review and meta-analysis. *Med Care.* 2010;48(10):923-933.

17. Dalton K, Byrne S. Role of the pharmacist in reducing healthcare costs: current insights. *Integr Pharm Res Pract.* 2017;6:37-46.

18. Gooen LG. Medication reconciliation in long-term care and assisted living facilities: opportunity for pharmacists to minimize risks associated with transitions of care. *Clin Geriatr Med.* 2017;33:225-239.

19. Hughes CM, Lapane KL. Pharmacy interventions on prescribing in nursing homes: from evidence to practice. *Ther Adv Drug Saf.* 2011;2(3):103-112.

20. Lee JK, Alsheri S, Kutbi H, Martin JR. Optimizing pharmacotherapy in elderly patients: the role of pharmacists. *Integr Pharm Res Pract.* 2015;4:101-111.

21. American Society of Consultant Pharmacists. Who we are: empowering pharmacists, transforming aging. Available at https://www.ascp.com/page/whoweare. Accessed April 19, 2020.

22. Elliott RA. Geriatric medicine and pharmacy practice: a historical perspective. *J Pharm Pract Res.* 2016;46:169-177.

23. Board of Pharmacy Specialties. Geriatric pharmacy. Available at https://www.bpsweb.org/bps-specialties/geriatric-pharmacy/. Accessed April 23, 2020.

24. Bonner A, Flaherty E, Hyer K, Karlin B, Fulmer T. Team care. In: Halter JB, Ouslander JG, Studenski S, High KP, Asthana S, Supiano MA, Ritchie C, eds. *Hazzard's Geriatric Medicine and Gerontology.* 7th ed. New York, NY: McGraw-Hill; 2017.

25. Sleeper RB. Chapter 1: Challenges in geriatric care. In: Hutchison LC, Sleepr RB, eds. *Fundamentals of Geriatric Pharmacotherapy.* 2nd ed. Bethesda, MD: American Society of Health-System Pharmacists; 2015:3-28.

26. Ambrosi C, Zaiontz C, Peragine G, Sarchi S, Bona F. Randomized controlled study on the effectiveness of animal-assisted therapy on depression, anxiety, and illness perception in institutionalized elderly. *Psychogeriatrics.* 2019;19(1):55-64.

27. Ching-Teng Y, Ya-Ping Y, Yu-Chia C. Positive effects of art therapy on depression and self-esteem of older adults in nursing homes. *Soc Work Health Care.* 2019;58(3):324-338.

28. Lyu J, Zhang J, Mu H, et al. The effects of music therapy on cognition, psychiatric symptoms, and activities of daily living in patients with Alzheimer's disease. *J Alzheimers Dis.* 2018;64(4):1347-1358.

29. Rivera JA, Reeves S, Aronson L. The interprofessional team. In: Williams BA, Chang A, Ahalt C, et al., eds. *Current Diagnosis & Treatment: Geriatrics.* 2nd ed. New York, NY: McGraw-Hill; 2014.

30. Baldwin SM, Zook S, Sanford J. Implementing posthospital interprofessional care team visits to improve care transitions and decrease hospital readmission rates. *Prof Cas Manag.* 2018;23(5):264-271.

31. Alhossan A, Kennedy A, Leal S. Outcomes of annual wellness visits provided by pharmacists in an accountable care organization associated with a federally qualified health center. *Am J Health Syst Pharm.* 2016;73(4):225-228.

32. Hohmann LA, Hastings TJ, Qian J, Curran GM, Westrick SC. Medicare Annual Wellness Visits: a scoping review of current practice models and opportunities for pharmacists. *J Pharm Pract.* 2019;897190019847793.

33. Zorek JA, Subash M, Fike DS, et al. Impact of an interprofessional teaching clinic on preventive care services. *Fam Med.* 2015;47(7):558-561.

34. Rankin A, Cadogan CA, Patterson SM, et al. Interventions to improve the appropriate use of polypharmacy for older people. *Cochrane Database Syst Rev.* 2018;9:CD008165.

35. Marcum ZA, Hanlon JT, Murray M. Improving medication adherence and health outcomes in older adults: an evidence-based review of randomized controlled trials. *Drugs Aging.* 2017;34(3):191-201.

36. Conn VS, Ruppar TM, Chan KC, Dunbare-Jacob J, Pepper GA, De Geest S. Packaging interventions to increase medication adherence: systematic review and meta-analysis. *Curr Med Res Opin.* 2015;31(1):145-160.

37. Schneider PJ, Murphy JE, Pederson CA. Impact of medication packaging on adherence and treatment outcomes in older ambulatory patients. *J Am Pharm Assoc.* 2008;48(1):58-63.

38. Furmidge DS, Stevenson JM, Schiff R, Davies JG. Evidence and tips on the use of medication compliance aids. *BMJ.* 2018;362:k2801.

39. Davies EA, O'Mahony MS. Adverse drug reactions in special populations—the elderly. *Br J Clin Pharmacol.* 2015;80(4):796-807.

40. Nair NP, Chalmers L, Peterson GM, Bereznick BJ, Castelino RL, Bereznick LR. Hospitalization in older patients due to adverse drug reactions—the need for a prediction tool. *Clin Interv Aging.* 2016;11:497-505.

41. Oconoa TJ, Lizaraso F, Carvajal A. Hospital admissions due to adverse drug reactions in the elderly. A meta-analysis. *Eur J Clin Pharmacol.* 2017;73(6):759-770.

42. Hanlon JT, Pieper CF, Hajjar ER, et al. Incidence and predictors of all and preventable adverse drug reactions in frail elderly persons after hospital stay. *J Gerontol.* 2006;61A(5):511-515.

43. Sun R, Karaca Z, Wong HS. Healthcare cost and utilization project (HCUP): trends in hospital stays by age and payer, 2000-2015. Available at https://www.hcup-us.ahrq.gov/reports/statbriefs/sb235-Inpatient-Stays_Age-Payer_trends.jsp. Accessed April 20, 2020.

44. Rui P, Okeyode T. National Ambulatory Medical Care Survey: 2016 National Summary Tables. Available at https://www.cdc.gov/nchs/data/ahcd/namcs_summary/2016_namcs_web_tables.pdf. Accessed April 20, 2020.

45. Lee JK, Slack MK, Martin J, Ehrman C, Chisholm-Burns M. Geriatric care by US pharmacists in healthcare teams: systematic review and meta-analysis. *J Am Geriatr Soc.* 2013;61:1119-1127.

46. Campbell AM, Coley KC, Corbo JM, et al. Pharmacist-led drug therapy problem management in an interprofessional geriatric care continuum: a subset of the PIVOTS group. *Am Health Drug Benefits.* 2018;11(9):469-478.

47. Hartford Healthcare Center for Healthy Aging: patient stories. Pharmacist's home visit helps older woman manage her medications. Available at https://hhcseniorservices.org/services/center-for-healthy-aging/patient-stories. Accessed April 9, 2020.

48. Cardelli M, Marchegiani F, Corsonello A, Lattanzio F, Provinciali M. A review of pharmacogenetics of adverse drug reactions in elderly people. *Drug Saf.* 2013;35(suppl 1):3-20.

49. Bain KT, Schwartz EJ, Knowlton OV, Knowlton CH, Turgeon J. Implementation of a pharmacist-led pharmacogenomics service for the program of all-inclusive care for the elderly (PHARM-GENOME-PACE). *J Am Pharm Assoc.* 2018;58:281-289.

50. Program of All-Inclusive Care for the Elderly (PACE). Available at https://www.cms.gov/Medicare-Medicaid-Coordination/Medicare-and-Medicaid-Coordination/Medicare-Medicaid-Coordination-Office/PACE/PACE. Accessed April 20, 2020.

51. American Society of Health-System Pharmacists. Residency information. Available at https://www.ashp.org/Professional-Development/Residency-Information. Accessed April 22, 2020.

52. Alvis BD, Hughes CG. Physiology considerations in the geriatric patient. *Anesthesiol Clin.* 2015;33(3):447-456.

53. Mangoni AA, Jackson SHD. Age-related changes in pharmacokinetics and pharmacodynamics: basic principles and practical applications. *Br J Clin Pharmacol.* 2004;57(1):6-14.

54. McLean AJ, Le Couteur LE. Aging biology and geriatric clinical pharmacology. *Pharmacol Rev.* 2004;56(2):163-184.

55. Cameron KA. Caregiver's guide to medications and aging. Available at https://www.caregiver.org/caregiver%CA%BCs-guide-medications-and-aging. Accessed April 29, 2020.

56. Anticholinergic drugs. In: Butterworth IV JF, Mackey DC, Wasnick JD, eds. *Morgan & Mikhail's Clinical Anesthesiology.* 6th ed. New York, NY: McGraw-Hill; 2018.

57. Kharimi S, Dharia SP, Flora DS, Slattum PW. Anticholinergic burden: clinical implications for seniors and strategies for clinicians. *Consult Pharm.* 2012;27(8):564-82.

58. Lieberman JAIII. Managing anticholinergic side effects. *Prim Care Companion J Clin Psychiatry.* 2004;6(suppl2):20-23.

59. Lopez-Alvarez J, Sevilla-Llewellyn-Jones J, Aguera-Ortiz L. Anticholinergic drugs in geriatric psychopharmacology. *Front Neurosci.* 2019;13:1-15.

60. Arena JM. *Poisoning: Toxicology-Symptoms-Treatments.* 3rd ed. Springfield, IL: C.C. Thomas; 1974:345.

61. Lozano-Ortega G, Johnston K, Cheung A, et al. A review of published anticholinergic scales and measures and their applicability in database analyses. *Arch Gerontol Geriatr.* 2020;87:103-885.

62. Naples JG, Marcum ZA, Perera S, et al. Concordance among anticholinergic burden scales. *J Am Geriatr Soc.* 2015;63(10):2120-2124.

63. Levy HD. Polypharmacy reduction strategies: tips on incorporating American Geriatrics Society Beers and screening tool of older people's prescriptions criteria. *Clin Geriatr Med.* 2017;33:177-187.

64. Masnoon N, Shakib S, Kalisch-Ellete L, Caughley GE. What is polypharmacy? A systematic review of definitions. *BMC Geriatrics.* 2017;17:230.

65. Sherman JJ, Davis L, Daniels K. Addressing the polypharmacy conundrum. *US Pharmacist.* 2017;42(6):HS14-HS20.

66. Rochon PA, Gurwitz J. The prescribing cascade revisited. *Lancet.* 2017;389:1778-1780.

67. Starr JM. Cholinesterase inhibitor treatment and urinary incontinence in Alzheimer's disease. *J Am Geriatr Soc.* 2007;55(5):800-801.

68. Gorina Y, Schappert S, Bercovitz A, Elgaddal N, Kramarow E. Prevalence of incontinence among older Americans. *Vital Health Stat 3.* 2014;(36):1-33.

69. Carnahan RM, Lund BC, Perry PJ, Pollock BG, Kulp KR. The anticholinergic drug scale as a measure of the drug-related anticholinergic burden: association with serum anticholinergic activity. *J Clin Pharmacol.* 2006;46:1481-1486.

70. Garfinkel D, Birkan I, Bahat G. Routine deprescribing of chronic medications to combat polypharmacy. *Ther Adv Drug Saf.* 2015;616:212-233.

71. Scott IA, Gray LKC, Martin JH, Pillans PI, Mitchell CA. Deciding when to stop: towards evidence-based deprescribing of drugs in older populations. *Evid Based Med.* 2013;18(4):121-124.

72. O'Mohony D, O'Sullivan D, Byrne S, et al. STOPP/START criteria for potentially inappropriate prescribing in older people: version 2. *Age Ageing.* 2015;44:213-218.

73. Hanlon JT, Schmader KE. The medication appropriateness index at 20: where it started, where it has been and where it may be going. *Drugs Aging.* 2013;30(11):893-900.

74. Curtin D, Gallagher PF, O'Mohony D. Explicit criteria as clinical tools to minimize inappropriate medication use and its consequences. *Ther Adv Drug Saf.* 2019;10:1-10.

75. National Center for Health Statistics. National Health Interview Survey, Family Core Component, 2018. Available at https://public.tableau.com/profile/nhis#!/vizhome/FIGURE12_2/Dashboard12_2. Accessed April 20, 2020.

76. Look KA, Stone JA. Medication management activities performed by informal caregivers of older adults. *Res Social Adm Pharm.* 2018;14(5):418-426.

77. Blaszczyk AT, Hutchison LC. Chapter 12: Central nervous system disorders. In: Hutchison LC, Sleeper RB, eds. *Fundamentals of Geriatric Pharmacotherapy.* 2nd ed. Bethesda, MD: American Society of Health-System Pharmacists; 2015:333-376.

78. What is Alzheimer's disease. Available at https://www.alz.org/alzheimers-dementia/what-is-alzheimers. Accessed April 23, 2020.

79. Brannon WL. Alois Alzheimer (1864–1915). I. Contributions to neurology and psychiatry. *J S C Med Assoc.* 1994;90(9):399-401.

80. Schaffer C, Sarad N, DeCrumpe A, et al. Biomarkers in the diagnosis and prognosis of Alzheimer's disease. *J Lab Autom.* 2015;20(5):589-600.

81. Jack CRJr, Bennett DA, Blennow K, et al. NIA-AA research framework: toward a biological definition of Alzheimer's disease. *Alzheimers Dement.* 2018;14(4):535-562.

82. Morinago A, Ono K, Ikeda T, et al. A comparison of the diagnostic sensitivity of MRI, CBF-SPECT, FDG-PET and cerebrospinal fluid biomarkers for detecting Alzheimer's disease in a memory clinic. *Dement Geriatr Cogn Disord.* 2010;30(4):285-292.

83. Fiest KM, Roberts JI, Maxwell CJ, et al. The prevalence and incidence of dementia: a systematic review and meta-analysis. *Can J Neurol Sci.* 2016;43(suppl 1):S3-S50.

84. Livingston G, Sommerlad A, Orgeta V, et al. Dementia prevention, intervention, and care. *Lancet.* 2017;390(10113):2673-2734.

85. Dementia Care Central. Early, middle & late stage Alzheimer's disease & the caregiver's role in each stage. Available at https://www.dementiacarecentral.com/aboutdementia/alzheimers/stages/. Accessed April 23, 2020.

86. Quetiapine. In: Lexi-Drugs [database on the Internet]. Hutson, OH: Wolters Kluwer Clinical Drug Information, Inc.; 2020. Accessed April 19, 2020.

87. Cerejeira J, Lagarto L, Mukaetova-Ladinska EB. Behavioral and psychological symptoms of dementia. *Front Neurol.* 2012;3:Article 73.

88. Kales HC, Gitlin LN, Lyketsos CG. Assessment and management of behavioral and psychological symptoms of dementia. *BMJ.* 2015;350:h369.

89. Ballard C, Waite J. The effectiveness of atypical antipsychotics for the treatment of aggression and psychosis in Alzheimer's disease. *Cochrane Database Syst Rev.* 2006; (1):CD003476.

90. Schneider LS, Tariot PN, Dagerman KS, et al. Effectiveness of atypical antipsychotic drugs in patients with Alzheimer's disease. *N Engl J Med.* 2006;355(15):1525-1538.

91. Centers for Medicare & Medicaid Services. State Operations Manual: Appendix PP—guidance to surveyors for long term care facilities. Available at https://www.cms.gov/Regulations-and-Guidance/Guidance/Manuals/downloads/som107ap_pp_guidelines_ltcf.pdf. Accessed April 23, 2020.

92. Silverman JJ, Galanter M, Jackson-Triche M, et al. The American Psychiatric Association practice guidelines for the psychiatric evaluation of adults. *Am J Psychiatry.* 2015;172(8):798-802.

93. Livingston G, Kelly L, Lewis-Holmes E, et al. Non-pharmacological interventions for agitation in dementia: systematic review of randomised controlled trials. *Br J Psychiatry.* 2014;205(6):436-442.

94. Becker C, Rapp K. Fall prevention in nursing homes. *Clin Geriatr Med.* 2010;26:693-704.

95. Seppala LJ, Wermelink A, de Vries M, et al. Fall-risk-increasing drugs: a systematic review and meta-analysis: II. psychotropics. *J Am Med Dir Assoc.* 2018;19(4):371.e11-371.e17.

96. Seppala LJ, van de Glind E, Daams JG, et al. Fall-risk-increasing drugs: a systematic review and meta-analysis: III. Others. *J Am Med Dir Assoc.* 2018;19(4):372.e1-372.e8.

97. Dwyer LL, Han B, Woodwell DA, Rechtsteiner EA. Polypharmacy in nursing home residents in the United States: results of the 2004 National Nursing Home Survey. *Am J Geriatr.* 2010;8(1):63-72.

98. Centers for Medicare & Medicaid Services. Description of antipsychotic medication quality measures on nursing home compare. Available at https://www.cms.gov/Medicare/Provider-Enrollment-and-Certification/CertificationandComplianc/Downloads/AntipsychoticMedicationQM.pdf. Accessed April 23, 2020.

99. Lucas JA, Chakravarty S, Bowblis JR, et al. Antipsychotic medication use in nursing homes: a proposed measure of quality. *Int J Geriatr Psychiatry.* 2014;29(10):1049-1061.

100. Center for Medicare & Medicaid Services. National Partnership to Improve Dementia Care in Nursing Homes: Antipsychotic Medication Use Data Report (April 2019). Available at https://www.cms.gov/Medicare/Provider-Enrollment-and-Certification/SurveyCertificationGenInfo/Downloads/Antipsychotic-Medication-Use-Data-Report.pdf. Accessed April 23, 2020.

101. Center for Medicare & Medicaid Services. National Partnership—dementia care resources. Available at https://www.cms.gov/Medicare/Provider-Enrollment-and-Certification/SurveyCertificationGenInfo/National-Partnership-Dementia-Care-Resources#h5sk24snrky1bo8kqz1pf0k39ygnm8r. Accessed April 23, 2020.

102. Code of Federal Regulations. 42 CFR §483.60(c). Requirements for states and long term care facilities—pharmacy services. Available at https://www.govinfo.gov/app/details/CFR-2011-title42-vol5/CFR-2011-title42-vol5-sec483-60. Accessed May 31, 2020.

103. Lee SWH, Mak VSL, Tang YW. Pharmacist services in nursing homes: a systematic review and meta-analysis. *Br J Clin Pharmacol.* 2019;85(12):2668-2688.

104. High KP, Bradley SF, Gravenstein S, et al. Clinical practice guideline for the evaluation of fever and infection in older adult residents of long-term care facilities: 2008 update by the Infectious Diseases Society of America. *J Am Geriatr Soc.* 2009;57(3):375-394.

105. Woodford HJ, George J. Diagnosis and management of urinary tract infection in hospitalized older people. *J Am Geriatr Soc.* 2009;57:107-114.

106. Stone ND, Ashraf MS, Calder J, et al. Surveillance definitions of infections in long-term care facilities: revisiting the McGeer criteria. *Infect Control Hosp Epidemiol.* 2012;33(10):965-977.

CHAPTER 8

Infectious Diseases
Featuring the Illustrated Case Studies "Wounded" & "Superinfection"

Authors

Warren E. Rose, Susanne G. Barnett, & Joseph A. Zorek

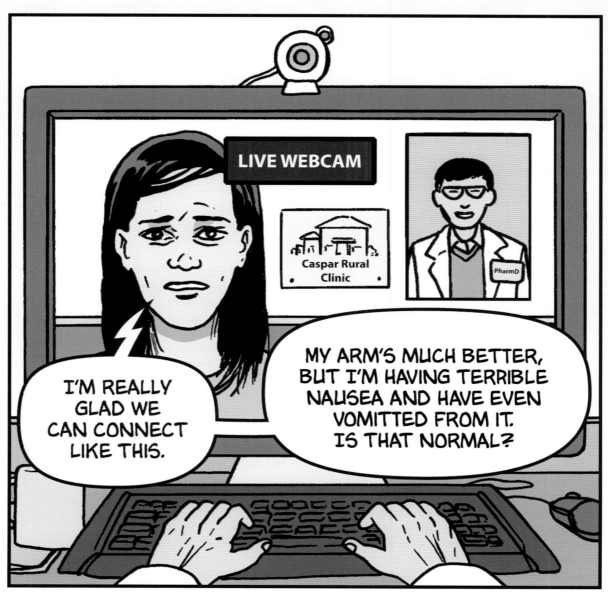

Illustration by George Folz, © 2019 Board of Regents of the University of Wisconsin System

BACKGROUND

The term *infectious diseases* is used to describe illnesses caused by microorganisms, such as viruses, bacteria, parasites, or fungi, that can be transmitted by animals, insects, food, or other people.[1] Although tremendous strides have been made toward controlling and treating infectious diseases, this broad category of disease still ranks as the second leading cause of death worldwide.[2] In the United States, it ranks third collectively.[3] While death rates have declined since the 1980s, substantial differences exist according to geographic region.[4,5] Patients of any age, background, gender, or ethnicity can be at risk of acquiring an infectious disease. That said, those who are at highest risk of infections and their complications include young children and the elderly, people with compromised immune systems caused by medications or secondary to another health condition (e.g., cancer, human immunodeficiency virus [HIV]), and individuals who engage in high-risk behaviors such as those depicted in Illustration 8-1.

Due to the frequency of infectious diseases, all health professionals should be capable of recognizing common infections, such as respiratory and skin infections, and have the requisite knowledge to refer patients for specialty care when warranted. Infectious diseases (ID) specialists play an important role in the study, treatment, control, and prevention of complicated cases.[6] Pharmacists in ID can serve as clinical specialists within the interprofessional ID team, as depicted in the illustrated cases "Wounded" and "Superinfection" in this chapter, and/or *antimicrobial* stewardship pharmacists. Pharmacists who run *antimicrobial* stewardship programs (ASPs) coordinate the safe, effective, and judicious use of *antimicrobial* medications used throughout entire healthcare organizations.[7] Broadly speaking, the term *antimicrobial* is used to capture all medications intended to treat infectious diseases; this includes antibiotics (antibacterials), antifungals, antivirals, and antiparasitic agents.

From the early 1900s until now, there has been a nearly 30-year increase in life expectancy in the United States.[8] Improvements in public health, coupled with the discovery, development, and commercialization of *antimicrobial* medications are the key reasons for this positive change. *Antimicrobials* have ushered in the modern era of medicine and are now essential to perform both general and sophisticated patient care; for example, childbirth, surgery, treatment of cancer, and solid organ or bone marrow transplantation. However, the rising and rapid spread of *antimicrobial* resistance worldwide and limited development of new *antimicrobial* medications have combined to become a significant threat to global health.[9]

Antimicrobial resistance describes the unfortunate situation whereby a once-effective *antimicrobial* medication ceases to work.[10] This has long been recognized as a consequence of unnecessary and inappropriate *antimicrobial* use. The World Health Organization estimates that 10 million deaths will be attributable to *antimicrobial* resistance every year by 2050.[11] In 2019, the US Centers for Diseases Control and Prevention (CDC) reported that more than 2.8 million *antimicrobial*-resistant infections occur in the United States annually, and that more than 35,000 people die as a result.[12] To highlight the importance of the emerging problem and frame a national action plan, the CDC created the *Antimicrobial Resistance Threats Report*.[13] This report categorizes specific types of microorganisms that have developed drug or multi-drug resistance according to whether they pose an urgent, serious, or concerning threat to the population.

Further aggravating the issue of *antimicrobial* resistance is the lack of discovery and development of new *antimicrobials* from the pharmaceutical industry.[14,15] As a result, there are very few effective options for patients with drug-resistant infections. There are several reasons for this troubling trend; chief among them being the scientific challenge of finding novel *antimicrobials*, developmental delays, regulatory issues, and lack of financial incentives for the industry compared to treatment of diseases in other fields such as oncology and cardiology.[16] Researchers have demonstrated that clinically detectable resistance to new antibiotics occurs within 1 to 2 years following introduction into clinical practice, which may jeopardize the economic viability of a new antibiotic. The reluctance to pursue development of new *antimicrobial* medications is understandable considering the millions of investment dollars necessary to bring a new medication to market.[16] Pharmacists practicing in ID and *antimicrobial* stewardship are positioned to understand the utility of new *antimicrobials* when approved by the US Food and Drug Administration (FDA) and to provide guidance for how to use them appropriately and judiciously to prevent the development of resistance.

ASPs have risen to meet the challenge of providing appropriate, optimal *antimicrobial* therapy and minimizing the spread of *antimicrobial* resistance within the healthcare environment.[17] These programs were initially developed and implemented in hospitals, and well-established evidence exists for the importance of these programs to improve *antimicrobial* use and patient care. Therefore, the structure, members, and accountability of ASPs discussed in this chapter will focus largely on the hospital setting. However, long-term care and outpatient (i.e., non-hospital) stewardship are areas of important new growth for ID pharmacists.[18,19] In 2014, the CDC endorsed the importance of ASPs by creating *Core Elements of Hospital Antibiotic Stewardship Programs*.[20] These *Core Elements* include the following:

1. Hospital Leadership Commitment
2. Accountability
3. Pharmacy Expertise
4. Action
5. Tracking
6. Reporting
7. Education

The Pharmacy Expertise *Core Element* specifically recommends appointing a pharmacist as the co-leader of the ASP to improve *antimicrobial* use and to engage the pharmacy department in this effort.[20] The other *Core Element* requirements involve pharmacists in some capacity, including monitoring and reporting *antimicrobial* use and resistance, and importantly, the education of other health professionals about *antimicrobials* and their optimization. Similar CDC *Core Elements* or ASP guidance documents are available for other settings, including nursing homes, outpatient settings, critical access hospitals (i.e., rural hospital settings with less than 25 beds), and resource-limited settings, which include low- and middle-income countries.[21] Each of these recommendations highlight the importance of pharmacy and ID pharmacists in implementing and managing ASPs. A pharmacist working on or leading an ASP in any of these healthcare environments must have high-level knowledge in infectious diseases and antibiotics, as well as strong leadership, communication, and collaboration skills given the large and diverse number of health professionals and patients involved.

Members of the Interprofessional Infectious Diseases Team

Infectious diseases and *antimicrobial* stewardship embody the interprofessional model of healthcare delivery. The recommendation to prioritize, even require, interprofessional care within ASPs comes from the Infectious Diseases Society of America (IDSA) and the Society of Healthcare Epidemiology of America (SHEA). Two guidelines for ASPs have been developed by experts in the field and endorsed by both IDSA and SHEA.[17,22] The first describes developing an institutional program for *antimicrobial* stewardship,[22] while the second focuses on recommendations related to implementation.[17] Both rely heavily upon interprofessional care as a fundamental principle for effectiveness.

The core members of the interprofessional ASP team include an ID physician and a clinical pharmacist trained in infectious diseases.[22] Administrative commitment is demonstrated through dedicated funding for, and investment in, one or more pharmacists in this role. ASPs are also recommended to include a medical laboratory scientist (i.e., clinical microbiologist) to survey and report *antimicrobial* resistance patterns at the institution. Since preventing the spread of resistant microorganisms is a key element to improving *antimicrobial* use, a representative from infection control and prevention, commonly an experienced nurse, as well as a hospital epidemiologist, should also be included on the ASP team. Other health and non-health professionals contribute to the success of ASPs in important ways, albeit in a less direct manner. Health informaticists, including pharmacy informaticists, work to leverage information systems and electronic health records to improve the efficiency and quality of programs.[23–25] Custodial staff responsible for cleaning and disinfecting facilities are also vitally important contributors to successful interprofessional ASP teams. Because ASPs are an institution-wide program, approval and endorsement from hospital medical staff, departments, chiefs, and institutional administration are essential.[22]

Role of Pharmacists within the Interprofessional Infectious Diseases Team

Pharmacists have unique training and skill sets in order to meet the diverse demands of an interprofessional ID team and ASP. Pharmacists in ID interact with individuals of various medical and professional backgrounds in both direct (face-to-face) and indirect ways (electronic and telephone). As the recognized medication expert, the role of the pharmacist involves recommendations to the interprofessional team on aspects of *antimicrobial* dosing, *antimicrobial* delivery (oral, intravenous, or other), audit and feedback of *antimicrobial* prescribing and use, guideline development, and implementation of diagnostic testing for microorganisms in order to direct *antimicrobial* therapy. Several of these roles are highlighted in the illustrated cases "Wounded" and "Superinfection" in this chapter.

Since the function of ASPs is driven by the regulatory standards for *antimicrobial* stewardship in the inpatient and long-term-care settings, the role of pharmacists will first be discussed around those recommendations. However, the overarching goal of any patient receiving *antimicrobials* is to optimize patient outcomes while minimizing or preventing *antimicrobial* resistance and adverse events. For this, pharmacists, regardless of ID specialty training or practice setting, can review *antimicrobial* regimens for appropriateness of use, dosing, delivery, and duration of therapy. In addition, pharmacists screen for adverse events to *antimicrobials*, which occur more commonly with higher dosing and longer durations of therapy.[26,27]

There are two strategies ID pharmacists use to optimize *antimicrobial* use in an ASP, and both approaches demonstrate improvement in not only appropriate *antimicrobial* use, but also patient outcomes.[17] The first is implementing strategies for prospective audit with intervention and feedback. This strategy involves interacting with providers after an *antimicrobial* order is placed. Pharmacists evaluate patients who are taking specific *antimicrobials*, and they interact with providers either directly or electronically to advocate for improvements. This approach involves interprofessional collaboration, uses evidence-based recommendations, provides opportunities for *antimicrobial* de-escalation (i.e., reducing spectrum of activity), reduces duration of therapy, and overall is less restrictive. However, the review process can be labor intensive, and recommendations are voluntary. Although improvements in patient outcomes can vary, reductions in *antimicrobial* use and resistance consistently occur.[28,29] Pharmacists have been key in innovating prospective audit and feedback by working within the electronic health record to automate some of these interventions or to flag high-risk patients for feedback.[23–25] An alternative approach is to restrict prescribing of select *antimicrobials* or to require authorization prior to use. ID pharmacists working in this capacity develop guidelines and pathways for appropriate use in the healthcare setting, and they discuss specific patients with providers prior to *antimicrobial* approval. This is seen as a more restrictive, less collaborative approach, but it does successfully reduce prescribing of targeted *antimicrobials*.[30] Regardless of the method used, pharmacists are a critically important health professional for the design, implementation, and management of a comprehensive ASP strategy.[17]

Nearly half of patients in hospital settings receive antibiotics, and 50% of this antibiotic use is considered unnecessary.[31] That said, the need for *antimicrobial* stewardship is vast. With these statistics, it is very difficult for a single pharmacist in medium-to-large healthcare organizations to perform all essential duties of *antimicrobial* stewardship. Therefore, an important role of ID pharmacists is to provide *antimicrobial* and stewardship education to physicians, nurses, physician assistants, other pharmacists, and other health professionals in the patient care setting. This is especially important in academic medical centers and teaching hospitals since students and trainees in multiple professions indicate that more education is necessary for appropriate antibiotic use.[32,33] In a recent study of pharmacy students throughout the United States, 94% of respondents believed strong knowledge of *antimicrobials* was important for their careers, and 89% indicated a desire for more education.[33] Commonly, this additional education comes in the patient care setting. Pharmacist-provided education must accompany stewardship activities to be successful.[30] The appropriateness of *antimicrobial* prescribing has been shown to improve by 11% to 43% using this educational approach.

Although reducing cost is not an objective of *antimicrobial* stewardship, ASPs work within budgetary constraints established by healthcare organizations. As a therapeutic class, *antimicrobials* consistently rank as one of the highest drug expenditures.[34,35] As a result of previously discussed strategies to optimize patient outcomes while minimizing or preventing *antimicrobial* resistance and adverse events, the pharmacist-led ASP initiatives consequently reduce *antimicrobial* costs.[35] Pharmacists in this setting monitor and report changes in *antimicrobial* costs, and they have developed novel strategies to minimize excess waste of prepared medications. This can result in significant savings for healthcare organizations.[37]

As experts in pharmacology, ID pharmacists provide high-level knowledge of drug dosing and therapeutic drug monitoring. Specific *antimicrobials* require monitoring of drug levels for safety and efficacy; this includes vancomycin and a class of *antimicrobials* called aminoglycosides (e.g., gentamicin, tobramycin, amikacin), along with occasional therapeutic drug-level monitoring of select antifungal agents. At a national level, pharmacists author guidelines on therapeutic antibiotic monitoring and novel applications.[38,39] ID pharmacists then use these recommendations to provide therapeutic drug monitoring guidelines for their specific organization and implement these new approaches for treatment. In addition to drug levels, ID pharmacists use expert drug knowledge to better understand how changing drug concentrations impact *antimicrobial* activity. Beta-lactam antibiotic infusions, for example, can be infused over longer periods (e.g., 3 hours instead of 30 minutes) in order to maximize *antimicrobial* activity. Pharmacists have implemented new infusion schemes like this within specific patient populations or even entire hospitals, and they have reported significant improvements in patient outcomes.[40,41]

Patient safety is one of the foundational pillars of ASPs. Although a representative from a healthcare organization's dedicated patient safety group may be included in ASPs, pharmacists as co-leaders of the ASP work to ensure patient safety with *antimicrobial* use. One of the most commonly reported allergies in patients is a reaction to penicillin or other beta-lactam antibiotics. This may cause a provider to forgo a beta-lactam antibiotic even though this *antimicrobial* class is often the treatment of choice.[42] Pharmacists involved in ASPs consult with patients about the type and severity of the reported *antimicrobial* allergy, correct the patient's health record, and, if needed, select agents in the same class with less allergy risk. Another approach is to implement *antimicrobial* desensitization so that patients can tolerate the *antimicrobial* for treatment of the infection.[43] Other important patient safety objectives of ASPs that rely upon pharmacy expertise include preventing *antimicrobial* adverse events, minimizing resistance development by selecting appropriate durations of therapy, and reducing *Clostridioides difficile* infection (CDI) from antibiotic therapy by avoiding CDI high-risk antibiotics. The illustrated case "Superinfection" describes the important role of any pharmacist, regardless of training or practice setting, in reducing CDI risk.

A significant amount of the medical and pharmacy literature supports the necessity of pharmacists to improve *antimicrobial* use. The growth of pharmacists in scholarship and research in the clinical setting has increased substantially, and ID pharmacists perform and publish important studies demonstrating these benefits.[44] Therefore, pharmacists are increasingly encouraged and expected to perform scholarship and research as another key role/responsibility connected to management of ASPs. With this scholarship, individual ID pharmacists are performing essential duties for *antimicrobial* stewardship, and they are increasingly recognized nationally for their novel contributions and findings.

INFECTIOUS DISEASES PHARMACISTS IN ACTION

Catching an Antibiotic Adverse Event

Adverse events from antibiotics can occur in patients without risk factors, or they can be exacerbated by other drugs that cause similar effects. Therefore, pharmacists must perform a thorough review of a patient's other medications and health conditions. In one report, a 46-year-old female presented to a hospital in Mississippi with a 1-week history of pain, swelling, and drainage from a foot wound following toe amputations.[45] Her past medical history of diabetes was a risk for lower leg wound ulcers and infections.[46] She was treated initially with two antibiotics based on the likely pathogens: oral ciprofloxacin and IV vancomycin. After hospital discharge, ciprofloxacin was continued but the vancomycin was changed to IV daptomycin, which is well-suited for the outpatient setting because it can be given once daily.[47] After 9 days, the patient returned to the emergency department complaining of aches and pains in her neck, shoulders and extremities; however, she was sent home when all laboratory tests (i.e., labs) and exams were normal. Five days later, during her outpatient ID follow-up visit, and still complaining of similar persistent pain, new labs revealed elevated serum creatinine (kidney dysfunction), creatine kinase (skeletal muscle toxicity), and liver enzymes (liver dysfunction). At this point, she was re-admitted to the hospital and the ID pharmacist recommended replacing daptomycin with doxycycline and continuing ciprofloxacin. Labs returned to near normal levels by day 3; during follow-up a few weeks later, they were back to normal and the infection had cleared. Daptomycin therapy was noted but never considered as a potential cause when the patient initially presented with symptoms. This report concluded that "routine education, critique, and feedback of pharmacists, nurses, and physicians is essential to improving awareness of adverse events." Other drugs can also cause skeletal muscle toxicity, which can lead to a condition called rhabdomyolysis, defined by release of intracellular muscle components, including creatine kinase, that can result in muscle pain and kidney failure when severe.[48] The most notorious of these are the statin medication class used to lower cholesterol.[49] Although daptomycin can cause creatine kinase leading to rhabdomyolysis, patients also on statins while receiving daptomycin have a five-fold greater risk of this event.[50] Therefore, ID pharmacists frequently recommend stopping statin therapy if/when daptomycin is used.[51]

Improving Use of Diagnostics

Several studies demonstrate that delayed or inappropriate *antimicrobial* therapy leads to worse patient outcomes, including death, in severe infections.[52] On the contrary, rapid and appropriate therapy has been shown to improve several patient outcomes and reduce hospital costs in these infections.[53,54] Therefore, the impact of rapid pathogen identification using advanced diagnostics (described in more detail in the illustrated case "Wounded") has promise to improve *antimicrobial* stewardship. Pharmacists quickly identified the potential novelty of these diagnostics systems, and designed studies to evaluate their utility for *antimicrobial* stewardship. In one of these examples, an experimental study was performed at the University of Michigan to assess the impact of mass spectrometry, a technique that can identify a pathogen within minutes among thousands of different types of microorganisms, when paired with *antimicrobial* stewardship interventions. The *antimicrobial* stewardship team involved two ID physicians, three ID pharmacists, and an ID pharmacy resident (i.e., trainee). One team member received an alert, through the electronic health record, notifying him/her of a positive blood culture with pathogen. This was then relayed to the patient's ID physician. Using this intervention, ID pharmacists improved time to effective antibiotic therapy by almost 6 hours, which allowed for rapid optimization of therapy. Death from bloodstream infections was reduced almost 30% and patient length of stay in the hospital was also reduced. This example highlights ID pharmacists improving population health. With this and similar studies, ID pharmacists have been successful in justifying new technologies, aligning computer algorithms, and improving patient care systematically. Rapid diagnostic tests are now the standard at many healthcare organizations, and some are now being implemented in outpatient clinics and community pharmacies.[55–57]

BECOMING AN INFECTIOUS DISEASES PHARMACIST

Antimicrobials are ubiquitous throughout healthcare. Therefore, immediately after completion of a Doctor of Pharmacy (PharmD) program accredited by the Accreditation Council for Pharmacy Education (ACPE) and successfully obtaining a pharmacist license, pharmacists can, and do, improve *antimicrobial* use in patients. However, practice as an ID pharmacist, either as a clinical specialist or an *antimicrobial* stewardship pharmacist, requires post-graduate training beyond the PharmD degree. Most individuals interested in ID pharmacy careers pursue a postgraduate year 1 (PGY-1) residency accredited by the American Society of Health-System Pharmacists (ASHP) focusing on acute care, which provides ample patient care experiences with a range of ID complications. Since all hospitals in the United States are required to have an ASP to receive federal funding, opportunities exist for a PGY-1 trained pharmacist to work in this area. Often, these individuals pursue on-the-job workshops or other professional development opportunities to enhance their skills in *antimicrobial* stewardship. Professional development opportunities are provided primarily by two organizations through certificate programs: the Society of Infectious Diseases Pharmacists (SIDP) and Making A Difference in Infectious Diseases (MAD-ID).[58,59] These certification programs provide a mix of self-learning modules and live interactive sessions along with submission of an ASP project for final certification.

Many employers require completion of an ID-focused PGY-2 residency, also accredited by ASHP. These PGY-2 residencies combine a mix of ID training to provide expert-level knowledge of this specialty area along with fundamental training in ASP development. Individuals completing ID-focused PGY-2 residencies may still choose to seek further training with the two organizations mentioned above for additional ASP certification based on personal or employer preference. The Board of Pharmacy Specialties recently approved a nationally recognized credential called the Board Certified Infectious Diseases Pharmacist (BCIDP).[60] Candidate eligibility requirements include graduation from an ACPE-accredited program (or international equivalent) and current active pharmacist license. Candidates must also demonstrate practice experience in one of three pathways: four years of practice experience with 50% or more of that time spent practicing in ID, completion of a PGY-1 residency plus 2 additional years of practice experience with at least 50% of time practicing in ID, or completion of a PGY-2 residency in ID pharmacy. In order to maintain BCIDP certification, individuals must earn 100 hours of professional development credit offered by SIDP and/or the joint program offered by ASHP and the American College of Clinical Pharmacy (ACCP) within the 7-year recertification cycle. Pharmacists interested in a research career in ID or *antimicrobial* stewardship can bolster their skills via pursuit of fellowship research training in academia or academic medical centers.[61] ACCP maintains a registry of accredited programs, but high-quality research training can be obtained in non-accredited programs as well. As displayed here, the ID specialty in pharmacy is robust, and it offers diverse practice opportunities and long-term career potential.

WOUNDED: An Illustrated Case Study

Story by Warren E. Rose & Joseph A. Zorek
Illustrations by George Folz, © 2019 Board of Regents of the University of Wisconsin System

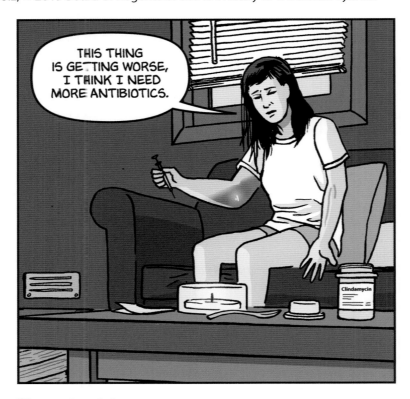

Illustration 8-1

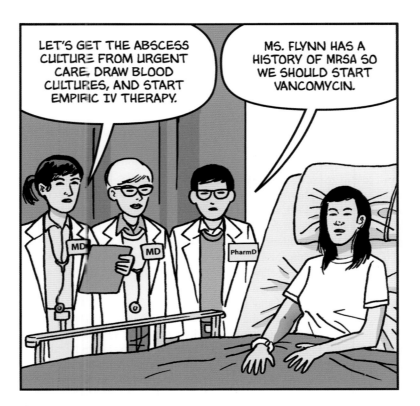

Illustration 8-2

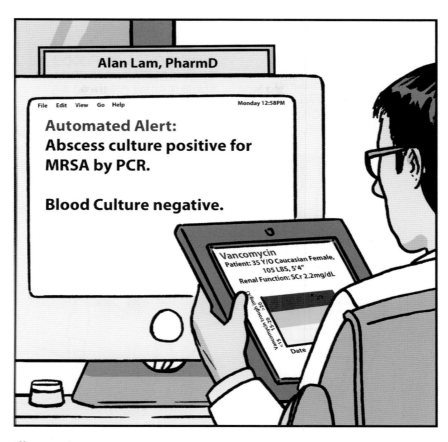

Illustration 8-3

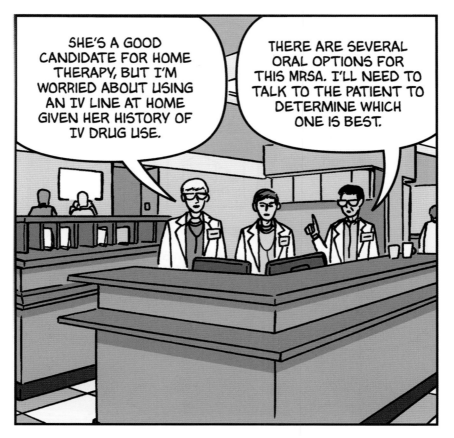

Illustration 8-4

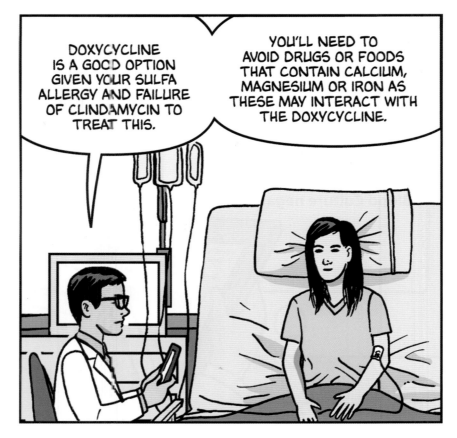

Illustration 8-5

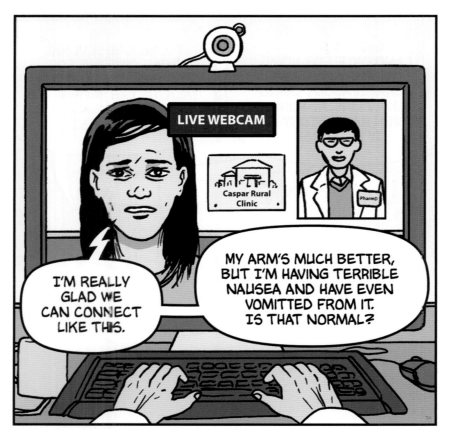

Illustration 8-6

Thoughts on "Wounded"

Infections often arise from a breakdown of host defenses. In other words, some mechanisms in humans that normally prevent microorganisms like bacteria, viruses, and fungi from taking root fail, and this failure leads to an infection. The breakdown of host defense mechanisms can come in many forms, including alteration of the immune response through aging, medications, or disease (e.g., multiple sclerosis, cancer). Some microorganisms can even affect the natural immune response, weakening a host's ability to fight infections from other microorganisms; human immunodeficiency virus, HIV, is a well-known example of this where a viral infection undermines immune defenses, making the person more susceptible to bacteria, fungi, and parasites.[62]

The best human defense against infection is the physical barrier of our skin and mucous membranes, which coat the linings of cavities in the body with a protective layer of mucous.[62] Many tracts that transport key substances vital to survival are lined with mucous membranes, such as the respiratory (air), gastrointestinal (food), and urinary tracts (urine). Breakdowns in these protective barriers, either through aging, disease, or the implantation or insertion of medical devices, represent a major risk factor for infection. Medical devices may be inserted through the skin for a variety of reasons, such as delivering medications directly into a vein. Other examples include tubes inserted into a patient's lungs or bladder to assist with breathing or voiding urine, respectively. Respiratory and urinary tract manipulations like these lead to some of the most common sites of infection in several healthcare settings.[63] For examples of such medical interventions, or downstream infections caused by them, see the illustrated cases "Shocking" and "Type 1" in Chapter 11 Critical Care, "Sleuth" in Chapter 7 Geriatrics, and "Superinfection" in this chapter.

In the illustrated case "Wounded," IV drug use is the culprit (Illustration 8-1). Use of illicit (i.e., illegal) IV drugs is one of the biggest risk factors for recurrent skin and soft tissue infections (SSTI), along with more complicated infections such as sepsis (bloodstream) and endocarditis (heart).[64,65] Escalating substance use disorders in the United States, including some described in the illustrated case "Gasping" in Chapter 12 Mental Health, further put patients at risk for recurrent skin infections and challenge the healthcare system for appropriate *antimicrobial* treatment and patient management. The following reflections on "Wounded" provide a contemporary summary of pharmacists' critical value in managing antibiotic therapy throughout the continuum of care.

SSTIs are among the most common types of infection in the United States in both the community and hospital environments.[66] In addition, SSTIs are responsible for high *antimicrobial* medication use throughout these settings.[67] Several studies indicate that SSTIs are both on the rise in the United States and becoming more severe, a trend underscored by a doubling in the amount of hospitalizations from SSTIs during a recent eight-year period.[68] The microorganisms responsible for SSTIs are highly diverse. However, nearly 80% are caused by gram-positive bacteria.[69]

Bacteria are broadly categorized through a method called Gram staining, named for the scientist who developed it in the late 1800s.[70] A sample from the source of the infection is taken, prepared using the stain, and placed under a microscope. Samples that appear purple are categorized as "gram-positive"; those that appear red, "gram-negative."[70] For serious infections, samples are also sent to a microbiology laboratory to be cultured (i.e., grown in a petri dish), identified, and tested for antibiotic susceptibility/resistance. The majority of gram-positive SSTIs are caused by a bacterial species called *Staphylococcus aureus* (*S. aureus*).[69,71,72] Many readers will be familiar with its most menacing, antibiotic resistant form called methicillin-resistant *S. aureus*, commonly referred to as MRSA (Illustration 8-2). SSTIs caused by MRSA are now commonplace, and the consequences for some have been dire and life-threatening.[69] A healthy 21-year-old football player in college contracted a MRSA skin infection, presenting initially as a pimple on his buttocks, which then spread to his blood and lungs. The failure of available antibiotics to treat this infection ultimately led to sepsis, end organ failure, and death. Within 1 week, he went from playing on the football field to being in the intensive care unit and dying from the infection. This and additional distressing patient stories are available on the IDSA website[73] to highlight the problem of antibiotic resistance in the United States and advocate for new antibiotic development.

Historically, one of the complexities in identifying SSTI pathogens is that routine culturing is not recommended because of difficulties in sample collection and lack of rapid identification in the settings where most SSTIs occur (i.e., outside of hospitals).[74] Patient risk factor assessment often helps to identify those who might have a higher risk of antibiotic-resistant organisms.[75] Risk factors include *S. aureus* in the nose or other areas (i.e., colonization), or contact with someone colonized, antibiotic therapy and/or hospitalization within the previous 12 months, history of previous infection, current housing in a long-term care facility (i.e., nursing home), and previous stay in an intensive care unit.[76] In addition, several patient conditions are risk factors for antibiotic-resistant pathogens, including diabetes, cirrhosis, and chronic kidney disease. Patients who require dialysis, who have implanted medical devices, or who use illicit IV drugs are also at increased risk.[76]

The burden of SSTIs on the healthcare system is substantial, with *S. aureus* SSTI alone accounting for over $4.5 billion in hospitalization costs.[77] An estimated 40% to 50% of patients are hospitalized merely to receive IV antibiotics, resulting in excessive and often unnecessary healthcare expenditures.[78] Therefore, tremendous opportunity exists for ID pharmacists to positively impact the healthcare system by contributing to and improving SSTI identification, antibiotic selection, patient management, and use of lower-cost SSTI treatments. This may also translate to many other acute infectious diseases caused by other microorganisms.

Due to the high incidence of SSTI in comparison to other infectious diseases, many developers of new antibiotics aim first for approval by the FDA for use in the treatment of SSTI.[79] As a result, several antibiotic options currently exist to treat SSTI. According to the most recent SSTI treatment guidelines from IDSA, several options exist for patients with various types of SSTI.[74] The patient in "Wounded" initially presented with a red, swollen infection on her arm that was discharging a yellowish pus (Illustration 8-1). In medical terminology, this would be described as an abscess focal point of infection with surrounding cellulitis. According to the most recent treatment guideline, a classification as moderate to severe purulent SSTI would be warranted.[74] As displayed in Table 8-1,[8] health professionals can choose among a variety of agents for management depending on patient characteristics, and if available, organism susceptibility. This demonstrates the value of a pharmacist in that setting to identify the best antibiotic to both treat the organism effectively and provide convenience to the patient.

Perhaps the most important innovation in the treatment of infectious diseases in the 21st century has been the development of rapid diagnostic testing (RDT) and its introduction into the clinical setting. Multiple RDT technologies can identify specific bacteria causing an infection and, in select organism types, identify antibiotic resistance. The speed with which RDTs achieve these results has changed how clinicians manage infections. Importantly, it has also improved *antimicrobial* use. Traditional microbiology laboratory work may take up to 3 to 5 days for results to be reported.[81] This delay can be problematic, as antibiotics active against the offending bacteria need to be initiated early in the course of an infection to prevent severe complications.[54,82,83] RDTs have provided a mechanism to do this with accuracy. RDT platforms detect unique genetic and molecular signatures from pathogens within hours of obtaining a patient sample.[56,84]

Pharmacists continually integrate new technologies into their practices. In recent years, the proliferation of ASPs has emerged as a prime example of this. Broadly speaking, such programs exist to ensure the appropriate use of *antimicrobials* throughout healthcare organizations.[55] Infectious disease pharmacists working in these programs are essential, and according to recommendations from the IDSA, pharmacists are recommended as co-leaders with physicians.[17] The value of ASPs for healthcare institutions and patients is highlighted by a plethora of literature. This includes reducing inappropriate *antimicrobial* use, preventing superinfections such as *Clostridioides difficile* (see the illustrated case "Superinfection"), reducing adverse drug events and drug interactions, providing precision care through therapeutic drug monitoring and dose adjustments, and lowering *antimicrobial* and healthcare costs.[85]

Research has shown that pharmacists play a critical role communicating microbiology results to the healthcare team and helping to optimize antibiotic therapy selection, which improves the quality of care.[86,87] As depicted in Illustration 8-3, pharmacists frequently review electronic health records, including microbiology culture results. In this illustration, the RDT from the patient culture detects MRSA; fortunately, this is present in the abscess only and has not progressed into a bloodstream

Table 8-1. Categories and Examples of Antibiotics Commonly Used in the Treatment of Moderate to Severe Purulent Skin and Soft Tissue Infections		
Infection Category	**Medication Examples***	**Antibacterial Action**
Moderate purulent infection	▪ cephalexin (Keflex)	Inhibits the cross-linking of peptidoglycan*****
	▪ doxycycline** (Monodox, Vibramycin)	Inhibits protein synthesis***
	▪ trimethoprim/sulfamethoxazole** (Bactrim, Septra)	Inhibits synthesis of folate, an essential compound for bacteria to live and replicate
Severe purulent infection	▪ cefazolin (Ancef)	Inhibits the cross-linking of peptidoglycan*****
	▪ nafcillin or oxacillin	
	▪ ceftaroline** (Teflaro)	
	▪ clindamycin** (Cleocin)	Inhibits protein synthesis***
	▪ daptomycin** (Cubicin)	Depolarizes the bacterial cell membrane
	▪ linezolid** (Zyvox)	Inhibits protein synthesis***
	▪ vancomycin** (Vancocin)	Inhibits cell wall transpeptidase*****
FDA-approved for SSTI consistent with moderate/severe purulent infection after treatment guidelines published	▪ dalbavancin** (Dalvance)	Inhibits cell wall transpeptidase*****
	▪ delafloxacin** (Baxdela)	Inhibits topoisomerase and gyrase, enzymes needed for bacterial DNA synthesis
	▪ omadacycline** (Nuzyra)	Inhibits protein synthesis***
	▪ oritavancin** (Orbactiv)	Inhibits cell wall transpeptidase***** and depolarizes the bacterial cell membrane
	▪ tedizolid** (Sivextro)	Inhibits protein synthesis***

*Medication examples presented in alphabetical order as "generic name (Brand Name)."
**Covers methicillin-resistant *Staphylococcus aureus*.
***Protein synthesis is needed for bacteria to replicate.
****Peptidoglycan is a substance used to form bacterial cell walls.
*****Transpeptidase is a bacterial enzyme needed to form cross-linkages of peptidoglycan.

infection. In Illustration 8-4, the pharmacist relays this information to the medical team in order to select an antibiotic capable of killing the identified resistant pathogen (MRSA). In clinical practice, this is either done through medical team rounds, as as depicted in Illustration 8-2, or via communication through the electronic health record. Both activities are central to ASPs.[23,24]

Although advances in diagnostic testing have mostly applied to hospitalized patients, new diagnostic technologies are beginning to be introduced in outpatient settings, such as clinics. Point-of-care (POC) tests, as they are called, can detect a range of host and pathogen signals for infection. Most POC tests currently in the clinic detect microorganism antigens, which are substances unique to microorganisms that trigger the immune system to react. Tests currently in use include Group A Streptococcus (e.g., strep throat), mononucleosis, *Helicobacter pylori*, influenza A and B, respiratory syncytial virus, HIV, Lyme disease, Hepatitis C, syphilis, as well as other select organisms.[88] The potential for pharmacists to incorporate the use and interpretation of POC tests into their practices provides a rich opportunity for the profession to impact public health through improved *antimicrobial* use in their communities.[89]

The hospital setting is a major driver of healthcare costs, and discharging patients home, or to other outpatient settings, with planning and intervention has resulted in reduced healthcare spending.[90] Importantly, quality of care and patient satisfaction have also been shown to improve with this transition.[47,91] However, transitioning patients from the hospital to the outpatient setting poses many risks and challenges; chief among these, at least from the perspective of pharmacy, include preventing medication errors and performing needed follow-up laboratory tests to monitor the safety and efficacy of *antimicrobial* treatments.[92]

For infectious diseases, significant attention to the transition of care process has provided new opportunities for pharmacists with home infusion services and *antimicrobial* stewardship practices. Many patients receive discharge antibiotics that are inappropriate as it relates to antibiotic selection, dose, and/or duration of therapy.[93] These are all contributors to *antimicrobial* resistance and potential adverse effects in patients. Among *antimicrobials* prescribed at discharge, up to 70% are found to be inappropriate.[93,94] In the largest surveillance study in the inpatient-to-outpatient transition setting, 40% of total days of antibiotic therapy were given in the outpatient setting.[95] Pharmacist intervention at the point of discharge reduces unnecessary antibiotic prescribing, selection, and duration of therapy.[96]

Illustrations 8-4 and 8-5 reveal that the pharmacist has identified several options for treating the patient's SSTI, and he recommends tailoring therapy from IV vancomycin to oral doxycycline (see Table 8-1). While not explicitly stated in "Wounded," hidden in Illustration 8-1 is a very important clue that informs the pharmacist's recommendation; namely, that the patient was already given oral clindamycin, which obviously failed to treat the infection. Additionally, the medical team prefers to use oral therapy and aims to transition from IV therapy in the hospital to oral therapy at home. With oral doxycycline, the patient is able to be managed in the outpatient setting without the need for a more difficult-to-manage indwelling central line and IV drug administration.

Although the interprofessional team was able to use oral antibiotics in the outpatient setting in "Wounded," patients are increasingly managed with outpatient parenteral (i.e., IV) *antimicrobial* therapy (OPAT) due to severity of infections and lack of oral alternatives in many instances. A focus and growth of many ASPs is the development and management of OPAT. The primary goal of an OPAT program is to facilitate patient treatment safely and effectively at home or another outpatient setting. The secondary goals include reducing inconvenience, evading hospital pathogens, and lowering healthcare costs.[97] The pharmacist's role in OPAT includes designing policies and procedures, assessing patients, selecting antibiotics, developing care plans, educating patients, monitoring response to therapy, communicating with other health professionals, and screening for adverse events, among other patient and administrative responsibilities.[97] Studies demonstrate that pharmacist monitoring of patients on OPAT is a cost-effective approach that may reduce hospital readmission rates and improve health outcomes.[98]

The infectious diseases specialty in pharmacy is currently at a crossroads of supply and demand. Due to the approval of a new standard for *antimicrobial* stewardship for hospital accreditation,[99] there is a significant need for pharmacists trained in infectious diseases.[100,101] However, the hospitals without ASPs are likely located in rural areas,[102] so highly trained pharmacists are greatly needed in these rural hospital settings. Technological advances are helping to close this gap with telemedicine or telehealth being used to address complex cases. Pharmacists work with other providers in *antimicrobial* stewardship telemedicine to provide care to resource-limited populations where traditional, direct specialty services are difficult to sustain.[103]

There are numerous applications of infectious diseases telehealth services, including infections like the SSTI portrayed in "Wounded," tuberculosis, and HIV. Telehealth can also be leveraged to advance *antimicrobial* stewardship initiatives, OPAT, and infection control and prevention activities. Pharmacists have an important role in the telehealth setting to ensure medication adherence and monitor for antibiotic efficacy and potential toxicity. In "Wounded," the pharmacist interacts with the patient in Illustration 8-6 through a telehealth format. From the convenience of a patient's home or, as in "Wounded," the patient's local clinic (i.e., Caspar Rural Clinic), pharmacists can address medication questions and patient concerns while monitoring adherence and managing side effects.

Telehealth services have shown similar health outcomes to traditional, in-person services, as well as high patient satisfaction.[103] In addition to individual patient telehealth, ASPs use telehealth for stewardship consultation.[104] This typically is for an established stewardship program to provide consultation to a smaller hospital setting without a formal stewardship program to share tools and best practices, patient

---

DISCUSSION QUESTIONS FOR "WOUNDED"

1. The pharmacist's tablet in Illustration 8-3 shows laboratory results from a test of the patient's blood; specifically, an elevated drug concentration for the antibiotic vancomycin. There is a clue embedded that the patient's kidney function may be contributing to this problem. What is this clue, and what role do you think kidney function plays in the appropriate dosing of antibiotics?

2. The patient has a history of MRSA, which increases her risk of having a drug-resistant pathogen. What other questions can the pharmacist ask the patient to assess her risk of antibiotic resistance?

3. The patient is experiencing nausea and vomiting from doxycycline therapy, as depicted in Illustration 8-6. What information do you think the pharmacist should collect during the telehealth appointment and what measures can be taken to minimize this in the future?

4. The pharmacist initially recommends intravenous vancomycin for treatment in the hospital due to the severity of the infection. What other intravenous agents might be an option for this patient that would cover the MRSA infection?

5. The pharmacist discusses potential drug interactions with doxycycline. What information should the pharmacist obtain about the patient's diet and other medications?

6. The treatment duration recommendation for SSTIs is generally 7 to 10 days of antibiotics. How might having other sites of infection (i.e., in addition to the patient's arm), such as blood, bone, or lung, change what the pharmacist recommended in terms of length of treatment?

---

care, and review of performance and *antimicrobial* use.[103,104] Implementation of telehealth for *antimicrobial* stewardship may decrease inappropriate *antimicrobial* use, increase infectious diseases consults, and reduce *antimicrobial* costs.[104] This improves equitable care for patients among hospitals with both large and limited resources.

Health professionals need to direct therapy toward infecting pathogens, but also need to be cognizant of the unintended consequences of *antimicrobial* use. Bacteria in the human gastrointestinal tract, or gut microbiome, are increasingly being recognized for their role in human health. A variety of conditions have been linked to the microbiome including autoimmune diseases, metabolic disorders, cancer, neuropsychiatric disorders, kidney disease, and infectious diseases.[105] The illustrated case "Superinfection" in this chapter highlights infectious disease complications with a patient who experiences *Clostridioides difficile* infection as a consequence of antibiotic treatment. *Antimicrobial* exposure early in life has been associated with obesity, allergies, behavior problems, and autoimmune disease in both children and adults.[106] The effect of a two-course antibiotic regimen on disrupting the gut microbiome can last for up to a year,[107] and the physical effects from this alteration may last for several years.[108] In Illustration 8-6, the patient reveals to the pharmacist that she is experiencing nausea and vomiting from the antibiotic. Almost all oral antibiotics have the potential to disrupt the gut microbiome. Probiotics may be used to restore healthy bacteria to the gut following antibiotic use; however, results in patients have been mixed and may come with potential adverse effects.[109-111] In addition, a recent study found that probiotics may slow the re-establishment of the native microbiome in the patient.[112] There remains much to understand about the role and maintenance of the microbiome on human health, and the judicious use of *antimicrobials* is important to minimize disrupting this important environment.

In summary, the illustrated case "Wounded" provides a contemporary example of the impact of an infectious diseases pharmacist on patient care throughout the inpatient, outpatient, and telehealth settings. This illustrated case features the pharmacist working within an interprofessional team, providing high-level therapeutic drug knowledge, and using technological innovations through the electronic health record, rapid diagnostic testing, and telehealth to optimize *antimicrobial* therapy for the patient. The impact of pharmacists and pharmacist-driven interventions on improving the outcome of patients, reducing inappropriate antibiotic use and resistance is supported by the medical literature. Pharmacists in the infectious diseases field will continue to lead innovation in *antimicrobial* stewardship to combat the perpetual threat of *antimicrobial* resistance.

SUPERINFECTION: An Illustrated Case Study

Story by Susanne G. Barnett & Joseph A. Zorek
Illustrations by George Folz, © 2019 Board of Regents of the University of Wisconsin System

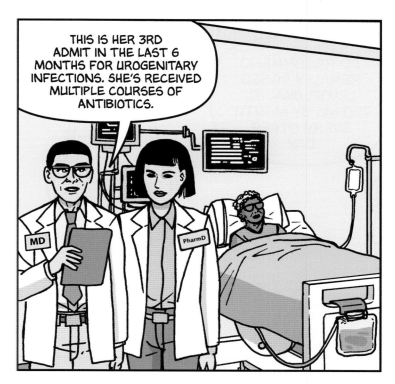

Illustration 8-7

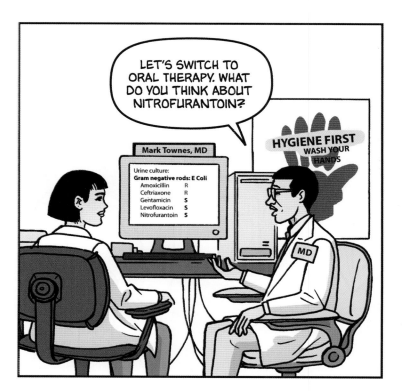

Illustration 8-8

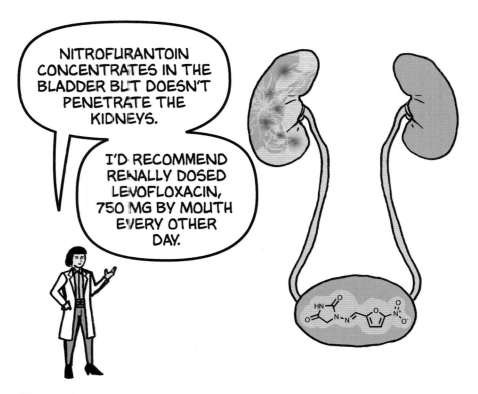

Illustration 8-9

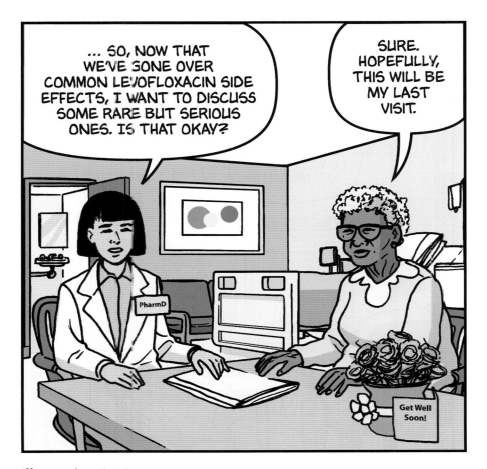

Illustration 8-10

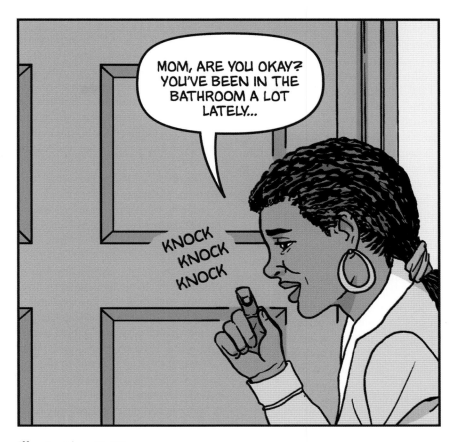

Illustration 8-11

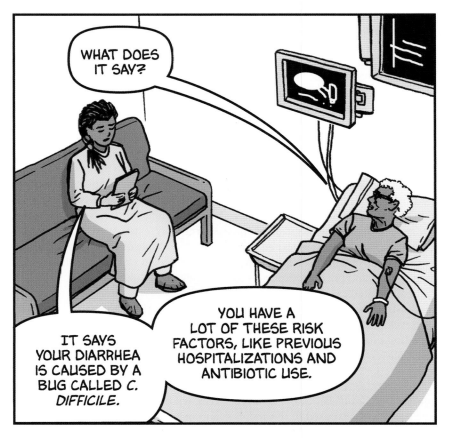

Illustration 8-12

Thoughts on "Superinfection"

Superinfections were first described in the late 1940s and early 1950s as a new infection that occurs in addition to a preexisting infection, or immediately following the treatment of an initial infection with antibiotics.[113,114] The human body plays host to an incredible array of microorganisms (e.g., bacteria, fungi, viruses) that, collectively, constitute what is referred to as our microbiome.[115] The balance of microorganisms within any one person's microbiome is in a constant state of flux that is influenced by a variety of factors, such as the food we eat or the drugs we take. When antibiotics are used to treat an infection, like we see in the illustrated case "Superinfection," bacteria within the microbiome that are susceptible to the antibiotic are eliminated (i.e., killed). It is important to note that antibiotics kill all bacteria that are susceptible to them; this includes non-harmful bacteria, as well as the bacteria causing the infection. As a result, use of antibiotics can lead to a marked change in the balance of microorganisms within the microbiome. Sometimes, this change allows for bacteria that are resistant to the antibiotic used (i.e., not killed by it) to flourish, become pathogenic, and cause a new infection. In this manner, antibiotic administration is directly linked to the development and spread of drug-resistant microorganisms.[13] For additional discussion of microbiomes and antibiotic resistance, readers are encouraged to explore the previous illustrated case in this chapter, "Wounded."

Clostridioides difficile, also known as *C. difficile* or *C. diff*, is a bacterium that causes severe, watery diarrhea and inflammation of the colon.[116] Infection severity can range from mild to severe, with severe disease having the possibility to result in toxic megacolon (swelling and inflammation of the large intestine), sepsis (bloodstream infection that results in malfunction of multiple organ systems), and death.[117] *C. difficile* infection (CDI) has been estimated to cause nearly 500,000 illnesses in the United States annually, at a cost of approximately $1 billion, and it is a common and known cause of superinfections.[116,117] Due to the clear association of CDI with antibiotic use, its large economic impact, and the ease of *C. diff* to be transmitted from one individual to another, the CDC has designated *C. diff* an urgent public health threat.[13]

Antibiotic use is the strongest risk factor for the development of CDI. In fact, an individual taking an antibiotic is 8 to 10 times more likely to develop CDI than an individual without antibiotic exposure.[118] Additional well-known risk factors associated with development of CDI include recent hospitalization, age greater than 65, a weakened immune system, and previous exposure to or infection with *C. diff*.[119] The illustrated case "Superinfection" opens with a physician in Illustration 8-7 revealing that his patient, who later goes on to develop CDI, has multiple risk factors for its development, including three admissions to the hospital in the last 6 months, multiple recent courses of antibiotics, and older age.

Although community acquisition of *C. diff* is becoming more common, it is most likely the patient was exposed to the spores of this bacterium during one of her previous hospitalizations.[120] Spores are an inactive form of *C. diff* capable of living outside the body due to a protective coating that allows survival in harsh environments.[121] *C. diff* is transmitted from one person to another through the fecal-oral route.[119] Once a spore is ingested, it can be activated in the intestine, causing either colonization or infection. *C. diff* spores have been documented to survive outside the body for several months, acting as a reservoir for transmission.[122] Within healthcare settings, equipment (e.g., stethoscopes, thermometers), toilets, phones, and clinic or hospital room surfaces have been known to harbor and transmit spores.[119]

The hands of healthcare personnel can also transfer *C. diff* spores from one patient to another, which has resulted in a global effort to educate health professionals about proper hand hygiene.[119] Recent national and international campaigns focused on hand hygiene include the CDC's *Clean Hands Count*, and the World Health Organization's *SAVE LIVES: Clean Your Hands*. Both of these campaigns aim to improve health professionals' compliance with hand hygiene recommendations. Downloadable promotional materials are available online for use in clinics, hospitals, and other healthcare settings.[123,124] In Illustration 8-8, we see a poster inspired by these campaigns hanging on the wall. This poster serves to remind the physician and pharmacist collaborating on drug selection of the importance of hand hygiene, and it also serves as a clue for readers who may wonder how the patient developed her CDI superinfection. Unlike the majority of bacteria and viruses, *C. diff* spores are not killed on exposure to alcohol-based hand gels employed throughout patient care areas; physical removal of *C. diff* spores by washing hands with running water and soap is required.[119,125]

In addition to proper hand hygiene, infection control processes are important considerations to prohibit the transmission of *C. diff*. Hospitalized patients with CDI should be kept in isolation, with a private hospital room and toilet, for the duration of their illness and at least 48 hours after diarrhea has subsided.[125] Additional recommendations to minimize the spread of *C. diff* include guidance for healthcare personnel and visitors to wear a gown and gloves when entering a patient's room.[125] This can be seen later in the case, with the patient's daughter donning these protective barriers while visiting her mother in a private hospital room. It is important to note that, given the durability of *C. diff* spores, bleach-containing solutions should be used to decontaminate both hospital and private dwellings where these spores may exist, such as the patient's home bathroom.[121,125] For an example of CDI in the setting of cancer care, readers are encouraged to explore the illustrated case "Compromising" in Chapter 9 Oncology.

Despite the risks associated with antibiotic use, including the development of CDI, antibiotics are incredible life-saving medications that play a critical role in healthcare. In "Superinfection," the patient was hospitalized due to a serious infection caused by the bacteria *Escherichia coli*, or *E. coli* (Illustrations 8-7 and 8-8). The term "urogenital" is used to describe the urogenital system, which is essentially a grouping of the reproductive organs and urinary tract due to their proximity to one another within the body.[126] In terms of basic anatomy and physiology, depicted in Illustration 8-9, urine is created in the kidneys through the filtering of blood, then transported via ureters to the bladder where it is stored until it is eliminated from the body.[126]

Urinary tract infections (UTIs) are the second most common type of infection in the United States, with more than half of all women reporting one or more UTIs in their lifetime.[127] Painful, frequent, and/or urgent urination are the most common signs of a developing UTI. In many, infection may be isolated to the bladder (i.e., cystitis); however, bacteria can travel up the ureter to cause infection and inflammation in one or both kidneys (i.e., pyelonephritis). This is depicted in Illustration 8-9, where one kidney is discolored and slightly enlarged due to infection. Despite adequate treatment with antibiotics, some patients may be predisposed to acquiring UTIs and experience recurrent infections. In fact, as the physician in Illustration 8-7 described, this is this patient's third admission to the hospital for the treatment of urogenital infections requiring antibiotics in the previous 6 months. Risk factors associated with recurrent UTIs in post-menopausal women include estrogen deficiency, lack of control during urination (incontinence), the presence of urine in the bladder after voiding, a structural abnormality, and medical comorbidities such as diabetes.[128] Those interested in diabetes are encouraged to explore the illustrated cases "Holistic" in Chapter 3 Primary Care, "Screen" in Chapter 4 Prevention & Wellness, and "Type 1" in Chapter 11 Critical Care. For an additional UTI example, see the illustrated case "Sleuth" in Chapter 7 Geriatrics.

Antibiotics commonly used to treat UTIs can be found in Table 8-2.[129,130] The decision to recommend one antibiotic over another is complex, and a pharmacist must consider multiple patient-specific factors to ensure appropriate therapy is chosen. Many of these considerations are captured in Illustrations 8-7 through 8-9. After a patient is assessed by a provider and the decision to treat an infection is made, antibiotic therapy is chosen empirically; meaning, without the knowledge of the specific bacterium causing the infection or its susceptibilities. Medication allergies/intolerances, how well the kidneys are currently functioning, and recent antibiotic exposure are important considerations to maximize therapy effectiveness and minimize adverse effects. As previously described, when a patient is exposed to an antibiotic, susceptible organisms are killed, allowing resistant bacteria to grow. The *E. coli* causing the current infection are therefore likely to be resistant to antibiotics which have recently been administered. In order to have the best chance of eliminating infection, an antibiotic should be chosen that a patient has not been recently exposed to. In Illustration 8-7, we see the physician and pharmacist discussing the patient's past antibiotic exposure as they consider appropriate therapy for the current infection.

In hospitalized patients, a sample of infected urine is often sent to a microbiology laboratory for identification of bacterial species causing the infection and determination of antibiotics to which the microorganism is susceptible. When available, review of this data is paramount to ensuring therapy appropriateness. Results of the patient's urine culture are shown in Illustration 8-8, with the pharmacist and physician jointly reviewing antibiotic susceptibilities as they consider a change from IV to oral therapy. Additional examples of medication selection based

Table 8-2. Categories and Examples of Antibiotics Commonly Used in the Treatment of Urinary Tract Infections

Category	Medication Examples*	Antibacterial Action
Cephalosporins	■ cefaclor (Ceclor, Raniclor) ■ cefdinir (Omnicef) ■ cefpodoxime (Banan, Vantin) ■ cefuroxime (Ceftin, Zinacef)	Inhibit the cross-linking of peptidoglycan, a substance used to form bacterial cell walls
Folate antagonists	■ trimethoprim/ sulfamethoxazole (Bactrim, Septra)	Block folate synthesis and the creation of bacterial DNA
Fluoroquinolones	■ ciprofloxacin (Cipro) ■ levofloxacin (Levaquin)	Inhibit DNA topoisomerases, enzymes involved in bacterial DNA synthesis
Nitrofurans	■ nitrofurantoin (Macrobid, Macrodantin)	Inhibit bacterial protein synthesis; however, the exact mechanism has not been well described
Penicillins	■ amoxicillin (Amoxil) ■ amoxicillin-clavulanate (Augmentin)	Inhibit the cross-linking of peptidoglycan and bacterial cell wall synthesis
Phosphoenolpyruvate synthetase inhibitors	■ fosfomycin (Monurol)	Block the creation of peptidoglycan and bacterial cell wall synthesis by inhibiting the formation of N-acetylmuramic acid

*Medication examples presented in alphabetical order as "generic name (Brand Name)."

on bacterial cultures and antibiotic susceptibilities can be seen in the illustrated cases "All In" in Chapter 6 Pediatrics and "Wounded" in this chapter.

Transition from IV to oral therapy is considered standard of practice when a patient is not critically ill, is improving on current therapy, and can swallow and tolerate oral medications.[131] Patients see many individual benefits of oral versus IV therapy; for example, decreased bloodstream infections associated with IV lines, decreased hospitalization costs due to use of less expensive medications, avoidance of supplies and staffing for administration of IV medications, and earlier hospital discharge.[131]

Treatment success is dependent on administration of an antibiotic that can penetrate the site of infection. In Illustration 8-9, we see the pharmacist consider and dismiss the use of nitrofurantoin, an antibiotic commonly used to treat cystitis (i.e., UTI from bladder infection), because it concentrates in the bladder. Nitrofurantoin does not reach detectable concentrations in the kidneys, and it is therefore ineffective for the treatment of pyelonephritis.[132] Based on these considerations and results of the urine culture, the pharmacist recommends a fluoroquinolone antibiotic called levofloxacin (see Table 8-2). Levofloxacin reaches adequate concentrations in the kidney to effectively treat pyelonephritis caused by susceptible organisms, and it is excreted by the kidneys and eliminated in urine from the body.[133] Patients with impaired kidney function do not excrete/eliminate levofloxacin effectively and are at an increased risk of developing toxicities.[133] Pharmacists must consider a patient's ability to process and eliminate an antibiotic when making drug selection and dosing recommendations. While not explicitly described in the illustrated case, the pharmacist recognized, perhaps through a review of other lab results, that the patient's kidney function was impaired. To account for the expected decrease in levofloxacin elimination, and hence to avoid accumulation of levofloxacin to toxic levels, the pharmacist recommends extending the dosing interval to every other day (versus daily, which is advised for patients with normal kidney function).

Medication dose and/or interval adjustment is a strategy that can be used to limit the development of adverse effects. Nevertheless, adverse effects can occur with administration of any medication, and it is the pharmacist's responsibility to educate patients on what to expect from their medications.[134] To accomplish this, pharmacists in hospital settings routinely perform discharge counseling prior to a patient's release from the hospital.[135] Discharge counseling efforts largely focus on the role of each medication in a patient's recovery or management of a chronic condition. Goals include increasing adherence to prescribed medications, teaching patients to identify and react to adverse effects should they occur, and preparing patients to transition to care outside of the hospital. For a more in-depth discussion of the role of pharmacists in transitions of care, readers are encouraged to explore the illustrated case "Support" in Chapter 3 Primary Care.

Illustration 8-10 of "Superinfection" depicts discharge counseling in preparation for a seamless transition home. Both common and rare, but serious, side effects associated with levofloxacin would have been covered during this interaction, including the possibility of developing CDI after levofloxacin administration (Illustrations 8-11 and 8-12).[136] Levofloxacin is classified as a high-risk antibiotic in its association to CDI and is avoided when alternative options exist.[137,138] Although not explicitly described in the illustrated case, the physician and pharmacist's clinical decision-making process included evaluation of the risk of adverse effects, such as CDI. Unfortunately, alternative antibiotics to effectively treat the patient's kidney infection were not available. The E. coli causing the patient's infection was resistant to two antibiotics, likely due to previous antibiotic exposure. Nitrofurantoin could not be used due to its inability to reach the site of infection (Illustration 8-9), and the final antibiotic to which the E. coli is reported as susceptible is only available in an IV form. Given the risks associated with IV antibiotic administration and the patient's readiness to transition home, the physician and pharmacist settled on levofloxacin as the best option. To minimize the risk of CDI, it is recommended to prescribe levofloxacin for the shortest effective duration possible, which was done for the patient in "Superinfection."[139]

The illustrated case "Superinfection" highlights the complexities associated with the antibiotic treatment of recurrent infections, as well as the value of an infectious diseases pharmacist's knowledge and expertise. The pharmacist plays a vital role in minimizing the risk of patient infection due to *Clostridioides difficile* through impacting antibiotic prescribing, patient education, and following/ensuring infection control processes.[140] Unfortunately for the patient, recent hospitalizations and exposure to *C. diff* spores, coupled with alterations to her microbiome through repeated use of antibiotics, conspired to result in a poor outcome. The physician and pharmacist must now regroup to determine the best course of action to treat the new *C. diff* infection. This will likely involve 10 additional days of antibiotic treatment, leading to further unpredictable changes in the patient's microbiome, as well as additional risks to manage associated with new adverse effects.[125,141] Undoubtedly, the pharmacist will again work to empower the patient, as well as her daughter, to play an active role in this process by counseling them on what to expect from the new antibiotic, when to contact a provider, how to avoid transmission of *C. diff* to others, and what steps they can take to prevent another bout of CDI in the future.[142]

DISCUSSION QUESTIONS FOR "SUPERINFECTION"

1. The illustrated case "Superinfection" focuses on pharmacist interventions to ensure appropriate antibiotic therapy for hospitalized patients. What role might a community pharmacist play to ensure appropriate and effective antibiotic therapy when antibiotic prescriptions are taken to them to be filled?

2. Prescribing antibiotics to individuals with viral infections (e.g., the common cold) contributes to the unnecessary development of antibiotic resistance. What are some ways pharmacists might change this practice?

3. Illustrations 8-7 and 8-3 show the physician and pharmacist collaborating to provide the best care possible to their patient. What other health professionals might contribute to the care of patients with *C. diff*? What non-health professionals might contribute?

4. What preventive measures could be employed in the patient's home to limit the transmission of *C. diff* spores from the mother to the daughter in this case?

5. Recurrent urinary tract infection and repeated exposure to antibiotics contributed to the patient developing *C. diff* infection. What lifestyle changes might be recommended to minimize the patient's risk of developing another urinary tract infection?

CHAPTER SUMMARY

- *Antimicrobial* resistance is a significant threat to public health and modern healthcare.

- *Antimicrobial* stewardship programs (ASPs) aim to provide appropriate, optimal *antimicrobial* therapy and minimize the spread of *antimicrobial* resistance within the healthcare environment.

- ASPs consist of physicians, pharmacists, clinical microbiologists, nurses, information technologists, and infection control and quality representatives.

- The US Centers for Disease Control and Prevention recommends that pharmacists should be co-leaders of ASPs to improve *antimicrobial* use.

- Infectious diseases (ID) pharmacists work to develop ASPs and use systematic approaches to monitor patients, guide prescriber practices, and report *antimicrobial* use and resistance.

- ID pharmacists provide patient care as clinical specialists by optimizing *antimicrobial* selection, dose, route, and duration, as well as screening for drug interactions and adverse events.

- Following completion of the Doctor of Pharmacy (PharmD) degree, 2 years of post-graduate residency training are required to become an ID pharmacist, and there are certificate programs available for additional credentialing.

- Healthcare systems are required to have pharmacist-guided ASPs, so pharmacist careers in this field will likely be in high demand for years to come.

REFERENCES

1. Relman DA, Falkow S, Ramakrishnan L. *A Molecular Perspective of Microbial Pathogenicity*. In: Bennett JE, Dolin R, Blaser MJ, eds. 9th ed. Philadelphia, PA: Saunders; 2020:1-11.

2. The top 10 causes of death. Available at https://www.who.int/news-room/fact-sheets/detail/the-top-10-causes-of-death. Published 2018. Accessed February 15, 2020.

3. Leading causes of death. https://www.cdc.gov/nchs/fastats/leading-causes-of-death.htm. Published 2017. Accessed February 15, 2020.

4. El Bcheraoui C, Mokdad AH, Dwyer-Lindgren L, et al. Trends and Patterns of Differences in Infectious Disease Mortality Among US Counties, 1980-2014. *JAMA*. 2018;319(12):1248-1260.

5. University of Minnesota Center for Infectious Disease Research and Policy. Infectious disease deaths decline across US, but not evenly. Available at http://www.cidrap.umn.edu/news-perspective/2018/03/infectious-disease-deaths-decline-across-us-not-evenly. Accessed January 15, 2020.

6. Infectious Diseases Society of America. Available at https://www.idsafoundation.org/about/. Accessed February 15, 2020.

7. ASHP statement on the pharmacist's role in *antimicrobial* stewardship and infection prevention and control. *Am J Health Syst Pharm*. 2010;67(7):575-577.

8. CDC on Infectious Diseases in the United States: 1900–99. *Population and Development Review*. 1999;25(3):635-640.

9. Jee Y, Carlson J, Rafai E, et al. *Antimicrobial* resistance: a threat to global health. *Lancet Infect Dis*. 2018;18(9):939-940.

10. Tenover FC. Mechanisms of *antimicrobial* resistance in bacteria. *Am J Med*. 2006;119(6 Suppl 1):S3-S10; discussion S62-70.

11. World Health Organization. No time to wait: securing the future from drug-resistant infections. Available at https://www.who.int/antimicrobial-resistance/interagency-coordination-group/final-report/en/. Accessed May 31, 2020.

12. University of Minnesota Center for Infectious Disease Research and Policy. CDC spotlights 'deadly threat' of antibiotic resistance. Available at http://www.cidrap.umn.edu/news-perspective/2019/11/cdc-spotlights-deadly-threat-antibiotic-resistance. Accessed January 14, 2020.

13. Centers for Disease Control and Prevention. Antibiotic resistance threats in the United States, 2019. Atlanta, GA. U.S. Department of Health and Human Services. Available at https://www.cdc.gov/drugresistance/pdf/threats-report/2019-ar-threats-report-508.pdf. Published 2019. Accessed May 31, 2020.

14. Talbot GH, Jezek A, Murray BE, et al. The Infectious Diseases Society of America's 10 × '20 Initiative (10 new systemic antibacterial agents US Food and Drug Administration approved by 2020): Is 20 × '20 a possibility? *Clin Infect Dis*. 2019;69(1):1-11.

15. Infectious Diseases Society of A. The 10 × '20 Initiative: pursuing a global commitment to develop 10 new antibacterial drugs by 2020. *Clin Infect Dis*. 2010;50(8):1081-1083.

16. Hogberg LD, Heddini A, Cars O. The global need for effective antibiotics: challenges and recent advances. *Trends Pharmacol Sci*. 2010;31(11):509-515.

17. Barlam TF, Cosgrove SE, Abbo LM, et al. Implementing an antibiotic stewardship program: guidelines by the Infectious Diseases Society of America and the Society for Healthcare Epidemiology of America. *Clin Infect Dis*. 2016;62(10):e51-77.

18. Kullar R, Yang H, Grein J, Murthy R. A roadmap to implementing *antimicrobial* stewardship principles in long-term care facilities (LTCFs): collaboration between an acute-care hospital and LTCFs.. *Clin Infect Dis*. 2018;66(8):1304-1312.

19. Rivera CG. Outpatient *antimicrobial* stewardship: field of dreams or land of opportunity for pharmacists? Available at https://www.contagionlive.com/publications/contagion/2019/june/outpatient-antimicrobial-stewardship-field-of-dreams-or-land-of-opportunity-for-pharmacists. Accessed January 5, 2020.

20. Pollack LA, Srinivasan A. Core elements of hospital antibiotic stewardship programs from the Centers for Disease Control and Prevention. *Clin Infect Dis*. 2014;59(Suppl 3):S97-S100.

21. Centers for Disease Control and Prevention. Core elements of antibiotic stewardship. Available at https://www.cdc.gov/antibiotic-use/core-elements/index.html. Accessed May 31, 2020.

22. Dellit TH, Owens RC, McGowan JE Jr, et al. Infectious Diseases Society of America and the Society for Healthcare Epidemiology of America guidelines for developing an institutional program to enhance *antimicrobial* stewardship. *Clin Infect Dis*. 2007;44(2):159-177.

23. Forrest GN, Van Schooneveld TC, Kullar R, Schulz LT, Duong P, Postelnick M. Use of electronic health records and clinical decision support systems for *antimicrobial* stewardship. *Clin Infect Dis*. 2014;59(Suppl 3):S122-S133.

24. Kullar R, Goff DA, Schulz LT, Fox BC, Rose WE. The "epic" challenge of optimizing *antimicrobial* stewardship: the role

of electronic medical records and technology. *Clin Infect Dis.* 2013;57(7):1005-1013.

25. Pogue JM, Potoski BA, Postelnick M, et al. Bringing the "power" to Cerner's PowerChart for *antimicrobial* stewardship. *Clin Infect Dis.* 2014;59(3):416-424.

26. Lodise TP, Lomaestro B, Graves J, Drusano GL. Larger vancomycin doses (at least 4 grams per day) are associated with an increased incidence of nephrotoxicity. *Antimicrob Agents Chemother.* 2008;52(4):1330-1336.

27. Narita M, Tsuji BT, Yu VL. Linezolid-associated peripheral and optic neuropathy, lactic acidosis, and serotonin syndrome. *Pharmacotherapy.* 2007;27(8):1189-1197.

28. Buising KL, Thursky KA, Robertson MB, et al. Electronic antibiotic stewardship—reduced consumption of broad-spectrum antibiotics using a computerized *antimicrobial* approval system in a hospital setting. *J Antimicrob Chemother.* 2008;62(3):608-616.

29. Pakyz AL, Oinonen M, Polk RE. Relationship of carbapenem restriction in 22 university teaching hospitals to carbapenem use and carbapenem-resistant *Pseudomonas aeruginosa. Antimicrob Agents Chemother.* 2009;53(5):1983-1986.

30. Davey P, Brown E, Charani E, et al. Interventions to improve antibiotic prescribing practices for hospital inpatients. *Cochrane Database Syst Rev.* 2013(4):CD003543.

31. Baggs J, Fridkin SK, Pollack LA, Srinivasan A, Jernigan JA. Estimating National trends in inpatient antibiotic use among US hospitals from 2006 to 2012. *JAMA Intern Med.* 2016;176(11):1639-1648.

32. Abbo LM, Cosgrove SE, Pottinger PS, et al. Medical students' perceptions and knowledge about *antimicrobial* stewardship: how are we educating our future prescribers? *Clin Infect Dis.* 2013;57(5):631-638.

33. Justo JA, Gauthier TP, Scheetz MH, et al. Knowledge and attitudes of doctor of pharmacy students regarding the appropriate use of *antimicrobials. Clin Infect Dis.* 2014;59 (Suppl 3):S162-S169.

34. Schumock GT, Li EC, Suda KJ, et al. National trends in prescription drug expenditures and projections for 2015. *Am J Health Syst Pharm.* 2015;72(9):717-736.

35. Schumock GT, Stubbings J, Hoffman JM, et al. National trends in prescription drug expenditures and projections for 2019. *Am J Health Syst Pharm.* 2019;76(15):1105-1121.

36. Day SR, Smith D, Harris K, Cox HL, Mathers AJ. An Infectious Diseases Physician-Led *Antimicrobial* Stewardship Program at a Small Community Hospital Associated With Improved Susceptibility Patterns and Cost-Savings after the First Year. *Open Forum Infect Dis.* 2015;2(2):ofv064.

37. Goff DA, Bauer KA, Reed EE, Stevenson KB, Taylor JJ, West JE. Is the "low-hanging fruit" worth picking for *antimicrobial* stewardship programs? *Clin Infect Dis.* 2012;55(4):587-592.

38. Rybak MJ, Lomaestro BM, Rotschafer JC, et al. Vancomycin therapeutic guidelines: a summary of consensus recommendations from the infectious diseases Society of America, the American Society of Health-System Pharmacists, and the Society of Infectious Diseases Pharmacists. *Clin Infect Dis.* 2009;49(3):325-327.

39. Nicolau DP, Freeman CD, Belliveau PP, Nightingale CH, Ross JW, Quintiliani R. Experience with a once-daily aminoglycoside program administered to 2,184 adult patients. *Antimicrob Agents Chemother.* 1995;39(3):650-655.

40. Rhodes NJ, Liu J, O'Donnell JN, et al. Prolonged infusion piperacillin-tazobactam decreases mortality and improves outcomes in severely ill patients: results of a systematic review and meta-analysis. *Crit Care Med.* 2018;46(2):236-243.

41. Vardakas KZ, Voulgaris GL, Maliaros A, Samonis G, Falagas ME. Prolonged versus short-term intravenous infusion of antipseudomonal beta-lactams for patients with sepsis: a systematic review and meta-analysis of randomised trials. *Lancet Infect Dis.* 2018;18(1):108-120.

42. Sakoulas G, Geriak M, Nizet V. Is a reported penicillin allergy sufficient grounds to forgo the multidimensional *antimicrobial* benefits of beta-lactam antibiotics? *Clin Infect Dis.* 2019;68(1):157-164.

43. Gauthier T. 5 things to know about patients labeled with penicillin allergy. Available at https://www.idstewardship.com/5-things-know-patients-labeled-penicillin-allergy/. Accessed January 20, 2020.

44. Pagels CM, McCreary EK, Rose WE, Dodds Ashley ES, Bookstaver PB, Dilworth TJ. Designing *antimicrobial* stewardship initiatives to enhance scientific dissemination. *J Am Coll Clin Pharm.* 2020;3(1):109-115

45. King ST, Walker ED, Cannon CG, Finley RW. Daptomycin-induced rhabdomyolysis and acute liver injury. *Scand J Infect Dis.* 2014;46(7):537-540.

46. Lavery LA, Armstrong DG, Wunderlich RP, Mohler MJ, Wendel CS, Lipsky BA. Risk factors for foot infections in individuals with diabetes. *Diabetes Care.* 2006;29(6):1288-1293.

47. Norris AH, Shrestha NK, Allison GM, et al. 2018 Infectious Diseases Society of America clinical practice guideline for the management of outpatient parenteral *antimicrobial* therapy. *Clin Infect Dis.* 2019;68(1):e1-e35.

48. Torres PA, Helmstetter JA, Kaye AM, Kaye AD. Rhabdomyolysis: pathogenesis, diagnosis, and treatment. *Ochsner J.* 2015;15(1): 58-69.

49. Mosshammer D, Schaeffeler E, Schwab M, Morike K. Mechanisms and assessment of statin-related muscular adverse effects. *Br J Clin Pharmacol.* 2014;78(3):454-466.

50. Dare RK, Tewell C, Harris B, et al. Effect of statin coadministration on the risk of daptomycin-associated myopathy. *Clin Infect Dis.* 2018;67(9):1356-1363.

51. University of Nebraska Medical Center. Daptomycin (Cubicin). Available at https://www.nebraskamed.com/for-providers/asp/restrictions/daptomycin. Accessed February 17, 2020.

52. Kollef MH. Inadequate *antimicrobial* treatment: an important determinant of outcome for hospitalized patients. *Clin Infect Dis.* 2000;31(Suppl 4):S131-S138.

53. Barenfanger J, Graham DR, Kolluri L, et al. Decreased mortality associated with prompt Gram staining of blood cultures. *Am J Clin Pathol.* 2008;130(6):870-876.

54. Lodise TP, McKinnon PS, Swiderski L, Rybak MJ. Outcomes analysis of delayed antibiotic treatment for hospital-acquired *Staphylococcus aureus* bacteremia. *Clin Infect Dis.* 2003;36(11):1418-1423.

55. Bauer KA, Perez KK, Forrest GN, Goff DA. Review of rapid diagnostic tests used by *antimicrobial* stewardship programs. *Clin Infect Dis.* 2014;59(Suppl 3):S134-S145.

56. Beganovic M, McCreary EK, Mahoney MV, Dionne B, Green DA, Timbrook TT. Interplay between rapid diagnostic tests and *antimicrobial* stewardship programs among patients with bloodstream and other severe infections. *J Appl Lab Med.* 2019;3(4):601-616.

57. Klepser DG, Klepser ME. Point-of-care testing in the pharmacy: how is the field evolving? *Expert Rev Mol Diagn.* 2018;18(1):5-6.

58. Society of Infectious Diseases Pharmacists. *Antimicrobial stewardship certificate programs.* Available at https://sidp.org/Stewardship-Certificate. Accessed February 15, 2020.

59. Making a Difference in Infectious Diseases. *Antimicrobial stewardship programs.* Available at https://mad-id.org/*antimicrobial*-stewardship-programs/. Accessed February 15, 2020.

60. Board of Pharmacy Specialties. Infectious diseases pharmacy. Available at https://www.bpsweb.org/bps-specialties/infectious-diseases-pharmacy/. Accessed February 15, 2020.

61. Society of Infectious Diseases Pharmacists. Fellowships. Available at https://sidp.org/Fellowships. Accessed February 15, 2020.

62. Levinson WE. *Review of Medical Microbiology & Immunology: A Guide to Clinical Infectious Diseases.* 14th ed. New York, NY: McGraw-Hill.

63. Haque M, Sartelli M, McKimm J, Abu Bakar M. Health care-associated infections—an overview. *Infect Drug Resist.* 2018;11:2321-2333.

64. Fowler VGJr, Miro JM, Hoen B, et al. *Staphylococcus aureus* endocarditis: a consequence of medical progress. *JAMA.* 2005;293(24):3012-3021.

65. Fowler VG Jr, Olsen MK, Corey GR, et al. Clinical identifiers of complicated Staphylococcus aureus bacteremia. *Arch Intern Med.* 2003;163(17):2066-2072.

66. Miller LG, Eisenberg DF, Liu H, et al. Incidence of skin and soft tissue infections in ambulatory and inpatient settings, 2005–2010. *BMC Infect Dis.* 2015;15:362.

67. Hersh AL, Chambers HF, Maselli JH, Gonzales R. National trends in ambulatory visits and antibiotic prescribing for skin and soft-tissue infections. *Arch Intern Med.* 2008;168(14):1585-1591.

68. Kaye KS, Petty LA, Shorr AF, Zilberberg MD. Current epidemiology, etiology, and burden of acute skin infections in the united states. *Clin Infect Dis.* 2019;68(Supplement_3):S193-S199.

69. Moran GJ, Krishnadasan A, Gorwitz RJ, et al. Methicillin-resistant *S. aureus* infections among patients in the emergency department. *N Engl J Med.* 2006;355(7):666-674.

70. O'Toole GA. Classic spotlight: how the gram stain works. *J Bacteriol.* 2016;198(23):3128.

71. Ray GT, Suaya JA, Baxter R. Incidence, microbiology, and patient characteristics of skin and soft-tissue infections in a U.S. population: a retrospective population-based study. *BMC Infect Dis.* 2013;13:252.

72. Zervos MJ, Freeman K, Vo L, et al. Epidemiology and outcomes of complicated skin and soft tissue infections in hospitalized patients. *J Clin Microbiol.* 2012;50(2):238-245.

73. Infectious Diseases Society of America. Patient stories: the faces of *antimicrobial* resistance. Available at https://www.idsociety.org/es/public-health/patient-stories/patient-stories/. Accessed February 12, 2020.

74. Stevens DL, Bisno AL, Chambers HF, et al. Practice guidelines for the diagnosis and management of skin and soft tissue infections: 2014 update by the infectious diseases society of America. *Clin Infect Dis.* 2014;59(2):147-159.

75. Zilberberg M, Micek ST, Kollef MH, Shelbaya A, Shorr AF. Risk factors for mixed complicated skin and skin structure infections

76. Russo A, Concia E, Cristini F, et al. Current and future trends in antibiotic therapy of acute bacterial skin and skin-structure infections. *Clin Microbiol Infect.* 2016;22(Suppl 2):S27-S36.

77. Suaya JA, Mera RM, Cassidy A, et al. Incidence and cost of hospitalizations associated with *Staphylococcus aureus* skin and soft tissue infections in the United States from 2001 through 2009. *BMC Infect Dis.* 2014;14:296.

78. Wiseman JT, Fernandes-Taylor S, Barnes ML, et al. Predictors of surgical site infection after hospital discharge in patients undergoing major vascular surgery. *J Vasc Surg.* 2015;62(4):1023-1031 e1025.

79. Miller LG. Another New antibiotic for skin infections and why infectious disease specialists are hypocrites. *Clin Infect Dis.* 2019;68(7):1223-1224.

80. Golan Y. Current treatment options for acute skin and skin-structure infections. *Clin Infect Dis.* 2019;68(Supplement_3):S206-S212.

81. Tenover FC. Potential impact of rapid diagnostic tests on improving *antimicrobial* use. *Ann N Y Acad Sci.* 2010;1213:70-80.

82. Lodise TP, Zhao Q, Fahrbach K, Gillard PJ, Martin A. A systematic review of the association between delayed appropriate therapy and mortality among patients hospitalized with infections due to *Klebsiella pneumoniae* or *Escherichia coli*: how long is too long? *BMC Infect Dis.* 2018;18(1):625.

83. Fraser A, Paul M, Almanasreh N, et al. Benefit of appropriate empirical antibiotic treatment: thirty-day mortality and duration of hospital stay. *Am J Med.* 2006;119(11):970-976.

84. Singhal N, Kumar M, Kanaujia PK, Virdi JS. MALDI-TOF mass spectrometry: an emerging technology for microbial identification and diagnosis. *Front Microbiol.* 2015;6:791.

85. File TM Jr, Srinivasan A, Bartlett JG. *Antimicrobial* stewardship: importance for patient and public health. *Clin Infect Dis.* 2014;59(Suppl 3):S93-S96.

86. Wenzler E, Wang F, Goff DA, et al. An automated, pharmacist-driven initiative improves quality of care for *Staphylococcus aureus* bacteremia. *Clin Infect Dis.* 2017;65(2):194-200.

87. Bauer KA, West JE, Balada-Llasat JM, Pancholi P, Stevenson KB, Goff DA. An *antimicrobial* stewardship program's impact with rapid polymerase chain reaction methicillin-resistant *Staphylococcus aureus/S. aureus* blood culture test in patients with *S. aureus* bacteremia. *Clin Infect Dis.* 2010;51(9):1074-1080.

88. Kozel TR, Burnham-Marusich AR. Point-of-care testing for infectious diseases: past, present, and future.. *J Clin Microbiol.* 2017;55(8):2313-2320.

89. Gubbins PO, Klepser ME, Adams AJ, Jacobs DM, Percival KM, Tallman GB. Potential for pharmacy-public health collaborations using pharmacy-based point-of-care testing services for infectious diseases. *J Public Health Manag Pract.* 2017;23(6):593-600.

90. Kansagara D, Chiovaro JC, Kagen D, et al. So many options, where do we start? An overview of the care transitions literature. *J Hosp Med.* 2016;11(3):221-230.

91. Allen J, Hutchinson AM, Brown R, Livingston PM. Quality care outcomes following transitional care interventions for older people from hospital to home: a systematic review. *BMC Health Serv Res.* 2014;14:346.

92. Keller SC, Ciuffetelli D, Bilker W, et al. The impact of an infectious diseases transition service on the care of outpatients on parenteral *antimicrobial* therapy. *J Pharm Technol.* 2013;29(5):205-214.

93. Scarpato SJ, Timko DR, Cluzet VC, et al. An evaluation of antibiotic prescribing practices upon hospital discharge. *Infect Control Hosp Epidemiol.* 2017;38(3):353-355.

94. Yogo N, Haas MK, Knepper BC, Burman WJ, Mehler PS, Jenkins TC. Antibiotic prescribing at the transition from hospitalization to discharge: a target for antibiotic stewardship. *Infect Control Hosp Epidemiol.* 2015;36(4):474-478.

95. Dyer A, Ashley ED, Anderson DJ, et al. Inpatient plus post-discharge durations of therapy to identify *antimicrobial* stewardship opportunities at transitions of care. *Open Forum Infect Dis.* 2017;4(Suppl 1):S19-S20.

96. Barnett SG, Lata P, Kavalier M, Crnich C, Balasubramanian P. Antibiotic assessment at hospital discharge—room for stewardship intervention. *Infect Control Hosp Epidemiol.* 2020;41(2):209-211.

97. Tice AD, Rehm SJ, Dalovisio JR, et al. Practice guidelines for outpatient parenteral *antimicrobial* therapy. IDSA guidelines. *Clin Infect Dis.* 2004;38(12):1651-1672.

98. Sheridan K, Shields RK, Falcione B, Glowa T. Pharmacist monitoring in an OPAT program can lead to a reduction in 30-day readmission rates. *Open Forum Infect Dis.* 2015;2(suppl_1).

99. Joint Commission on Hospital A. Approved: New *antimicrobial* stewardship standard. *Jt Comm Perspect.* 2016;36(7):1, 3-4, 8.

100. Owens RC Jr, Shorr AF, Deschambeault AL. *Antimicrobial* stewardship: shepherding precious resources. *Am J Health Syst Pharm.* 2009;66(12 Suppl 4):S15-S22.

101. Ragucci KR, O'Bryant CL, Campbell KB, et al. The need for PGY2-trained clinical pharmacy specialists. *Pharmacotherapy.* 2014;34(6):e65-73.

102. Trivedi KK, Rosenberg J. The state of *antimicrobial* stewardship programs in California. *Infect Control Hosp Epidemiol.* 2013;34(4):379-384.

103. Young JD, Abdel-Massih R, Herchline T, et al. Infectious Diseases Society of America position statement on telehealth and telemedicine as applied to the practice of infectious diseases. *Clin Infect Dis.* 2019;68(9):1437-1443.

104. Shively NR, Moffa MA, Paul KT, et al. Impact of a telehealth-based *antimicrobial* stewardship program in a community hospital health system. *Clin Infect Dis.* 2019.

105. Kho ZY, Lal SK. The human gut microbiome—a potential controller of wellness and disease. *Front Microbiol.* 2018;9:1835.

106. Neuman H, Forsythe P, Uzan A, Avni O, Koren O. Antibiotics in early life: dysbiosis and the damage done. *FEMS Microbiol Rev.* 2018;42(4):489-499.

107. Dethlefsen L, Relman DA. Incomplete recovery and individualized responses of the human distal gut microbiota to repeated antibiotic perturbation. *Proc Natl Acad Sci USA.* 2011;108(Suppl 1):4554-4561.

108. Korpela K, Salonen A, Virta LJ, Kekkonen RA, de Vos WM. Association of early-life antibiotic use and protective effects of breastfeeding: role of the intestinal microbiota. *JAMA Pediatr.* 2016;170(8):750-757.

109. Hempel S, Newberry SJ, Maher AR, et al. Probiotics for the prevention and treatment of antibiotic-associated

110. Olek A, Woynarowski M, Ahren IL, et al. Efficacy and safety of *Lactobacillus plantarum* DSM 9843 (LP299V) in the prevention of antibiotic-associated gastrointestinal symptoms in children—randomized, double—blind, placebo—controlled study. *J Pediatr.* 2017;186:82-86.

111. Allen SJ, Wareham K, Wang D, et al. Lactobacilli and bifidobacteria in the prevention of antibiotic-associated diarrhoea and *Clostridium difficile* diarrhoea in older inpatients (PLACIDE): a randomised, double-blind, placebo-controlled, multicentre trial. *Lancet.* 2013;382(9900):1249-1257.

112. Suez J, Zmora N, Zilberman-Schapira G, et al. Post-antibiotic gut mucosal microbiome reconstitution is impaired by probiotics and improved by autologous FMT. *Cell.* 2018;174(6):1406-1423.e1416.

113. Appelbaum E, Leff WA. Occurrence of superinfections during antibiotic therapy. *J Am Med Assoc.* 1948;138(2):119-121.

114. Superinfections during antibiotic treatment. *Br Med J.* 1952;1(4757):537-538.

115. Amon P, Sanderson I. What is the microbiome? *Arch Dis Child Educ Pract Ed.* 2017;102(5):257-250.

116. Centers for Disease Control and Prevention. What is C. diff? Available at https://www.cdc.gov/cdiff/what-is.html. Accessed May 31, 2020.

117. Centers for Disease Control and Prevention. *Clostridioides difficile* (C. diff): Your risk of C. diff. Available at https://www.cdc.gov/cdiff/risk.html. Accessed May 31, 2020.

118. Hensgens MP, Goorhuis A, Dekkers OM, Kuijper EJ. Time interval of increased risk for *Clostridium difficile* infection after exposure to antibiotics. *J Antimicrob Chemother.* 2012;67(3):742-748.

119. Czepiel J, Drozdz M, Pituch H, et al. *Clostridium difficile* infection: review. *Eur J Clin Microbiol Infect Dis.* 2019;38(7):1211-1221.

120. Kim G, Zhu NA. Community-acquired Clostridium difficile infection. *Can Fam Physician.* 2017;63(2):131-132.

121. Centers for Disease Control and Prevention. Prevent the spread of C. diff. Available at https://www.cdc.gov/cdiff/prevent.html. Accessed May 31, 2020.

122. Hensgens MP, Keessen EC, Squire MM, et al. *Clostridium difficile* infection in the community: a zoonotic disease? *Clin Microbiol Infect.* 2012;18(7):635-645.

123. Centers for Disease Control and Prevention. Clean hands count campaign. Available at https://www.cdc.gov/handhygiene/campaign/index.html. Accessed May 31, 2020.

124. World Health Organization. Infection prevention and control. SAVE LIVES: Clean your hands. Available at https://www.who.int/infection-prevention/campaigns/clean-hands/en/. Accessed May 31, 2020.

125. McDonald LC, Gerding DN, Johnson S, et al. Clinical practice guidelines for *Clostridium difficile* infection in adults and children: 2017 update by the Infectious Diseases Society of America (IDSA) and Society for Healthcare Epidemiology of America (SHEA). *Clin Infect Dis.* 2018;66(7):e1-e48.

126. Moses KP, Banks JC, Nava PB, Petersen DK. Pelvis Viscera. In: Moses KP, Banks JC, Nava PB, Petersen DK, eds. *Atlas of Clinical Gross Anatomy.* 2nd ed. Philadelphia, PA Saunders; 2015:460-477.

diarrhea: a systematic review and meta-analysis. *JAMA.* 2012;307(18):1959-1969.

127. U.S. Department of Health & Human Services. Office on women's health. Urinary tract infections. Available at https://www.womenshealth.gov/a-z-topics/urinary-tract-infections. Accessed May 31, 2020.

128. Arnold JJ, Hehn LE, Klein DA. Common questions about recurrent urinary tract infections in women. *Am Fam Physician.* 2016;93(7):560-569.

129. Gallagher JC, MacDougall C. *Antibiotics Simplified.* 4th ed. Burlington, MA: Jones & Bartlett Learning; 2016.

130. Horton JM. Urinary tract agents: Nitrofurantoin, fosfomycin, and methenamine. In: *Mandell, Douglas, and Bennett's Principles and Practice of Infectious Disease.* 8th ed. Philadelphia, PA: Saunders; 2015.

131. Cyriac JM, James E. Switch over from intravenous to oral therapy: a concise overview. *J Pharmacol Pharmacother.* 2014;5(2):83-87.

132. Squadrito FJ, del Portal D. Nitrofurantoin. In: *StatPearls.* Treasure Island (FL)2020.

133. Levaquin package insert. Available at https://www.accessdata.fda.gov/drugsatfda_docs/label/2018/020634s069lbl.pdf. Published 2018. Accessed May 31, 2020.

134. The consensus of the Pharmacy Practice Model Summit. *Am J Health Syst Pharm.* 2011;68(12):1148-1152.

135. Bonetti AF, Reis WC, Mendes AM, et al. Impact of pharmacist-led discharge counseling on hospital readmission and emergency department visits: a systematic review and meta-analysis. *J Hosp Med.* 2020;15(1):52-59.

136. Owens RC Jr, Donskey CJ, Gaynes RP, Loo VG, Muto CA. Antimicrobial-associated risk factors for *Clostridium difficile* infection. *Clin Infect Dis.* 2008;46(Suppl 1):S19-S31.

137. Vardakas KZ, Trigkidis KK, Boukouvala E, Falagas ME. *Clostridium difficile* infection following systemic antibiotic administration in randomised controlled trials: a systematic review and meta-analysis. *Int J Antimicrob Agents.* 2016;48(1):1-10.

138. Brown KA, Khanafer N, Daneman N, Fisman DN. Meta-analysis of antibiotics and the risk of community-associated *Clostridium difficile* infection. *Antimicrob Agents Chemother.* 2013;57(5):2326-2332.

139. Kavanagh K, Pan J, Marwick C, et al. Cumulative and temporal associations between antimicrobial prescribing and community-associated *Clostridium difficile* infection: population-based case-control study using administrative data. *J Antimicrob Chemother.* 2017;72(4):1193-1201.

140. Blanchette L, Gauthier T, Heil E, et al. The essential role of pharmacists in antibiotic stewardship in outpatient care: an official position statement of the Society of Infectious Diseases Pharmacists. *J Am Pharm Assoc.* 2018;58(5):481-484.

141. Isaac S, Scher JU, Djukovic A, et al. Short- and long-term effects of oral vancomycin on the human intestinal microbiota. *J Antimicrob Chemother.* 2017;72(1):128-136.

142. Eyre DW, Walker AS, Wyllie D, et al. Predictors of first recurrence of *Clostridium difficile* infection: implications for initial management. *Clin Infect Dis.* 2012;55(Suppl 2):S77-S87.

CHAPTER 9

Oncology
Featuring the Illustrated Case Studies "Compromising" & "Compassion"

Authors

Cameron L. Ninos, Paul R. Hutson, & Joseph A. Zorek

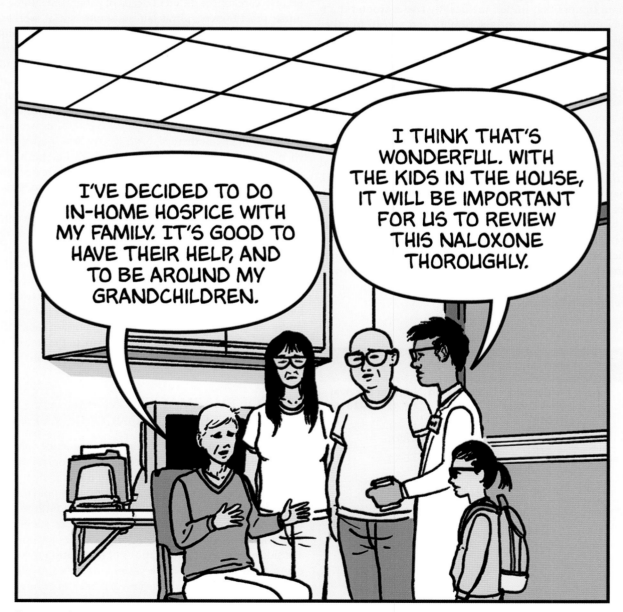

Illustration by George Folz, © 2019 Board of Regents of the University of Wisconsin System

BACKGROUND

Oncology is the branch of medicine that specializes in the diagnosis and treatment of cancer.[1] There are over 100 different types of cancer, each named for either their location in the body (e.g., breast cancer, colon cancer) or for the individual who first discovered or described it (e.g., Hodgkin's lymphoma, Kaposi's sarcoma). The uncontrolled growth of cells within the body is the defining feature of all cancers. Healthy cells regularly grow and divide. When they become old or damaged, they die and are replaced by new cells. In cancer, genetic changes within cells accumulate, which leads to uncontrolled growth and tumor formation. These genetic changes can have a multitude of different causes such as the chemicals in tobacco smoke, radiation from the sun's rays, or inheritance from one's parents. Some tumors are benign. These cells grow and divide in an atypical manner but are not considered cancerous as they do not spread to other parts of the body and are rarely life-threatening. On the contrary, cancer consists of malignant tumors that invade the healthy tissue around them and may metastasize (form new tumors and spread to other parts of the body). Cancer is classified in many ways and may broadly be divided into cancers of the blood, which include leukemias and lymphomas, and solid tumors, which include breast, lung, prostate, and colon cancers. Table 9-1 lists common cancers, including estimated and reported data regarding new diagnoses, deaths caused, and 5-year survival from the time of diagnosis.[2]

Depending on the patient, as well as the cancer type, stage, and location, a variety of treatment modalities may be employed. This may involve surgery to physically remove the tumor, radiation or chemotherapy to destroy cancerous cells using high energy x-rays or toxic medications, respectively, or a combination of all three. Newer ways of treating cancer include targeted therapies and immunotherapies. The former use medications that target a specific part of the cancer cell, effecting its growth and survival, while the latter boosts the body's natural immunologic defenses to fight and destroy cancer cells.

Members of the Interprofessional Oncology Team

Due to the high level of complexity associated with the care of patients with cancer, a multitude of health professionals are involved.[3] The physician expert who often coordinates a patient's care is the medical oncologist.[1] This is someone who specializes in diagnosing and treating cancer in adults using chemotherapy, hormonal therapy, biological therapy, and targeted therapy. Medical oncologists frequently collaborate with radiation oncologists or surgical oncologists who use radiation or surgery, respectively, to treat cancer. Other physicians who may assist with oncology patients' care include hematologists, who specialize in diagnosing and treating blood disorders (including cancers of the blood), palliative care physicians, who focus on improving a patient's quality of life, and pathologists, who study cells and tissues under a microscope in order to develop a diagnosis.

Aside from physicians, many other health professionals collaborate to care for the different needs of patients including nurses, nurse practitioners, physician assistants, social workers, and dietitians/nutritionists. One example of this is the close cooperation between pharmacists and nurses. In a hospital setting, this may entail coordinating chemotherapy infusions around complicated medication administration schedules, or problem solving when chemotherapy infusions are delayed or interrupted. In a clinic setting, pharmacists may work with nurses to identify when and how to obtain laboratory (i.e., lab) draws to ensure the safety of chemotherapy, or to discuss how best to reinforce chemotherapy education in a patient with low health literacy. An additional role that is emerging in oncology care is that of a patient navigator.[3] This individual follows a patient longitudinally from diagnosis through survivorship, and works to coordinate a patient's care to assist with counseling, finances, rehabilitation, and other services as needed. A pharmacist's practice setting will influence the amount and types of interactions with other health professionals.[4] Hospital-based pharmacists will have different interactions with other health professionals than those housed in a clinic-, infusion-, or community pharmacy-based setting. Due to the complexity of care, the large number of other health professionals involved, and the vitally important role of medications, pharmacists in all settings will share in the care of patients with cancer through interprofessional collaboration.

ROLE OF PHARMACISTS WITHIN THE INTERPROFESSIONAL ONCOLOGY TEAM

Due to the broad scope of oncology practice, pharmacists may have a wide variety of roles and responsibilities within the oncology team.[4] These range from direct patient care roles to developing healthcare organization-wide policies, such as determining which medication regimens should be preferred for certain cancers, which cancer medications should be used and stocked by an organization, or guidelines for how to manage side effects and complications of medication therapies. The commonality between these various roles lies in pharmacists contributing their knowledge and expertise to ensure the safest and most effective use of medications in the treatment of cancer.

Table 9-1. Common Cancers and Their Impact on American Lives			
Type	Estimated New Cases (2019)	Estimated Deaths (2019)	5-Year Survival % (2009–2015)
Breast	271,270	42,260	89.8
Colon and rectum	145,600	51,020	64.4
Leukemia	61,780	22,840	62.7
Lung and bronchus	228,150	142,670	19.4
Non-Hodgkin lymphoma	74,200	19,970	72.0
Pancreas	56,770	45,750	9.3
Prostate	174,650	31,620	98.0

One of the key professional activities shared by oncology pharmacists is chemotherapy order review.[5,6] Prior to dispensing a chemotherapeutic medication, oncology pharmacists review the patient's profile to ensure its appropriateness. This is a multistep process that begins with an assessment of indication; in other words, that the patient, his/her diagnosis, and the chemotherapy regimen all match.[7] This includes confirmation that the regimen prescribed has published literature to support its efficacy and safety for the particular type of patient. For example, pertuzumab (Perjeta) is a targeted agent shown to have benefit in certain early-stage breast cancer patients, but its toxicities can include heart dysfunction.[8] Prior to a patient receiving pertuzumab, an oncology pharmacist would ensure that the patient (1) fits the group profile shown to benefit from this therapy, and (2) lacks any characteristics that would make the patient more likely to be harmed by pertuzumab than to benefit from its use (e.g., pre-existing heart failure).

Another key component of the patient's profile that oncology pharmacists review is lab results.[5] Oncology pharmacists must ensure that the patient's kidneys and liver are working well enough to handle the chemotherapy. If not, chemotherapeutic medications can accumulate in the body, leading to life-threatening toxicities such as organ damage. Oncology pharmacists also confirm that the patient's blood counts have recovered enough from prior chemotherapy treatments; for example, white blood cells and platelets. This reduces the likelihood of life-threatening infections or bleeding events, respectively.

Once oncology pharmacists are certain that the chemotherapy ordered for the patient is appropriate based on published literature and lab results, they then perform calculations to ensure the dose ordered is accurate and optimal.[6] Chemotherapies are typically dosed based on height and weight, and patient weights can fluctuate significantly throughout the course of treatment, leading to significant toxicity if an inappropriate weight is used.[5] Finally, pharmacists evaluate dosing and appropriateness of medications ordered alongside chemotherapy as supportive care.[6] These medications are intended to mitigate expected side effects; a few examples include intravenous fluids to prevent kidney dysfunction, white blood cell growth factors to ensure blood count recovery, or anti-infectives, such as antibiotics or antifungals, to prevent opportunistic infections.[9–11]

Another critical area of pharmacist involvement is toxicity management and monitoring.[12] Some chemotherapy regimens, for example, will cause over 90% of patients to vomit (otherwise known as emesis) without medication support. With appropriate anti-emetic therapy, however, the number of patients who experience this side effect can be greatly reduced, decreasing the percentage of patients experiencing significant nausea to as little as 26% to 45%.[13,14] Despite the efficacy of initial anti-emetic therapy, patients should be evaluated for breakthrough nausea and vomiting throughout the course of treatment, and their anti-emetic regimens should be tailored to their needs.[15] Oncology pharmacists are in an excellent position to assess a patient's nausea and emesis after each chemotherapy treatment, and, based upon medications being used and comorbidities, recommend additional agents to be used at a regular interval or as backup medications.[16]

An emerging area where pharmacists improve patient care is oral oncolytics.[17] This is a broad class of medications including traditional chemotherapy agents, as well as small molecular inhibitors that target specific proteins or receptors in cancer cells. Best practices now recommend that oncology pharmacists participate in comprehensive patient education prior to the initiation of oral oncolytic therapy. Also, pharmacists should be involved in the regular monitoring and follow-up of patients on these therapies, including symptom management, adherence assessment, and leveraging collaborative practice agreements. Working in a coordinated fashion with a physician or group of physicians, such agreements permit oncology pharmacists to order labs and supportive care medications directly based on their assessment of patient needs, and have been shown to prevent medication errors, identify adverse reactions, and increase patient adherence.[18]

Pharmacists are also key members of interprofessional teams for complex procedures and immunotherapies such as hematopoietic transplantation (otherwise known as bone marrow transplant or BMT) or chimeric antigen receptor (CAR) T-cell therapy. These specialized therapies may be used in patients with certain types of cancer, the mechanisms of which are discussed in the illustrated case "Compromising" in this chapter. Responsibilities unique to pharmacists in these fields include managing immune suppression therapies, including dosing and monitoring drug levels in order to prevent the immune system from becoming overactive and attacking an individual, while preventing medication toxicities.[19] Pharmacists also recommend anti-infective therapy and vaccinations in these patients, who are at high risk of infectious complications due to their compromised immune systems. Pharmacists in CAR-T therapy assist with managing the unique immune toxicities of that therapy, and the use of unique drugs in the treatment of toxicity, such as immune system-specific antibodies.[20] Accreditation standards also require pharmacist involvement in the development of guidelines for the pharmaceutical management of transplant patients.[19] Like many other areas of oncology, pharmacists benefit BMT and CAR T-cell therapy patients throughout their care through direct medication management and institutional policy development.

The professional activities of oncology pharmacists have also been shown to improve the health of patient populations.[17] For example, Sweiss and colleagues found that having a pharmacist meet with every patient in a myeloma clinic (a type of blood cancer) increased adherence to prescribing of recommended blood thinners from 83% to 100%, and reduced the percentage of patients experiencing delays in obtaining oral chemotherapy from 85% to 21%.[21] The utilization of oncology pharmacist-developed chemotherapy plans that include recommended dosing, lab monitoring, and supportive care required to safely use a chemotherapy regimen has led to population-level improvements in cancer care.[6,7,22,23] Oncology pharmacists also shape population-level use of chemotherapy and supportive care agents via the development of guidelines, as well as participation in formulary decisions that drive prescribing patterns throughout healthcare organizations.[4,24,25] For more information on the impact of pharmacy services on populations, see Chapter 14 Population Health.

Oncology-trained pharmacists can practice in a variety of different areas based upon their personal interests and preferences.[4] Inpatient oncology pharmacists care for hospitalized patients who are suffering from acute medical issues, such as a pain crisis or a lung infection, or who are admitted to hospital for a chemotherapy regimen that requires 24-hour supervision. Pharmacists choosing this practice setting may do so for the opportunity to help patients who are very sick, or because they enjoy the complexity and interactions of working within a large interprofessional oncology team. Conversely, clinic-based oncology pharmacists have the opportunity to form relationships with patients as they travel through diagnosis, treatment initiation, toxicities, and survivorship. These pharmacists play a pivotal role in patient education, medication adherence, and medication optimization to prevent hospitalizations from occurring. Other practice settings include chemotherapy infusion centers or specialty pharmacies, where, due to the complexity of chemotherapeutic medications, the expertise of oncology pharmacists is required to ensure safe and effective medication use. Due to the wide variety of oncology pharmacy positions, many pharmacists may fulfill several of these roles within their job based upon their interests and expertise.

ONCOLOGY PHARMACISTS IN ACTION

Easing in the Immune System, One Drip at a Time

Anaphylaxis is defined as a serious type of hypersensitivity reaction (i.e., allergic reaction) that can be life-threatening or fatal, and typically involves an inability to breathe or an unsafe drop in blood pressure.[26] At an academic health center in Kentucky, a patient with a rare form of leukemia had experienced recurrent anaphylactic reactions to alemtuzumab (Campath), an antibody used in leukemia treatment, which led to changing the chemotherapy regimen to a more traditional approach.[27] However, the patient's leukemia became resistant to traditional options. At this time, the oncology pharmacist presented a potential solution to the interprofessional team; specifically, desensitization. Desensitization works by introducing very small doses of a medication (in this case 1/20,000 of the full dose of the medication), and then slowly escalating exposures to the full dose of the medication. In this way, the immune system learns to tolerate the medication, which can prevent anaphylactic reactions from occurring. As may be expected, this is a complicated process requiring coordination of multiple health professionals, and this can only be completed in an intensive care unit within a hospital. In

this case, oncology pharmacists were vital in designing the protocol that determined which medications the patient should receive prior to starting the desensitization process, which doses should be administered, the duration of each infusion, and which medications needed to be available in case an anaphylactic reaction did occur. They also coordinated with compounding pharmacists to ensure such miniscule doses could be accurately compounded. Thanks to the oncology pharmacists' diligence, attention to detail, and creativity, this patient tolerated the desensitization, which allowed her to receive infusions of alemtuzumab three times weekly in order to treat her leukemia.

Caution! Interaction Alert!

In France, a patient with mantle cell lymphoma on treatment with ibrutinib (Imbruvica), was admitted to the hospital following a fall and loss of consciousness lasting several minutes.[28] He reported nausea, dizziness, fatigue, and severe diarrhea that had started the previous day. Ibrutinib is a targeted oral chemotherapy agent that is used for the treatment of several lymphomas. It works by inhibiting cancerous B cell replication and survival. It is metabolized (i.e., broken down in the body) via a common drug pathway in the liver, and is therefore susceptible to multiple drug interactions. On review, the oncology pharmacist identified that the patient was also taking verapamil, a blood pressure medication known to interfere with the same drug metabolism pathway used by ibrutinib. As a result of this interaction, ibrutinib accumulated in the patient's body, leading to ibrutinib exposure up to nine times higher than the intended dose. The oncology pharmacist worked with the interprofessional team to change verapamil to an alternative, non-interacting blood pressure medication, and 5 days later ibrutinib was able to be restarted. Three months after this intervention, the patient was still tolerating the full dose of ibrutinib. This example underscores the importance of oncology pharmacists and their expert knowledge of medications, including the mechanisms of how drug interactions occur. Absent the oncology pharmacist's identification of the drug interaction, ibrutinib likely would have been discontinued altogether, abandoning one of the few effective therapies in treating this challenging type of cancer.

BECOMING AN ONCOLOGY PHARMACIST

Graduates of Doctor of Pharmacy (PharmD) programs accredited by the Accreditation Council for Pharmacy Education (ACPE) are educated to manage the pharmacotherapy of a broad range of patients.[29] Given the complexities associated with cancer and chemotherapies, most employment opportunities require specialized training and/or experience on top of the solid foundation provided during pharmacy school. Most individuals interested in an oncology career pursue a general post-graduate year 1 (PGY-1) residency to further develop generalized patient care, problem-solving, and leadership skills, followed by a PGY-2 residency with an oncology specialization.[30] PGY-2 oncology residencies are designed to transition PGY-1 residency graduates from generalist practice to specialized practice in oncology care. Many employers also require specific credentialing to demonstrate advanced knowledge and expertise in optimizing outcomes for patients with cancer beyond residency training. The Board of Pharmacy Specialties offers a nationally recognized credential called the Board Certified Oncology Pharmacist (BCOP).[31] To obtain BCOP status, pharmacists must attain a passing score on a written pharmacy specialty examination. In order to qualify for the examination, pharmacists are required to be actively licensed, have graduated from an ACPE-accredited program (or international equivalent), and to demonstrate practice experience via one of the following pathways: 4 years of oncology practice experience, completion of a PGY-1 residency plus 2 additional years of practice experience, or completion of a specialty residency in oncology pharmacy. Practice experience must include at least 50% of time spent within oncology. In order to maintain BCOP certification, individuals must either earn 100 hours of BCOP continuing education credit or achieve a passing score on a recertification exam in the seventh year following initial certification.

COMPROMISING: An Illustrated Case Study

Story by Cameron L. Ninos & Joseph A. Zorek
Illustrations by George Folz, © 2019 Board of Regents of the University of Wisconsin System

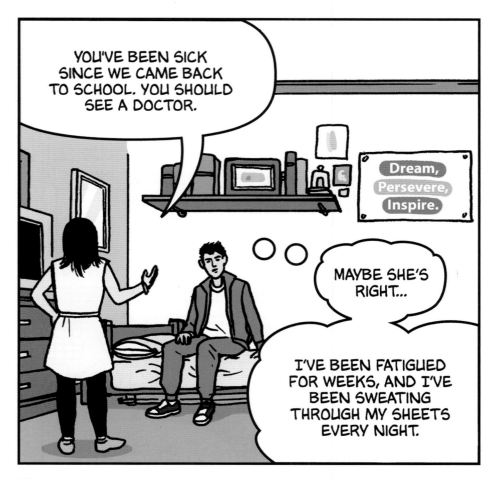

Illustration 9-1

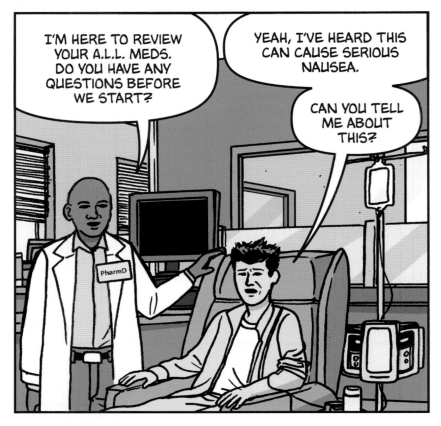

Illustration 9-2

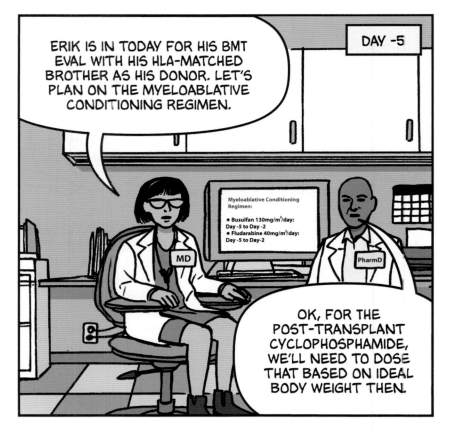

Illustration 9-3

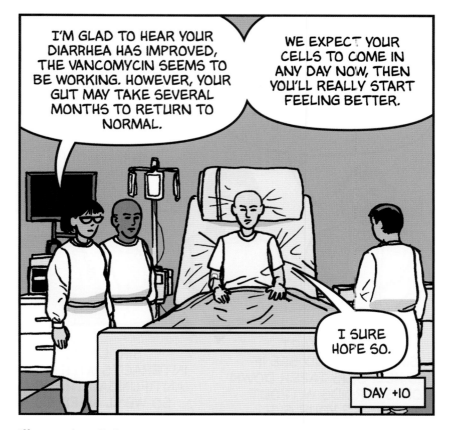

Illustration 9-4

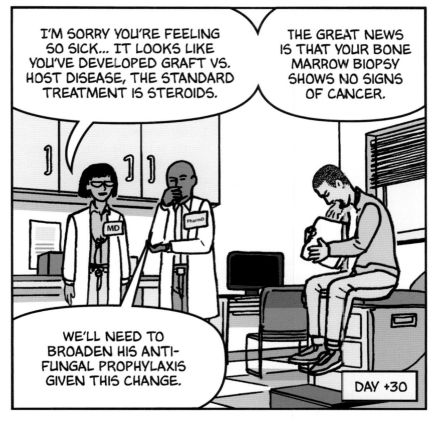

Illustration 9-5

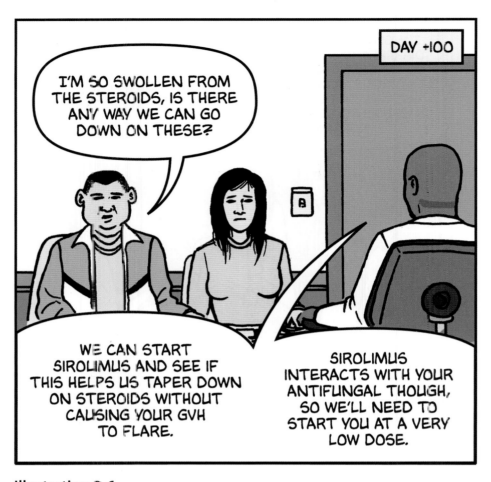

Illustration 9-6

Thoughts on "Compromising"

The illustrated case "Compromising" focuses on acute lympho-blastic leukemia (ALL), which is a type of blood cancer whereby the body produces too many of a certain type of white blood cell (WBC) called a lymphocyte.[32] A healthy immune system fights infections through the activity of different types of WBCs, and each plays a different role in the process: neutrophils, eosino-phils, basophils, lymphocytes, and monocytes (Table 9-2).[1,33] In addition to white blood cells, blood contains red blood cells that carry oxygen and platelets, which form clots to prevent bleed-ing. Most blood cells are produced in the bone marrow, which is a spongy tissue in the hollow center of bones, such as the skull, hips, shoulders, and breastbone.[34] Erik, the main character in the case, develops ALL and undergoes a BMT in an attempt to cure this disease. The important role of an oncology pharma-cist, from educating Erik about his medications to collaborat-ing with his oncologist to maximize the efficacy of medications used and manage their side effects, is highlighted throughout.

As depicted in Illustration 9-1, it may be difficult initially to differentiate symptoms of ALL from those of more common infectious causes, such as influenza. Fatigue, fever, and night sweats are common symptoms of infection, while other symp-toms, such as prolonged nosebleeds, weight loss, bone pain, or painless lumps in the neck, underarm, stomach, or groin, are

frequently seen in leukemia.[32] While not shown, the presence and persistence of these unique symptoms prompted Erik's phy-sician to pursue the cancer workup that led to his ALL diagnosis.

ALL is thought to arise from genetic alterations in the DNA of immature WBCs, which results in uncontrolled WBC growth.[34] Cancer is broadly defined by the uncontrolled replication of cells attributed to genetic alterations that are either inherited or acquired throughout someone's life.[35] Most patients do not have an obvious reason for developing cancer. However, as it relates to ALL, certain factors are known to increase risk, such as pre-vious exposure to chemotherapy or radiation therapy, certain genetic disorders (e.g., Down syndrome), and age (most com-mon in children/adolescents and in adults over 70 years old).[34]

Nearly 6000 new cases of ALL in the United States were expected to occur in 2019.[36] Once considered a fatal diagnosis, medical advances have led to childhood cure rates greater than 90%.[37] Unfortunately, the prognosis for adults is less impressive.[36,38] For younger adults (aged 15 to 39), the cure rate is roughly 70%, and this drops substantially to 10% to 15% in older adults (i.e., 60 years and older). There are multiple reasons for this disparity, includ-ing more aggressive, treatment-resistant disease experienced by older adults, as well as their inability to tolerate intensive treat-ments as well as children and younger adults. In the illustrated

Table 9-2. Types and Functions of White Blood Cells	
Cell Type	**Function**
Neutrophils	One of the first cells to travel to the site of infection. These cells ingest microorganisms and release enzymes[*] to kill them, which also activate other immune cells.
Eosinophils	Contain granules filled with enzymes and signaling molecules[**] that are released during infections, allergic reactions, and asthma.
Basophils	Contain granules filled with enzymes and signaling molecules[**] that are released during allergic reactions and asthma.
T Lymphocytes (T cells)	Part of the body's adaptive immune response,[***] divided into cytotoxic T cells, which directly kill invading pathogens, and helper T cells, which interact with B cells (and others) to enhance the immune response to pathogens.
B Lymphocytes (B cells)	Part of the body's adaptive immune response that produces antibodies[****] following exposure to foreign substances that cause harm, such as bacteria or viruses.
Monocytes	Immune cells that travel through the blood to tissues where they become macrophages, which surround and kill microorganisms, ingest foreign materials, remove dead cells, and boost the immune response.

[*]An enzyme is a protein that speeds up chemical reactions in the body.
[**]Signaling molecules carry information from one cell to another.
[***]Adaptive immunity refers to immune responses that are learned following exposure to harmful foreign substances, called antigens.
[****]Antibodies are immune proteins that bind to a specific foreign substance and attract the immune system to help destroy it. They may be made naturally in the body or manufactured and used as medications.

Table 9-3. Categories and Examples of Medications Commonly Used in Leukemia Treatment and Bone Marrow Transplant		
Category	**Medication Examples[*]**	**Physiologic Effect**
Chemotherapy	■ cyclophosphamide (Cytoxan) ■ cytarabine (ara-C) ■ doxorubicin (Adriamycin) ■ methotrexate ■ vincristine (Oncovin)	Stops the growth of cells by either directly inducing cell death or preventing cells from dividing
Radiation	not applicable	X-rays cause DNA breaks that induce cell death
Targeted therapy	■ inotuzumab ozogamicin (Besponsa)	Chemotherapy toxin attached to an antibody[**] that targets a protein expressed on cancer cells. Once the antibody interacts with the targeted cell, the chemotherapy is released into the cancer cell, killing it.
	■ dasatinib (Sprycel) ■ imatinib (Gleevec)	Targets a single protein that drives cell growth in a special type of leukemia. This prevents cancer replication and induces cell death, without many of the adverse effects of cytotoxic chemotherapy.
Immunotherapy	■ blinatumomab (Blincyto)	Antibody[**] that brings together T cells and cancer cells by binding a specific protein located on each type of cell, leading to immune destruction of the cancer cells.
	■ axicabtagene ciloleucel (Yescarta) ■ tisagenelecleucel (Kymriah)	T cells are removed from a patient, then have a receptor attached to them that targets a specific protein on cancer cells, and then are infused back into the patient where they multiply, seek out, and destroy cancer cells.

[*]Medication examples presented in alphabetical order as "generic name (Brand Name)."
[**]Antibodies are immune proteins that bind to a specific foreign substance and attract the immune system to help destroy it. They may be made naturally in the body or manufactured and used as medications.

case "Compromising," Erik is depicted as a college-aged young adult able to tolerate an intensive approach to treatment, which is what he receives beginning with Illustration 9-2.

In terms of treatment, ALL is targeted through a variety of different methods, including chemotherapy, radiation, targeted therapy, and immunotherapy (summarized in Table 9-3).[32] Chemotherapy is one of the most common approaches. This is a broad term that refers to the use of medications to slow or stop the replication of cells, commonly through effects on DNA and chromosomes.[39] This is also referred to as cytotoxic chemotherapy; cyto- meaning "cellular," -toxic meaning "damaging."

Cytotoxic chemotherapies target cells that are replicating, and cancerous cells replicate at a faster rate than healthy ones.[40] As a result, chemotherapy causes greater toxicity to cancerous cells than healthy ones. That said, healthy cells are also damaged, especially ones that replicate frequently; examples include hair follicles and cells in the oral cavity, gastrointestinal (GI) tract, and, importantly, the bone marrow. As a result, the most common side effects of chemotherapy are hair loss, mouth sores, loss of appetite, nausea, vomiting, and diarrhea.[32] The most common

dose-limiting toxicity (i.e., a side effect that leads to medications being reduced or stopped) of cytotoxic chemotherapy originates from suppression of the bone marrow, where decreased WBCs make patients more prone to serious infections and decreased platelets put patients at risk for bleeding. There are many different chemotherapy agents available that have varying activities in different cancers. Oncology pharmacists contribute to the interprofessional care of patients with cancer through expert knowledge of how to manage these medications.

In addition to cytotoxic medications, a multitude of novel, biologic therapies with unique mechanisms of action are emerging.[32] Biologic therapies work by manipulating the tumor environment and the patient's immune system to favor tumor destruction.[39] They may consist of antibodies that deliver toxins specifically to cancer cells (see Targeted therapy in Table 9-3) or block the ability of cancer cells to hide from the immune system (see Immunotherapy in Table 9-3).

Chimeric antigen receptor (CAR) T-cell directed therapy is one of the most exciting examples of novel biologic approaches.[41] In CAR-T therapy, a patient's own T cells are removed from his/her body, genetically modified in a lab to recognize and attack cancerous cells, then re-inserted into the body. Once re-inserted, the modified T cells replicate in the bone marrow, then attack and kill the cancerous cells. Early clinical trials of CAR-T therapy in patients whose cancers relapsed (i.e., returned) or proved refractory (i.e., resistant) to traditional treatments have shown impressive results.[42,43] In one study, response rates nearly doubled compared to standard therapy.[42] Importantly, the ongoing replication of the CAR-T cells can provide immune surveillance against cancer relapse in the future, much like antibodies produced during a viral illness provide protection if re-exposed at a future point in time.[43] Erik would likely be a candidate for CAR-T therapy should his cancer relapse following BMT.

For certain patients with high-risk leukemia, like Erik, replacing cancerous WBCs with those from a healthy donor, also known as allogeneic BMT, may be considered.[44] This type of transplant relies upon the restoration of an intact, healthy immune system to provide ongoing anticancer effects. A donor must first be found by comparing immune markers on the patient's WBCs with those of potential candidates. Donors may be related, like Erik's brother (Illustration 9-3), or unrelated. Unrelated donors are identified from national databases, such as the National Marrow Donor Program.[45] The more closely matched the donor's WBCs are to the patient's, the greater the likelihood of long-term success.[46] The type of donor used, including how closely matched their WBCs are, is often determined by donor availability, urgency of transplant, and the patient's disease status.[47]

BMT begins with a conditioning, or preparative, chemotherapy regimen. This is depicted in Illustration 9-3. The conditioning regimen is administered in the days immediately prior to the stem cell infusion, and typically consists of chemotherapy with or without the addition of radiation.[44] The purpose is to suppress the patient's immune system to make room for the donor cells, and to provide anticancer effects. Notice that the time stamp in Illustration 9-3 reads "Day -5." This indicates that the conditioning regimen for Erik is starting 5 days before his BMT. Subsequent time stamps use the "+" symbol to indicate the number of days after, or post-transplant.

Conditioning regimens vary in intensity and medications used.[48] As depicted in Illustration 9-3, Erik is scheduled to receive a myeloablative regimen, which is a high-dose, high-intensity regimen designed to kill healthy and diseased bone marrow cells alike. The rationale behind myeloablative conditioning is that wiping the bone marrow of all cells provides the best opportunity for donor cells to take root in the bone marrow, or engraft. These regimens are typically preferred for younger patients, who tend to tolerate the harsh side effects better than older adults. Reduced-intensity and nonmyeloablative regimens (i.e., where bone marrow cells are not completely depleted) have been developed to decrease the number of deaths associated with myeloablative conditioning. This has allowed for the broadening of the transplant recipient pool to older adults or those whose health is complicated by multiple comorbidities, or health conditions.

Engraftment takes place when donor stem cells have migrated to the host's bone marrow and begin producing new blood cells.[49] This typically occurs within the first 30 days after transplant, and represents the highest risk period of the transplant. During the time between conditioning and engraftment, a patient's blood cell counts drop to dangerously low levels, which puts them at risk for a variety of life-threatening complications; for example, anemia (red blood cells), bleeding (platelets), and infections (WBCs). As a result, BMT patients may require transfusions of red blood cells and platelets, as well as various anti-infective agents.[50]

Infections associated with transplant represent a major complication due to patients' impaired immune function both before and after engraftment.[44] The major culprits are from bacterial, viral, and fungal sources. Prophylactic therapies, where anti-infective medications are given before known BMT-associated infections take place, are routinely used to prevent bacterial infections, herpes virus infections, yeast infections, and a specific type of fungal-like pneumonia called *Pneumocystis* from occurring. Even despite these preventive therapies, infections are still the leading cause of non-relapse death after transplant.[44] Oncology pharmacists and infectious diseases pharmacists play a critical role reducing the likelihood of poor outcomes tied to infections. Those interested in the role of infectious diseases pharmacists are encouraged to explore Chapter 8 Infectious Diseases for more information.

One infection that frequently affects BMT patients, depicted in Illustration 9-4, is *Clostridioides difficile,* or *C. diff* for short.[51] Traditional risk factors for *C. diff* infection include a compromised immune system, older age, and antibiotic exposure. BMT patients commonly have all three of these risk factors; not surprisingly, studies have shown that as many as one in four BMT patients experience this infection.[51] *C. diff* is an infection of the GI tract that typically manifests as watery diarrhea multiple times a day. Anti-infective treatment is effective; however, recurrence has been documented to be as high as 20%. Pharmacists provide assistance with medication selection, dosing, and monitoring in this setting. Additional support provided by pharmacists include assistance with medication access. While not explicitly stated in Illustration 9-4, Erik was given fidaxomicin (Dificid) for this infection because he could not tolerate other, more commonly used oral antibiotics for *C. diff*. In preparation for leaving the hospital, the oncology team would have needed to ensure he could complete the course of fidaxomicin treatment at home. A 10-day course of fidaxomicin tablets is estimated to cost nearly $1800.[52] Oncology pharmacists frequently work with patients, insurance companies, pharmacy benefit management companies, and other health professionals to help patients obtain needed medications. For a more in-depth exploration of *C. diff*, see the illustrated case "Superinfection" in Chapter 8 Infectious Diseases. Those interested in medication access issues are encouraged to read the illustrated case "Holistic" in Chapter 3 Primary Care.

Another major complication for patients following transplant is graft versus host disease (GVHD). GVHD occurs when the immune cells of the donor react against host (or recipient) cells.[44] It is typically classified as either acute or chronic based on onset and duration of symptoms, with day +100 as the cut-off. Beyond timing, acute GVHD is also characterized by symptoms that affect the skin, GI tract, and liver. Illustration 9-5 shows Erik, at day +30, experiencing acute GVHD via severe upper GI symptoms (i.e., vomiting). What is not shown, but is also part of Erik's story, is that he is also experiencing lower GI symptoms at the same time in the form of profuse diarrhea. Confirmation that these lower GI symptoms were not due to a recurrence of *C. diff* (i.e., that the fidaxomicin eliminated the *C. diff* infection) also informed the acute GVHD diagnosis.

Early trials of allogeneic BMT were complicated by severe and life-threatening acute GVHD.[53] Advances have been made over the last several decades to prevent acute GVHD and minimize complications when it does occur. Nearly all BMT medication regimens now contain some form of GVHD prophylaxis.[53] One approach, first highlighted in Illustration 9-3, includes the use of high-dose cyclophosphamide as the backbone of acute GVHD prophylaxis, in combination with other immunosuppressive medications. Cyclophosphamide selectively destroys GVHD-causing immune cells while sparing other immune cells that aid in GVHD prevention.[54]

Chronic GVHD can affect a wider array of organs including the eyes, mouth, lungs, musculoskeletal, and genitourinary systems, in addition to those affected by acute GVHD.[55] On a cellular level, chronic GVHD is frequently associated with tissue scarring and inflammation leading to impaired organ function. This may manifest as limitations in joint motion, severe dry eyes, lichen-like plaques on the skin, or disruption of lung function. Some features resemble certain autoimmune diseases. Once chronic GVHD is diagnosed, patients frequently deal with the symptoms for years, and possibly for the rest of their lives. Unfortunately for Erik, as demonstrated in Illustration 9-6, his GVHD has continued to flare despite initial treatment, and is now transforming into chronic GVHD, indicating a poor prognosis for full recovery and likely years of immunosuppressive treatment to manage symptoms.[56]

For both acute and chronic GVHD, first-line treatment involves corticosteroids.[44] These medications slow the immune response of donor cells against the host. The goal is to alleviate symptoms by stopping donor immune cells from destroying healthy host cells. When used at high doses for prolonged periods of time, which is often required to bring GVHD under control, corticosteroids can have a wide array of undesired side effects.[57] Side effects that significantly affect patients include weight gain and fluid retention in their face, upper back, hands, and feet (Illustration 9-6). Other common side effects include anxiety, irritability, muscle wasting, high blood pressure, elevated blood sugar, and bone weakening. Perhaps the most dangerous corticosteroid-associated side effect involves increased vulnerability to certain fungal infections, which can become life-threatening.[58]

Illustrations 9-5 and 9-6 demonstrate the vital role pharmacists play helping to manage and/or prevent these side effects. The ultimate goal as it relates to GVHD is to withdraw immune suppression (i.e., stop the use of corticosteroids).[55] This may be accomplished via a slow corticosteroid taper or by leveraging

DISCUSSION QUESTIONS FOR "COMPROMISING"

1. In Illustration 9-2, Erik expresses concern over nausea as a potential side effect of chemotherapy. What other aspects related to chemotherapy do you think the pharmacist should counsel Erik on at this point in time?

2. Oncology pharmacists often interact with patients after an initial diagnosis or a change in treatment, as depicted in Illustrations 9-2 and 9-4. What concerns might the patient have in situations like these? How might oncology pharmacists alleviate some of these concerns?

3. Side effects of chemotherapy and steroids that impact a patient's physical appearance can be seen in Illustrations 9-4 and 9-6. Focusing on changes to/impact on physical appearance, what are some ways oncology pharmacists might help patients work through these side effects?

4. Beyond physically, in what ways might a cancer diagnosis impact a person's self-image? If not related to medications, do you think it would be appropriate for the oncology pharmacist to engage with the patient around such concerns?

5. The illustrated case "Compromising" demonstrates the necessity of interprofessional teamwork, but focuses almost exclusively on collaboration between pharmacists and physicians. What other types of health professionals can you think of who were likely involved in Erik's care? In what ways would they have contributed? And in what ways might they have collaborated with the oncology pharmacist?

other immunosuppressive medications, such as sirolimus (Illustration 9-6). Oftentimes a switch like this involves trading one set of problems for another, such as known drug interactions with essential anti-infectives.[53] Due to the complexities of medications used for GVHD, and the fact that they impact other medications critical to successful BMT, oncology pharmacists play a vital role in this interprofessional practice setting.

A cancer diagnosis is a life-changing event. Beyond the existential crisis created by the threat of losing one's life, anxieties associated with anticipating known treatment-related side effects, like nausea, vomiting, and hair loss, can be debilitating. In acute lymphoblastic leukemia, some patients must also face the daunting prospect of a bone marrow transplant. This involves having to cope with unique complications and medication-related side effects. Oncology pharmacists play a pivotal role helping patients and other health professionals navigate medication-related issues. This involves optimizing medication efficacy through correct medication dosing, as well as monitoring and troubleshooting toxicities associated with treatment. Though few patients have a perfect outcome, through their knowledge, expertise, and compassion, oncology pharmacists work hard to give patients the best possible chance at one.

COMPASSION: An Illustrated Case Study

Story by Paul R. Hutson & Joseph A. Zorek
Illustrations by George Folz, © 2019 Board of Regents of the University of Wisconsin System

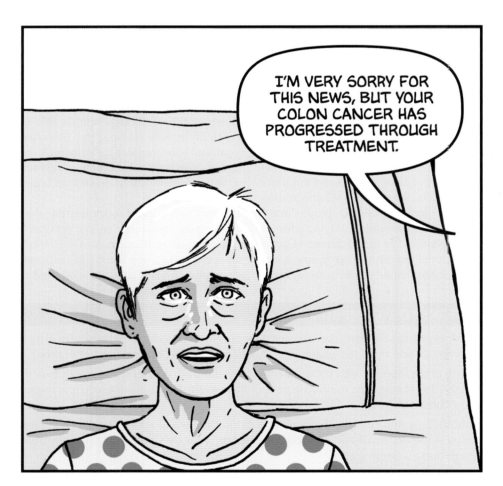

Illustration 9-7

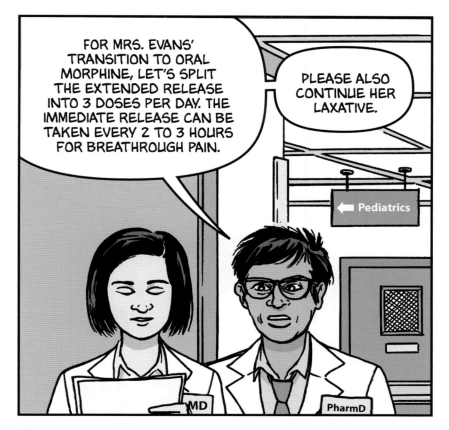

Illustration 9-8

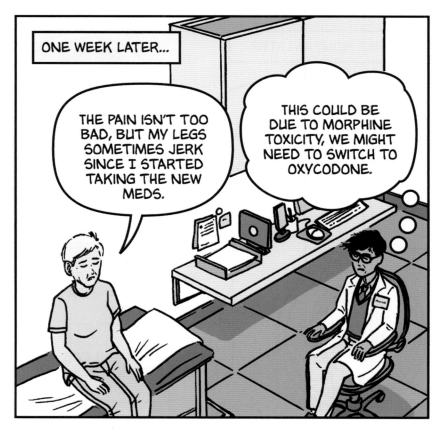

Illustration 9-9

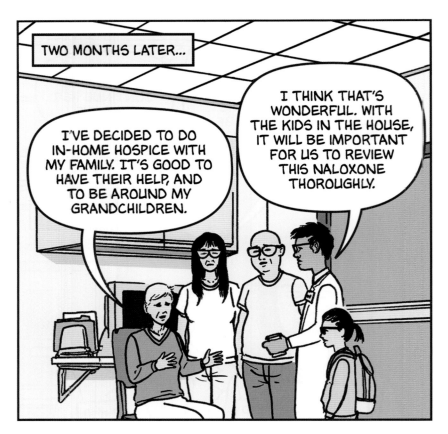

Illustration 9-10

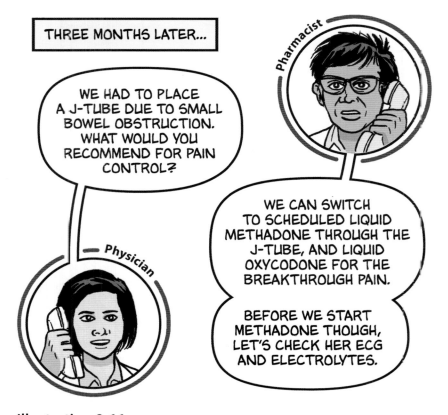

Illustration 9-11

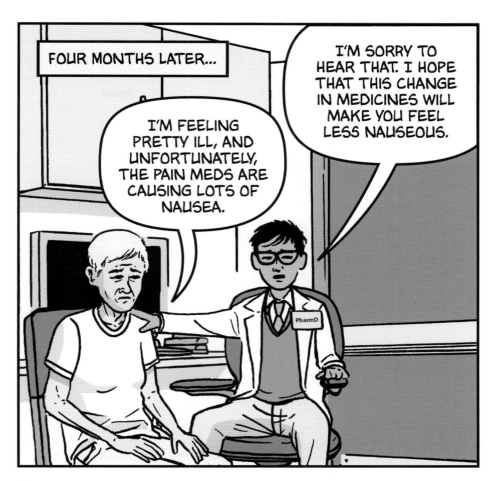

Illustration 9-12

Thoughts on "Compassion"

Perhaps no health professionals will walk alongside a patient with cancer longer than their pharmacists. The illustrated case "Compassion," for example, begins in the middle of this patient's journey, and the backstory that led to the unfortunate news she receives in Illustration 9-7 is unclear. Based on typical early signs and symptoms of colon cancer, however, such as diarrhea, constipation, and abdominal discomfort, it is quite easy to imagine her journey beginning inside a community pharmacy long before Illustration 9-7.[59] Assisting patients with gastrointestinal issues is a hallmark of community pharmacy practice, as evidenced by sales of associated over-the-counter medications.[60] It is equally easy to imagine the failure of over-the-counter remedies prompting the community pharmacist to recommend a medical consultation that would have led to the initial colon cancer diagnosis. Readers interested in learning more about community pharmacy are encouraged to visit Chapter 2 Community Pharmacy and the illustrated cases "Organized Chaos," "Transformation," and "Breathe."

Once diagnosed, an oncology pharmacist, like the one featured in "Compassion," would engage with other members of the interprofessional team to optimize use of chemotherapeutic medications targeting tumor cells, as well as adjunctive medications employed to support the patient's care (i.e., to control pain, relieve constipation, etc.). The community pharmacist, meanwhile, would continue to support the patient by filling prescriptions and providing counseling and advice to augment efforts of the interprofessional oncology team. Unfortunately, as depicted in "Compassion," many cancers prove resistant to available treatments, and planning for the end of life must begin. When this occurs, patients typically transition to palliative care, where more aggressive treatments to control pain and other symptoms are deployed in an attempt to make patients as comfortable as possible for their remaining time. The oncology pharmacist and community pharmacist would remain actively engaged with the patient during this phase as well, effectively closing the loop of pharmacist-provided care that began with the patient's initial gastrointestinal complaints.

Pharmacists engaged in the care of patients with cancer require knowledge and skills that stretch beyond the safe and effective use of medications. They must demonstrate an understanding of the emotional aspects associated with cancer and an ability to connect with patients on a human level throughout various phases of their care; for example, through empathy, sympathy, and compassion.[61,62] Empathy can be a shared sense of pain or distress, sometimes felt viscerally. One might anticipate how they might feel, for example, if they had severe nausea from disease or the side effect of a drug. Sympathy is an understanding of the distress that an individual is experiencing. This may be physical pain, or it may be the distress of facing advancing disease. Compassion builds upon empathetic and sympathetic responses, and is characterized by an individual's efforts to identify ways in which suffering and distress can be named, mitigated, and resolved. A pharmacist operating on this level might ask, "How are you handling your diagnosis and treatment?" or "What can I do to help?"

Simple demonstrations of empathy, sympathy, and compassion have been shown to produce therapeutic relief; for example, by setting aside other tasks for a moment to intentionally listen to, and engage with, a patient or caregiver.[53] Personal interactions like these are important to the patient-pharmacist relationship, and ensuring privacy is critical. Attempts to discuss intimate health details can be awkward in public spaces, such as the traditional pharmacy counter (see the illustrated case "Barriers" in Chapter 12 Mental Health for an example), and are better suited for consultation rooms such as those depicted in Illustrations 9-10 and 9-12 (see the illustrated case "Breathe" in Chapter 2 Community Pharmacy for another good example).

Illustration 9-7 opens with bad news from an unidentified clinician, presumably the oncologist leading the interprofessional team. The patient's colon cancer has progressed through treatment and her prognosis (i.e., most likely outcome), implied by her tears, is poor. It can be assumed from Illustration 9-7 that the patient's new diagnosis is metastatic colon cancer. The term *metastatic* means that the tumor has metastasized, or spread, from the primary (i.e., original) site to a distant location in the body. Unfortunately, for most cancers, metastasis likely means that the cancer is incurable. Later reference to in-home hospice confirms this situation.

As tumors invade healthy tissue, it is not uncommon for severe pain to develop. Much of the oncology pharmacist's interventions in "Compassion" revolve around pain control and mitigation of side effects associated with pain medications. Table 9-4 lists medications in alphabetical order by category that are commonly used in the setting of cancer-associated pain control, along with their physiologic effect.[64–66]

Much attention in recent years has been directed toward the overuse and abuse of opioids.[67,68] Readers are encouraged to explore the illustrated case "Gasping" in Chapter 12 Mental Health for an in-depth review of this topic. While the malicious and deliberate over-prescribing of opioids for profit has been well-documented, other, less nefarious factors, also contributed.[69] The pursuit of high patient satisfaction scores through pain relief is one such factor. In the late 1990s, for example, there was an emphasis in healthcare on assessing pain severity to the extent that a pain rating was referred to as the "5th vital sign," with hospital accreditation (and funding) requiring pain treatment similar to heart rate, blood pressure, respiratory

Table 9-4. Categories and Examples of Medications Commonly Used to Control Cancer-Related Pain in Palliative Care

Category	Medication Examples*	Physiologic Effect
Analgesics	- acetaminophen (Tylenol)	Decrease synthesis of prostaglandin, a pain signaling molecule, in the brain and spinal cord, impairing transmission of pain signals
Antidepressants	- amitriptyline (Elavil) - doxepin (Silenor) - duloxetine (Cymbalta) - venlafaxine (Effexor)	Increase the availability of certain signaling molecules (serotonin and/or norepinephrine) along nerve cells, resulting in decreased pain transmission
GABA analog, calcium channel blockers	- gabapentin (Neurontin) - pregabalin (Lyrica)	Decrease the activation of calcium channels leading to decreased transmission and perception of pain along nerve cells
NMDA receptor antagonists	- ketamine (Ketalar)	Block the action of signaling molecules at the NMDA receptor, decreasing pain transmission and perception
Non-steroidal anti-inflammatory drugs (NSAID)	- celecoxib (Celebrex) - diclofenac (Voltaren) - ibuprofen (Advil, Motrin) - ketorolac (Torado) - nabumetone (Relafen) - naproxen (Aleve, Naprosyn)	Decrease prostaglandin synthesis in the body, brain, and spinal cord, impairing transmission of pain signals. Also work outside of the brain and spinal cord to decrease inflammation at areas of injury that would otherwise sensitize nerves and amplify that level of perceived pain.
Opioids	- fentanyl (Duragesic) - hydrocodone (Vicodin, Norco)** - hydromorphone (Dilaudid) - methadone (Dolophine) - morphine (MS Contin) - oxycodone (OxyContin) - oxymorphone (Opana)	Bind to mu-opioid receptors in the brain and spinal cord to impair the transmission of pain impulses.
Sodium channel inhibitor anesthetics	- lidocaine (Lidoderm) - mexiletine (Mexitil)	Decrease the ability of pain impulses to be propagated by impairing nerve cell signaling

*Medication examples presented in alphabetical order as "generic name (Brand Name)."

**Vicodin and Norco are combination products with acetaminophen.

rate, and body temperature.[70] Though the method of pain treatment was not mandated, hospitals loosened opioid prescribing restrictions in order to meet accreditation standards, leading to significant increases in opioid prescribing.[71]

Large studies of patients suffering from common musculoskeletal pain (e.g., lower back pain, nerve pain) have shown that strong opioids do not provide a significant, long-term benefit.[72] Nevertheless, the majority of opioids are prescribed for such non-cancer pain.[73,74] Regardless of the purpose for which an opioid is prescribed, after 2 weeks of regular use the patient can be assumed to be physically dependent on opioids.[75] This does not necessarily mean that the patient is addicted, but rather that suddenly stopping opioids after this point will likely lead to a characteristic, unpleasant, and sometimes debilitating withdrawal syndrome.[76] An analogous, albeit much less severe, dependence can be seen in coffee drinkers who commonly develop a headache after a day of abstinence from caffeine.[77] Fear of, and aversion to, opioid withdrawal syndrome is thought to play a role in the inappropriate, chronic use of opioids.[76] It is also the basis for arguments that opioid use should be limited to as short a course as possible. Concerns of overuse of opioids in the general population, as well as increasing barriers to their use, have created challenges for the rational, appropriate, and justifiable use of opioids in the setting of palliative care, as well as for patients who suffer from other chronic pain syndromes.[78,79]

Opioid use in the palliative care setting is typically started on an as needed basis within set parameters; for example, to be taken every 4 to 6 hours, but only if pain is present and bothersome.[76] As needed dosing is used to determine how much drug is required to effectively control a patient's pain. If the need for the opioid is consistent, it is best to schedule the opioid; in other words, administer it every day at the same time or times, depending on the medication and the patient's needs. Drug formulations that release the medication over an extended period of time (e.g., over the course of 8 to 24 hours) are often used in this manner. As shown in Illustration 9-8, even with a scheduled opioid, such as morphine, it is routine for a separate, rapidly absorbed formulation to be available for the patient to use for breakthrough pain. Typically, the dose of opioid used for breakthrough pain is 10% to 20% of the daily dose of the scheduled opioid, and is made available to the patient on an as needed basis every 2 to 3 hours.[76,80] Effective education of the patient and caregiver is needed to help titrate the use of opioids and to make sure that the doses given as needed are not confused with those taken routinely on a scheduled basis.

Constipation is a common side effect of opioid therapy that affects a majority of cancer patients prescribed opioids, and may cause significant discomfort as well as negative impact on quality of life.[81] For this reason, laxatives are routinely recommended in patients starting opioid therapy to prevent this side effect.[82] The pharmacist's role in preventing opioid side effects, such as constipation, is demonstrated in Illustration 9-8. In patients for whom routine laxative use is not adequate to prevent constipation, pharmacists help patients by tailoring bowel regimens to their specific needs.

Illustration 9-9 shows the pharmacist assessing the adequacy of the patient's pain control, as well as side effects associated with her use of morphine. While pain control is good, the patient is complaining of muscle jerking. The pharmacist recognizes this as a side effect of morphine that has been documented in patients with decreased kidney function.[83] Muscle jerking, or twitching, has been attributed to the accumulation of a morphine metabolite called morphine-3-glucuronide (M3G). Morphine is broken down (i.e., metabolized) in the liver into metabolites, of which M3G is one. Most metabolites of morphine are eliminated from the body through urine produced by the kidneys. If a patient's kidneys are not functioning normally, or as efficiently as they should, metabolites like M3G can build up in the body.[83] In addition to muscle jerking, accumulation of M3G has been associated with delirium, bad dreams, and even hallucinations.[84] When M3G accumulation is suspected, a switch to a different opioid is advised. Several options are available, and oxycodone is a common choice with both sustained- and immediate-release formulations available. Pharmacists are frequently called upon to assist prescribers in converting from one opioid to another. Multiple factors need to be considered, including the condition of the patient's kidneys and liver, body size, current opioid dose and duration of use, and the concurrent use of drugs that may interact with the old or new opioid.[85]

After the passage of several months, it is revealed in Illustration 9-10 that the patient has decided to enroll in hospice care as her disease has progressed. Hospice care is home- or facility-based care focused on the management of symptoms in patients who are considered to have a life-limiting illness, and for whom life-prolonging treatments are usually discontinued.[86] Patients are eligible for hospice benefits if, based on a physician's judgement, their remaining survival is likely to be 6 months or less. While chemotherapy is stopped for hospice patients, they continue to receive palliative care. Broadly speaking, this refers to treatments that are intended to alleviate pain, maximize comfort, or otherwise improve the quality of the patient's remaining time. This can vary from patient to patient based upon his or her specific characteristics and values. For example, in two patients being treated for the same bloodstream infection, one patient may opt to continue anti-infective treatment in order to spend a few more days with loved ones, while the other patient may stop anti-infective therapy due to the nausea it causes, and instead focus on comfort therapies such as pain and nausea relief. Pharmacists play a vital role in identifying what medications can assist patients in meeting their goals, and how those medications can be administered. In addition to making patients more comfortable, patients with advanced cancer who received palliative care in some cases survived as long or longer than patients who continued to receive aggressive treatments.[87–89]

Patients can receive hospice care at home, as the patient in "Compassion" has elected to do, or in a number of institutionalized settings, such as long-term care or dedicated hospice facilities. Pharmacists are valued members of palliative care teams in hospice settings, and studies have shown that their inclusion leads to improved symptom management and reduced costs.[90–92] For care-continuity purposes, hospice patients will often continue receiving care from the same interprofessional oncology team, as evidenced in Illustrations 9-10 through 9-12. As the patient's symptoms and needs progress, so too do medication-related interventions from the oncology pharmacist.

Noting a change in the patient's living situation, and undoubtedly in preparation for expected increases in opioid doses as the patient's cancer progresses, the oncology pharmacist advocates for adding naloxone (Narcan) to the patient's medication list. Illustration 9-10 shows him preparing to educate the patient and her family on its use, which is intended to quickly reverse opioid toxicity/overdose symptoms. This is particularly important in a household with children, as analgesic medications are a common cause of accidental ingestions leading to poison control calls and emergency department visits.[93,94] Pharmacists train patients and caregivers how to recognize opioid overdose symptoms and administer naloxone when necessary. For more information on opioid overdose and naloxone, see the illustrated case "Gasping" in Chapter 12 Mental Health. Readers interested in learning more about accidental ingestions of medications are encouraged to explore the illustrated case "Accidental" in Chapter 6 Pediatrics.

In Illustration 9-11, the physician and pharmacist discuss pain control options following a further deterioration of Mrs. Evans' condition. One of several tumors in the patient's abdomen has grown around part of her small intestine, causing an obstruction in the normal flow of stomach contents and necessitating the insertion of a jejunostomy tube (J-tube) for feeding and medication administration. The J-tube is inserted through the skin of the abdomen directly into the jejunum (i.e., a specific segment of the small intestine), bypassing the obstruction. In these situations, pharmacists play an important role on the interprofessional team assisting with medication changes to ensure the effectiveness and compatibility of medications administered through the J-tube, and to avoid common errors associated with these changes.[95] For example, some orally administered drugs can be crushed or their contents opened, suspended or dissolved in water, and injected into the gut through such tubes. However, an increasing number of oral medications are formulated in such a way that they cannot be crushed for administration in this manner.[96]

To accommodate J-tube administration of medications, the pharmacist in Illustration 9-11 recommends replacing the patient's scheduled, extended-release oxycodone with liquid methadone. This circumvents the potentially life-threatening mistake of crushing and administering extended-release oxycodone, which could result in the medication being released at once, rather than over a 12-hour span, leading to an overdose. Methadone, in addition to its availability as an oral liquid, has additional benefits of use for pain control in this patient which include its low cost, effectiveness for neuropathic as well as somatic (i.e., musculoskeletal) pain, and the long elimination half-life that permits scheduled 8-hour dosing even for the oral liquid formulation.[97,98] Neuropathic pain arises from nerve damage or chronic, poorly treated somatic pain, and tends to be resistant to treatment with typical opioids.[99] In addition to methadone, other drugs such as ketamine, gabapentin, lidocaine, or duloxetine can be tried and combined to treat neuropathic pain (see Table 9-4).

There are important considerations associated with methadone use, including the frequency with which its dose can be adjusted, a variable conversion ratio between methadone and other opioids, and potentially serious adverse effects, such as changes in heart rhythm.[97] The pharmacist recommends obtaining a baseline electrocardiogram (ECG) prior to the switch to methadone for this reason. By doing so, the interprofessional team will be able to compare results of future ECGs with the baseline results and, importantly, allow therapies to be modified. For the same purpose, the pharmacist also recommends measuring levels of electrolytes (e.g., potassium, magnesium) because electrolyte abnormalities can also lead to heart rhythm abnormalities.[100]

The illustrated case "Compassion" closes in Illustration 9-12, where the patient's progressive physical deterioration is apparent. Based on the course of her disease, the patient's remaining time is likely limited. Knowing this, and in keeping with the compassionate approach to care that he and other members of the interprofessional team have demonstrated, the oncology pharmacist continues to search for ways to alleviate Mrs. Evans' pain and discomfort. It is unclear what change in medication has been made; perhaps a tweak to the opioid dose, perhaps the addition of an anti-nausea medication. The most important intervention at this point is not about medication therapy, but human connection, and it calls upon the pharmacist to be empathetic, sympathetic, and compassionate.

DISCUSSION QUESTIONS FOR "COMPASSION"

1. Have you ever experienced the loss of a family member or friend? If so, what lessons from this experience might shape your future career as a health professional?

2. Think about two to three individuals from your life you would consider to be compassionate. What makes them stand out in your mind? What can you learn from them that might help you demonstrate compassion in your future career?

3. What are some concerns a patient with cancer-related pain might express about taking opioid pain medications such as morphine? How would you address these concerns? How would you react if a patient with cancer experiencing severe pain refused to take an opioid for relief?

4. Family members are often heavily involved in the care of patients with cancer, including helping to manage medications. What challenges might caregivers experience in this role, and how can pharmacists help?

5. In the illustrated case "Compassion," as the patient's condition worsened and her needs increased, she moved in with her daughter, son-in-law, and grandchildren for help. What steps do you think the family could/should take to prevent opioids or other strong pain medications from being diverted (i.e., stolen)?

CHAPTER SUMMARY

- Chemotherapy order review is a vital safety process entrusted to pharmacists.

- The complicated nature of oncology care requires close collaboration with a multitude of health professionals, including physicians, nurses, nurse practitioners, physician assistants, social workers, and dietitians/nutritionists.

- Direct patient care provided by pharmacists frequently involves education, drug interaction monitoring, dosing recommendations, symptom management, and prophylactic therapy recommendations.

- Oncology pharmacists may practice in a wide variety of settings, including hospitals, clinics, infusion centers, and specialty pharmacies.

- Multiple opportunities are available for advanced training in oncology pharmacy including residencies, fellowships, and the opportunity to pursue board certification.

- Patients with leukemia face a barrage of potential complications and difficulties associated with their treatment. Oncology pharmacists use their knowledge of cancer treatment and patient characteristics to personalize treatment in order to maximize patient well-being and quality of life.

- Pharmacist engagement in palliative care demonstrates the importance of pharmacists forming personal relationships with patients, and the many ways pharmacists' medication expertise can provide comfort and relief to patients.

REFERENCES

1. National Cancer Institute. NCI dictionary of cancer terms. Available at https://www.cancer.gov/publications/dictionaries/cancer-terms/. Accessed May 31, 2020.

2. National Cancer Institute. Common cancer sites—cancer stat facts. Available at https://seer.cancer.gov/statfacts/html/common.html. Accessed May 31, 2020.

3. American Society of Clinical Oncology. The oncology team. Available at https://www.cancer.net/navigating-cancer-care/cancer-basics/cancer-care-team/oncology-team. Accessed May 31, 2020.

4. Further defining the scope of Hematology/Oncology Pharmacy Association. Available at http://www.hoparx.org/images/hopa/resource-library/guidelines-standards/HOPA18_Scope-2_Web2.pdf. Accessed May 31, 2020.

5. Crandell BC, Bates JS, Grgic T. Start using a checklist, PRONTO: recommendation for a standard review process for chemotherapy orders. *J Oncol Pharm Pract.* 2018;24(8):609-616.

6. Goldspiel B, Hoffman JM, Griffith NL, et al. ASHP guidelines on preventing medication errors with chemotherapy and biotherapy. *Am J Health Syst Pharm.* 2015;72(8):e6-e35.

7. Neuss MN, Gilmore TR, Belderson KM, et al. 2016 updated American Society of Clinical Oncology/Oncology Nursing Society chemotherapy administration safety standards, including standards for pediatric oncology. *J Oncol Pract.* 2016;12(12):1262-1271.

8. Ishii K, Morii N, Yamashiro H. Pertuzumab in the treatment of HER2-positive breast cancer: an evidence-based review of its safety, efficacy, and place in therapy. *Core Evid.* 2019;14:51-70.

9. Crona DJ, Faso A, Nishijima TF, McGraw KA, Galsky MD, Milowsky MI. A systematic review of strategies to prevent cisplatin-induced nephrotoxicity. *Oncologist.* 2017;22(5):609-619.

10. Smith TJ, Bohlke K, Lyman GH, et al. Recommendations for the use of WBC growth factors: American Society of Clinical Oncology clinical practice guideline update. *J Clin Oncol.* 2015;33(28):3199-3212.

11. Taplitz RA, Kennedy EB, Bow EJ, et al. Antimicrobial prophylaxis for adult patients with cancer-related immunosuppression: ASCO and IDSA clinical practice guideline update. *J Clin Oncol.* 2018;36(30):3043-3054.

12. Barbour M. Role of pharmacists in the management of chemotherapy-induced nausea and vomiting. Available at http://jhoponline.com/jhop-issue-archive/2019-issues/jhop-june-2019-vol-9-no-2/17788-role-of-pharmacists-in-the-management-of-chemotherapy-induced-nausea-and-vomiting. Accessed May 31, 2020.

13. Navari RM, Qin R, Ruddy KJ, et al. Olanzapine for the prevention of chemotherapy-induced nausea and vomiting. *N Engl J Med.* 2016;375(2):134-142.

14. Clemmons AB, Orr J, Andrick B, Gandhi A, Sportes C, DeRemer D. Randomized, placebo-controlled, phase III trial of fosaprepitant, ondansetron, dexamethasone (FOND) versus FOND plus olanzapine (FOND-O) for the prevention of chemotherapy-induced nausea and vomiting in patients with hematologic malignancies receiving highly emetogenic chemotherapy and hematopoietic cell transplantation regimens: the FOND-O trial. *Biol Blood Marrow Transplant.* 2018;24(10):2065-2071.

15. Hesketh PJ, Kris MG, Basch E, et al. Antiemetics: American Society of Clinical Oncology clinical practice guideline update. *J Clin Oncol.* 2017;35(28):3240-3261.

16. Jackson K, Letton C, Maldonado A, et al. A pilot study to assess the pharmacy impact of implementing a chemotherapy-induced nausea or vomiting collaborative disease therapy management in the outpatient oncology clinics. *J Oncol Pharm Pract.* 2019;25(4):847-854.

17. Mackler E, Segal EM, Muluneh B, Jeffers K, Carmichael J. 2018 Hematology/Oncology Pharmacist Association best practices for the management of oral oncolytic therapy: pharmacy practice standard. *J Oncol Pract.* 2019;15(4):e346-e355.

18. Battis B, Clifford L, Huq M, Pejoro E, Mambourg S. The impacts of a pharmacist-managed outpatient clinic and chemotherapy-directed electronic order sets for monitoring oral chemotherapy. *J Oncol Pharm Pract.* 2017;23(8):582-590.

19. Clemmons AB, Alexander M, DeGregory K, Kennedy L. The hematopoietic cell transplant pharmacist: roles, responsibilities, and recommendations from the ASBMT pharmacy special interest group. *Biol Blood Marrow Transplant.* 2018;24(5):914-922.

20. Langebrake C, Admiraal R, van Maarseveen E, Bonnin A, Bauters T. Consensus recommendations for the role and competencies of the EBMT clinical pharmacist and clinical pharmacologist involved in hematopoietic stem cell transplantation. *Bone Marrow Transplant.* 2020;55(1):62-69.

21. Sweiss K, Wirth SM, Sharp L, et al. Collaborative physician-pharmacist-managed multiple myeloma clinic improves guideline adherence and prevents treatment delays. *J Oncol Pract.* 2018;14(11):e674-e682.

22. Mulkerin DL, Bergsbaken JJ, Fischer JA, Mulkerin MJ, Bohler AM, Mably MS. Multidisciplinary optimization of oral

chemotherapy delivery at the University of Wisconsin Carbone Cancer Center. *J Oncol Pract.* 2016;12(10):e912-e923.

23. Maleki S, Alexander M, Fua T, Liu C, Rischin D, Lingaratnam S. A systematic review of the impact of outpatient clinical pharmacy services on medication-related outcomes in patients receiving anticancer therapies. *J Oncol Pharm Pract.* 2019;25(1):130-139.

24. Holle LM, Harris CS, Chan A, et al. Pharmacists' roles in oncology pharmacy services: results of a global survey. *J Oncol Pharm Pract.* 2017;23(3):185-194.

25. Gatwood J, Gatwood K, Gabre E, Alexander M. Impact of clinical pharmacists in outpatient oncology practices: a review. *Am J Health Syst Pharm.* 2017;74(19):1549-1557.

26. Aun MV, Kalil J, Giavina-Bianchi P. Drug-induced anaphylaxis. *Immunol Allergy Clin North Am.* 2017;37(4):629-641.

27. McKenzie MG, Bissell BD, Disselkamp MA, Hildebrandt GC, Cox JN. Sensitizing the interdisciplinary team to desensitizations: an alemtuzumab case report. *J Oncol Pharm Pract.* 2019:1078155219865313.

28. Lambert Kuhn E, Leveque D, Lioure B, Gourieux B, Bilbault P. Adverse event potentially due to an interaction between ibrutinib and verapamil: a case report. *J Clin Pharm Ther.* 2016;41(1):104-105.

29. Accreditation Council for Pharmacy Education. Available at https://www.acpe-accredit.org/about/. Accessed January 11, 2020.

30. American Society of Health-System Pharmacists. Residency information. Available at https://www.ashp.org/Professional-Development/Residency-Information/Residency-Directory. Accessed May 31, 2020.

31. Board of Pharmacy Specialties. Oncology pharmacy. Available at https://www.bpsweb.org/bps-specialties/oncology-pharmacy/. Published 2019. Accessed 27 Jan 2020.

32. National Cancer Institute. Adult Acute lymphoblastic leukemia treatment (PDQ®)–patient version. Available at https://www.cancer.gov/types/leukemia/patient/adult-all-treatment-pdq. Accessed May 31, 2020.

33. Haynes BF SK, Fauci AS. Introduction to the immune system. In: Jameson JL FA, Kasper DL, Hauser SL, Longo DL, Loscalzo J, ed. *Harrison's Principles of Internal Medicine.* 20th ed. United States: McGraw-Hill; 2019.

34. Leukemia and Lymphoma Society. Acute lymphoblastic leukemia. Available at https://www.lls.org/leukemia/acute-lymphoblastic-leukemia. Accessed May 31, 2020.

35. National Cancer Institute. What is cancer? Available at https://www.cancer.gov/about-cancer/understanding/what-is-cancer. Accessed May 31, 2020.

36. National Cancer Institute. Cancer stat facts: leukemia—acute lymphocytic leukemia (ALL). Available at https://seer.cancer.gov/statfacts/html/alyl.html. Accessed May 31, 2020.

37. Pui CH, Evans WE. A 50-year journey to cure childhood acute lymphoblastic leukemia. *Semin Hematol.* 2013;50(3):185-196.

38. Terwilliger T, Abdul-Hay M. Acute lymphoblastic leukemia: a comprehensive review and 2017 update. *Blood Cancer J.* 2017;7:e577.

39. Sausville SA, Longo DL. Principles of cancer treatment. In: Jameson JL, Fauci AS, Kasper DL, Hauser SL, Longo DL, Loscalzo J, eds. *Harrison's Principles of Internal Medicine.* 20th ed. McGraw-Hill Education; 2019.

40. Mayo Clinic. Chemotherapy. Available at https://www.mayoclinic.org/tests-procedures/chemotherapy/about/pac-20385033. Accessed May 31, 2020.

41. National Cancer Institute. CAR T cells: engineering immune cells to treat cancer. Available at https://www.cancer.gov/about-cancer/treatment/research/car-t-cells. Accessed May 31, 2020.

42. Park JH, Riviere I, Gonen M, et al. Long-Term follow-up of CD19 CAR therapy in acute lymphoblastic leukemia. *N Engl J Med.* 2018;378(5):449-459.

43. June CH, Sadelain M. Chimeric antigen receptor therapy. *N Engl J Med.* 2018;379(1):64-73.

44. Im A, Pavletic SZ. Hematopoietic stem cell transplantation. In: Niederhuber JE, Armitage JO, Kastan MB, Doroshow JH, Tepper JE, eds. *Abeloff's Clinical Oncology.* 6th ed. Philadelphia, PA: Elsevier; 2020.

45. Be The Match. How bone marrow donation works. Available at https://bethematch.org/transplant-basics/how-marrow-donation-works/. Accessed May 31, 2020.

46. Be The Match. How donors and patients are matched. Available at https://bethematch.org/transplant-basics/matching-patients-with-donors/how-donors-and-patients-are-matched/. Accessed May 31, 2020.

47. Heslop HE. Overview and choice of donor of hematopoietic stem cell transplantation—clinicalkey. In: Hoffman R, Benz EJ, Silberstein LE, et al., eds. *Hematology: Basic Principles and Practice.* Vol. 7. Philadelphia, PA: Elsevier; 2018.

48. Gyurkocza B, Sandmaier BM. Conditioning regimens for hematopoietic cell transplantation: one size does not fit all. *Blood.* 2014;124(3):344-353.

49. Be The Match. Engraftment. Available at https://bethematch.org/patients-and-families/life-after-transplant/physical-health-and-recovery/engraftment/. Accessed May 31, 2020.

50. McCollough J. Principles of transfusion support before and after hematopoietic cell transplantation. In: Forman SJ, Negrin RS, Antin JH, Appelbaum FR, eds. *Thomas' Hematopoietic Cell Transplantation.* 5th ed. Hoboken, NJ: John Wiley & Sons, Ltd; 2015.

51. Alonso CD, Marr KA. *Clostridium difficile* infection among hematopoietic stem cell transplant recipients: beyond colitis. *Curr Opin Infect Dis.* 2013;26(4):326-331.

52. Rajasingham R, Enns EA, Khoruts A, Vaughn BP. Cost-effectiveness of treatment regimens for *Clostridioides difficile* infection—an evaluation of the 2013 Infectious Diseases Society of America guidelines. *Clin Infect Dis.* 2019.

53. Chao NJ. Pharmacologic prevention of acute graft-versus-host disease. In: Forman SJ, Negrin RS, Antin JH, Appelbaum FR, eds. *Thomas' Hematopoietic Cell Transplantation.* 5th ed. Hoboken, NJ: John Wiley & Sons, Ltd; 2015.

54. Al-Homsi AS, Roy TS, Cole K, Feng Y, Duffner U. Post-transplant high-dose cyclophosphamide for the prevention of graft-versus-host disease. *Biol Blood Marrow Transplant.* 2015;21(4):604-611.

55. Flowers ME, Martin PJ. How we treat chronic graft-versus-host disease. *Blood.* 2015;125(4):606-615.

56. Sarantopoulos S, Cardones AR, Sullivan KM. How I treat refractory chronic graft-versus-host disease. *Blood.* 2019;133(11):1191-1200.

57. Oray M, Abu Samra K, Ebrahimiadib N, Meese H, Foster CS. Long-term side effects of glucocorticoids. *Expert Opin Drug Saf.* 2016;15(4):457-465.

58. Ullmann AJ, Lipton JH, Vesole DH, et al. Posaconazole or fluconazole for prophylaxis in severe graft-versus-host disease. *N Engl J Med.* 2007;356(4):335-347.

59. Mayo Clinic. Colon cancer. Available at https://www.mayoclinic.org/diseases-conditions/colon-cancer/symptoms-causes/syc-20353669. Accessed May 31, 2020.

60. Consumer Healthcare Products Association. OTC sales by category 2015-2018. Available at https://www.chpa.org/OTCsCategory.aspx. Accessed May 31, 2020.

61. Wollenburg KG. Leadership with conscience, compassion, and commitment. *Am J Health Syst Pharm.* 2004;61(17):1785-1791.

62. Fjortoft N, Zgarrick D. An assessment of pharmacists' caring ability. *J Am Pharm Assoc.* 2003;43(4):483-487.

63. Datta-Barua I, Hauser J. Four communication skills from psychiatry useful in palliative care and how to teach them. *AMA J Ethics.* 2018;20(8):E717-723.

64. McCrae JC, Morrison EE, MacIntyre IM, Dear JW, Webb DJ. Long-term adverse effects of paracetamol—a review. *Br J Clin Pharmacol.* 2018;84(10):2218-2230.

65. Challapalli V, Tremont-Lukats IW, McNicol ED, Lau J, Carr DB. Systemic administration of local anesthetic agents to relieve neuropathic pain. *Cochrane Database Syst Rev.* 2019;2019(10).

66. Abd-Elsayed A. *Pain.* Springer International Publishing; 2019. Available at http://dx.doi.org/10.1007/978-3-319-99124-5.

67. Chen Q, Larochelle MR, Weaver DT, et al. Prevention of prescription opioid misuse and projected overdose deaths in the United States. *JAMA Netw Open.* 2019;2(2):e187621.

68. IQVIA Institute for Human Data Science. Medicine use and spending in the US: a review of 2018 and outlook to 2023. Available at https://www.iqvia.com/insights/the-iqvia-institute/reports/medicine-use-and-spending-in-the-us-review-of-2017-outlook-to-2022. Accessed May 31, 2020.

69. The New York Times. Opioid epidemic. https://www.nytimes.com/spotlight/opioid-epidemic. Accessed May 31, 2020.

70. Scher C, Meador L, Van Cleave JH, Reid MC. Moving beyond pain as the fifth vital sign and patient satisfaction scores to improve pain care in the 21st century. *Pain Manag Nurs.* 2018;19(2):125-129.

71. Tompkins DA, Hobelmann JG, Compton P. Providing chronic pain management in the "fifth vital sign" era: historical and treatment perspectives on a modern-day medical dilemma. *Drug Alcohol Depend.* 2017;173(Suppl 1):S11-s21.

72. Busse JW, Wang L, Kamaleldin M, et al. Opioids for chronic noncancer pain: a systematic review and meta-analysis. *JAMA.* 2018;320(23):2448-2460.

73. Dowell D, Haegerich TM, Chou R. CDC guideline for prescribing opioids for chronic pain—United States, 2016. *JAMA.* 2016;315(15):1624-1645.

74. Pasricha SV, Tadrous M, Khuu W, et al. Clinical indications associated with opioid initiation for pain management in Ontario, Canada: a population-based cohort study. *Pain.* 2018;159(8):1562-1568.

75. Dumas EO, Pollack GM. Opioid tolerance development: a pharmacokinetic/pharmacodynamic perspective. *AAPS J.* 2008;10(4):537-551.

76. Scarborough BM, Smith CB. Optimal pain management for patients with cancer in the modern era. *CA Cancer J Clin.* 2018;68(3):182-196.

77. Shapiro RE. Caffeine and headaches. *Curr Pain Headache Rep.* 2008;12(4):311-315.

78. Dowell D, Haegerich T, Chou R. No shortcuts to safer opioid prescribing. *N Engl J Med.* 2019;380(24):2285-2287.

79. Paice JA. Navigating cancer pain management in the midst of the opioid epidemic. *Oncology.* 2018;32(8) 386-390, 403.

80. Fallon M, Giusti R, Aielli F, et al. Management of cancer pain in adult patients: ESMO clinical practice guidelines. *Ann Oncol.* 2018;29(Suppl 4):iv166-iv191.

81. Hjalte F, Ragnarson Tennvall G, Welin KO, Westerling D. Treatment of severe pain and opioid-induced constipation: an observational study of quality of life, resource use, and costs in Sweden. *Pain Ther.* 2016;5(2):227-236.

82. Boland JW, Boland EG. Pharmacological therapies for opioid induced constipation in adults with cancer. *BMJ.* 2017;358:j3313.

83. Sjogren P, Dragsted L, Christensen CB. Myoclonic spasms during treatment with high doses of intravenous morphine in renal failure. *Acta Anaesthesiol Scand.* 1993;37(8):780-782.

84. Waller SL, Bailey M. Hallucinations during morphine administration. *Lancet.* 1987;2(8562):801.

85. McPherson MLM. *Demystifying Opioid Conversion Calculations: A Guide for Effective Dosing.* 2nd ed. Bethesda, MD: American Society of Health-System Pharmacists; 2018.

86. American Cancer Society. What is hospice care? Available at https://www.cancer.org/treatment/end-of-life-care/hospice-care/what-is-hospice-care.html. Accessed May 31, 2020.

87. El-Jawahri A, Greer JA, Temel JS. Does palliative care improve outcomes for patients with incurable illness? A review of the evidence. *J Support Oncol.* 2011;9(3):87-94.

88. Temel JS, Greer JA, El-Jawahri A, et al. Effects of early integrated palliative care in patients with lung and GI cancer: a randomized clinical trial. *J Clin Oncol.* 2017;35(8):834-841.

89. Davis MP, Temel JS, Balboni T, Glare P. A review of the trials which examine early integration of outpatient and home palliative care for patients with serious illnesses. *Ann Palliat Med.* 2015;4(3):99-121.

90. DiScala SL, Onofrio S, Miller M, Nazario M, Silverman M. Integration of a clinical pharmacist into an interdisciplinary palliative care outpatient clinic. *Am J Hosp Palliat Care.* 2017;34(9):814-819.

91. Herndon CM, Nee D, Atayee RS, et al. ASHP guidelines on the pharmacist's role in palliative and hospice care. *Am J Health Syst Pharm.* 2016;73(17):1351-1367.

92. Richter C. Implementation of a clinical pharmacist service in the hospice setting: financial and clinical impacts. *J Pain Palliat Care Pharmacother.* 2018;32(4):256-259.

93. Gummin DD, Mowry JB, Spyker DA, et al. 2017 annual report of the American Association of Poison Control Centers' National Poison Data System (NPDS): 35th annual report. *Clin Toxicol.* 2018;56(12):1213-1415.

94. Lovegrove MC, Weidle NJ, Budnitz DS. Trends in emergency department visits for unsupervised pediatric medication exposures, 2004–2013. *Pediatrics.* 2015;136(4):e821-829.

95. Grissinger M. Preventing errors when drugs are given via enteral feeding tubes. *P T.* 2013;38(10):575-576.

96. Institute for Safe Medication Practices. Oral dosage forms that should not be crushed. Available at https://www.ismp.org/recommendations/do-not-crush. Accessed May 31, 2020.

97. Edmonds KP, Saunders IM, Willeford A, Ajayi TA, Atayee RS. Emerging challenges to the safe and effective use of methadone for cancer-related pain in paediatric and adult patient populations. *Drugs.* 2020;80(2):115-130.

98. McNicol ED, Ferguson MC, Schumann R. Methadone for neuropathic pain in adults. *Cochrane Database Syst Rev.* 2017;5:CD012499.

99. Gilron I, Baron R, Jensen T. Neuropathic pain: principles of diagnosis and treatment. *Mayo Clin Proc.* 2015;90(4):532-545.

100. McPherson ML, Walker KA, Davis MP, et al. Safe and appropriate use of methadone in hospice and palliative care: expert consensus white paper. *J Pain Symptom Manage.* 2019;57(3):635-645.e634.

CHAPTER 10

Emergency Medicine
Featuring the Illustrated Case Studies "Life & Death" & "One Day"

Authors

Emily M. Zimmerman, Ana F. Bienvenida, & Joseph A. Zorek

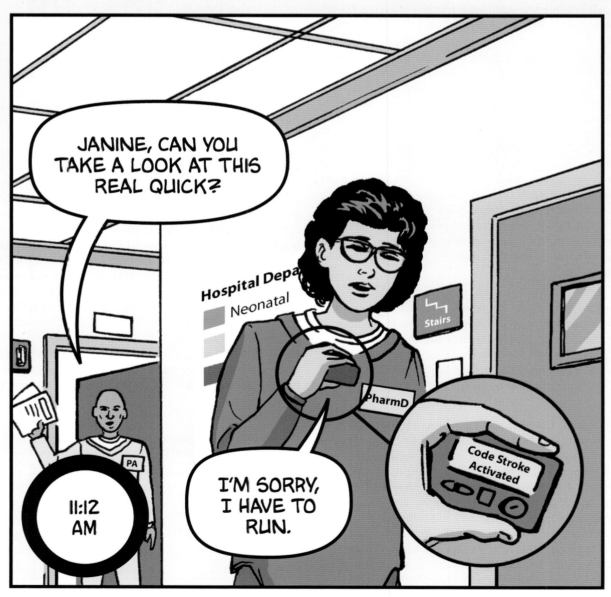

Illustration by George Folz, © 2020 McGraw-Hill Education

BACKGROUND

Emergency departments have been featured prominently on American television sets for decades, with drama and intrigue set against a backdrop of trauma and health crises. These shows highlight two trends that are noteworthy insofar as they ring true, at least from the perspective of pharmacy. First, interprofessional teamwork is the lifeblood of emergency departments (EDs). Good outcomes abound when first responders, nurses, physicians, and other health professionals effectively communicate and coordinate their efforts. Second, pharmacists very rarely make it on screen.

Historical comparisons provide a good explanation for these trends. As a distinct specialty practice area for physicians, emergency medicine (EM) was first recognized by the American Board of Medical Specialties in 1979.[1] As of 2020, there were over 2500 available positions for graduates of medical schools seeking the additional training required for this career path.[2]

EM pharmacy practice, by comparison, is relatively new. In 2006, there were only four EM pharmacy residency programs for graduates of pharmacy schools seeking specialty training in this area.[3] By 2020, this number had grown to 50, representing an increase of over 1100%. In recognition of this rapid growth, which underscores the value health systems and other health professionals place in pharmacists as members of EM teams, the Board of Pharmacy Specialties formally recognized EM pharmacy as its fourteenth official specialty practice area in 2020.[4] The American College of Clinical Pharmacy and the American Society of Health-System Pharmacists (ASHP) jointly submitted the petition to recognize EM pharmacy as a specialty. Importantly, during the public comment period, over 200 physicians and 70 nurses voiced their support. The petition included the following description:

> "Emergency medicine pharmacy practice focuses on rapid assessment of available patient data to optimize pharmacotherapy, improve patient safety, increase efficiency and cost-effectiveness of care, facilitate medication stewardship, educate patients and health care clinicians, and contribute to research and scholarly efforts."

Broadly speaking, EM pharmacists maximize the safe and effective use of medications within EDs. To fully appreciate this, a review of EM as a distinct branch within healthcare is warranted. EM involves the triage, stabilization, diagnosis, management, and disposition of patients who present to the ED.[5] The word "triage" has roots meaning "to sort," and the history of this process stems from mass casualty and battlefield situations.[6] When resources are limited, those who are most critical must be tended to sooner. This is why EDs do not operate on a "first come, first served" basis; instead, "sickest first" is more appropriate. Stabilization refers to care that is provided to ensure that the patient will not deteriorate if moved from one health facility to another.[7]

Diagnosis is typically led by an EM physician and is usually based on laboratory values taken from the patient's blood or urine, as well as vital signs (e.g., heart rate, blood pressure, temperature) and imaging (e.g., x-rays, computed tomography [CT] scans). Management of the patient's condition follows diagnosis. This can take on many forms, including surgery, use of medications, or watchful waiting. Finally, disposition refers to whether a patient will be admitted to the hospital, transferred to a different healthcare facility capable of providing additional specialty services, or discharged home.

As an example, if you were to break your wrist playing basketball, you may wait in the ED while others with complaints of chest pain or tingling are seen before you, even if you arrived first. When seen, you would be stabilized with pain medications and have a diagnosis obtained with the help of x-ray imaging to identify if a break occurred in the bone. Your disposition would likely be back to home with a cast, pain medications, return precautions, and an outpatient follow-up appointment.

Most emergencies can be categorized as either traumatic or medical.[8,9] Traumatic emergencies account for the death of nine patients per minute around the world.[9] In patients between the ages of 1 and 44 years old, trauma is the leading cause of death worldwide. Not surprisingly, motor vehicle accidents account for most of these deaths.[8] Health professionals in EDs are trained to systematically approach trauma patients and evaluate for injuries. Providers use the acronym ABCDE to guide their approach to such work, as described in Table 10-1.[8]

Medical emergencies differ from traumatic emergencies in that they do not involve a physical injury event. Instead, medical emergencies are tied to health crises that stem from either a new health issue or the deterioration of a patient's pre-existing health condition. For examples of new health issues leading to ED visits and subsequent transfer to intensive care units, readers are encouraged to explore the illustrated cases "Shocking" (pneumonia and septic shock) and "Type 1" (diabetic ketoacidosis from type 1 diabetes) in Chaper 11 Critical Care. Those interested in the deterioration of pre-existing health conditions leading to ED visits and subsequent hospitalization would benefit from reading the illustrated cases "Breakdown" (myocardial infarction [i.e., heart attack]) in Chapter 1 Interprofessional Practice

Table 10-1. The ABCDE Approach to Trauma Care

Focus	Definition	Description
A	Airway	Keep airway open and unobstructed
B	Breathing	Assist with breathing, if needed
C	Circulation	Control sources of bleeding and perform chest compressions to circulate blood if the heart has stopped
D	Disability	Assess all injuries from head to toe
E	Exposure	Ensure the patient is a normal temperature

in Pharmacy, and "Educator" (heart failure) in Chapter 5 Cardiology. Sometimes, a medical emergency can precipitate a traumatic emergency, such as when a patient has a myocardial infarction while driving a car. An example of this kind of situation is highlighted in the illustrated case "Innovator" in Chapter 13 Technology, where a young adult experiences a seizure that results in an automobile accident. Table 10-2 lists the most common traumatic and medical emergencies reported in the United States in 2018.[10]

The capacity to care for patients at a single hospital is dependent upon the number of hospital beds available. Once stabilized in the ED, patients who do not require additional care are discharged home. Those who need additional care, however, are admitted to designated parts of the hospital designed for their specific condition. These destinations are often referred to as floors, wards, or units; for example, general medicine ward, cardiology floor, or intensive care unit. Once admitted to the hospital, teams of health professionals care for patients until it is safe for them to be discharged. The most common discharge destination is the patient's home. Some patients, however, require additional care before they are able to manage their own condition at home. In this situation, patients are generally transferred for short-term transitional care at a rehabilitation facility, or a skilled nursing facility. Those who will never be able to manage their own care independently will often move into a long-term-care facility. For an example of pharmacist involvement in long-term care, readers are encouraged to explore the illustrated case "Sleuth" in Chapter 7 Geriatrics.

When visits to the ED increase, but the number of available hospital beds is limited, a bottleneck of sorts develops within the ED. This situation is called boarding, defined by patients who are technically admitted to a ward, floor, or unit, but who remain physically in the ED under the care of EM nurses and other EM health professionals. ED boarding is associated with an overall increased hospital length of stay, lower patient satisfaction, adverse events, and increased mortality.[11] Boarding creates a situation whereby EM pharmacists need to be competent in the medication management of not only traumatic and medical emergencies, but also a host of other health conditions ranging from cardiovascular and psychiatric conditions to infectious diseases and solid organ transplant. As a result, EM pharmacists must remain well-rounded in their knowledge and skills in order to remain adequately prepared.

Members of the Interprofessional Emergency Medicine Team

Due to the diverse complaints and complexity of needs of any given ED patient, many different health professionals make up the organized team required to optimize patient care. Patients can arrive to the hospital via personal vehicle, ambulance, or helicopter, and care begins at this transition point. In an emergency transport situation, first responders such as paramedics and emergency medical technicians (EMTs) communicate the patient's status and any anticipated needs with the receiving ED while en route. Examples of this can be seen in the illustrated case "Life & Death" discussed later in this chapter, as well as in the illustrated cases "Shocking" and "Type 1" in Chapter 11 Critical Care, and "Innovator" in Chapter 13 Technology.

Commonly, before a patient is seen by the attending, or lead, EM physician, a nurse or technician will document the patient's complaints and history of illness/injury, collect vitals (e.g., temperature, pulse, blood pressure), establish intravenous (IV) access (i.e., prepare the patient to receive liquid medications directly into a vein) if indicated, and triage the patient based on the severity of his or her symptoms. The attending physician will then meet with the patient to complete a physical examination after reviewing existing records and the nursing or technician notes. Attending physicians drive the care of patients through ordering labs and diagnostic imaging. In some practice settings, nurse practitioners and physician assistants with specialty training or experience in EM see patients prior to the attending physician.[12] Based on the patient's complaints, respiratory therapists may administer breathing treatments to the patient.[13] Social workers and case managers may also assist patients with resource issues such as transportation, food, and housing.[14] If available at the hospital where the ED is located, a consult with a specialty physician such as an oncologist (i.e., cancer), nephrologist (i.e., kidney disease), or orthopedist (i.e., musculoskeletal issues) may occur. Chaplains can be available for end-of-life and spiritual needs. Readers interested in the role of pharmacists in cancer treatment and end-of-life care are encouraged to explore the illustrated cases "Compromising" and "Compassion" in Chapter 9 Oncology.

EM pharmacists interact with these health professionals in different ways. Pharmacists may be present when patients are transferred from first responders to EM staff to hear first-hand the patient's chief complaint and vitals during his or her pre-hospital course of treatment. Pharmacists answer medication-related questions from nurses; for example, how fast a medication can be safely administered or whether two different medications can be given through the same IV line. Pharmacists assist respiratory therapists by obtaining inhaled medications for patients in respiratory distress, and by determining cost-effective options for patients who are stabilized and discharged home from the ED. Pharmacists work directly with attending physicians, medical residents, physician assistants, and nurse practitioners to select the best medication management strategy for the patient based on their condition(s).

Table 10-2. Top 5 Traumatic and Medical Emergencies Reported in 2018

Rank	Traumatic Emergencies	Medical Emergencies
1	Fall	Acute respiratory infection
2	Head injury	Urinary tract infection
3	Motor vehicle collision	Chest pain
4	Overexertion	Headache
5	Bite/sting	Abdominal pain

Pharmacists also help modify and optimize medication regimens based on the patient's weight, interacting medications, kidney and liver function, and allergies.[15]

Role of Pharmacists within Interprofessional Emergency Medicine Teams

The role of EM pharmacists has evolved over its relatively short history. Pharmacists originally served a primarily distributive role.[15,16] This involved acquiring medications and delivering them to the patient's nurse. As pharmacy technicians took on this role, EM pharmacists strengthened their involvement in the selection of the most appropriate and effective medications for patients, with added involvement in pharmacotherapy recommendations, resuscitation, direct patient care, medication information questions, and medication order review.[16,17] Practice patterns from one ED to another vary based on the ED's size and resources, as well as the communities they serve. As a result, some pharmacists practice in a medication specialist role and purely answer drug information questions, while others continue to focus on medication acquisition and dispensing; in many EDs, EM pharmacy practice models incorporate both approaches. In 2015, the American College of Emergency Physicians published a policy statement recommending that pharmacists should be well-integrated into the interprofessional EM team due to the complexity and breadth of patients seen in the ED, and the challenges associated with high-risk medications being used in a fast-paced environment.[18]

ASHP, the national organization representing pharmacists that co-sponsored the petition leading to EM pharmacy being recognized as a distinct specialty practice, recognizes several essential direct patient care roles for EM pharmacists.[16] Chief among these roles is the prospective verification and retrospective review of medication orders in the ED. Due to the emergency nature of this practice setting, medications cannot always be prospectively verified by a pharmacist before they are administered, as is customary across all other pharmacy practice settings.[19] To account for this reality, EM pharmacists review medication use patterns to develop protocols and guidance aimed at maximizing their safe and effective use during emergencies. EM pharmacists partner closely with physicians, other prescribers, and nurses to address medication questions as they arise. Importantly, EM pharmacists are intimately involved in the selection of medication products, as well as their real-time preparation at bedside for unstable patients.

As previously described, trauma management involves the ABCDE approach to care.[8] EM pharmacists are involved most commonly in the airway and circulation portion of the primary assessment for trauma patients. For example, pharmacists assist in the selection and preparation of medications used for establishing a breathing tube for patients in respiratory distress who are not able to adequately breathe. Two classes of medications are used for this procedure; induction medications that help patients become unaware of the procedure, and paralytic medications that remove the gag reflex to gain access into the

Table 10-3. Categories and Examples of Medications Commonly Used in the Protection of Patients' Airways

Category	Medication Examples*	Physiologic Effect
Induction agents	• etomidate (Amidate) • ketamine (Ketalar) • midazolam (Versed) • propofol (Diprivan)	Cause sedation and loss of memory
Neuromuscular blocking agents	• rocuronium (Zemuron) • succinylcholine (Anectine)	Paralyze the patient's muscles and allow breathing tubes to pass through the vocal cords

*Medication examples presented in alphabetical order as "generic name (Brand Name)."

trachea, in that order.[20] Table 10-3 includes examples of common medications used in this manner.[21]

Many medications have a narrow therapeutic index, which means that dosing those medications needs to be incredibly precise. One such example is the anticoagulant warfarin (Coumadin), which is used as a "blood thinner" to prevent blood clots that might lead to a stroke. The difference between a warfarin dose that will lead to insufficient anticoagulation, thus putting the patient at risk of stroke, and a warfarin dose that will lead to excessive anticoagulation, thus putting the patient at risk of major bleeding and harm, is small. In the case of the latter, EM pharmacists can be impactful in selecting appropriate reversal agents and ensuring their timely administration when patients arrive to the ED over-anticoagulated with uncontrollable bleeding.[22,23] Speedy reversal of anticoagulation, guided by a laboratory test called the International Normalized Ratio (INR), can help control bleeding and buy the trauma team time until the patient can get to the operating room for definitive management of bleeding. For a more in-depth discussion of anticoagulation, readers are encouraged to explore the illustrated case "Empowerment" in Chapter 5 Cardiology.

Several medications used in the ED are considered high-alert medications, meaning they have a high risk of causing patient harm, including death, if used in error.[24] EM pharmacists must demonstrate expert knowledge of high-alert medications, as their involvement in the selection, administration, dosing, monitoring, and management of these medications is considered a foundational, essential role. Succinylcholine and rocuronium, described in Table 10-3, are examples of high-alert medications. Table 10-4 includes a handful of additional examples.[24]

Two incredibly important roles EM pharmacists play involve management of vasopressors, thrombolytics, and other medications associated with Advanced Cardiac Life Support (ACLS) and emergency efforts to restore blood flow to the brain using "clot busting" drugs for patients experiencing an acute ischemic stroke. The illustrated cases "Life & Death" and "One Day" in this chapter cover these topics in depth. For additional examples, readers are encouraged to explore Chapter 5 Cardiology.

Table 10-4. Categories and Examples of High Alert Medications Commonly Used in Emergency Departments

Category	Medication Examples*	Physiologic Effect
Antiarrhythmics	▪ amiodarone (Cordarone) ▪ lidocaine (Xylocaine)	Control electrical activity in the heart, restoring a normal heartbeat rhythm
Anticoagulants	▪ enoxaparin (Lovenox) ▪ fondaparinux (Arixtra) ▪ unfractionated heparin	Prevent the formation of blood clots by blocking the action of proteins that lead to their formation
Osmotics	▪ mannitol (Osmitrol) ▪ sodium chloride 3%	Decrease swelling in the brain and also cause diuresis, where the kidneys produce urine to excrete excess fluid
Insulins	▪ insulin lispro (Humalog) ▪ insulin regular (Humulin R, Novolin R)	Decrease glucose (i.e., sugar) levels in blood by facilitating glucose uptake into cells; also, move potassium into cells when potassium levels in blood are dangerously high
Thrombolytics	▪ alteplase (Activase) ▪ tenecteplase (TNKase)	Rapidly break apart existing blood clots
Vasopressors	▪ epinephrine (Adrenalin) ▪ norepinephrine (Levophed)	Increase blood pressure, ensuring adequate oxygen delivery to vital organs

*Medication examples presented in alphabetical order as "generic name (Brand Name)."

EMERGENCY MEDICINE PHARMACISTS IN ACTION

Rat Poison Reversal

A 20-year-old male with a disheveled appearance and nervous demeanor arrived at an ED complaining of dizziness and blood in his urine, which he reported was occurring daily for the last week.[25] Reviewing the patient's laboratory results and nursing notes, which revealed low blood counts, an incredibly high INR, and a history of marijuana use, an EM pharmacist became intrigued. Recently, this pharmacist had learned through a listserv shared between local hospitals of a synthetic marijuana in the community that had been laced with brodifacoum, a potent blood thinner. Brodifacoum is commonly used as a household rodenticide, thinning the blood of rodents and then causing

cerebral hemorrhage and death when they squeeze into small spaces. Guided by the EM pharmacist's recommendations, the patient was started on an IV medication called phytonadione to reverse the effects of brodifacoum and given 1 unit of blood. He was discharged home with a 30-day supply of phytonadione tablets and instructions for periodic INR monitoring.

Drug-Induced and Life-Threatening

An Asian male in his early 30s arrived to an ED complaining of pain and blisters in his throat and on his lips, eyes, and the soles of his hands and feet.[26] The patient was seen the day before with influenza-like symptoms, a fever, and a sore throat. He was sent home with prescriptions for amoxicillin, an antibiotic, as well as a steroid. Blisters began to emerge shortly after the first doses of these medications. A serious adverse drug event attributed to amoxicillin called toxic epidermal necrolysis (TEN) was suspected by the EM team, which is a potentially life-threatening condition where portions of the skin become red and inflamed, often with widespread blistering, before dying (i.e., tissue necrosis). While researching the patient's medication history, the EM pharmacist discovered that the patient was prescribed a drug called allopurinol 10 days prior to this episode for a painful condition called gout, which occurs when crystals from high blood levels of uric acid form in one or more joints. Allopurinol is also known to cause TEN, especially in patients of Asian descent.[27] The EM pharmacist's efforts led to a quicker diagnosis and effective treatment plan, a time-sensitive intervention of significant value for a patient whose life was on the line.

BECOMING AN EMERGENCY MEDICINE PHARMACIST

Pharmacists who practice in the ED must have adequate preparation for this jack-of-all-trades setting; meaning, they must know a little about a lot of medications, as nearly all patients admitted to the hospital pass through the doors of the ED. Therefore, EM pharmacists can come from a variety of backgrounds. In recent years, the EM specialty route has become a popular pathway into this career. Broadly speaking, this includes successful completion of a Doctor of Pharmacy (PharmD) degree, followed by completion of a general post-graduate year 1 (PGY-1) residency program. After completion of a PGY-1 residency, pharmacists seeking specialty training complete a post-graduate year 2 (PGY-2) residency program in emergency medicine.[28] Beyond these specialized training routes, many EM pharmacists demonstrate their expertise via attainment of certification as a Board Certified Pharmacotherapy Specialist (BCPS) and/or Board Certified Critical Care Pharmacist (BCCCP).[29] Combined, BCPS and BCCCP cover the primary care and critical care health conditions commonly experienced in the ED. Board certification dedicated specifically to EM pharmacy will be available starting in 2022. Pharmacists interested in an EM career may also pursue fellowship training in clinical and applied toxicology, and those with qualifying experience can demonstrate their expertise by becoming a Diplomate of the American Board of Applied Toxicology (DABAT).[30]

LIFE & DEATH: An Illustrated Case Study

Story by Emily M. Zimmerman & Joseph A. Zorek
Illustrations by George Folz, © 2019 Board of Regents of the University of Wisconsin System

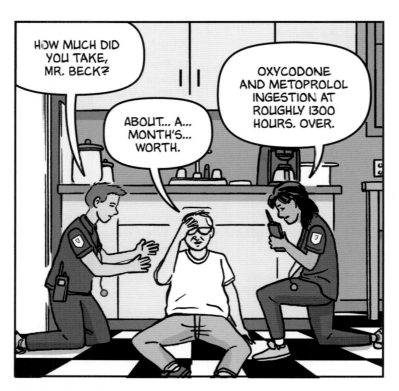

Illustration 10-1

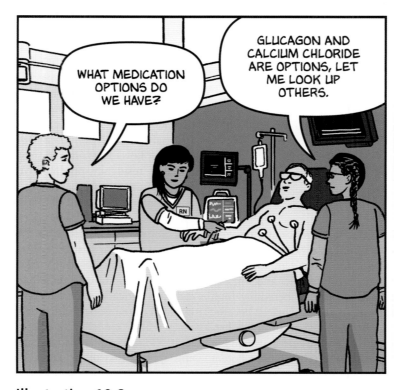

Illustration 10-2

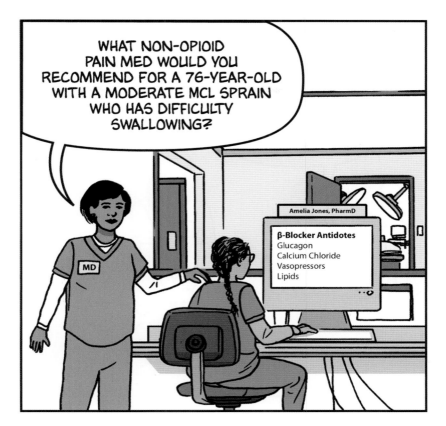

Illustration 10-3

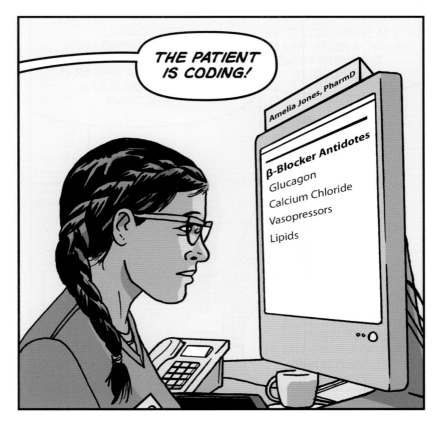

Illustration 10-4

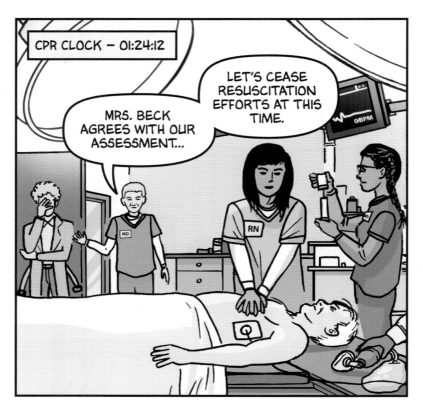

Illustration 10-5

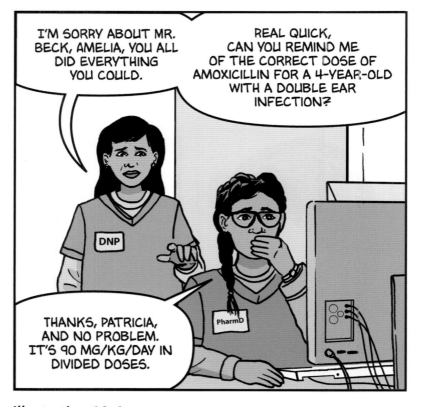

Illustration 10-6

Thoughts on "Life & Death"

According to the American Foundation for Suicide Prevention, suicide was the fourth-leading cause of death in patients 34 to 55 years of age in 2018.[31] In 2019, 1.4 million Americans attempted suicide. Self-inflicted gunshot wounds and asphyxiation (i.e., suffocation) were reported as the most frequent methods used, followed by poisoning.[32] Poisoning has been documented to occur more frequently in woman; whereas, in men, attempted suicide by firearm use is more common. As patients age, so too do the types of substances used in suicide attempts via poisoning; specifically, analgesics like oxycodone, sedatives like alprazolam, and cardiovascular drugs like metoprolol have been cited in reports of suicide attempts in older adults.[33] To get a sense of the economic impact, the combination of costs associated with medical bills and work lost from suicide and suicide attempts is estimated at nearly $70 billion annually.[31]

The main character in the illustrated case "Life & Death" is an elderly gentleman named James Beck. In Illustration 10-1, Mr. Beck reports to first responders that he intentionally ingested excessive amounts of oxycodone and metoprolol in an attempt to end his life. In recent years, a common challenge faced by EM pharmacists has been the management of medication-related issues stemming from misuse and overdose of opioid medications. Pharmacists across a variety of practice settings are involved in this effort, which includes contributing knowledge and expertise to the safe and appropriate use of opioids for acute and chronic conditions.[34] An additional important contribution includes assisting prescribers (e.g., physicians, physician assistants, nurse practitioners, and dentists) and patients to safely utilize prescription medications intended to reduce dependence on opioids, such as buprenorphine/naloxone (Suboxone), as well as the life-saving opioid reversal agent naloxone (Narcan).[35] Naloxone is used by first responders as well as EM nurses, pharmacists, and physicians to reverse the effects of an opioid overdose. Those interested in a more in-depth discussion of opioids and opioid use disorder are encouraged to read Chapter 12 Mental Health and the illustrated case "Gasping." For an example of a pharmacist intervention to support the safe use of opioids in the setting of end-of-life care, see the illustrated case "Compassion" in Chapter 9 Oncology.

Patients who present to the ED with a respiratory rate of less than 12 breaths per minute, constricted or smaller-than-normal pupils, and circumstantial evidence of opioid overdose can be considered for administration of naloxone.[36] Naloxone works by competing with the opioid to bind to the same receptor, which reverses the negative effects of opioid overdose.[37] As naloxone binds to these receptors and displaces the opioid from them, the undesired physiologic response from the overdose is reversed. Importantly, the duration of action of naloxone (i.e., the amount of time it will remain active in the body) is much shorter than most opioids.[37,38] As a result, patients in the ED must be closely observed, as additional naloxone doses may be required. For the same reason, administration of naloxone in the community requires transportation of the patient to a hospital for monitoring. This step has allowed the EM team to focus on antidotes for metoprolol toxicity, as depicted in Illustration 10-2.

In emergency situations like Mr. Beck's suicide attempt, pre-hospital personnel play a vital role stabilizing patients and relaying information to the receiving ED, as depicted in Illustration 10-1. When the cause of the emergency is poisoning, first responders may also retrieve the suspected substances for further evaluation by ED staff. In this manner, the process for treating patients who have overdosed on medications can start even before their physical arrival to the ED. Family members and citizens acting as Good Samaritans can also serve as important pre-hospital resources by calling the Poison Control Center (1-800-222-1222) for recommendations on early treatment or to determine what level of care a patient needs (e.g., urgent care, ED, and ambulance transport). As the radio report is transmitted to the ED, mobilization and planning begin in anticipation of the patient's arrival.

Pre-hospital preparation might include gathering the needed personnel, such as respiratory therapists, or organizing medications that the EM pharmacist believes might be helpful. As it relates to preparation for Mr. Beck's arrival, Dr. Amelia Jones, the EM pharmacist, already began researching toxicity of beta-blockers, of which metoprolol is one, and potential antidotes, which are shown pulled up on her computer screen in Illustrations 10-3 and 10-4. Since the formulation of Mr. Beck's metoprolol was unknown from the radio report transmitted (e.g., immediate release, delayed release, extended release), Amelia did not call the Poison Control Center for additional guidance yet. This is a step she will pursue as soon as this information becomes available, either from the pill bottles brought to the ED, via consultation with a family member, such as Mrs. Beck, or by calling Mr. Beck's community pharmacy. The formulation of the medication is important in an overdose situation such as this, as it will determine how quickly the ingested medications will enter the bloodstream and will determine the speed with which Mr. Beck's condition may, or may not, deteriorate. Knowledge about the formulation, in other words, will help the interprofessional EM team determine how long Mr. Beck should be observed, once stabilized, before the worst possible effects of the drug would be seen.

Illustration 10-2 shows the interprofessional EM team in action, composed of an EM physician, nurse, and pharmacist. This team comes together to hear the report from the first responders when they arrive. ED technicians typically obtain intravenous (IV) access upon patient arrival; however, in Mr. Beck's case, the first responders obtained access and began giving him IV fluids during transport in response to his low blood pressure. In this case, a second IV access point is obtained so that medications can be administered concurrently with fluids, and to avoid any issues of medication incompatibility. As depicted in Illustration 10-2, the EM nurse works to obtain vital signs such as blood pressure, heart rate, and oxygen saturation, and the EM physician positions himself at the foot of the patient's bed to direct the actions of the team. Amelia is present, as well, developing her own monitoring and treatment plan in order to anticipate potential medication needs, such as the antidotes being discussed.

Patients at high risk for rapid deterioration, such as Mr. Beck, or those whose conditions are already rapidly declining, require bedside assessment and many interventions simultaneously. However, other patients are concurrently being seen in the ED by other EM physicians, nurse practitioners, and physician assistants. Most EDs only have one EM pharmacist covering all of these patients, which puts a premium on their ability to multitask. Such behavior is highlighted in Illustration 10-3. Amelia, having just sat down to complete the task from Illustration 10-2, is immediately interrupted with a drug information question for a different patient; in this case, an older adult who has injured her knee after falling. Readers interested in the care of older adults and the role of pharmacists in the prevention of adverse drug events in this population are encouraged to read Chapter 7 Geriatrics and the illustrated cases "Burden" and "Sleuth."

With so many providers in the ED caring for a diverse patient population, one of the main non-clinical skills that Amelia must demonstrate is the ability to triage, prioritize, and compartmentalize. There will undoubtedly be a long list of tasks to complete during Amelia's shift, and as one is completed, others will be added. EM pharmacists must work efficiently to complete each task accurately and quickly. Illustration 10-3 introduces a situation whereby Amelia must research two drug information topics, one for Mr. Beck, and another for non-opioid pain medications that either come in liquid form or capsules that can be opened and sprinkled on food. Amelia prioritizes research for Mr. Beck, as his condition is more urgent. However, she is quickly interrupted in Illustration 10-4 with the announcement that Mr. Beck has coded. Amelia appropriately triages her two drug information tasks in order to attend to the more critical one.

The term *code* refers to a situation in which a patient has lost his or her pulse and is in cardiac arrest; meaning, their heart is no longer pumping in an organized rhythm that moves blood throughout the body. Cardiopulmonary resuscitation (CPR) is the act of performing chest compressions and breathing for a patient in an attempt to manually circulate oxygen-rich blood to the brain and other vital organs.[39] Most health professionals in hospital settings are trained in Advanced Cardiac Life Support, or ACLS.[40] An evidenced-based algorithm is used to treat the underlying heart rhythm that is found and medications and/or electrical current is administered to the patient.[41] The EM pharmacist's role in ACLS can range from one healthcare setting to the next.[42] Various activities reported include preparation of medications, keeping time, recording heart rhythms and medication administration times, guiding providers on next steps of the ACLS algorithm, and discussing reversable causes with the ACLS leader. Certain states allow pharmacists to administer medications via IV and intraosseous (i.e., through the bone) routes to patients in code situations.[9] Illustration 10-5 depicts Amelia drawing medication out of a vial and into a syringe. Over the course of the interprofessional EM team's long battle to save Mr. Beck's life, Amelia would have prepared many medication syringes like this one, ensuring each was

Table 10-5. Categories and Examples of Medications Commonly Used During Advanced Cardiovascular Life Support		
Category	**Medication Examples***	**Physiologic Effect**
Vasopressors	■ epinephrine (Adrenalin) ■ norepinephrine (Levophed)	Increase the ability of the heart to pump, which increases blood pressure
Antiarrhythmics	■ amiodarone (Cordarone) ■ lidocaine (Xylocaine)	Correct abnormal electrical activity in the heart
Reversal agents	■ flumazenil (Romazicon) ■ naloxone (Narcan)	Block the effects of either opioids or benzodiazepines to reverse their negative effects
Anti-hypoglycemic agents	■ dextrose 50% ■ dextrose 10%	Increase blood glucose levels, if low
Electrolytes	■ calcium chloride 10%	Stabilize electrical activity in the heart in situations where a patient has too much potassium in their blood
	■ magnesium sulfate	Terminate a life-threatening arrhythmia of the heart called Torsades de Pointes
	■ sodium bicarbonate 8.4%	Improve conditions for cardiac activity when a patient's blood pH is too low (i.e., acidic)

*Medication examples presented in alphabetical order as "generic name (Brand Name)."

labeled with the correct concentration of the medication and dose. Table 10-5 includes additional information on ACLS medications.[41,43,44]

CPR is the last option for patients, and if a patient does not respond to ACLS, they will die. Illustration 10-5 shows the EM physician sharing his assessment with Mrs. Beck that resuscitation efforts, which have been ongoing for nearly 1.5 hours, have failed. The decision to cease CPR on a patient is very difficult. Providers such as the EM physician depicted in this case take many factors into consideration, including duration of the resuscitation attempt, the patient's comorbidities (i.e., other health conditions), and past experience with similar clinical cases.[45] In the past, it was considered best practice to separate family members from their loved ones during resuscitation efforts, and to share the hardest news of all in a private location. However, recent studies have shown that having family members present during resuscitation efforts reduces the incidence of post-traumatic stress compared to not being present, without interfering with clinical efforts.[46] It is important to note that each family is unique, with different cultural and/or religious beliefs regarding life and death; hence, family preferences should be respected even if they conflict with the aforementioned evidence regarding post-traumatic stress.

For EM health professionals, like Amelia, transitioning back to daily tasks after the death of a patient can be difficult. Debriefing sessions may be scheduled for ED staff to review the timeline of events, share frustrations about the event, and provide support to those involved. This can be particularly helpful when patients pass away unexpectedly or, as in the case of children, prematurely. Illustration 10-6 highlights Amelia in the process of transitioning back to her normal ED workflow following Mr. Beck's death. Here, an EM nurse practitioner who was not involved in Mr. Beck's care approaches Amelia with a drug information request for a non-emergency situation. In a display of support and in recognition that Amelia has been emotionally impacted by Mr. Beck's passing, the nurse practitioner is depicted as understanding, empathetic, and supportive, demonstrating great interprofessional teamwork.

The illustrated case "Life & Death" is a complex story that begins with a suicide attempt by medication overdose of an older adult named James Beck. After ingesting about a month's worth of two different medications, Mr. Beck calls 9-1-1, which activates the emergency response system. First responders stabilize and transport him to a local emergency department, where the work of an interprofessional team that includes Dr. Amelia Jones, an emergency medicine pharmacist, is portrayed. In this fast-paced environment, the ability to multitask is emphasized as Mr. Beck's condition deteriorates and cardiopulmonary resuscitation with advanced cardiac life support efforts begin. Unfortunately, the team is unable to save Mr. Beck's life, and the emotional toll of his death are felt by all. The emergency department staff support one another as they continue to work through remaining tasks to deliver the highest quality of care.

DISCUSSION QUESTIONS FOR "LIFE & DEATH"

1. When first responders call into the hospital with a reported medication ingestion, as depicted in Illustration 10-1, what steps do you think the physicians, physician assistants, nurse practitioners, nurses, and pharmacists might take to prepare?

2. Reflect on how you would feel working in an environment with constant interruptions and change. Would this excite you? Or would this leave you feeling frustrated and/or upset? Why?

3. How might you determine if an unresponsive person suspected of substance abuse has overdosed on alcohol or an opioid medication?

4. Imagine a situation in which a family member is critically ill. How would you feel being in the room when the emergency medicine team stops resuscitation efforts, as they did with Mrs. Beck in the room in Illustration 10-5?

5. In the debrief with emergency department staff that will follow Mr. Beck's death in Illustration 10-5, what do you think will be discussed?

ONE DAY: An Illustrated Case Study

Story by Ana F. Bienvenida & Joseph A. Zorek
Illustrations by George Folz, © 2020 McGraw-Hill Education

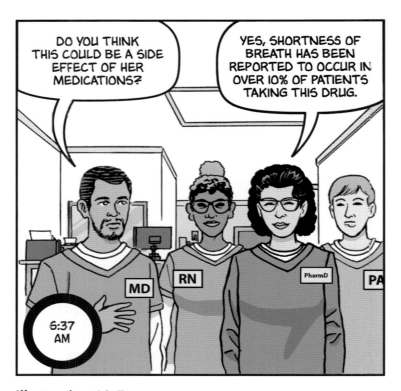

Illustration 10-7

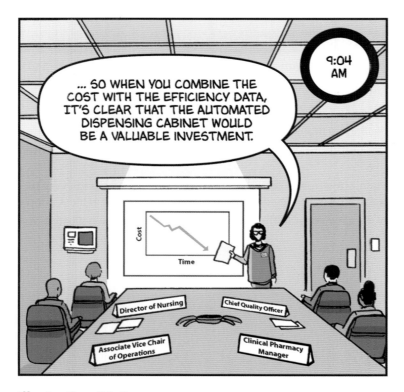

Illustration 10-8

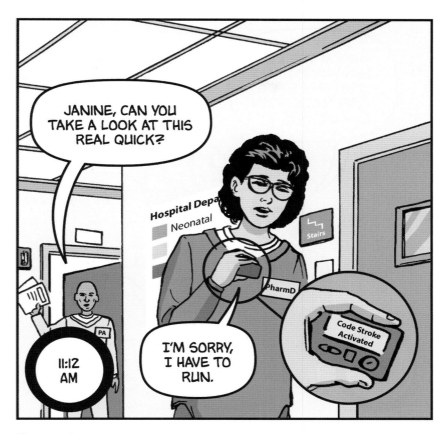

Illustration 10-9

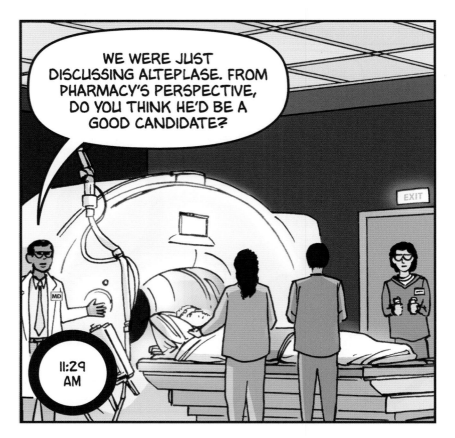

Illustration 10-10

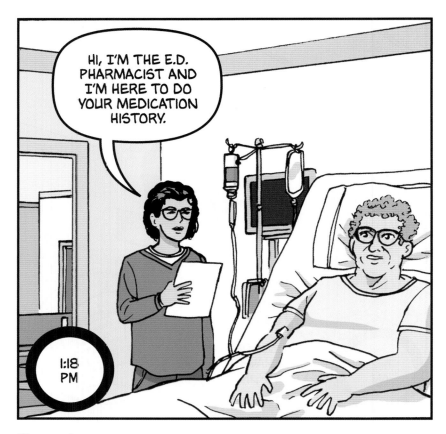

Illustration 10-11

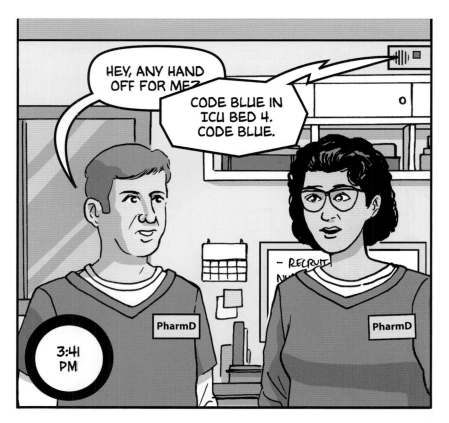

Illustration 10-12

Thoughts on "One Day"

The ability to prioritize, triage, and compartmentalize are essential skills that emergency medicine (EM) pharmacists, like Dr. Janine Ori in the illustrated case "One Day," must develop to succeed in the emergency department (ED). Throughout this single ED shift, Janine demonstrates these skills seamlessly as she bounces from interprofessional rounds (Illustration 10-7) and a formal presentation (Illustration 10-8) to a code situation (Illustrations 10-9 and 10-10) and a basic patient encounter (Illustration 10-11), propelled all the while by either obligations or time-dependent emergencies. Such is the inherent culture in the ED, where health professionals like nurses, nurse practitioners, pharmacists, physician assistants, physicians, respiratory therapists, and technicians are expected to leave trauma bays or resuscitation rooms and continue with their day in the face of either profound loss or the emotional high of a life-saving triumph.

This book is replete with examples of pharmacists balancing the human aspects of providing high quality care with the need to continue moving forward, touched but not hindered by human emotion.[47] While the extremes of this are depicted in the illustrated case "Life & Death," the ability to compartmentalize in order to balance multiple tasks efficiently throughout the course of a busy ED shift is further elucidated in the illustrated case "One Day." Health professionals working in EDs have had success extending this compartmentalization approach to their personal lives. In a survey exploring coping strategies of EM staff, for example, nearly half of responders reported that the ability to separate personal lives from work was critical to their success.[48] Compartmentalization to deal with adversity or extreme challenges is not unique to healthcare; in fact, it has been highlighted as a key factor for success in multiple sectors, including business.[47,49]

Lessons about compartmentalizing can be applied to any setting, but these are especially useful in the ED, where the stakes are high and the pace is fast. One key lesson is that different tasks should be isolated when possible, and then prioritized. Next, extreme focus should be dedicated to the task with the highest priority, and this should be done for as short a period of time as possible. Once the first priority task is completed, the ability to "close the compartment" and move to the next task on the priority list is essential. If a task cannot be completed in a timely manner due to competing priorities, then the task needs to be triaged and the prioritization list must be rearranged. Janine prioritizes, triages, and compartmentalizes throughout her ED shift. One example is provided in Illustration 10-9, which depicts her departing quickly in response to a medical emergency; namely, a code stroke. Unfortunately, due to the emergency nature of the stroke page, Janine is unable to assist the physician assistant shown in the background of this illustration. In a matter of moments, she has closed the compartment on that task and shifted attention to the care of this stroke patient.

EM pharmacy is unique insofar as the tasks and professional activities provided can range from one extreme to another over a short span of time. Medication history taking and reconciliation, depicted in Illustration 10-11, are two examples of constant, lower-stress, and rather universal activities of EM pharmacists. These tasks are completed to ensure that the EM team has accurate information about a patient's medications, upon which diagnoses and treatment plans can be built. Many EM pharmacists also contribute to the preparation and/or review of discharge prescriptions. In this role, they work in real time with prescribers to develop discharge medication plans for patients who do not require hospital admission. Incorporating EM pharmacists into the ED workflow in this manner has been shown to reduce medication errors and lead to optimization of medication use.[50,51]

On the higher-stress end of the spectrum, EM pharmacists also prepare medications urgently at the patient's bedside. An example of this is shown in the cardiac arrest depicted in Illustration 10-5 in the illustrated case "Life & Death." Within the illustrated case "One Day," while not explicitly stated in Illustration 10-9, one of the reasons that compelled Janine to abandon the task she was about to begin for the physician assistant is that, in this ED, it is the EM pharmacist's job to assist with the screening of stroke patients for the use of "clot busting" medications like alteplase (Activase). If the EM team decides to use this medication, Janine will prepare it at bedside to speed administration. What the illustrated case "One Day" captures well is the different roles that ED pharmacists play, and how they must balance acute, higher-stress activities such as these with non-acute, lower-stress ones to maximize their impact on patient care.

In recent years, the focus within EM pharmacy has shifted to preventing medication errors, optimizing medication management, and collaborating with prescribers to develop goal-directed medication therapy plans.[50] Illustration 10-7 highlights the importance of pharmacist involvement in medication management, where Janine is shown working within the EM team to troubleshoot a potential adverse drug event (ADE). It is estimated that 4 in 1000 patients in the United States present to the ED as a result of harm caused by medications.[52] In Illustration 10-7, the medication in question is ticagrelor (Brilinta), with the EM team working to identify a cause for the patient's shortness of breath. Ticagrelor is often used in patients who have undergone a procedure to open the arteries that deliver oxygenated blood to the heart.[53] For an in-depth discussion of this topic, readers are encouraged to explore the illustrated case "Breakdown" in Chapter 1 Interprofessional Practice in Pharmacy.

As part of their professional development, EM pharmacists regularly read new studies and case reports when they are published, like the one Janine refers to, scouring for data and associated trends, such as ADEs. Based on her behind-the-scenes reading and research, Janine is able to confirm the EM physician's hunch in Illustration 10-7 and help the team move in the right direction. Maintaining a current knowledge base is critical to maximizing impact, and EM pharmacists must be prepared to contribute to the team in a meaningful way when situations, like this one, arise. Readers interested in learning more about evidence-based decision making and ADEs are encouraged to explore the illustrated case "Support" in Chapter 3 Primary Care.

While less glamorous, EM pharmacists also lend their expert knowledge and professional opinions to important administrative discussions and decisions. Illustration 10-8 highlights this role, where Janine, after finishing up reviewing current patients in the ED, breaks away briefly to deliver a presentation to a committee of administrative leaders. This committee, led by the Chief Quality Officer, has been tasked with identifying solutions that will improve medication use and patient safety, while decreasing costs to the organization. Janine was asked to develop a presentation about the use of automated dispensing cabinets to inform this committee's decisions about upcoming investments within the ED. Janine's research on this topic indicates that such technology would benefit patients and the organization, increasing efficiency in medication use and decreasing costs over time. Readers interested in the interface of pharmacy and technology are encouraged to explore the illustrated cases "Leverage," "Integrated," and "Innovator" in Chapter 13 Technology. Those who would benefit from an in-depth review of leadership roles within pharmacy are encouraged to delve into the illustrated cases "Opportunities" and "Relationships" in Chapter 15 Administration.

After her brief presentation, Janine is right back to work within the ED, participating in goal-directed therapy and medication management activities before being interrupted by the code stroke described earlier. A more detailed description of stroke treatment highlights the importance of EM pharmacist's contributions to the use of high-risk medications. As stated in the Background section, high-risk medications can cause significant patient harm or death when used in error.[24] EM pharmacists ensure that high-risk medications like alteplase are administered appropriately. Many of these medications can be described as having a narrow therapeutic index; essentially, a small difference between a dose that will produce the desired effect and one that will lead to toxicity and potential harm.[54,55] In these situations, benefits and risks must be weighed against one another without the luxury of time to perform extensive research.

In high-income countries like the United States, stroke ranks second only to heart disease in terms of number of years lost to disability and premature death.[56] A stroke is a sudden interruption in the blood supply to the brain.[57] Most strokes, like the one experienced by the patient in this illustrated case, are classified as ischemic; meaning, they are caused by a blockage in one of the arteries in the brain that carries oxygen-rich blood, depriving that area of the brain of oxygen. Brain cell death from ischemia is rapid, hence the time pressures associated with a code stroke. Acute ischemic stroke is characterized by the sudden onset of focal neurological symptoms, such as impaired consciousness, difficulty speaking, and weakness.

In the ED, once a code stroke is paged out to the appropriate health professionals, a neurologist will conduct an assessment of the patient and lead the team's decision-making process and treatment strategy. The role of the EM pharmacist in these situations can vary based on the ED; generally speaking, though, it is to provide pertinent background information about the patient, such as pre-existing health conditions, medications the patient takes, and an assessment of the appropriateness of clot busting medication therapies such as alteplase. However, a cerebral clot cannot be distinguished from clinical signs and symptoms alone. In patients with suspected ischemic stroke, computed tomography (i.e., CT scan) or magnetic resonance imaging (i.e., MRI) of the brain is required to make the final diagnosis.[57] Illustration 10-4 is set in the CT room of the ED, where presumably a diagnosis of an ischemic stroke is made after imaging has been performed.

The American Heart Association (AHA) and the American Stroke Association (ASA) provide recommendations for the care of patients with suspected ischemic stroke.[58] Recommendations include several important goals related to time; for example, time from ED arrival to physician evaluation, time to activation of the code stroke, time to completion of CT scan, and time to initiation of thrombolytic (i.e., clot busting) therapy.[55] Since patients with suspected stroke are frequently managed within the ED, the role of the EM pharmacist is extremely important. Pharmacists are critical team members within the code stroke team, as they help facilitate timely assessment of the patient and timely administration of thrombolytic therapy.

Alteplase is a prime example of a medication with an extremely narrow therapeutic index that is also time dependent. This medication works by activating the conversion of an enzyme inside the body that is responsible for clot breakdown.[59] The clinical trial that led to alteplase's approval by the US Food and Drug Administration demonstrated that patients with acute ischemic stroke who received alteplase within 3 hours of symptom onset were less likely to be disabled at 3 months compared to patients who did not receive alteplase. However, alteplase use was also associated with intracranial hemorrhage for patients with certain characteristics, such as more severe neurological deficits at baseline and increased brain swelling.[60] It is critical for the EM team to evaluate patients with ischemic stroke for these risk factors, and to mitigate them when identified, in order to reduce the life-threatening risks associated with intracranial hemorrhage.

Absolute contraindications to receiving alteplase (i.e., reasons that would preclude its use) for acute ischemic stroke include the findings of significant bleeding in the brain, severe uncontrolled high blood pressure, a serious head trauma or stroke in the past 3 months, certain blood clotting disorders, and the recent use of any blood thinning medications that may still be having an effect in the body.[62] Relative contraindications to alteplase (i.e., reasons that should lead health professionals to exercise caution when considering its use) also exist, including advanced age, mild or improving stroke symptoms, recent major surgery, or dementia.[58,51–63] Difficult decision-making like this within the ED occurs frequently, and EM pharmacists must learn how to operate and be confident with their contributions to these decisions.

The illustrated case "One Day" closes with a process that is critical to the success of ED operations; namely, an effective hand-off.[64] The constant arrival, transfer, and discharge of patients in the ED persists on a 24/7 basis. When Janine's shift comes to an end in Illustration 10-12, she must collaborate with the incoming EM pharmacist who is replacing her. Several studies have shown that ineffective hand-offs increase opportunities for medical errors.[65,66] The objective of the hand-off is to provide accurate information about a patient's care, treatment or services, current condition, and any recent or anticipated changes.[64,66–68] Hand-offs can be completed using a variety of methods, including in writing through the electronic health record and verbally, as depicted in Illustration 10-12.

Interestingly, this EM pharmacist hand-off is interrupted by a code blue through the intercom system. The patient in question has experienced sudden cardiac arrest, and the emergency response team must head to the intensive care unit (ICU) to support Advanced Cardiac Life Support. Those interested in learning more about cardiovascular conditions and the role of cardiology pharmacists are encouraged to explore Chapter 5 Cardiology and the illustrated cases "Underlying Cause," "Educator," and "Empowerment." For more information and examples focused on ICUs and the role of critical care pharmacists, see Chapter 11 Critical Care and the illustrated cases "Shocking" and "Type 1."

For critically ill patients, initially treated and triaged in the ED who are about to transfer to another team or service within the hospital, the transfer process is essential to ensuring continuity of effective patient care. The absence of a structured transfer could lead to critical incidents or omissions in delivery of care. For critically ill patients who might be on various medications for sedation or pain, or started on antibiotics, timing and coordination of medications is critical. Pharmacists in the ED and ICU collaborate closely to minimize medication errors during the transfer process. It is important to note that initial ED care has downstream effects on subsequent care patients will receive after they are admitted to the hospital. The importance of effective communication at this stage of the process cannot be overstated.

Emergency medicine pharmacists are an integral part of the patient care team in emergency departments across the United States. The illustrated case "One Day" captures several high-impact practices of Dr. Janine Ori, one such EM pharmacist. Throughout the course of this single day, Janine leverages her knowledge and skills to identify an adverse drug event, support the work of administrative leaders, and contribute to the safe and effective use of medications. At the end of Janine's shift, during her hand-off to the incoming EM pharmacist, a new emergency paged over the ED intercom reinforces that, to succeed in this environment, EM pharmacists must remain flexible and calm as they prioritize, triage, and compartmentalize tasks in one of the fastest-paced environments in healthcare.

DISCUSSION QUESTIONS FOR "ONE DAY"

1. Interprofessional collaboration involving a nurse, pharmacist, physician, and physician assistant is shown in Illustration 10-7. What other health professionals can you identify who also work to improve patient care in the emergency department?

2. In Illustration 10-8, the pharmacist Janine is shown advocating for automated dispensing cabinets to leaders within the hospital tasked with improving quality of care and patient safety. After reading this illustrated case, what are some other initiatives you think an emergency medicine pharmacist might advocate for to improve quality and safety?

3. The emergency department can be a stressful environment with life and death situations occurring on a regular basis. Imagine for a moment that you are an emergency medicine pharmacist. What kinds of thoughts and/or emotions might you experience? Would you be able to compartmentalize, like the pharmacist Janine? Or is this something that might require additional education and/or training?

4. Many medications used in the emergency department, like alteplase in this illustrated case, have a narrow therapeutic index; meaning, there is a small difference between the dose required to produce a desired effect and one that will produce a toxic, potentially harmful one. As a result, the pressure on emergency medicine pharmacists to ensure the use of correct doses can be high. Reflect on this pressure; is this something that might motivate and excite you, or does it terrify you? Or both?

5. Illustration 10-12 depicts a pharmacist hand-off that is interrupted by a new emergency. It is implied that the hand-off will not be able to be completed. Brainstorm three possible negative consequences of this interruption for the patients in this illustrated case? How might Janine and her colleague prevent those from occurring?

CHAPTER SUMMARY

- Emergency medicine is a specialty field within healthcare dedicated to the prevention, diagnosis and treatment of unforeseen illness or injury affecting patients of all age groups.

- Emergency medicine pharmacy practice is a relatively new, distinct, and unique specialty area within pharmacy that focuses on rapid assessment of available patient data to optimize medication use in one of the most fast-paced environments in healthcare.

- Interprofessional teamwork in the emergency department provides the backbone for safe, effective, and efficient patient care.

- Emergency medicine pharmacists play many important roles as contributing members of interprofessional teams, ranging from consultative services at the patient's bedside to administrative tasks dedicated to optimizing emergency department workflows.

- While emergency medicine pharmacists are experts in the appropriate and safe use of high-risk medications that have little room for dosing errors, they must also keep up to date on a wide range of other disease states and medication therapies.

- EM pharmacists experience life or death situations routinely and manage the emotional and physical stress of these situations through various coping strategies.

- Multitasking and prioritization are essential skills to manage the challenging and unpredictable nature of the emergency department, from which many emergency medicine pharmacists derive energy and professional satisfaction.

REFERENCES

1. American Board of Emergency Medicine: ABEM history. Available at https://www.abem.org/public/about-abem/abem-history. Accessed February 11, 2020.

2. Ramsay N. EMRA match 2020 by the numbers. Available at https://www.emra.org/students/newsletter-articles/em-match-2020-by-the-numbers/. Accessed May 5, 2020.

3. American Society of Health-System Pharmacists. Participating PGY2-emergency medicine programs. Available at https://natmatch.com/ashprmp/directory-archive/pharm69-ph1.html. Accessed May 5, 2020.

4. Board of Pharmacy Specialties. Emergency medicine pharmacy recognized as new specialty. Available at https://www.bpsweb.org/2020/02/21/emergency-medicine-pharmacy-recognized-as-new-specialty/. Accessed May 5, 2020.

5. Yale School of Medicine. What is emergency medicine? Available at https://web.archive.org/web/20101119080037/http://medicine.yale.edu/emergencymed/whatis.aspx. Accessed February 11, 2020.

6. Robertson-Steel IRS. Evolution of triage systems. *Emerg Med J.* 2006;23(2):154-155.

7. Zibulewsky J. The emergency medical treatment and active labor act (EMTALA): What It Is and What It Means for Physicians. *Baylor Univ Med Cent Proc.* 2001;14(4):339-346.

8. Gwinnutt CL, Driscoll P. Advanced trauma life support. *Anaesthesia.* 1993;48(5):441-442, author reply 442-443.

9. Green NA, Durani Y, Brecher D, DePiero A, Loiselle J, Attia M. Emergency Severity Index version 4: a valid and reliable tool in pediatric emergency department triage. *Pediatr Emerg Care.* 2012;28(8):753-757.

10. HealthData.gov. Hospital emergency department—diagnosis, procedure, and external cause codes. Available at https://healthdata.gov/dataset/hospital-emergency-department-diagnosis-procedure-and-external-cause-codes. Accessed May 28, 2020.

11. Kobayashi KJ, Knuesel SJ, White BbA, et al. Impact on length of stay of a hospital medicine emergency department boarder service. *J Hosp Med.* 2019;14:E1-E7.

12. Shareef M, Craine PL, Bern AI. Ch. 17—Advanced practice providers in the ED. In: Emergency Medicine Advocacy Handbook. Available at https://www.emra.org/books/advocacy-handbook/advanced-providers/. Accessed May 28, 2020.

13. American Association for Respiratory Care. What it's like to be an emergency department RT. Available at https://www.aarc.org/careers/career-advice/professional-development/like-rt-ed/. Accessed May 28, 2020.

14. Van Pelt J. Making care connections, cutting costs—social work in the emergency department. *Soc Work Today.* 2010;10(6):12.

15. Rudis MI, Attwood RJ. Emergency medicine pharmacy practice. *J Pharm Pract.* 2011;24(2):135-145.

16. Eppert HD, Reznek AJ. Overview of ASHP guidelines on emergency medicine pharmacist services. *Am J Heal Pharm.* 2011;68(23):2296.

17. Morgan SR, Acquisto NM, Coralic Z, et al. Clinical pharmacy services in the emergency department. *Am J Emerg Med.* 2018;36(10):1727-1732.

18. American College of Emergency Physicians. Clinical pharmacist services in the emergency department. Available at https://www.acep.org/globalassets/new-pdfs/policy-statements/clinical-pharmacist-services-in-the-emergency-department.pdf. Accessed May 28, 2020.

19. Sin B, Lau K, Tong R, et al. The feasibility and impact of prospective medication review in the emergency department. *J Pharm Pract.* 2018;31(1):22-28.

20. Reynolds SF, Heffner J. Airway management of the critically ill patient: rapid-sequence intubation. *Chest.* 2005;127(4):1397-1412.

21. Stollings JL, Diedrich DA, Oyen LJ, Brown DR. Rapid-sequence intubation: a review of the process and considerations when choosing medications. *Ann Pharmacother.* 2014;48(1):62-76.

22. Masic D, Hidalgo DC, Kuhrau S, Chaney W, Rech MA. Pharmacist presence decreases time to prothrombin complex concentrate in emergency department patients with life-threatening bleeding and urgent procedures. *J Emerg Med.* 2019;57(5):620-628.

23. Frontera JA, Lewin JJ, Rabinstein AA, et al. Guideline for reversal of antithrombotics in intracranial hemorrhage: a statement for healthcare professionals from the neurocritical care society and society of critical care medicine. *Neurocrit Care.* 2016;24(1):6-46.

24. Institute for Safe Medication Practices. High-alert medications in acute care settings. Available at https://www.ismp.org/recommendations/high-alert-medications-acute-list. Accessed May 28, 2020.

25. Panigrahi B, Jones BC, Rowe SP. Brodifacoum-contaminated synthetic marijuana: clinical and radiologic manifestations of a public health outbreak causing life-threatening coagulopathy. *Emerg Radiol.* 2018;25(6):715-718.

26. Wang F, Ma Z, Wu X, Liu L. Allopurinol-induced toxic epidermal necrolysis featuring almost 60% skin detachment. *Medicine.* 2019;98(25):e16078.

27. Yu KH, Yu CY, Fang YF. Diagnostic utility of HLA-B*5801 screening in severe allopurinol hypersensitivity syndrome: an updated systematic review and meta-analysis. *Int J Rheum Dis.* 2017;20(9):1057-1071.

28. American society of health-system pharmacists. Residency information. Available at https://www.ashp.org/Professional-Development/Residency-Information?loginreturnUrl=SSO CheckOnly. Accessed May 20, 2020.

29. Board of pharmacy specialties. Available at https://www.bpsweb.org. Accessed May 28, 2020.

30. American board of clinical toxicology (ABAT). American academy of clinical toxicology. Available at https://www.clintox.org/resources/abat. Accessed May 28, 2020.

31. American foundation for suicide prevention. Suicide facts & figures: United States 2020. Available at https://chapterland.org/wp-content/uploads/sites/13/2017/11/US_FactsFigures_Flyer.pdf. Accessed May 28, 2020.

32. National institute of mental health. Suicide. Available at https://www.nimh.nih.gov/health/statistics/suicide.shtml. Accessed May 28, 2020.

33. Gummin DD, Mowry JB, Spyker DA, et al. 2018 annual report of the American association of poison control centers' national poison data system (NPDS): 36th annual report. *Clin Toxicol.* 2019;57(12):1220-1413.

34. Cobaugh DJ, Gainor C, Gaston CL, et al. The opioid abuse and misuse epidemic: Implications for pharmacists in hospitals and health systems. *Am J Heal Pharm.* 2014;71(18):1539-1554.

35. Chisholm-Burns MA, Spivey CA, Sherwin E, Wheeler J, Hohmeier K. The opioid crisis: origins, trends, policies, and the roles of pharmacists. *Am J Heal Pharm.* 2019;76(7):424-435.

36. Hoffman JR, Schriger DL, Luo JS. The empiric use of naloxone in patients with altered mental status: a reappraisal. *Ann Emerg Med.* 1991;20(3):246-252.

37. Narcan (naloxone hydrochloride) nasal spray [package insert]. Radnor, PA: Adapt Pharma, Inc.; 2020.

38. Chou R, Korthuis PT, McCarty D, et al. Management of suspected opioid overdose with naloxone by emergency medical services personnel [Internet]. Rockville (MD): Agency for Healthcare Research and Quality (US); 2017 Nov. (Comparative Effectiveness Reviews, No. 193.) Introduction. Available at https://www.ncbi.nlm.nih.gov/books/NBK487465/. Accessed May 28, 2020.

39. Neumar RW, Shuster M, Callaway CW, et al. Part 1: Executive summary: 2015 American Heart Association guidelines update for cardiopulmonary resuscitation and emergency cardiovascular care. *Circulation.* 2015;132(18 Suppl 2):S315-S367.

40. American Heart Association. Highlights of the 2015 American Heart Association guidelines update for CPR and ECC. Available at https://eccguidelines.heart.org/wp-content/uploads/2015/10/2015-AHA-Guidelines-Highlights-English.pdf. Accessed May 28, 2020.

41. American Heart Association. Highlights of the 2018 focused updates to the American Heart Association guidelines for CPR and EEC: advanced cardiovascular life support and pediatric advanced life support. Available at https://eccguidelines.heart.org/wp-content/uploads/2018/10/2018-Focused-Updates_Highlights.pdf. Accessed May 28, 2020.

42. Draper HM, Eppert JA. Association of pharmacist presence on compliance with advanced cardiac life support guidelines during in-hospital cardiac arrest. *Ann Pharmacother.* 2008;42(4):469-474.

43. Moskowitz A, Ross CE, Andersen LW, Grossestreuer AV, Berg KM, Donnino MW. Trends over time in drug administration during adult in-hospital cardiac arrest. *Crit Care Med.* 2019;47(2):194-200.

44. Velissaris D, Karamouzos V, Pierrakos C, Koniari I, Apostolopoulou C, Karanikolas M. Use of sodium bicarbonate in cardiac arrest: current guidelines and literature review. *J Clin Med Res.* 2016;8(4):277-283.

45. Lockey AS, Hardern RD. Decision making by emergency physicians when assessing cardiac arrest patients on arrival at hospital. *Resuscitation.* 2001;50(1):51-56.

46. Jabre P, Belpomme V, Azoulay E, et al. Family presence during cardiopulmonary resuscitation. *N Engl J Med.* 2013;368(11):1008-1018.

47. Lycette J. Making Room. *JAMA.* 2018;319(24):2479-2480.

48. Abraham LJ, Thom O, Greenslade JH, et al. Morale, stress and coping strategies of staff working in the emergency department: A comparison of two different-sized departments. *Emerg Med Australas.* 2018;30(3):375-381.

49. Blair R. 5 steps of compartmentalization: the secret behind successful entrepreneurs. Available at https://www.forbes.com/sites/ryanblair/2012/06/26/5-steps-of-compartmentalization/#57c9ed4d1a62. Accessed May 20, 2020.

50. American Society of Health-System Pharmacists. Draft ASHP guidelines on emergency medicine pharmacist services. Available at https://www.ashp.org/-/media/assets/policy-guidelines/docs/draft-guidelines/draft-guidelines-emergency-medicine-pharmacy-services.ashx?la=en&hash=E4D3618CEAEAD7786377053970D4EF81E8DF2EED. Accessed May 28, 2020.

51. Johnston R, Saulnier L, Gould O. Best possible medication history in the emergency department: comparing pharmacy technicians and pharmacists. *Can J Hosp Pharm.* 2010;63(5):359-365.

52. De winter S, Spriet I, Indevuyst C, et al. Pharmacist- versus physician-acquired medication history: a prospective study at the emergency department. *Qual Saf Health Care.* 2010;19(5):371-375.

53. Lombardi N, Lucenteforte E, Torrini M, et al. Ticagrelor-related late-onset dyspnea as cause of emergency department visit: a 3-year outpatient study. *J Cardiovasc Med.* 2018;19(6):284-289.

54. Tamargo J, Le heuzey JY, Mabo P. Narrow therapeutic index drugs: a clinical pharmacological consideration to flecainide. *Eur J Clin Pharmacol.* 2015;71(5):549-67.

55. Cesarz JL, Steffenhagen AL, Svenson J, Hamedani AG. Emergency department discharge prescription interventions by emergency medicine pharmacists. *Ann Emerg Med.* 2013;61(2):209-214.

56. Lopez AD, Mathers CD, Ezzati M, Jamison DT, Murray CJ. Global and regional burden of disease and risk factors, 2001: systematic analysis of population health data. *Lancet.* 2006;367:1747-1757.

57. Brott T, Adams HP Jr, Olinger CP, et al. Measurements of acute cerebral infarction: a clinical examination scale. *Stroke.* 1989;20:864-870.

58. Powers WJ, Rabinstein AA, Ackerson T, et al. 2018 Guidelines for the early management of patients with acute ischemic

stroke: A guideline for healthcare professionals from the american heart association/american stroke association. *Stroke.* 2018;49(3):e46-e110.

59. National institute of neurological disorders and stroke rt-PA stroke study group. Tissue plasminogen activator for acute ischemic stroke. *N Engl J Med.* 1995;333(24):1581-1587.

60. Fugate JE, Rabinstein AA. Absolute and relative contraindications to IV rt-PA for acute ischemic stroke. *Neurohospitalist.* 2015;5(3):110-121.

61. Demaerschalk BM, Kleindorfer DO, Adeoye OM, et al. Scientific rationale for the inclusion and exclusion criteria for intravenous alteplase in acute ischemic stroke: a statement for healthcare professionals from the American heart association/american stroke association. *Stroke.* 2016;47(2):581-641.

62. Micieli G, Marcheselli S, Tosi PA. Safety and efficacy of alteplase in the treatment of acute ischemic stroke. *Vasc Health Risk Manag.* 2009;5(1):397-409.

63. Van der worp HB, Van gijn J. Clinical practice. Acute ischemic stroke. *N Engl J Med.* 2007;357(6):572-579.

64. Arora V, Johnson J. A model for building a standardized hand-off protocol. *Jt Comm J Qual Patient Saf.* 2006;32(11):646-655.

65. Gephart SM. The art of effective handoffs: what is the evidence? *Adv Neonatal Care.* 2012;12(1):37-39.

66. Sutcliffe KM, Lewton E, Rosenthal MM. Communication failures: an insidious contributor to medical mishaps. *Acad Med.* 2004;79(2):186-194.

67. Volpp KG, Grande D. Residents' suggestions for reducing errors in teaching hospitals. *N Engl J Med.* 2003;348(9):851-855.

68. Mcfetridge B, Gillespie M, Goode D, Melby V. An exploration of the handover process of critically ill patients between nursing staff from the emergency department and the intensive care unit. *Nurs Crit Care.* 2007;12(6):261-269.

CHAPTER 11

Critical Care

Featuring the Illustrated Case Studies "Shocking" & "Type 1"

Authors

Jeffrey T. Fish, Chloe R. Schmidt, & Joseph A. Zorek

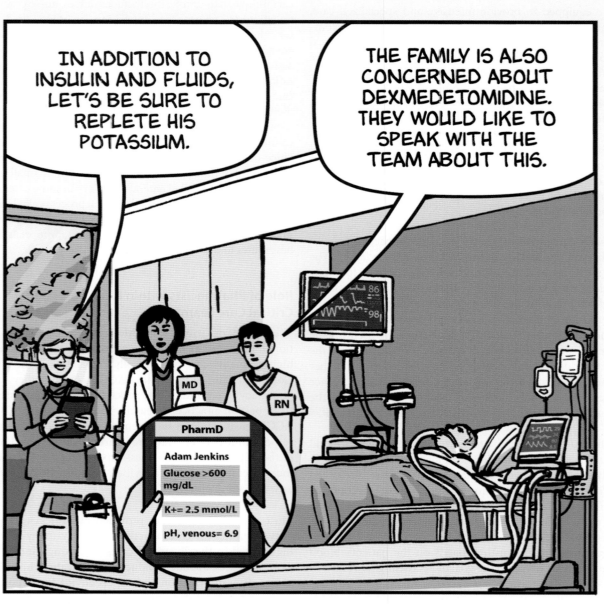

Illustration by George Folz, © 2020 McGraw-Hill Education

BACKGROUND

Critical care is a field in healthcare devoted to managing patients having, or at risk of having, acute life-threatening failure of organs, such as the lungs, heart, and kidneys.[1] The terms "critical care" and "intensive care" are used interchangeably to describe this specialized area of practice. Essentially, critical care specialists from a host of different professions provide care for the sickest of all patients. The most prevalent health conditions treated in this setting are respiratory failure, acute myocardial infarction (i.e., heart attack), and head bleed or stroke.[2] The primary goals are to stabilize the patient (i.e., prevent their condition from worsening), determine the underlying causes of the illness/problem if unknown, and begin treatment to correct identified issues.[1]

Critically ill patients are cared for in intensive care units (ICUs), which are areas of the hospital dedicated to the management and monitoring of patients with life-threatening conditions. ICUs are equipped to provide intensive and specialized care, including organ support.[1,3] Several types of equipment are commonly used in ICUs to accomplish this, including mechanical ventilators to support breathing, extracorporeal membrane oxygenators (ECMOs) to maintain heart and lung function, and hemodialysis machines to filter the blood when kidney function declines or stops.[1] Patients with severe head injuries due to an accident may have a monitor placed inside their head, while patients with other conditions may have tubes inserted into their chest attached to suction to drain excessive fluid buildup.[1] As shown in the illustrated cases "Shocking" and "Type 1" later in this chapter, bedside monitors display real-time data on blood pressure, heart rate, breathing rate, amount of oxygen in the blood, and body temperature.

Use of such equipment can have profound impacts on medication therapy, particularly in the setting of kidney failure. The kidneys are a major route of elimination from the body for many medications used in critically ill patients, particularly antibiotics.[4] Underdosing antibiotics is associated with treatment failure, and overdosing antibiotics is associated with adverse effects.[5] Cefepime (Maxipime) is an antibiotic commonly used for the treatment of severe infections, and 85% of it is cleared from the body by the kidneys.[6] Patients with kidney failure are at a higher risk of adverse effects including confusion and seizures.[7] Since cefepime is cleared by hemodialysis machines, determining the right dose in critically ill patients with kidney failure is difficult.[7,8]

The ability to monitor real-time data on blood pressure and heart rate has important implications for drug therapy, as well. Critically ill patients can develop low blood pressure, also called shock, from certain diseases; for example, severe infections or heart failure.[9] Patients who develop shock are at an increased risk of dying.[9] Medications called vasopressors are used to increase blood pressure.[9] Bedside monitors allow nurses to titrate vasopressors in real-time based on the patient's blood pressure and heart rate with the goal of decreasing mortality.[9]

Working as a critical care pharmacist is challenging and rewarding. The life-or-death circumstances within which the ICU team operates drives a sense of unity and tends to bring out the best in people, particularly those who thrive under pressure. As recognized medication experts with access to an incredible amount of real-time data, from both the life-saving machines and monitors mentioned above, to frequent blood tests that reveal clues about the effects of various medications, critical care pharmacists have many opportunities throughout the course of a single day to contribute meaningfully to patient care. There is great satisfaction derived by all team members when a critically ill patient recovers and is able to leave the ICU with their loved ones.

Members of the Interprofessional Critical Care Team

ICU teams are typically led by a specialty-trained physician called an intensivist.[10,11] Other members of the ICU team come from a host of health professions, each with specialized training in critical care unique to their role; this includes nurses, nurse practitioners, nutritionists, pharmacists, physician assistants, and respiratory therapists.[1,2] High-level ICUs usually have intensivists and advanced practice providers (e.g., nurse practitioners, physician assistants) in the hospital 24 hours a day, with nurse-to-patient ratios of 1:1 or 1:2 at all times to account for the amount of nursing care ICU patients require.[1] Respiratory therapists contribute their expertise in support of ventilator management for patients requiring breathing support, including assistance with insertion (intubation) and removal (extubation) of tubes into the lungs.[12] Since intubated patients cannot swallow food, they are usually fed through a tube placed into their stomach or small intestines through a process called enteral nutrition. In some cases, patients are fed directly into their vein through a process called parenteral nutrition. ICU nutritionists contribute their expertise by determining needs as it relates to caloric intake, appropriate diet, and best routes to deliver nutrition.

Role of Pharmacists within Interprofessional Critical Care Teams

The Society of Critical Care Medicine (SCCM) is an international, interprofessional organization that seeks to achieve the highest quality care for critically ill patients.[13] The American College of Clinical Pharmacy (ACCP), on the other hand, is a pharmacy organization that seeks to help pharmacists achieve their best in practice, research, and education.[14] SCCM and ACCP released a joint statement detailing recommended roles/responsibilities of critical care pharmacists as valued members of the ICU team.[15] These roles/responsibilities are divided into four different pharmacy activities: clinical, educational, scholarly, and administrative.[16]

Most patient care services provided by critical care pharmacists fall under the clinical activity category, many of which are highlighted in the illustrated cases "Shocking" and "Type 1."[15] Core activities include conducting medication histories, providing drug information and expert advice to support clinical decision making, intervening to optimize medication therapies, determining effective routes of medication delivery and, when patients are stabilized, transitioning to medications and formulations suitable for non-ICU settings (e.g., general care hospital floors, home).

During hospitalization, medication administration can be complicated by several factors. Often, pharmacists play a key role in determining alternative routes to administer drugs and figuring out which home medications to hold versus resume. For example, a mechanically ventilated, sedated patient will not be able to swallow tablets and capsules orally. Typically, a tube is temporarily inserted through either the nose or mouth directly into the patient's stomach (nasogastric or orogastric, respectively). Many medications can be crushed, mixed with water, and administered down these tubes. There are times, however, when administering medications directly into a patient's stomach is not advised. Additionally, some drugs are not safe to crush and deliver via tube.[17] In other situations, drug manufacturers advise against opening capsules. When faced with these situations, critical care pharmacists must put their knowledge, skills, and creativity to work to identify alternative routes of delivery for medically necessary medications. One example involves isavuconazole (Cresemba), a broad-spectrum antifungal medication. At one hospital, physicians and pharmacists reviewed patients who had isavuconazole capsules opened and given via nasogastric tube and found that administration of the opened capsule produced drug levels comparable to patients swallowing the capsule whole.[18] Data like these help pharmacists determine which capsules can be opened and administered nasogastrically, as well as those that need to be given via another route of administration.

Critical care pharmacists assess medication routes on a daily basis. Generally speaking, patients whose conditions require treatment in the ICU will receive most medications intravenously (i.e., directly into the patient's blood through their vein, also referred to as IV). One reason is that medications start working faster via this route, as the time spent waiting for absorption into the blood through the intestines is bypassed. Studies have also shown that orally administered medications are poorly absorbed in critically ill patients; meaning, much of the drug that is swallowed (or delivered directly to the stomach via a tube) does not get absorbed into the blood.[19]

Some medications, such as the antiepileptic levetiracetam (Keppra), which is used to treat and prevent seizures, have excellent oral absorption.[20] In these cases, medication doses can be converted from oral to IV or from IV to oral using a 1:1 conversion. For example, a 500 mg tablet of levetiracetam is approximately equivalent to a 500 mg IV-administered dose. That said, this is not the case for the vast majority of medications. Furosemide, a medication used to eliminate excess fluid retention in many critical care situations, is only partially absorbed when given orally. Critical care pharmacists, therefore, must ensure a 50% reduction in furosemide dose when switching from oral to IV.[21] Likewise, when transitioning from IV to oral furosemide, critical care pharmacists must ensure

Table 11-1. Common Routes of Medication Administration in the Critical Care Setting	
Route	**Description**
Intranasal	Delivered onto the nasal mucosa
Intramuscular	Injected into the muscle
Intraosseous	Injected into the bone marrow
Intrathecal	Injected into the spinal canal
Nasogastric	Delivered via tube through the nose into the stomach
Orogastric	Delivered via tube through the mouth into the stomach
Rectal	Placed into the rectum
Subcutaneous	Injected below the skin
Sublingual	Placed under the tongue

that the dose gets doubled to account for partial absorption via the oral route. Other medication routes that are employed in the ICU setting are shown in Table 11-1.[22] Critical care pharmacists must develop a deep knowledge base of each of these routes, as well as the requisite dose conversions when changing from one route to another.

Critical care pharmacists also respond to resuscitation events throughout the hospital when a patient does not have a pulse or when their blood pressure drops to a level that is insufficient to perfuse and sustain organ function. During these events, the pharmacist is responsible for managing medications, which includes recommending optimal therapies, determining appropriate doses, and preparing medications so they can be administered. Those interested in a more in-depth exploration of advanced cardiac life support (ACLS), including the role of pharmacists, are encouraged to read the illustrated case "Life & Death" in Chapter 10 Emergency Medicine.

Optimizing medication therapies based on real-time data is another core function of critical care pharmacists. This activity is exemplified by a process called pharmacokinetic monitoring.[23] Broadly speaking, the term *pharmacokinetics* refers to how a drug moves in the body, which determines how much of it is in the blood at a given time and, thus, able to exert the desired effect. Certain medications have a narrow therapeutic index; in other words, there is a small difference between a dose that will provide the desired response and a dose that will cause toxicity. Critical care pharmacists perform pharmacokinetic calculations using a host of variables to figure out the safest dose possible. These variables include the half-life of the drug (i.e., the amount of time it takes for half of the drug to be eliminated from the body), the time it was administered, the time the blood sample was drawn to measure the amount of drug present, and the patient's kidney function.

Critical care pharmacists also serve on hospital committees designed to optimize ICU medication use through the development of guidelines and protocols.[15,16] These tools help prescribers order the most beneficial medications to maximize patient outcomes and minimize the risk of side effects. Critical care pharmacists provide education about these guidelines and protocols, as well as other medication-related topics, to other health professionals on the ICU team. This includes health professionals in training, such as students, residents, and fellows. Such educational activities can be informal, such as a bedside discussion during interprofessional rounds, or formal, such as a lecture to Doctor of Pharmacy (PharmD) students. Since the ICU offers many opportunities for learning, critical care pharmacists train a lot of pharmacy students, residents, and fellows during rotations in the ICU. Some critical care pharmacists also teach about medications in ACLS classes certified by the American Heart Association.

It is important for health professionals in the ICU to systematically study their activities and interventions, in order to share impactful practices with colleagues throughout the United States and globally via professional presentations and publications.[15,16] Critical care pharmacists play an important role in such scholarly activities, which may include the supervision of investigational medications (i.e., medications actively being studied for potential approval by the US Food and Drug Administration). Pharmacists in the ICU also conduct their own research projects, where they design studies, collect and analyze data, and publish results in the pharmacy and/or biomedical literature. These research projects are used locally and elsewhere to improve the care of critically ill patients.

CRITICAL CARE PHARMACISTS IN ACTION

Decreasing Use of ICU Medications at Discharge

Critically ill intubated patients have an increased risk of developing a gastrointestinal bleed, called a stress ulcer, during their ICU stay.[24] These stress ulcers may be associated with coughing up blood, decreased blood pressure, increased heart rate, and potentially the need for a blood transfusion.[24] Experts suggest using medications that decrease stomach acid in intubated patients to prevent stress ulcers.[25] It is also recommended that these medications be discontinued once the patient is extubated. Long-term use of these medications is associated with health risks, such as the development of an infectious diarrhea caused by the bacteria *Clostridioides difficile*, also known as *C. difficile* or *C. diff*, and pneumonia.[25] An early study showed that nearly 25% of patients who had medications started for stress ulcer prophylaxis in the ICU were discharged home on these medications without a reason to continue them.[26] A critical care pharmacist led an initiative to decrease the continuation of stress ulcer prophylaxis medications at discharge, which included direct communication with physicians and pharmacists in the hospital, development of educational resources describing best practices, and delivery of presentations to all pharmacists within the hospital.[27] After the initiative, inappropriate prescribing of stress ulcer prophylaxis medications decreased by over 60%.

Protecting Patients' Kidneys

Critically ill patients on mechanical ventilation may need medications to keep them calm.[28] One of the calming medications

that can be used is lorazepam (Ativan). Lorazepam is administered intravenously. In order to be administered via this route, lorazepam is dissolved in a substance called propylene glycol. A critical care pharmacist, in the course of regular drug monitoring, noticed a pattern in which eight patients receiving IV lorazepam developed kidney failure. Case reports within the published biomedical literature suggested that high levels of propylene glycol in IV lorazepam were likely associated with kidney failure. Based on this literature, lorazepam was switched to other calming agents that were dissolved using substances other than propylene glycol. After this intervention, seven of the eight patients had their kidney function return to normal. New ICU protocols within the institution were developed as a result, whereby all patients receiving IV lorazepam for ventilator-associated sedation were required to have their blood drawn to monitor kidney function and prevent such kidney injury.[29]

BECOMING A CRITICAL CARE PHARMACIST

All critical care pharmacists practice in hospital settings. After graduating from a PharmD program accredited by the Accreditation Council for Pharmacy Education (ACPE), most pharmacists interested in critical care complete a general post-graduate year 1 (PGY-1) residency gearing their rotations toward critical care.[30,31] These rotations include different types of ICUs within the hospital (medical, surgical, cardiac, pediatric, and neurology), as well as the emergency department and training in infectious diseases. The PGY-1 residency builds on education received during the PharmD degree to contribute to the advanced development of clinical pharmacists. Most PGY-1 residents interested in a career in critical care complete a post-graduate year 2 (PGY-2) residency dedicated exclusively to critical care.[31] This 1-year residency provides intense training under the guidance of an experienced critical care pharmacist.

Many employers also look for specific credentialing to demonstrate advanced knowledge and expertise to optimize critical care patient outcomes.[32] The Board of Pharmacy Specialties offers a nationally recognized credential called the Board Certified Critical Care Pharmacist (BCCCP).[32] To obtain BCCCP status, pharmacists must achieve a passing score on the Critical Care Pharmacy Specialty Certification Examination. In order to qualify for the examination, pharmacists must have graduated from an ACPE-accredited program (or international equivalent) and have a current license/registration to practice pharmacy in the United States or another jurisdiction. They must also demonstrate practice experience via one of the following pathways: 4 years of critical care practice experience, completion of a PGY-1 residency plus 2 additional years of practice experience, or completion of a PGY-2 residency in critical care pharmacy. Practice experience must include at least 50% of time spent in critical care. In order to maintain BCCCP certification, individuals must either earn 100 hours of BCCCP continuing education credit or achieve a passing score on a recertification exam in the seventh year following initial certification.

SHOCKING: An Illustrated Case Study

Story by Jeffrey T. Fish & Joseph A. Zorek
Illustrations by George Folz, © 2019 Board of Regents of the University of Wisconsin System

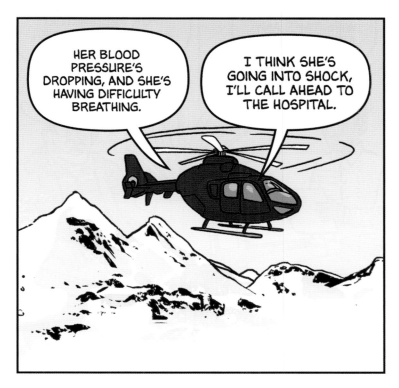

Illustration 11-1

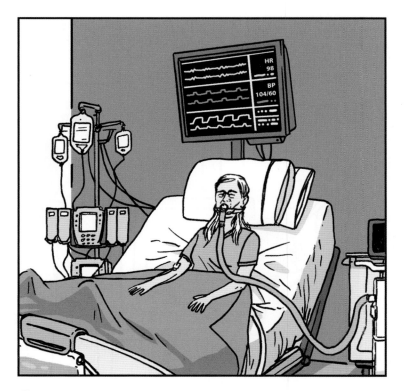

Illustration 11-2

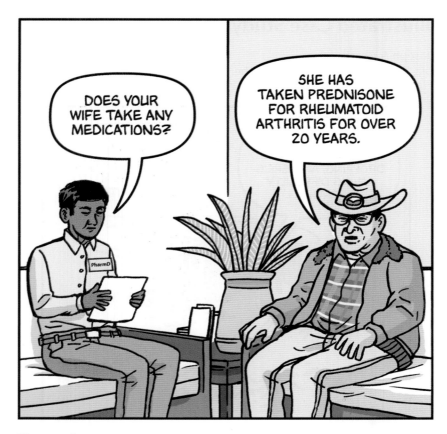

Illustration 11-3

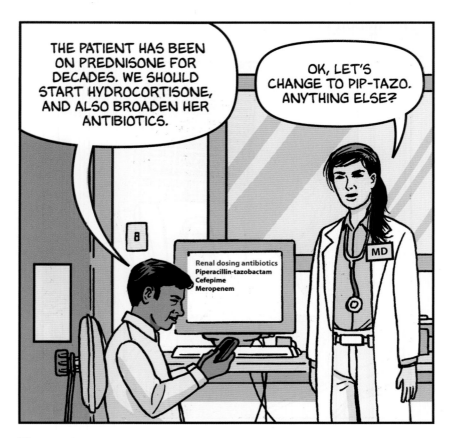

Illustration 11-4

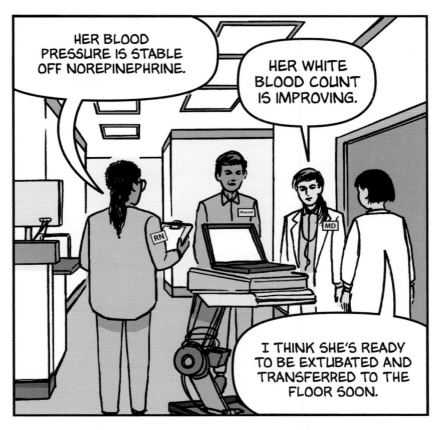

Illustration 11-5

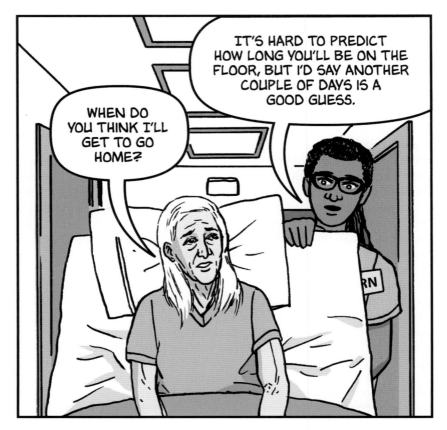

Illustration 11-6

Thoughts on "Shocking"

The illustrated case "Shocking" tells the story of a couple in their 70s from a rural part of the United States. Unexpectedly, they find themselves being life-flighted to a city with a hospital capable of treating the most severe, complex conditions. Unbeknownst to the couple, what started as a mild cough for the wife had quickly progressed to pneumonia, a bacterial infection of the lungs. By the time the couple arrived at their local hospital for care, the wife was experiencing some difficulty breathing and was feeling dizzy and disoriented. Fortunately, the physician and nurse at their local hospital recognized symptoms consistent with sepsis. Fearful that their patient's condition might further deteriorate, they made the difficult decision to transfer her to a hospital in a large urban setting. Illustration 11-1 picks up the story mid-flight, where the crew radios into the receiving hospital their assessment that the wife is developing septic shock. While not depicted, the husband is understandably terrified that he may be witnessing the end of his wife's life.

In US rural hospitals, 3% of all emergency department visits result in transfer to another hospital.[33] Rural hospitals are defined by their location in nonmetropolitan counties and include rural towns with populations less than 2500 people and areas with populations of 2500 to 49,999 that are not part of larger labor market areas.[34] The main reasons patients are transferred include advanced heart issues, strokes and head injuries, trauma, and other conditions necessitating critical care.[35] For those who become critically ill, rural hospitals serve a vitally important role stabilizing patients and starting time-sensitive therapies. For more information on the role of pharmacists in rural settings, readers are encouraged to explore the illustrated case "Breathe" in Chapter 2 Community Pharmacy.

Advanced care begins as soon as the patient boards the transport aircraft, as the medical crew on board usually consist of a specialty trained critical care nurse and a paramedic or physician, essentially bridging the specialized critical care needed in these emergency situations until arriving at the destination.[36] Patients, like the main character in "Shocking," are transferred to be cared for by physicians called intensivists and a team of health professionals who also have specialized training in their respective professions; this includes advanced practice providers, nurses, pharmacists, respiratory therapists, nutritionists, and social workers.[2] The provision of critical care by intensivist-led interprofessional teams is associated with up to $13 million in annual hospital cost savings.[2] High-level intensivist staffing is associated with a 30% reduction in death in the hospital and a 40% reduction in death in the intensive care unit (ICU).[37] Patients with severe infections have better outcomes when treated in facilities that treat higher numbers of critically ill patients; hence, the importance of helicopter transport for the main character in "Shocking."[38]

The main character in this illustrated case is suffering from septic shock, a severe form of sepsis.[39,40] Sepsis is a life-threatening condition that occurs when a localized infection (i.e., one that is isolated to one part of the body, such as the lungs, kidneys, skin, abdomen, or elsewhere) escapes into the bloodstream. In response, the body mounts a major defense, essentially triggering a chain reaction in the patient's body that can result in severe injury to tissues and organs. One of the characteristic markers of sepsis is lactate, a substance released by tissues and organs when they are not getting enough oxygen.[39,40] The "shock" component enters into the equation when this chain reaction is so severe that the patient experiences an inability to maintain a blood pressure high enough to adequately perfuse (i.e., oxygenate) vital organs. Septic shock substantially increases the risk of death, and immediate action is required to save patients' lives. Each year, at least 1.7 million American adults develop sepsis, and nearly 270,000, or roughly 16%, die. Staggeringly, of all patients who die in hospitals, one in three have sepsis as a contributing factor.[40] The main risk factors associated with the development of sepsis include the following:

1. Adults over 65 years old or children less than 1 year old
2. People with chronic health issues like diabetes, cancer, lung disease, or kidney disease
3. People whose immune systems are weakened by the medications they take

The signs and symptoms of sepsis include increased heart rate, fever, confusion, shortness of breath, extreme pain, and clammy or sweaty skin.[40] To diagnose sepsis, clinicians will look at the patient's signs and symptoms, and they will draw blood to look for increased white blood cells and lactate. White blood cells are one part of the immune system, and these can become extremely elevated in the setting of sepsis.[40] A sample from the primary site of infection is taken to determine the causative organism; in other words, the type of microorganism (bacteria, virus, fungi) that is causing the sepsis.[40] Sometimes samples are obtained by swabbing an external skin infection. When the infection is growing under the skin (e.g., in the abdomen or inside of a kidney), a needle is inserted into the area in order to pull out, or aspirate, the sample. Samples are called cultures and health professionals called medical laboratory scientists test them in a hospital laboratory. See the illustrated cases "Wounded" and "Superinfection" in Chapter 8 Infectious Diseases for more information on infections and the complexities associated with antibiotic therapies. For a more in-depth exploration of the immune system, read the illustrated case "Compromising" in Chapter 9 Oncology.

An international initiative called the Surviving Sepsis Campaign (SSC) was started to decrease high death rates associated with sepsis.[41] SSC promotes the "Hour-1 Bundle," which is a short set of guidelines intended to improve outcomes.[42] For patients with sepsis or septic shock, time is of the essence; hence, the wise decision by the rural hospital staff to initiate helicopter transport of the main character in "Shocking" for intensivist care. Importantly, while not explicitly stated, all of the following elements of the Hour-1 Bundle were also started in the rural hospital prior to her transport, which likely contributed to the ultimately positive outcome:

1. Measure a lactate level in the blood;

2. Obtain blood cultures prior to giving medications to treat the infection (e.g., antibiotics);

3. Administer antibiotics that treat multiple different organisms (i.e., broad-spectrum antibiotics);

4. Begin giving fluid rapidly into the patient's blood to treat low blood pressure (i.e., IV fluid resuscitation); and

5. Start medications to raise blood pressure (i.e., vasopressors) if the patient's blood pressure is low during or after fluid resuscitation.

The importance of appropriate medication selection, dosing, and monitoring in the setting of septic shock cannot be overstated (Table 11-2).[43] Critical care pharmacists, therefore, perform vitally important roles on the interprofessional critical care team.

A lot has happened to the main character between Illustrations 11-1 and 11-2. In addition to receiving fluid resuscitation with lactated ringers at the rural hospital prior to transport, staff there also drew blood cultures and started broad-spectrum antibiotics in the form of ceftriaxone and vancomycin. In response to the precipitous drop in blood pressure experienced

en route to the urban hospital during transport, the flight crew also started norepinephrine. This team also gave her oxygen via a mask to assist with breathing. Fortunately, Illustration 11-2 depicts the patient in a stable condition, one in which her situation is no longer life-threatening. Hanging on the medication poles in Illustration 11-2 are bags of IV lactated ringers, norepinephrine, and vancomycin, all of which are flowing into a vein in her arm. Review Table 11-1 for other routes of medication administration.

Illustration 11-2 also includes important clues about the main character's condition. The monitor above the bed displays her blood pressure, heart rate, breathing rate, and the amount of oxygen in her blood. The ICU team uses these readings to adjust therapeutic decisions in real time. It is also important to note that our patient has been intubated; meaning, a tube was inserted through her mouth, down her throat, and into her lungs. A breathing machine called a ventilator is delivering air directly into her lungs at a rate established by the ICU team, informed by the expert opinion of a respiratory therapist. Patients may need medications for pain and anxiety when they are on the ventilator, and the critical care pharmacist will assist with mediation selection, dosing, and monitoring. Generally, a patient will stay on the ventilator until the ICU team feels she/he has recovered enough to breath independently without difficulty. At this point, the tube is removed from the lungs in a process called extubation.

Critical care pharmacists are responsible for conducting medication histories of new patients.[15] This task is complicated in the ICU because many patients, either due to the severity of their illness or secondary to mechanical ventilation, are unable to speak directly to the pharmacist. As a result, obtaining an accurate medication history often involves some detective work, as depicted in Illustration 11-3, which shows the critical care pharmacist interviewing the main character's husband. Telephone calls to other hospitals or local pharmacies where the patient fills her/his prescriptions may also be required. For a non-ICU example of medication history development, readers are encouraged to explore the illustrated case "Burden" in Chapter 7 Geriatrics.

An accurate medication history is vital to the work of the ICU team. It is important to know, for example, whether a specific medication needs to be restarted. Similarly, as is the case for the main character in "Shocking," home medications may have important implications for care and treatment decisions. Some medications that are important to restart include those for thyroid dysfunction and for heart vessel stents.[44] Medications that influence how patients are cared for in the ICU include chemotherapy agents for cancer and steroids used for a variety of conditions, such as rheumatoid arthritis.[25,45] Patients receiving chemotherapy medications and steroids may have a suppressed immune system, which can make them more vulnerable to infections.[46] These patients are also at a higher risk of being infected with drug-resistant organisms. Broadly

Table 11-2. Categories and Examples of Medications Commonly Used in the Treatment of Septic Shock		
Category	**Medication Examples***	**Physiologic Effect**
Vasopressors	▪ dopamine (Intropin) ▪ epinephrine (Adrenalin) ▪ norepinephrine (Levophed) ▪ vasopressin (Vasostrict)	Increase blood pressure, ensuring adequate oxygen delivery to vital organs
Antibiotics	▪ cefepime (Maxipime) ▪ ceftriaxone (Rocephin) ▪ piperacillin-tazobactam (Zosyn) ▪ vancomycin (Vancocin)	Kill the bacteria causing the infection
Steroids	▪ hydrocortisone (Solu-Cortef)	Enhance the body's natural steroids to help fight the infection
Fluids	▪ lactated ringers ▪ normal saline	Increase the volume of blood, which increases blood pressure, ensuring adequate oxygen delivery to vital organs

*Medication examples presented in alphabetical order as "generic name (Brand Name)."

speaking, drug resistance refers to a situation where a once-effective antibiotic loses its ability to kill targeted bacteria. Besides having a suppressed immune system, patients taking steroids could also have suppressed adrenal gland function, which further weakens their ability to fight off infections.[45] Illustration 11-4 shows the critical care pharmacist and intensivist collaborating on antibiotic and steroid therapy selection based on the information gathered in Illustration 11-3. The computer monitor in the background provides a clue that the critical care pharmacist, in addition to troubleshooting implications from long-term prednisone therapy, is also preparing to provide appropriate antibiotic dosing recommendations based on decreased kidney function.

Research has shown that including critical care pharmacists as part of the interprofessional ICU team is associated with decreases in adverse drug reactions and medication order-writing mistakes.[47] Of the recommendations made by critical care pharmacists in this single study, 99% were accepted by intensivists. This is important because patients in the ICU are also at high risk of adverse drug reactions.[16] Reasons for this increased risk include how unstable they are, the frequency of kidney and liver dysfunction experienced by ICU patients, and the sheer number of medications used to treat ICU patients. It has been estimated that, on average, critically ill patients receive 15 medications per day.[48]

Critical care pharmacists are trained to keep a close eye on medications removed from the body by the kidneys and/or the liver, as dosing of these medications needs to be adjusted if these organs begin to fail. In patients who develop sepsis, over half develop acute kidney failure.[2] Kidney function is monitored daily by ICU pharmacists because it is constantly changing depending on how the patient is doing (Illustration 11-4). Without this level of medication vigilance and corresponding adjustments for fluctuating organ function/dysfunction, patients would be at risk of developing serious adverse drug events like seizures and bone marrow suppression.[49]

Approximately 10% to 29% of patients admitted to an ICU do not survive.[2] Risks for poor outcomes include older age, multiple pre-existing conditions, and how sick the patient is when they get to the ICU. For patients admitted to the hospital with sepsis, the average ICU length of stay is nearly 7 days and the average hospital length of stay is 12 days.[50] Fortunately, the main character in "Shocking" has survived her brush with death, in no small part due to the quick thinking of many health professionals along the way. Of the septic patients who survive their hospitalization, about 3% get transferred to another hospital, while nearly 8% are sent to hospice care for end-of-life treatment.[50] Approximately 30% of surviving sepsis patients go to a long-term-care or rehabilitation facility, while roughly 60% go home. For additional details on end-of-life and/or long-term care, see the illustrated cases "Compassion" in Chapter 9 Oncology and "Sleuth" in Chapter 7 Geriatrics, respectively.

One final, important note that is not explicitly stated in "Shocking" is that patients diagnosed with sepsis receive antibiotics for 7 to 10 days to treat the infection that caused their illness.[25] Illustrations 11-5 and 11-6 depict the main character's transition from the ICU to a general medicine floor within the hospital. While she is understandably anxious to go home, we can predict that she is about halfway through the course of her hospital stay.

The main character in the illustrated case "Shocking" presented to her hometown hospital in distress and became unstable, necessitating transfer to a larger hospital to be cared for by experts in critical care. The interprofessional critical care team at the accepting hospital made several important interventions to save her life. These interventions included intubation, starting blood pressure medications, continuing antibiotics for her pneumonia, and continuing steroids since she was on them prior to admission. The critical care pharmacist played a vitally important role in medication selection, dosing, and monitoring throughout the main character's time in the ICU, and this effort contributed meaningfully to her recovery. Through the work of the interprofessional critical care team, the patient improved dramatically and, thankfully, is well on her way to getting back home to her normal daily life.

DISCUSSION QUESTIONS FOR "SHOCKING"

1. Illustration 11-1 shows a critically ill patient being transferred to a larger hospital so she can be cared for by a team of health professionals with expertise in treating certain conditions. Take a moment to view this scenario from the patient's perspective. What kinds of thoughts and emotions do you think she is having/experiencing?

2. The patient has a breathing tube in Illustration 11-2, which prevents her from being able to talk. What are some other ways patients in this situation might be able to communicate with members of the interprofessional team, as well as their family, in this situation?

3. The interprofessional critical care team most likely has never met the patients for whom they are providing care. Especially in situations where patients are unable to communicate, what are some ways members of this team might be able to learn important past medical information to guide their decision-making?

4. Understandably, intensive care units can become stressful at times. What are some ways members of the interprofessional critical care team can remain calm when stress/tensions rise?

5. Critically ill patients tend to express a strong desire to return home once their conditions are stabilized. What are some reasons these patients may have to remain in the hospital for several days after getting transferred out of the ICU?

TYPE 1: An Illustrated Case Study

Story by Chloe R. Schmidt & Joseph A. Zorek
Illustrations by George Folz, © 2020 McGraw-Hill Education

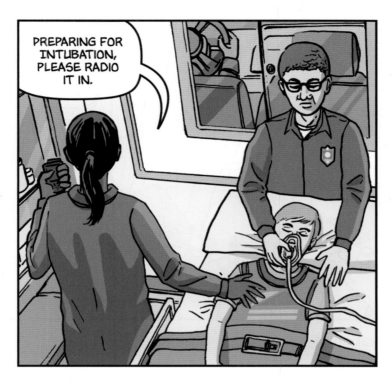

Illustration 11-7

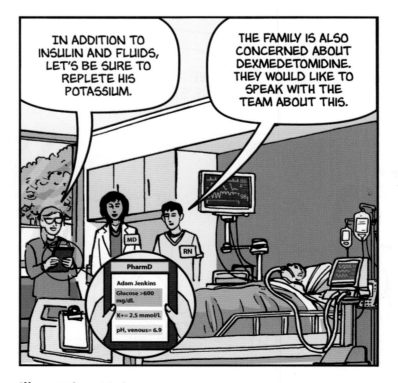

Illustration 11-8

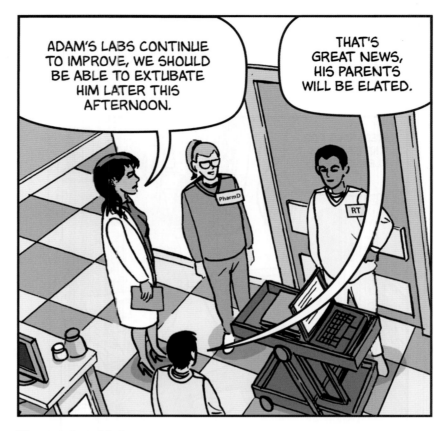

Illustration 11-9

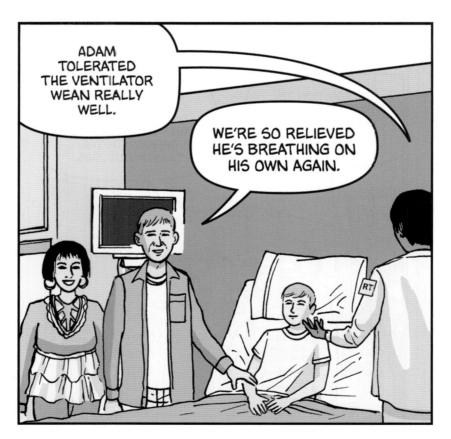

Illustration 11-10

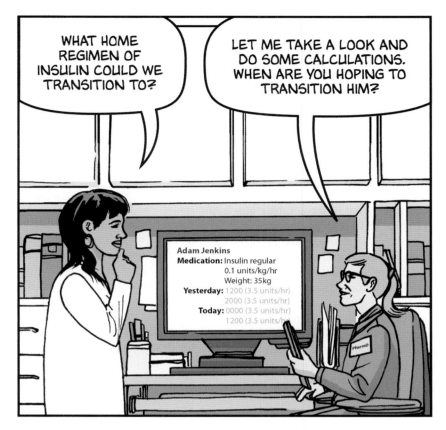

Illustration 11-11

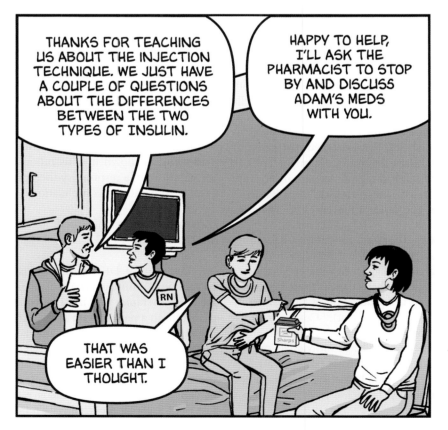

Illustration 11-12

Thoughts on "Type 1"

Type 1 diabetes develops when the cells that make insulin, the β-cells of the pancreas, are inappropriately destroyed by the body's immune system.[51] This is thought to be triggered by a combination of genetics and the environment.[52] β-cells cease to function when they are damaged, which typically leads to absolute insulin deficiency; meaning, no insulin production at all. Insulin is a vitally important hormone, a substance produced by one part of the body that impacts how cells, tissues, or organs in other parts of the body function. If insulin production stops, as in type 1 diabetes, catastrophic effects on metabolism ensue.[53]

Metabolism is a term used to describe all of the complex biochemical processes that take place inside our bodies to derive and use energy, and to process the byproducts that are created along the way. Our primary energy source is glucose, a simple sugar produced through digestion of food. Changes to metabolic processes as a result of certain diseases can result in wide-ranging negative effects. The absence of insulin is one example, where the body essentially loses its ability to appropriately utilize glucose. Insulin acts as a gatekeeper, allowing glucose to enter the body's cells from the blood. Without this gatekeeping role from insulin, glucose remains in the blood and cells must resort to alternative energy sources (e.g., fat, protein) to continue functioning. The end result is the accumulation of abnormal metabolic by-products, as well as elevated blood glucose levels. As depicted in Illustrations 11-7 and 11-8, this situation can be life-threatening if it is left untreated for an extended period of time.[53]

Type 1 and type 2 diabetes both result in high blood glucose levels. Unlike type 1 diabetes, however, insulin production by the β-cells of the pancreas remains stable in type 2 diabetes. What changes is the body's ability to use insulin; in other words, the cells become resistant to insulin's gatekeeping function. Over time, the effectiveness of glucose transport into the cells decreases, and the pancreas is unable to make enough insulin to overcome this resistance. Likewise, the causes of type 2 diabetes are different than type 1 diabetes. For a detailed discussion of type 2 diabetes, including causes, diagnosis, treatment, and the role of pharmacists in this health condition, readers are encouraged to explore the illustrated cases "Holistic" in Chapter 3 Primary Care and "Screen" in Chapter 4 Prevention & Wellness.

Type 1 diabetes is most often diagnosed early in life. According to the US Centers for Disease Control and Prevention (CDC), approximately 18,000 children are diagnosed with type 1 diabetes each year.[54] Children with type 1 diabetes usually present with the classic symptoms of polyuria (i.e., production of large amounts of urine) and polydipsia (i.e., excessive thirst).[51] Common symptoms also include nausea, vomiting, weight loss, and abdominal pain. However, approximately one-third of individuals present with a condition called diabetic ketoacidosis (DKA).[51] DKA is characterized by a triad of high blood glucose, ketones in the blood, and increased blood acidity (i.e., acidosis).[55]

The shift from glucose to fat as an energy source leads to the creation of a metabolic by-product called ketones.[55] As ketones accumulate, the acidity of the blood increases, causing a metabolic condition called acidosis. The pH value is used to measure acidity of the blood; the lower the pH, the higher the acidity level. Accumulation of ketones can induce acidosis (i.e., ketoacidosis), which leads to widespread cell damage throughout the body. The body attempts to compensate for this increase in acidity by buffering with bicarbonate. However, the body only carries a finite amount of bicarbonate, and when it runs low, this buffering capacity gets overwhelmed. Severity of DKA is primarily determined by blood pH and mental status.[56] As DKA unfolds, severe dehydration, imbalances in electrolytes (e.g., potassium, sodium) and swelling of the brain (i.e., cerebral edema) can cause marked confusion. Cerebral edema is one of the most severe complications. This may clinically manifest as headache, irritability, altered mental status and/or trouble getting enough oxygen. Additional symptoms of DKA may include fast heart rate, deep/fast breathing, vomiting, blurry vision, drowsiness, and, in the worst-case scenario, coma (i.e., complete loss of consciousness).[56] Most patients who meet criteria for severe DKA require treatment in an ICU so that their mental status can be closely monitored. Critical care pharmacists must be familiar with diagnostic criteria, as many of these are used to classify conditions, which directly influences drug selection and monitoring.[5,57]

The main character in "Type 1" is Adam Jenkins, a 12-year-old boy. Adam had not been feeling well for weeks. He and his parents thought he had come down with a bug and was having a hard time shaking it. Adam became difficult to arouse one afternoon, and his mother called 9-1-1. En route to the hospital (Illustration 11-7), first responders were unsuccessful in their attempts to arouse Adam and help him breathe with a non-invasive oxygen mask. Ultimately, concerned by Adam's inability to breathe, they made the difficult decision to intubate him. In addition to Adam's poor mental status and inability to breathe, Illustration 11-8 reveals his glucose and pH to be >600 mg/dL and 6.9, respectively. Adam's DKA, thus, would be classified as severe. The interprofessional critical care team, as shown in Illustrations 11-9 and 11-10, rely on the expertise of a respiratory therapist to help manage Adam's associated breathing complications.

Medications commonly used in the treatment of DKA are presented in Table 11-3.

The mainstay of DKA treatment is the administration of a continuous IV infusion of regular insulin.[56,58,59] However, there are a few therapies that must be considered prior to initiation of insulin in a patient with DKA. First, the patient's hydration status needs to be assessed and addressed. Often, children presenting with DKA are dehydrated due to excess urine production, which occurs because the body is attempting to get rid of the glucose that has built up in the blood.[60] If there are signs of dehydration (e.g., dry mucus membranes, inelastic skin), lost fluid must be replaced (i.e., fluid resuscitation), generally via fast administration of an IV fluid like normal saline. Once rehydrated, patients are then transitioned to maintenance IV

Table 11-3. Categories and Examples of Medications Commonly Used in the Acute Treatment of Diabetic Ketoacidosis

Category	Medication Examples*	Physiologic Effect
Intravenous fluids	• sodium chloride/normal saline	Increase the blood volume
Electrolytes	• phosphate • potassium	Regulate nerve and muscle function
Insulin: U-100 short-acting	• human regular (Humulin R, Novolin R)	Facilitates glucose uptake into cells so glucose can be used for energy, lowering blood glucose levels and restoring normal metabolic pathways

*Medication examples presented in alphabetical order as "generic name (Brand Name)."

fluids, essentially a continuous rate of IV fluids to make sure the patient remains hydrated throughout the course of treatment.

Prior to and during insulin administration, electrolytes must be assessed and repleted (i.e., deficiencies corrected) as necessary. Electrolytes help conduct electrical nerve impulses, and they play a quintessential role in fluid balance in the body. Profound electrolyte abnormalities can be dangerous because they can lead to impaired heart contractility, brain dysfunction, and respiratory failure due to diaphragm weakness. Normal saline, a common fluid used for resuscitation, contains sodium and chloride, which are the body's primary electrolytes in the blood. Children with DKA often suffer from potassium and phosphate losses, as depicted in Illustration 11-8, which shows Adam's potassium level at 2.5 mmol/L (normal range: 3.5 to 5.0).[61] To complicate the situation, when insulin therapy is initiated, potassium gets pushed intracellularly (i.e., from the blood into the cells), which further decreases the potassium in the blood that is available to the muscles. To help maintain potassium and phosphate, these electrolytes are often added into the continuous infusion of maintenance IV fluids after they are replaced acutely. Critical care pharmacists, like the one depicted in Illustration 11-8, are trained to keep a close eye on electrolyte status given this interplay with insulin.

Insulin therapy in DKA is crucial to help restore normal cellular metabolism, stop the utilization of fat and protein as a primary energy source, and restore normal levels of glucose in the blood.[56,59] Insulin therapy is continued for life in people with type 1 diabetes.[62] When blood glucose levels fall, IV dextrose (another form of sugar) is initiated to ensure the patient's blood glucose does not get too low.[63] It is recommended for patients to be maintained on an insulin infusion until their DKA has resolved; in other words, until the pH and electrolyte levels have normalized.[64-66] This typically takes longer than normalization of blood glucose. When DKA resolves, patients are switched to subcutaneous insulin therapy that can be continued when they go home, as shown in Illustrations 11-11 and 11-12. See the illustrated case "Holistic" in Chapter 3 Primary Care for a detailed description of long-term treatment of diabetes, including common medications.

Critical care pharmacists are well positioned to collaborate within the interprofessional team to manage patients with DKA. Illustration 11-8 provides a good example, where the pharmacist is depicted working with the intensivist (i.e., critical care physician) and nurse to address Adam's electrolyte abnormality that, if left unresolved, will worsen upon initiation of insulin therapy. Pharmacists in the ICU are relied upon not only to be familiar with all medications patients are receiving, but also for daily interventions to address or prevent medication-related issues; examples include drug interactions, adverse drug events, medication reconciliation, and medication optimizations like adjustments to dosing or switching to alternative/more effective therapies.

Illustration 11-8 shows Adam mechanically ventilated and on a sedative medication called dexmedetomidine (Precedex). Dexmedetomidine works in the brainstem to cause semi-arousable (light to moderate) sedation.[67] SCCM's pain, agitation, and delirium guidelines recommend using light sedation in mechanically ventilated patients to prevent agitation associated with mechanical ventilation, and use of dexmedetomidine still allows patients to respond to stimuli (unlike deep sedation caused by other medications).[28] Ideally, a lighter level of sedation improves tolerance to ventilation, while allowing the patient to continue to participate in their care. For example, on light sedation, a patient can communicate if they are in pain (facilitating appropriate treatment) and participate in neurologic exams performed by members of the interprofessional team. Like many drugs, literature surrounding the use of dexmedetomidine in the pediatric population is limited, though based on current evidence it is considered a safe and effective therapy for several indications, including Adam's condition.[68]

During care transitions, when a patient's condition has stabilized and they are ready to step down to a lower level of care (e.g., from intensive to intermediate, or from intermediate to general), pharmacists attempt to transition medication regimens to reflect what they will be taking at home. It is complicated and costly, for example, for a patient to be discharged from the hospital on an IV medication. As depicted in Illustrations 11-11 and 11-12, critical care nurses, pharmacists, and physicians regularly collaborate in anticipation of these transitions.

Subcutaneous insulin is the most common administration route and medication for patients, like Adam, with type 1 diabetes.[1] This is dosed according to units, which differs from other conventions readers are likely more familiar with, such as grams or milligrams. A typical starting dose of subcutaneous insulin is 0.3 to 0.5 units/kg/day (read as "units per kilogram per day"). Adam weighs 77 pounds (lb), which is equivalent to 35 kilograms (kg) as there are 2.2 lb in 1 kg. The recommended starting dose for Adam's subcutaneous insulin, therefore, is in the range of 10.5 to 17.5 units per day. It is also recommended for half of this daily dose (i.e., 5.25 to 8.75 units) to be given as a single injection of a long-acting insulin formulation, which will work continuously throughout the day to provide blood glucose control. This is referred to as basal dosing.

The other half, called bolus dosing, is recommended to be divided out and administered at or around mealtimes to control spikes in blood glucose associated with food intake and digestion. It is important to note that subcutaneous insulin doses are rounded to the nearest unit to facilitate accurate measurement. While basal-bolus insulin dosing is also used in type 2 diabetes, the calculation of daily requirements is very different for patients with type 1 diabetes.[65,69] It is this calculation that the pharmacist references in Illustration 11-11. Readers are encouraged to review the illustrated case "Holistic" and Table 3-5 in Chapter 3 Primary Care, as well as the illustrated case "Screen" in Chapter 4 Prevention & Wellness, for more detailed information on long-term management of diabetes.

While it is the nurse who teaches Adam and his parents how to administer subcutaneous insulin in Illustration 11-12, pharmacists in hospital settings and those working in the community are well positioned to provide this education, as well.[70,71] Ensuring that insulin is delivered into the correct tissue in the proper way is essential to optimize blood glucose and to prevent adverse drug events.[72] If insulin is injected too deep, for example, or at the incorrect angle, the drug may instead be injected intramuscularly. Absorption into the bloodstream differs between subcutaneous tissue and muscle; as a result, incorrectly administered insulin may result in increased absorption and therefore low blood glucose levels (i.e., hypoglycemia).[72] Hypoglycemia is a dangerous condition, and pharmacists also play an important role educating patients and caregivers on how to manage this.

Appropriate sites in which subcutaneous insulin may be administered include the abdomen, thighs, buttocks, and upper arms. To inject subcutaneously, needle length should be relatively short, about 4 millimeters.[73] Insulin should be injected perpendicular to the skin (i.e., straight up and down) using a lifted skinfold or injected at a 45-degree angle without lifting a skinfold to ensure subcutaneous administration.[73] Another important component to insulin administration is injection site rotation. If insulin is injected into the same place repeatedly, it can lead to the buildup of subcutaneous fat and may contribute to less predictable insulin absorption and inappropriately controlled diabetes. Proper insulin administration helps ensure that the benefits of the insulin therapy are maximized, and side effects are minimized.

Type 1 diabetes is a life-altering diagnosis to which there is no curative therapy. With the rising cost of medications, it can also be a diagnosis with grave financial implications for patients and their families.[74,75] Adam Jenkins, the main character in the illustrated case "Type 1," will have to manage this new condition for the rest of his life. Through interprofessional collaboration in this illustrated case, the critical care nurse, pharmacist, physician, and respiratory therapist have helped Adam and his family take their first important step. Next steps will include developing expert knowledge about nutrition, as the interplay between food and insulin requirements is strong.[76] Assistance from a registered dietitian nutritionist, working in concert with Adam's interprofessional pediatric primary care team and his diabetes specialist (i.e., endocrinologist), will further help with their transition to what will soon become the Jenkins family's new normal.

DISCUSSION QUESTIONS FOR "TYPE 1"

1. In Illustration 11-8, the critical care pharmacist is shown using a tablet to look at the patient's labs in real-time while the rest of the interprofessional team is assessing the patient at bedside. In what other ways might technology be useful in a setting such as this?

2. Assume for a moment that Adam was using an inhaler and taking a capsule by mouth every day for other health conditions prior to his hospitalization. What options might be available for medication administration while he is intubated and unable to swallow?

3. What health professional shown in this case specializes in breathing problems? Aside from assisting with the management of mechanically ventilated patients, what other health conditions involving the lungs might this person help manage?

4. One of the side effects of insulin is low potassium, as insulin drives potassium from the blood into cells. If someone came into the hospital with high potassium, do you think insulin could be used to lower this into a normal range? If so, what kinds of complications might you need to account for or consider?

5. In Illustration 11-12, Adam is shown administering his insulin via subcutaneous injection. How do you think having to inject insulin several times each day will affect Adam's everyday life?

CHAPTER SUMMARY

- The terms *critical care* and *intensive care* are used interchangeably, and they describe the management of patients having, or at risk of having, acute life-threatening failure of organs, such as the lungs, heart, and kidneys.

- Critical care pharmacists practice within interprofessional teams that also include intensivists (i.e., physicians), nurses, nurse practitioners, nutritionists, physician assistants, and respiratory therapists, among others.

- Intensive care units (ICUs) have specialized equipment to provide organ support for critically ill patients, including mechanical ventilators (lungs), extracorporeal membrane oxygenators (heart and lungs), and hemodialysis machines (kidneys).

- Critical care pharmacists are experts in the use of medications to treat life-threatening conditions, including those featured in this chapter (septic shock, diabetic ketoacidosis), and they incorporate real-time data and information to support medication decisions within the interprofessional team that contribute to patient care.

- Critically ill patients are at an increased risk for adverse drug events due to the instability and complexity of their conditions, including frequent kidney and liver dysfunctions that impact medication use.

- Pharmacists in the ICU make daily medication-related interventions, including assessing for drug interactions, monitoring for adverse drug events, completing medication reconciliation, and optimizing medication dosing.

- Critical care pharmacists derive great professional satisfaction through meaningful contributions to team-based care that result in patients recovering and being able to leave the ICU with loved ones.

REFERENCES

1. Marshall JC, Bosco L, Adhikari NK, et al. What is an intensive care unit? A report of the task force of the World Federation of Societies of Intensive and Critical Care Medicine. *J Crit Care.* 2017;37:270-276.

2. Society of Critical Care Medicine. Critical care statistics. Available at https://www.sccm.org/Communications/Critical-Care-Statistics. Accessed April 2, 2020.

3. The Faculty of Intensive Care Medicine and the Intensive Care Society. Core standards for intensive care units. Edition 1; 2013.

4. Crass RL, Rodvold KA, Mueller BA, Pai MP. Renal dosing of antibiotics: are we jumping the gun? *Clin Infect Dis.* 2019;68(9):1596-1602.

5. Heintz BH, Matzke GR, Dager WE. Antimicrobial dosing concepts and recommendations for critically ill adult patients receiving continuous renal replacement therapy or intermittent hemodialysis. *Pharmacotherapy.* 2009;29(5):562-577.

6. Maxipime (cefepime) [package insert]. Lake Forest, IL: Hospira Inc; 2012.

7. Huwyler T, Lenggenhager L, Abbas M, et al. Cefepime plasma concentrations and clinical toxicity: a retrospective cohort study. *Clin Microbiol Infect.* 2017;23(7):454-459.

8. Maynor LM, Carl DE, Matzke GR, et al. An in vivo-in vitro study of cefepime and cefazolin dialytic clearance during high-flux hemodialysis. *Pharmacotherapy.* 2008;28(8):977-983.

9. Gamper G, Havel C, Arrich J, et al. Vasopressors for hypotensive shock. *Cochrane Database Syst Rev.* 2016;2:CD003709.

10. Leapfrog Hospital Survey. Factsheet: ICU Physician Staffing. Available at www.leapfroggroup.org/survey. Accessed April 2, 2020.

11. Guidelines Committee, Society of Critical Care Medicine. Guidelines for the definition of an intensivist and the practice of critical care medicine. *Crit Care Med.* 1992;20(4):540-542.

12. Haupt MT, Bekes CE, Brilli RJ, et al. Guidelines on critical care services and personnel: Recommendations based on a system of categorization of three levels of care. *Crit Care Med.* 2003;31(11):2677-2683.

13. Society of Critical Care Medicine. Available at https://www.sccm.org/Home. Accessed April 2, 2020.

14. American College of Clinical Pharmacy. Available at https://www.accp.com/. Accessed April 2, 2020.

15. Society of Critical Care Medicine and American College of Clinical Pharmacy. Position paper on critical care pharmacy services. *Pharmacotherapy.* 2000;20(11):1400-1406.

16. Preslaski CR, Lat I, MacLaren R, Poston J. Pharmacist contributions as members of the multidisciplinary ICU team. *Chest.* 2013;144(5):1687-1695.

17. Bradnam V, White R. *Handbook of Drug Administration via Enteral Feeding Tubes.* Vol. 3. Pharmaceutical Press; 2015.

18. McCreary EK, Borlagdan J, Andes DR, Kinn P, Schulz LT, Lepak AJ. Achievement of clinical isavuconazole (ISA) serum and plasma drug concentrations in two patients with isavuconazoium capsules administered via nasogastric feeding tube (NGT). *Open Forum Infect Dis.* 2018;5:S156.

19. Smith BS, Yogaratnam D, Levasseur-Franklin KE, Forni A, Fong J. Introduction to drug pharmacokinetics in the critically ill patient. *Chest.* 2012;141(5):1327-1336.

20. Keppra (levetiracetam) [package insert]. Smyrna, GA: UCB, Inc.; 2009.

21. Lasix (furosemide) [package insert]. Shirley, NY: American Regent Inc; 2011.

22. U.S. Food and Drug Administration. Route of administration. Available at https://www.fda.gov/drugs/data-standards-manual-monographs/route-administration. Accessed November 7, 2020.

23. Touw DJ, Neef C, Thomson AH, Vinks AA. Cost-effectiveness of therapeutic drug monitoring: a systematic review. *Ther Drug Monit.* 2005;27(1):10-17.

24. Cook DJ, Fuller HD, Guyatt GH, et al. Risk factors for gastrointestinal bleeding in critically ill patients. Canadian Critical Care Trials Group. *N Engl J Med.* 1994;330(6):377-381.

25. Rhodes A, Evans LE, Alhazzani W, et al. Surviving Sepsis Campaign: international guidelines for management of sepsis and septic shock: 2016. *Intensive Care Med.* 2017;43(3):304-377.

26. Wohlt PD, Hansen LA, Fish JT. Inappropriate continuation of stress ulcer prophylactic therapy after discharge. *Ann Pharmacother.* 2007;41(10):1611-1616.

27. Hatch JB, Schulz L, Fish JT. Stress ulcer prophylaxis: reducing non-indicated prescribing after hospital discharge. *Ann Pharmacother.* 2010;44(10):1565-1571.

28. Devlin JW, Skrobik Y, Gélinas C, et al. Executive summary: clinical practice guidelines for the prevention and management of pain, agitation/sedation, delirium, immobility, and sleep disruption in adult patients in the ICU. *Crit Care Med.* 2018;46(9):1532-1548.

29. Yaucher NE, Fish JT, Smith HW, Wells JA. Propylene glycol-associated renal toxicity from lorazepam infusion. *Pharmacotherapy.* 2003;23(9):1094-1099.

30. Accreditation Council for Pharmacy Education. Available at https://www.acpe-accredit.org/. Accessed March 27, 2020.

31. American Society of Health System Pharmacists. Residency information. Available at https://www.ashp.org/Professional-Development/Residency-Information. Accessed March 27, 2020.

32. Board of Pharmacy Specialties. Available at https://www.bpsweb.org/. Accessed March 27, 2020.

33. Kindermann D, Mutter R, Pines JM. Emergency department transfers to acute care facilities, 2009. May 2013. Statistical Brief #155.

34. Hall MJ, Owings M. Rural and urban hospitals' role in providing inpatient care, 2010. *NCHS Data Brief.* 2014;147:1-8.

35. Feazel L, Schlichting AB, Bell GR, et al. Achieving regionalization through rural interhospital transfer. *Am J Emerg Med.* 2015;33(9):1288-1296.

36. The Association of Air Medical Services. Air Med "101." Available at https://aams.org/. Accessed April 2, 2020.

37. Pronovost PJ, Angus DC, Dorman T, Robinson KA, Dremsizov TT, Young TL. Physician staffing patterns and clinical outcomes in critically ill patients: a systematic review. *JAMA.* 2002;288(17):2151-2162.

38. Gaieski DF, Edwards JM, Kallan MJ, Mikkelsen ME, Goyal M, Carr BG. The relationship between hospital volume and

mortality in severe sepsis. *Am J Respir Crit Care Med.* 2014;190(6):665-674.

39. Singer M, Deutschman CS, Seymour CW, Shankar-Hari M, Annane D. The third international consensus definitions for sepsis and septic shock (Sepsis-3). *JAMA.* 2016;315(8):801-810.

40. Centers for Disease Control and Prevention. Sepsis. Available at https://www.cdc.gov/sepsis/index.html. Accessed March 27, 2020.

41. Surviving Sepsis Campaign. Available at https://www.sccm.org/SurvivingSepsisCampaign/Home. Accessed March 27, 2020.

42. Levy MM, Evans LE, Rhodes A. The Surviving Sepsis Campaign Bundle: 2018 Update. *Crit Care Med.* 2018;46(6):997-1000.

43. Lexicomp. Available at https://online.lexi.com/lco/action/home/switch. Accessed March 27, 2020.

44. Levine GN, Bates ER, Bittl JA, et al. 2016 ACC/AHA guideline focused update on duration of dual antiplatelet therapy in patients with coronary artery disease: a report of the American College of Cardiology/American Heart Association Task Force on Clinical Practice Guidelines. *J Thorac Cardiovasc Surg.* 2016;152(5):1243-1275.

45. Metlay JP, Waterer GW, Long AC, et al. Diagnosis and treatment of adults with community-acquired pneumonia. An official clinical practice guideline of the American Thoracic Society and Infectious Diseases Society of America. *Am J Respir Crit Care Med.* 2019;200(7):e45-e67.

46. Taplitz RA, Kennedy EB, Flowers CR. Antimicrobial prophylaxis for adult patients with cancer-related immunosuppression: ASCO and IDSA clinical practice guideline update summary. *J Oncol Pract.* 2018;36(30):3043-3054.

47. Leape LL, Cullen DJ, Clapp MD, et al. Pharmacist participation on physician rounds and adverse drug events in the intensive care unit. *JAMA.* 1999;282(3):267-270.

48. Camiré E, Moyen E, Stelfox HT. Medication errors in critical care: risk factors, prevention and disclosure. *CMAJ.* 2009;180(9):936-943.

49. Hammond DA, Gurnani PK, Flannery AH, et al. Scoping review of interventions associated with cost avoidance able to be performed in the intensive care unit and emergency department. *Pharmacotherapy.* 2019;39(3):215-231.

50. Rhee C, Dantes R, Epstein L, et al. Incidence and trends of sepsis in US hospitals using clinical vs claims data, 2009-2014. *JAMA.* 2017;318(13):1241-1249.

51. American Diabetes Association. Standards of medical care in diabetes. *Diabetes Care.* 2020;43:1-212.

52. American Diabetes Association. Genetics of diabetes. Available at https://www.diabetes.org/diabetes/genetics-diabetes. Accessed January 3, 2020.

53. Wolfsdorf J, Glaser N, Sperling MA, Association AD. Diabetic ketoacidosis in infants, children, and adolescents: a consensus statement from the American Diabetes Association. *Diabetes Care.* 2006;29(5):1150-1159.

54. Centers for Disease Control and Prevention. Type 1 diabetes. Available at https://www.cdc.gov/diabetes/basics/type1.html. Accessed January 2, 2020.

55. Kitabchi AE, Umpierrez GE, Murphy MB, Kreisberg RA. Hyperglycemic crises in adult patients with diabetes: a consensus statement from the American Diabetes Association. *Diabetes Care.* 2006;29(12):2739-2748.

56. Wolfsdorf JI, Glaser N, Agus M, et al. ISPAD clinical practice consensus guidelines 2018: diabetic ketoacidosis and the hyperglycemic hyperosmolar state. *Pediatr Diabetes.* 2018;19(27):155-177.

57. Kraut JA, Madias NE. Serum anion gap: its uses and limitations in clinical medicine. *Clin J Am Soc Nephrol.* 2007;2(1):162-174.

58. Tran TTT, Pease A, Wood AJ, et al. Review of evidence for adult diabetic ketoacidosis management protocols. *Front Endocrinol.* 2017;8:106.

59. Kamel KS, Schreiber M, Carlotti AP, Halperin ML. Approach to the treatment of diabetic ketoacidosis. *Am J Kidney Dis.* 2016;68(6):967-972.

60. Jayashree M, Williams V, Iyer R. Fluid therapy for pediatric patients with diabetic ketoacidosis: current perspectives. *Diabetes Metab Syndr Obes.* 2019;12:2355-2361.

61. Elisaf MS, Tsatsoulis AA, Katopodis KP, Siamopoulos KC. Acid-base and electrolyte disturbances in patients with diabetic ketoacidosis. *Diabetes Res Clin Pract* 1996;34(1):23-27.

62. Wood J, Peters A. *The Type 1 Diabetes Self-Care Manual: A Complete Guide to Type 1 Diabetes Across the Lifespan for People with Diabetes, Parents, and Caregivers.* Arlington, VA: American Diabetes Association; 2018.

63. Kapellen T, Vogel C, Telleis D, Siekmeyer M, Kiess W. Treatment of diabetic ketoacidosis (DKA) with 2 different regimens regarding fluid substitution and insulin dosage (0.025 vs. 0.1 units/kg/h). *Exp Clin Endocrinol Diabetes.* 2012;120(5):273-276.

64. Westerberg DP. Diabetic ketoacidosis: evaluation and treatment. *Am Fam Physician.* 2013;87(5):337-346.

65. Weant KA, Ladha A. Conversion from continuous insulin infusions to subcutaneous insulin in critically ill patients. *Ann Pharmacother.* 2009;43(4):629-634.

66. American Diabetes Association. Insulin basics. Available at https://www.diabetes.org/diabetes/medication-management/insulin-other-injectables/insulin-basics. Accessed May 31, 2020.

67. Keating GM. Dexmedetomidine: a review of its use for sedation in the intensive care setting. *Drugs.* 2015;75(10):1119-1130.

68. Plambech MZ, Afshari A. Dexmedetomidine in the pediatric population: a review. *Minerva Anestesiol.* 2015;81(3):320-332.

69. Schmeltz LR, DeSantis AJ, Schmidt K, et al. Conversion of intravenous insulin infusions to subcutaneously administered insulin glargine in patients with hyperglycemia. *Endocr Pract.* 2006;12(6):641-650.

70. Arcebido R, Wong E, Cohen V, Likourezos A. Pharmacist-led discharge counseling on subcutaneous insulin use and administration. *Am J Health Syst Pharm.* 2013;70(16):1371-1373.

71. Tripathi S, Crabtree HM, Fryer KR, Graner KK, Arteaga GM. Impact of clinical pharmacist on the pediatric intensive care practice: an 11-year tertiary center experience. *J Pediatr Pharmacol Ther.* 2015;20(4):290-298.

72. American Diabetes Association. Insulin administration. *Diabetes Care.* 2003;26(suppl 1):s121-s124.

73. Frid AH, Kreugel G, Grassi G, et al. New insulin delivery recommendations. *Mayo Clin Proc.* 2016;91(9):1231-1255.

74. Magge E. Diabetes brings constant worries—especially when deductibles reset. *The Washington Post.* Published December 30, 2019.

75. Ferguson E. US citizens are dying and we can save them. Available at https://www.nytimes.com/2019/05/04/learning/us-citizens-are-dying-and-we-can-save-them.html. Accessed May 31, 2020.

76. Adragna A. Pricks and needles: what living with type 1 diabetes is like. Available at https://www.theatlantic.com/health/archive/2012/06/pricks-and-needles-what-living-with-type-1-diabetes-is-like/258399/. Accessed May 31, 2020.

CHAPTER 12

Mental Health

Featuring the Illustrated Case Studies "Gasping" & "Barriers"

Authors

Cody J. Wenthur, Casey E. Gallimore, & Joseph A. Zorek

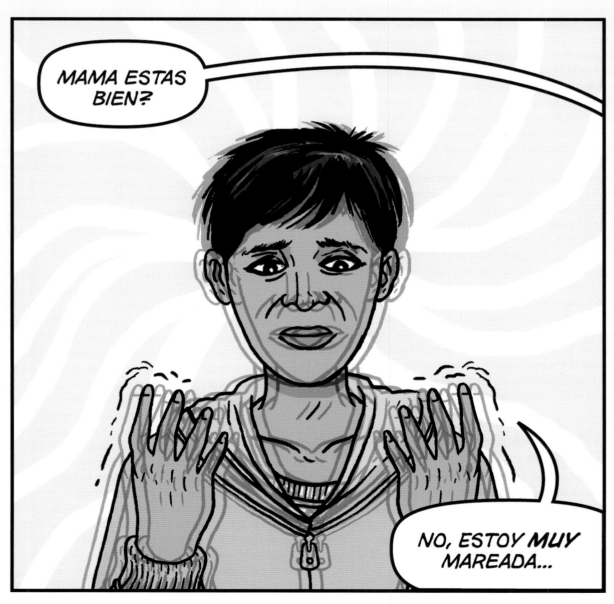

Illustration by George Folz, © 2019 Board of Regents of the University of Wisconsin System

BACKGROUND

Mental healthcare, also called psychiatric care, is an essential component of overall wellness that is focused on supporting social, psychological, and emotional health.[1] Although some people may consider physical and mental health to be separate concerns, they are actually two highly interconnected systems that influence each other constantly.[2] Just as poor mental health can worsen the quality of physical health, good physical health can support positive mental health outcomes. Considering this irreducible biological connectivity, it should come as no surprise that full integration of physical and mental health services throughout all practice settings, for all patients, is a frequent goal of modern healthcare systems.[3]

In the past, psychiatric diseases had been considered to arise from defects in personality, or even as the result of supernatural causes. Today, they are largely considered to be a consequence of underlying genetic and biological dysfunction in the brain, although the complexity of the central nervous system makes the identification of exact causes an ongoing challenge for many psychiatric conditions.[4] Nevertheless, this biologically oriented viewpoint has led to the development of numerous medications that can help treat the symptoms and progression of these diseases. The act of using these medications is known as providing pharmacologic treatment. Pharmacologic treatment is one major component of mental healthcare, and often the area where psychiatric pharmacists employ the majority of their expertise.[5]

However, in light of the close connection between the brain and body, ongoing psychosocial factors frequently play a shared role alongside biological dysfunction in the development and progression of ongoing mental health issues. Therefore, the other major component of mental healthcare is non-pharmacologic treatment, which is frequently provided in the form of ongoing counseling and behavioral and lifestyle support.[6] The concept of behavioral health encompasses these two components, most frequently referring to the intersection of traditional mental health topics, substance use concerns, and behavioral and lifestyle factors that contribute to health and wellness. The need for close integration of these two components of treatment is a practical manifestation of the brain-body connection that serves to define modern mental healthcare, and is the foundation for the diverse membership of the interprofessional mental health team.

Members of the Interprofessional Mental Health Team

Many of the important members of the interprofessional mental health team will be familiar from other areas of healthcare, including primary care physicians, nurses, physician assistants, nurse practitioners, and pharmacists.[7] Given that mental health concerns are a common part of everyday life and healthcare, most health professionals will interact with mental health patients on a regular basis.

That being said, there are also multiple health professionals who specialize in the treatment of mental health concerns, and are thus more likely to be regularly encountered by a psychiatric pharmacist. Psychiatrists and psychiatric nurse practitioners are two major categories of mental health-focused prescribers who work closely with psychiatric pharmacists in the provision of pharmacologic treatment. Psychologists and other behavioral health professionals (e.g., social workers, mental health counselors, marriage and family counselors) are also important members of the interprofessional team. Psychologists are often a major source of non-pharmacologic treatment, and social workers are frequently invaluable for securing patient access to needed treatment facilities and supporting patient success through the entire lifetime of care. Depending on a psychiatric pharmacist's practice setting and patient population, they may also interact with substance abuse counselors, who provide specialized care to individuals with substance use disorders. More frequent interactions with specialists focused on other aspects and/or integrative functions of the nervous system, such as neurologists and neuropsychiatrists, can also be expected, given the common occurrence of comorbidities between psychiatric and neurologic disorders.[8]

Role of Pharmacists within Interprofessional Mental Health Teams

As important members of the interprofessional mental health team, psychiatric pharmacists have many inter-related responsibilities—all directed toward the improvement of human health at either the individual or population level. As with many pharmacy practice areas, core direct patient care activities include the selection and optimization of medication therapy, monitoring of ongoing therapy for the emergence of adverse effects or treatment failure, and educating patients and their caregivers on the nature of their diagnoses and the medications that are used to treat them.[5]

When providing direct patient care, the mental health conditions most likely to be encountered by a psychiatric pharmacist are depression and anxiety.[9] In any given year, roughly 19% of the US adult population experiences a mental health condition, and 4.5% experience a serious mental illness (SMI).[10] SMI has been defined as a "mental, behavioral, or emotional disorder resulting in serious functional impairment, which substantially interferes with or limits one or more major life activities."[11] Examples of SMI that a psychiatric pharmacist is likely to encounter in their daily work include bipolar disorder, psychotic disorders such as schizophrenia, and severe depression.[12] Additionally, individuals with mental health diagnoses often have co-occurring substance use disorders, although issues arising from unsafe drug use also frequently arise in isolation.[13] The presence of SMI frequently results in the prescription of a psychotropic medication (medications capable of altering someone's mental state); in fact, psychotropic medications can account for nearly a quarter of the top 100 drugs prescribed in the United States.[14] Commonly encountered psychotropic medications include antidepressants like sertraline (Zoloft), benzodiazepines like alprazolam (Xanax), opioids like oxycodone (OxyContin), hypnotics like zolpidem (Ambien), and antipsychotics like aripiprazole (Abilify).[15]

Some of those medications may sound familiar, while others may not. Yet, they only represent a small selection of the possible therapeutic options available. Indeed, because psychiatric medication regimens can be highly complex, with multiple medications being used together, the ability to understand and manage drug interactions is often an especially important skill in mental health pharmacy.[16] Likewise, many medication classes that are used as first line treatments in psychiatry are sensitive to genetic variations that exist across the population, which requires careful dose selection and monitoring to maximize medication benefits for a particular patient.[17] Adherence to therapy is often another area of challenge for patients with psychiatric diagnoses, so the ability to engage with patients and achieve mutually agreeable methods and goals for their treatment plan is another crucial skill for pharmacists who primarily practice in mental health.[18]

Beyond direct patient care responsibilities, psychiatric pharmacists will often be responsible for making decisions and engaging in activities that can promote mental health at the level of entire populations. Some common responsibilities for psychiatric pharmacists at the population level include making decisions about which psychiatric medications will be included on an institutional formulary (a standardized drug availability and payment list); engagement with peer recovery and patient advocacy groups; evaluation of the current state of medical literature in their specialty area; pursuit of independent research and publication in the medical literature; and teaching of peer groups, students and pharmacy residents, as well as members of the public.[19-21] Given the persistent myths and misconceptions that surround mental health and psychiatric conditions, expansion of pharmacy services in this area continues to be extremely important in terms of access to care, as well as improvement of population-level outcomes.[22] Major employment sites for psychiatric pharmacists include inpatient adult or pediatric psychiatry facilities, outpatient facilities like primary and ambulatory care clinics, forensic psychiatry services, state psychiatric facilities, academia, and the pharmaceutical industry.[23]

MENTAL HEALTH PHARMACISTS IN ACTION

Teaming Up to Tackle Opioid Overdose

Because overdose from risky use of illicit opioids like heroin and misuse of prescription opioids like oxycodone continue to cause tens of thousands of deaths in the United States each year, mental health professionals, including pharmacists, have an enormous opportunity to save lives every day through their actions. For example, in Philadelphia, there is an innovative mobile health clinic prescribing buprenorphine (a medication used to treat addiction to opioids) to individuals who want to get help. However, due to challenges with stocking the medication, concerns related to diversion, and disparate teachings of how the medication should be used between medical and pharmacy schools, patients were often having a hard time getting these prescriptions filled. Fortunately, as reported by National Public Radio, a group of local physicians and pharmacists were able to reconcile differences in their past training, and work together to overcome these hurdles to make an immediate difference in their community by improving medication access and preventing fatal opioid overdoses. As one pharmacist said, "I've heard firsthand from patients—'that saved my life.' You know, that's something that … you can't really put a price tag on."[24]

Good Model, Great Medicine

For members of the Eastern Band of Cherokee, taking an integrative approach to healthcare came naturally. According to one member, "an integrated approach is more consistent with traditional healing. We don't separate our physical, mental, spiritual, and emotional health the way we do in modern specialized health care." When they elected to decentralize from the Indian Health Service, the health system they built, including everything from the interprofessional teams, to the building itself, embraced this philosophy. Patients are now assigned core teams with a primary care physician or family nurse practitioner, a pharmacist, a behavioral health specialist, a nutritionist, a case manager, and a scheduler. This holistic approach has improved patient satisfaction and buy-in, and it has allowed the hospital to become a top performer in many preventive health quality measures. Considering that Native American populations overall have historically had elevated rates of physical and mental illnesses in comparison to the US average, this culturally informed mandate to treat the whole individual has been a clear success.[25]

Finding a Niche, Filling a Need

In Regina, Saskatchewan, there was a pressing need for expanded access to care for patients with mental health concerns. As noted previously, patients with psychiatric diagnoses were having trouble engaging with primary care and getting the long-term, stable care they needed. In response, a local board-certified psychiatric pharmacist opened her own mental health-focused pharmacy, the first of its kind in a province the size of Texas. The pharmacy not only focuses on providing support for the notably complex psychiatric regimens of their patients and administering injectable treatments that are otherwise difficult to access, but also strives to provide an atmosphere where mental health patients feel comfortable enough to continue coming back time and time again. "We really focus on having no stigma here. That's a deal breaker when hiring staff. When [patients] encounter barriers, they just decide, 'I'm not going to take my medications.'" By training and mentoring pharmacists and pharmacy students interested in psychiatric pharmacy, this community-based site will certainly continue to expand their already outstanding impact on the reduction of barriers to care and improvement of long-term health for their patients.[26]

BECOMING A MENTAL HEALTH PHARMACIST

Any actively licensed graduate of an Accreditation Council for Pharmacy Education (ACPE)–accredited pharmacy program will have demonstrated the ability to care for patients with a broad range of illnesses, including mental health concerns, and the degree to which any particular individual will specialize in knowledge in this area often depends on the patient population they interact with in the course of their day-to-day duties. However, for those individuals who desire specific additional training beyond that provided in the core Doctor of Pharmacy (PharmD) curriculum, they may choose to pursue a general post-graduate year 1 (PGY-1) residency, followed by a specialty post-graduate year 2 (PGY-2) residency in psychiatric pharmacy. This specialty residency focus continues to be a growth area, as both the need for mental healthcare, and the complexity of mental health treatment regimens continue to expand.[27] Additionally, fellowship opportunities are available to those individuals seeking specific training in research methods and practice innovations at the forefront of psychiatric care.

For pharmacists who desire specific credentialing to demonstrate their expertise in the treatment of mental health, the Board of Pharmacy Specialties (BPS) has a dedicated program for becoming a Board Certified Psychiatric Pharmacist (BCPP). Written examination for this certification is available to actively licensed individuals who have graduated from an ACPE-accredited PharmD program (or its international equivalent), and have either (1) completed 4 years of practice experience with at least 50% of time focused on psychiatric and related disorders; (2) completed a PGY-1 residency, plus 2 years of practice experience with at least 50% of time focused on psychiatric and related disorders; or (3) completed a PGY-2 residency in psychiatric pharmacy. After passing the Psychiatric Pharmacy Specialty Certification Examination, individuals are certified as BCPPs for a period of 7 years, with recertification contingent upon either (1) earning 100 hours of continuing education credit provided by a BPS-approved program, or (2) passing a 100-item recertification examination administered by BPS.[28]

Regardless of whether an individual is a student just beginning the process of considering psychiatric pharmacy, or has been an actively practicing BCPP, applying for membership in a professional organization like the College of Psychiatric and Neurologic Pharmacists is an open opportunity to get involved with a community of like-minded individuals supporting this important, fascinating, and growing practice area within pharmacy.

GASPING: An Illustrated Case Study

Story by Cody J. Wenthur & Joseph A. Zorek
Illustrations by George Folz, © 2019 Board of Regents of the University of Wisconsin System

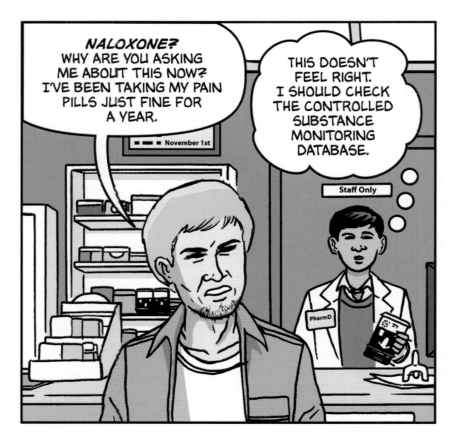

Illustration 12-1

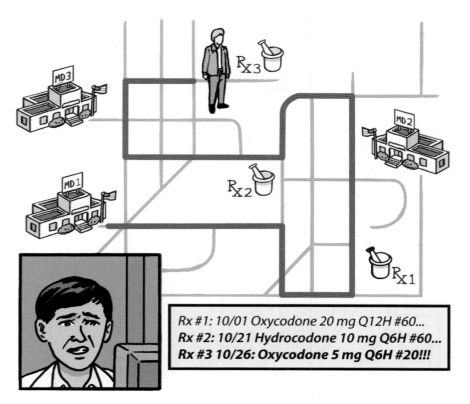

Illustration 12-2

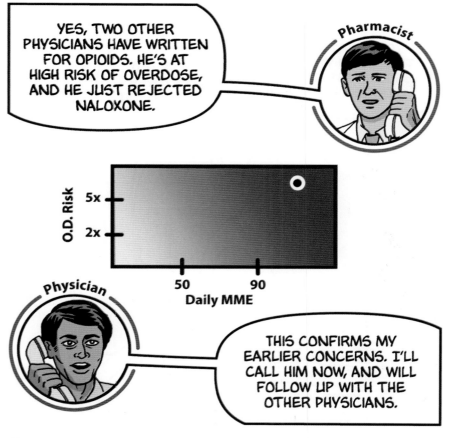

Illustration 12-3

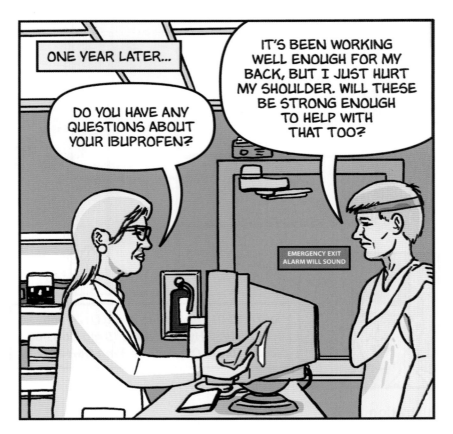

Illustration 12-4

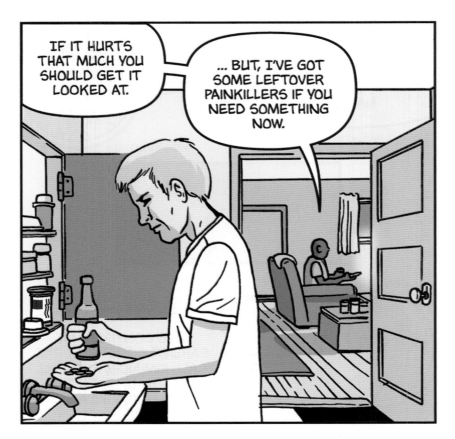

Illustration 12-5

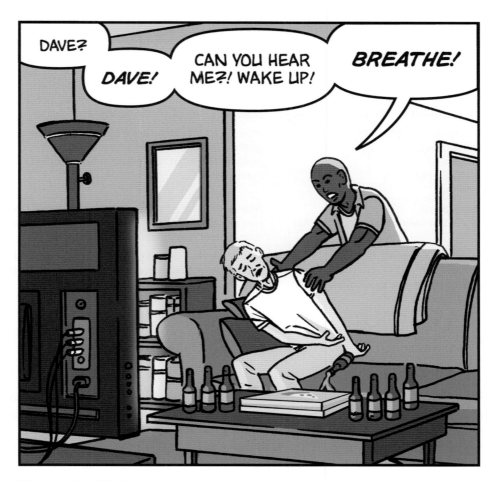

Illustration 12-6

Thoughts on "Gasping"

Addiction, or substance use disorder (SUD), is a common mental illness that arises in approximately 10% of individuals during their lifetime.[29] Individuals with SUD can become addicted to many kinds of substances, including depressants, stimulants, cannabinoids, or opiates (Table 12-1).

Pharmacists play a role in the care of patients with SUD through screening and collaboration with/referral to other health professionals, as well as through interventions designed to help patients manage withdrawal and craving symptoms using medications and targeted counseling services. Indeed, these interventions are often provided across a period of many years, as SUD is a chronic, often relapsing condition.[30]

Importantly, pharmacists also help to prevent and treat drug overdoses by dispensing overdose-reversal medications and teaching patients how to appropriately use prescription medications that carry a risk for addiction and overdose. This is an especially important task considering how common the use of opioid painkillers remains in the United States. In 2018 alone, there were 168.9 million prescriptions written for opioid painkillers, enough for every adult in the country to have received 34 tablets.[31]

Pharmacists routinely impact the care of individuals who are at risk for opioid misuse, including those diagnosed with opioid use disorder (OUD). The illustrated case "Gasping" highlights some of the important roles that pharmacists play in the treatment of patients with SUD in general, and OUD in particular, by presenting one possible trajectory for an individual who has been prescribed the opioid painkiller oxycodone (OxyContin) for treatment of his chronic back pain.

Oxycodone is an opioid medication that relieves pain by turning on, or activating, mu-opioid receptors in the brain. When these receptors are activated, patients not only report decreased sensitivity to pain, but many also report feeling a highly pleasurable, or euphoric sensation.[32] That being said, it is easy to understand why these medications can be overused.[33] However, over-activation of these mu-opioid receptors can lead to life-threatening complications. Opioids slow down, or depress, the automatic drive we all have to breathe. In an overdose situation, this can lead to severe respiratory depression, suffocation, and death.

Unfortunately, drug overdoses are now more common than they have ever been in the United States, with almost 400,000 individuals having died from an opioid overdose since 1999.

Table 12-1. Categories and Examples of Commonly Used Addictive Substances

Category	Substance Examples*	Physiologic Effect
Depressants	■ alcohol ■ alprazolam (Xanax) ■ ketamine (Ketalar) ■ pentobarbital (Nembutal)	Slow down the mind and body by inhibiting normal functioning in the central nervous system. Effects include sedation, dizziness, discoordination, disinhibition, relaxation, memory impairment, and confusion.
Stimulants	■ amphetamine (Adderall) ■ cathinones (i.e., Bath Salts) ■ cocaine ■ methamphetamine ■ nicotine	Increase activity in the brain by stimulating the central nervous system. Effects include insomnia, upset stomach, increased blood pressure and heart rate, enhanced concentration, restlessness, and nervousness.
Cannabinoids	■ marijuana ■ synthetic cannabinoids (i.e., Spice/K2)	Alter normal brain function to result in a range of effects which may include discoordination, disorientation, memory impairment, relaxation, sensory impairment, and inattention.
Opiates	■ fentanyl (Duragesic) ■ heroin ■ hydrocodone (Lortab, Vicodin) ■ morphine (MS Contin) ■ oxycodone (OxyContin)	Modify nervous system responses in the brain and body that contribute to pain perception, mood, reward responses, digestion, and respiration.

*Substance examples listed in alphabetical order with prescription medications presented as "generic name (Brand Name)."

Tragically, that number is likely to continue to rise rapidly for the next several years.[34] In 2017 alone, nearly 50,000 people died from an opioid overdose; an average of 130 every day.[35] About half of these deaths were caused by misuse of prescription medications, with the other half arising from the use of illicit, or illegal, drugs like heroin, which is increasingly being contaminated with another very powerful opioid called fentanyl.[36] High-profile coverage of multi-million-dollar lawsuits and celebrity deaths may make it easy to imagine that the opioid overdose crisis is a remote issue being played out in far-off halls of power and opulent mansions of the rich and famous; the reality is that the overwhelming majority of the problems and solutions related to this epidemic occur in the lives of everyday Americans and the health professionals with whom they interact.[37]

Fortunately, these health professionals now have access to more treatment options for OUD than ever before. For example, naloxone (Narcan) is a life-saving medication that can rapidly block activity at opioid receptors to reverse overdose symptoms. Pharmacists in nearly every part of the United States have the authority to directly dispense naloxone injectors or nasal sprays without a prescription if they believe it is necessary.[38] Although more progress is needed, routine dispensing of these life-saving emergency medications alongside all opioid prescriptions is becoming increasingly common, as shown in Illustration 12-1. Unfortunately, just as with other health conditions, there is substantial social stigma surrounding addiction. The fear of being negatively labeled or shamed in some way can increase patient resistance to accepting naloxone.[39] Such resistance is certainly present for the patient in "Gasping," as indicated by his negative reaction to the pharmacist's offer to discuss naloxone. Pharmacists address this stigma and other barriers by educating patients that naloxone is a life-saving medication for use as an emergency safety measure, and that overdose and respiratory depression are potential risks for all individuals taking opioids, not just individuals with SUD.[40]

Nevertheless, some individuals are predisposed to develop SUD upon exposure to rewarding medications such as opioids.[41] These individuals eventually develop physical and psychological dependence that can lead to drug-seeking behavior, which is highlighted in Illustration 12-2. Drug-seeking behavior is SUD's distinguishing symptom and frequently takes place despite ongoing negative consequences (e.g., loss of employment, relationship distress, legal troubles).[42] Pharmacists have an important role in identifying "red flags" for SUD, or behaviors that may signal worsening of the patient's condition.[43] For patients taking prescription medications like opioids, red flag behaviors may include use of multiple prescribers and pharmacies, or altered/forged prescriptions.

Red flag behaviors may help pharmacists distinguish true drug-seeking behavior from the need for simple dose increases due to tolerance. The human body adapts to repeated opioid exposure by requiring higher doses to produce the same response, sensation, or effect.[32] As a result, a patient whose pain was relieved by a single opioid tablet at the start of treatment may require multiple tablets to produce the same effect months later. For example, professional athletes who had been using opioids for years reported that they were taking up to 200 tablets per day at the height of their misuse, which is around 33 times the number of tablets a person with no previous opioid exposure would be prescribed.[44]

As depicted in Illustrations 12-1 and 12-2, pharmacists routinely access electronic databases that track the distribution of controlled substances that are legally dispensed by pharmacies to monitor for red flag behaviors. Such databases include detailed information about prescribers, medications dispensed, dosages, quantities, dispensing locations, and dates filled.[45] Controlled substances are those medications considered by the US Drug Enforcement Administration to have a high risk for misuse and diversion.[46] The map in Illustration 12-2 is intended to be a mental representation of what the pharmacist is thinking about as he reviews the patient's recent controlled substance use in a database such as this. Although illicit drug use often occurs alongside legal prescription medication misuse in individuals with SUD, such information is not captured in these monitoring databases.

For most individuals with SUD, the combination of tolerance, psychological dependence, and persistent cravings results in ongoing dose escalation for their substance of choice. This often puts patients at substantially increased risk of overdose. There are many different types of opiates (Table 12-1), and each has a different level of activity at the mu-opioid receptor. In other words, some are stronger than others. This influences the overall dose needed to achieve the desired effect, as well as the likelihood of inducing overdose.

To help patients manage their medications, pharmacists frequently conduct patient interviews, record medication histories, and work with other health professionals to improve medication use. This book is replete with examples of these professional activities. Since there are usually many similar medications within a given drug class (i.e., category), pharmacists often use dose conversion calculations or reference dose conversion tables in completing their work. In OUD, where patients may be taking multiple types of opiates with different strengths, pharmacists often use a strategy of converting all opiate use into morphine milligram equivalents (MME).[47] The daily MME, as depicted in Illustration 12-3, is directly related to a patient's level of overdose risk. The patient's daily MME in the illustrated case "Gasping" exceeds 90 due to taking multiple different opioid prescriptions as a consequence of his drug-seeking behavior. This puts him at a four-fold increased risk of overdose compared to individuals taking less than 20 MME daily.[48] Keep in mind, however, that this increased risk would be present even in a patient who does not have OUD and is simply taking a 90 MME daily opioid dose exactly as prescribed.

As demonstrated in Illustration 12-3, when patient safety concerns related to overdose are identified, pharmacists work with prescribers and other health professionals to discuss their treatment options. In the case of prescription substances like opioids, this will often include a plan to reduce the patient's dose of the medication according to a defined taper regimen. Tapering involves steadily reducing medication intake in a strategic manner in order to safely lower a patient's dose while minimizing withdrawal symptoms.[49] Even a well-designed taper regimen, however, can induce withdrawal symptoms. Pharmacists are responsible for providing advice regarding appropriate medications to reduce such symptoms. Likewise, where ongoing treatment of the underlying condition (e.g., chronic pain) still needs to be addressed, pharmacists will make recommendations to patients and other health professionals about alternative medication options.[50] While it is not explicitly stated in the case, the result of the pharmacist's intervention in Illustration 12-3 led to his primary care physician transitioning him to ibuprofen, a non-steroidal anti-inflammatory drug (NSAID), to treat his chronic back pain. Data from current studies indicate that NSAIDs are likely to have equivalent or improved benefit for the patient, without the risks associated with opioids.[51]

While treatment modification to reduce overall drug burden will be taken whenever an overdose risk is present, there are additional steps that pharmacists should take when the presence of SUD is known or suspected to be involved. Depending on the practice setting, these may include formal or informal screening of the patient for SUD risk factors, direct discussion of readiness to change, referral to specialty care through an inpatient or outpatient addiction medicine or counseling program, management of co-morbid or complicating health conditions, and provision of ongoing medication support for the patient.[52] For individuals with OUD, Tobacco Use Disorder, or Alcohol Use Disorder, pharmacist expertise is frequently employed in the selection and provision of maintenance medications that can reduce cravings and decrease the risk of relapse. Indeed, pharmacists continuously help patients with OUD through their critical participation in the use of medication-assisted therapies (MAT) like buprenorphine, as one facet of a long-term integrated care plan. For more information on readiness to change and management of co-morbid conditions, readers are encouraged to explore the illustrated cases "Change Talk" in Chapter 4 Prevention & Wellness and "Wounded" in Chapter 8 Infectious Diseases, respectively.

Unfortunately, although MAT is often a life-saving intervention, not all patients are aware of this care option. As implied in Illustration 12-4, proper access to documentation of SUD-related treatment considerations can be critical. This is the case for improving patient access to not only MAT, but all types of treatment resources. While progress has been made to increase shared documentation across pharmacies in some places, different businesses often continue to maintain separate records, and this fragmentation can lead to missed opportunities.[53] In the illustrated case "Gasping," one year following the pharmacist-initiated intervention that reduced the patient's opioid overdose risk, he returned to the same pharmacy with a new injury to fill his prescription-strength ibuprofen. The pharmacist in Illustration 12-4 is new to this pharmacy. Without any explicit documentation in the local records or input from other members of the team providing this patient's care, she is unaware of the patient's history with opioid misuse. As a result, she misses a critical opportunity to provide customized education for the patient about the safe use of pain medications.

Pharmacists also serve as a key source of non-medication support by providing information regarding community resources for addiction recovery, such as 12-step treatment programs like Alcoholics Anonymous (AA) and Narcotics Anonymous (NA).[54] Pharmacists should also be vigilant for potential relapse triggers like increased pain, as the patient indicates in Illustration 12-4. When pharmacists notice these triggers, they can support patient application of learned behavioral coping mechanisms to reduce the risk of patients returning to problematic patterns of medication use.[55]

A less direct, though still crucially important, facet of pharmacist care in relation to SUD and overdose is public education regarding the safe storage and disposal of controlled substances. As exemplified in Illustration 12-5, the majority of misused controlled substances are either provided by a friend or family member or taken from their unsecured supply.[56] Pharmacists have an active role in not only providing counseling regarding the secure storage and effective disposal of controlled substances, but also through direct efforts to support drug take-back programs. Many pharmacies have assumed responsibility for managing disposal programs for unused medications.[57]

Where unsecured controlled substances are misused, the risks of overdose are dramatically increased compared to individuals previously using opioids as prescribed.[58] While an SUD diagnosis, or a history of SUD, is one factor increasing an individual's risk of overdose, there are many other possibilities; these include concurrent use of other drugs, prior drug use and tolerance, and a host of individual factors like genetic variations in drug metabolism and co-morbid health conditions.[59] In "Gasping," we see the patient and a friend in Illustration 12-5 drinking alcohol together. The patient's ibuprofen is not relieving his symptoms, possibly due to an acute flare-up following a sports injury, and he is poised to take five tablets of a painkiller from his friend's leftover supply. Perhaps recognizing these as similar to the previously received oxycodone 5-mg tablets, he would be taking a dose that is less than half of what he was using one year ago. However, even use of a previously "safe" amount of an opioid medication can be disastrous if factors in the patient's life have been modified. One important example from this patient's case would be his decreased tolerance to opioids due to an extended period of abstinence. Another critical consideration is the simultaneous consumption of alcohol, another central nervous system depressant.

As revealed in Illustration 12-6, the combination of these factors have increased the potency and effects of the painkiller the patient took in Illustration 12-5 and have resulted in an unintentional opioid overdose. Opioid overdose is characterized by the individual appearing sleepy or unresponsive, with breathing that is absent or shallow with sputtering, choking, or gasping. While pharmacists will optimally use their expertise to identify at-risk patients and educate these individuals, their friends, family, and other caregivers on specific medication-related risks to prevent overdoses from occurring, the impact of pharmacist interventions on behalf of these patients is far from over even after overdoses occur. Pharmacists are not only a major source of public education regarding how to recognize and respond to an overdose, but are also directly involved in the provision of emergency care when accidental or intentional drug overdoses happen. See the illustrated cases "Accidental" in Chapter 6 Pediatrics and "Life & Death" in Chapter 10 Emergency Medicine for additional examples of drug overdoses. In opioid overdose situations similar to this case, without immediate access to naloxone, patient survival depends on whether family members, friends, or bystanders in the vicinity have been trained to (1) identify the hallmarks of opioid overdose and (2) to perform life-saving interventions such as immediately contacting emergency services and performing rescue breathing until support arrives.

DISCUSSION QUESTIONS FOR "GASPING"

1. In Illustrations 12-1 and 12-2, it is not shown whether the pharmacist ever dispensed the prescription opioid medication to the patient. What do you think the appropriate decision would be in this case?

2. Between Illustrations 12-3 and 12-4, the patient has switched from oxycodone to ibuprofen for treatment of his back pain. What other treatment changes do you think could have been made in the past year? Why?

3. In Illustration 12-5, we do not see what the patient is thinking. Given your impressions of individuals with substance use disorder, what is your interpretation?

4. In Illustration 12-6, the patient is in the midst of an overdose, but the outcome of the case is not shown. What single pharmacist intervention would you add, remove, or change to maximize the probability of a positive resolution?

5. Throughout this illustrated case, no one explicitly mentions substance use disorder. At which point, if any, do you think each character should have broached this concept?

6. Physician-pharmacist interprofessional collaboration is shown in Illustration 12-3. What other health professionals can you identify whose expertise could have been leveraged to improve the care of this patient? What would each have contributed?

BARRIERS: An Illustrated Case Study

Story by Casey E. Gallimore & Joseph A. Zorek
Illustrations by George Folz, © 2019 Board of Regents of the University of Wisconsin System

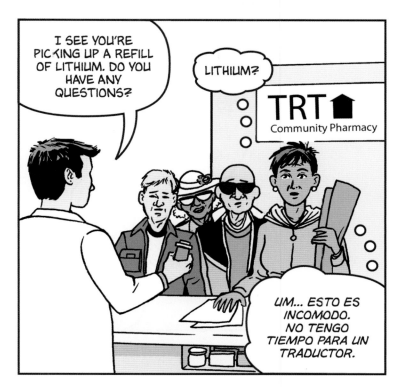

Illustration 12-7

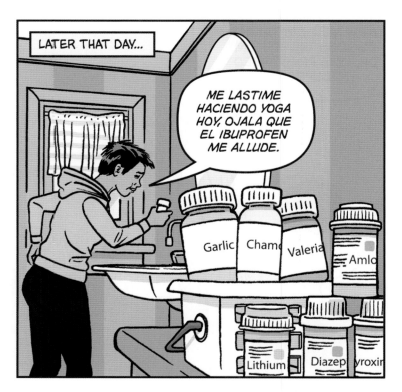

Illustration 12-8

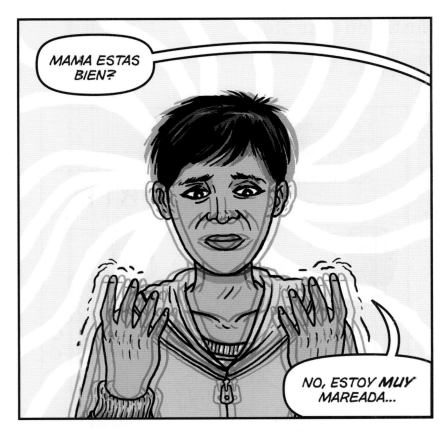

Illustration 12-9

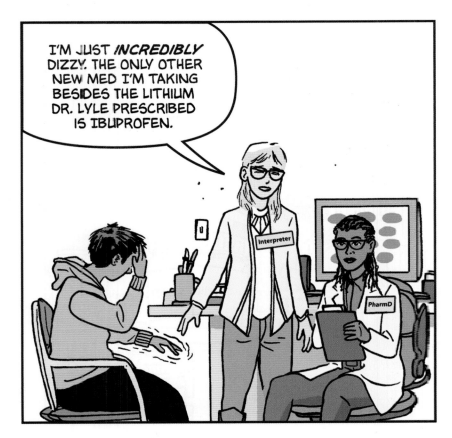

Illustration 12-10

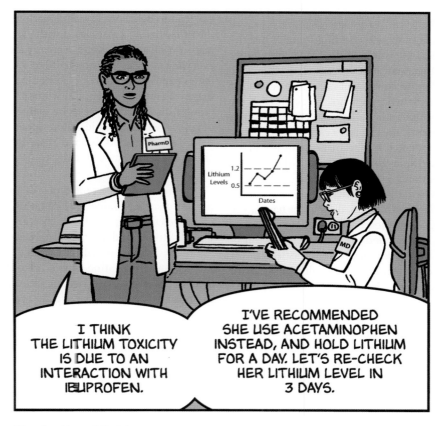

Illustration 12-11

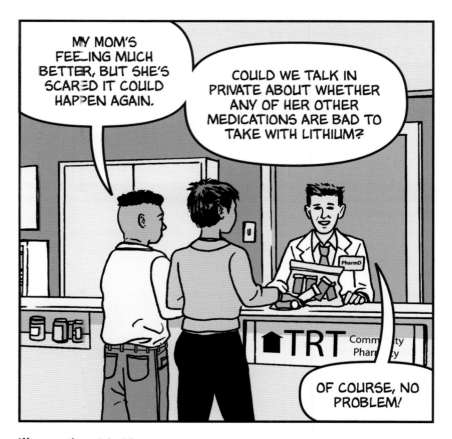

Illustration 12-12

Thoughts on "Barriers"

There are numerous obstacles to safe and high-quality healthcare in the United States, with some of the most frequently noted difficulties including unaffordable care, lack of access to care, and lack of culturally competent care.[60] Experienced through the lens of a patient who does not speak English, or one whose cultural background and beliefs may differ from the majority of American patients, the last issue can be particularly problematic.[61] A study conducted by the Institute of Medicine identified that racial and ethnic disparities in healthcare exist independent of health insurance coverage, income, age, or type of health condition.[62] When these challenges are combined with the presence of mental health issues, difficulties navigating the complexities of the US healthcare system grow exponentially.[12,63] The illustrated case "Barriers" is a fictional account of one patient's experience dealing with such complexities. In this case, a lack of culturally competent mental healthcare leads to a serious adverse drug event, which is reversed through interprofessional teamwork in a primary care setting, ending with an opportunity for redemption, which the patient's community pharmacist eagerly takes advantage of.

Indeed, because psychotropic medications are so commonly used, community pharmacists are often the most regular point of interaction with the healthcare system for individuals experiencing mental health challenges. As an example, Illustration 12-7 of the illustrated case "Barriers" introduces a patient picking up lithium from a local community pharmacy. Dosed carefully and monitored closely, lithium can be a safe and effective medication for treating bipolar disorder. Individuals with bipolar disorder experience shifts in mood from extreme highs to intense lows. These shifts go beyond simply being "moody" from the normal ups and downs of day-to-day life. Mood shifts in the context of bipolar disorder are dramatic and disabling, and involve episodes of mania or depression.[64] Manic episodes are characterized by abnormally elevated, expansive, or irritable mood and drastically increased activity or energy. Severe mania

can lead to delusions or hallucinations.[42] Bipolar depression, on the other hand, is associated with extreme sadness or hopelessness, as well as reductions in energy and motivation to complete everyday tasks. It is estimated that 4.4% of adults in the United States experience bipolar disorder in their lifetime, with similar diagnosis rates for men and women.[65] The underlying cause of bipolar disorder has yet to be identified, but given patterns of diagnosis within families, there appears to be a genetic component. Left untreated, bipolar disorder can be very debilitating and is a risk factor for suicide.[64]

There are many different types of medications used to treat bipolar disorder (Table 12-2).[66] Lithium is an older medication compared to antipsychotics such as aripiprazole (Abilify), lurasidone (Latuda), and the mood stabilizer lamotrigine (Lamictal). However, lithium is still considered a first-line, or preferred, medication for treating bipolar disorder due to the wealth of evidence supporting its benefit and safety when used over long periods of time. Furthermore, it is relatively inexpensive when compared to newer antipsychotics.

It is important to note that pharmacists play a critically important role on interprofessional mental health teams ensuring the safe use of psychotropic medications. This frequently involves monitoring drug concentrations (i.e., levels) in the body to ensure they remain in a range that is likely to produce the desired effect without causing toxicity. This is referred to as therapeutic drug monitoring (TDM), and it is a professional activity highlighted several times throughout this book, including its use in outpatient settings similar to "Barriers." Readers are encouraged to explore the illustrated cases "Underlying Cause" in Chapter 5 Cardiology and "Integrated" in Chapter 13 Technology for additional examples. Lithium requires TDM at regular intervals to ensure its safe use. As demonstrated in Illustration 12-11, the therapeutic range for lithium is 0.5 mg/dL to 1.2 mg/dL, which the main character's concentration far exceeds.[67]

Category	Medication Examples*	Physiologic Effect
Mood stabilizers	<ul><li>carbamazepine (Tegretol)</li><li>divalproex (Depakote)</li><li>lamotrigine (Lamictal)</li><li>lithium (Lithobid)</li></ul>	Promote euthymic mood by preventing or minimizing episodes of depression and mania.
Antipsychotics	<ul><li>aripiprazole (Abilify)</li><li>asenapine (Saphris)</li><li>cariprazine (Vraylar)</li><li>lurasidone (Latuda)</li><li>olanzapine (Zyprexa)</li><li>paliperidone (Invega)</li><li>quetiapine (Seroquel)</li><li>risperidone (Risperdal)</li><li>ziprasidone (Geodon)</li></ul>	Treat or prevent episodes of psychosis (hallucinations, delusions, disorganized speech, and thoughts) by changing the effect certain chemicals have in the brain. These chemicals include dopamine, serotonin, noradrenaline, and acetylcholine.

Table 12-2. Categories and Examples of Medications Commonly Used in the Treatment of Bipolar Disorder

*Medication examples presented in alphabetical order as "generic name (Brand Name)."

Early signs and symptoms of lithium toxicity include, but are not limited to, tremor, dizziness, nausea, vomiting, confusion, and slurred speech. As one might imagine, symptoms of lithium toxicity can be terrifying for patients. This fear is captured in Illustration 12-9, which depicts the patient as extremely dizzy. We also meet for the first time the patient's son, whom we later learn serves as an informal guide/healthcare navigator for his mother. He asks, "Mom, are you okay?" to which she replies, "No, I'm really dizzy ..."

To complicate the illustrated case "Barriers" further, many medications interact with lithium, including some commonly purchased over-the-counter ones. Community pharmacists can play a significant role in helping patients avoid drug interactions, but they need to develop trusting relationships with patients to do so. Patients regularly make self-care decisions without all the necessary information to do so safely, and without informing health professionals of their decisions. In Illustration 12-8, we encounter such a situation. The patient states, "Yoga did a number on my back ... hope this ibuprofen helps." Unfortunately, the patient does not realize that ibuprofen is one of the many medications that interacts negatively with lithium. Lithium is primarily eliminated by the body through the kidneys. When ibuprofen is taken simultaneously, it limits the kidneys' ability to filter and get rid of lithium through the urine. When this happens, the concentration of lithium in the body begins to increase.

It is the responsibility of all health professionals to provide information that empowers people to be informed consumers, able to use and interpret information on their own to make decisions. The illustrated case "Empowerment" in Chapter 5 Cardiology provides a good example. Due to the frequency with which many people visit pharmacies and purchase self-care products like ibuprofen, pharmacists play an especially important role in supporting patients in making informed self-care decisions. It is important to recognize that patients from different backgrounds may utilize medications differently. For example, it is common in some cultures to rely heavily on natural products or herbal medications. Indeed, a scene common in many households unfolds in the patient's bathroom in Illustration 12-8. Here we see that the patient has on hand at least three other prescription medications in addition to lithium (diazepam for anxiety, levothyroxine for hypothyroidism, and amlodipine for high blood pressure), several herbal medications (garlic, used for a wide range of purposes; chamomile, used most commonly to promote sleep or treat stomach upset; and valerian, used most commonly to promote sleep or treat anxiety), and a bottle of ibuprofen, which she has unfortunately selected without consulting any health professional.[68]

Although this lack of consultation may occur for any number of reasons, in this case, an initial lack of culturally competent care played a significant role. Cultural competence is a combination of behaviors, attitudes, and policies that enable health professionals and organizations to provide care in a manner that respects diversity in patient populations. It does so by taking into consideration cultural factors that can affect health and healthcare, such as language, communication styles, customs, beliefs, values, attitudes, and behaviors.[69] While providing care that is culturally competent across diverse patient populations is challenging in many care settings, certain characteristics common to community pharmacies can make this especially difficult. The layout and workflow within many community pharmacies, for example, are not conducive to supporting private conversations between pharmacists and patients. This is demonstrated in Illustration 12-7, where the pharmacist inadvertently reveals the patient's health condition due to the proximity of the line of patients queued behind her.

Additionally, lack of privacy in community pharmacies is particularly problematic in instances of stigmatizing mental health diagnoses and associated medications. Guarding against stigma and helping patients navigate stigmatized health conditions is an important role for pharmacists. Readers are encouraged to explore the illustrated case "Swish" in Chapter 3 Primary Care for another example. Within the general population there are preconceived ideas or stereotypes of what a person diagnosed with bipolar disorder or schizophrenia or severe depression looks like and how they think and behave. Individuals experiencing mental health challenges are often viewed negatively and treated differently.[12] Recurring discussions linking mental illness to mass shootings and other violence in the United States have likely added to the fear and stigmatization surrounding mental health.[70] As a result, individuals may fear negative consequences in their relationships, work prospects, and status in the community should others find out about their diagnosis.[12] This is apparent in the patient's reaction to the inadvertent revelation of her diagnosis in Illustration 12-7, as she thinks to herself "Uh, this is awkward."

Language barriers also challenge the ability of health professionals to provide culturally competent care. As the United States continues to become more diverse, the healthcare system must be able to provide high-quality care to patients from diverse backgrounds who may not speak English. Unfortunately, many healthcare facilities in the United States are not set up in a manner to do this. In addition to thinking about the awkwardness of discussing lithium therapy in a public space, the patient is in a hurry and thinks "I don't have time for an interpreter." This suboptimal experience ultimately results in the dangerous drug interaction and negative outcome she experiences.

Of course, language barriers are not unique to community pharmacies. In Illustration 12-10, we meet a clinical pharmacist working in a primary care setting with access to on-site medical interpreters who are able to provide in-person, real-time translation. Medical interpreting is its own field within healthcare and interpreters go through training and certification in order to provide their services, although specific requirements vary by state.[71] Several key aspects of communication through an interpreter are shown in Illustration 12-10; for example, the interpreter is positioned off to the side and the pharmacist maintains eye contact with the patient, speaking directly to her. In addition to interprofessional teamwork with the medical interpreter, Illustration 12-11 demonstrates collaborative practice between the pharmacist and primary care physician to address the patient's pain while safely reversing the toxicity from the drug interaction.

Efforts have been underway for many years to expand pharmacy services and interprofessional teamwork across a range of practice settings, including in community pharmacies. Medication therapy management (MTM) is the systematic review of a patient's regimen to ensure all medications are indicated, safe, and effective.[72] During an MTM interaction, pharmacists often provide medication education and may send recommendations to the patient's prescriber. Legislation at the federal level in 2006 allowed pharmacists to be reimbursed for providing MTM services for patients meeting certain criteria.[73] In schools and colleges of pharmacy across the nation, pharmacy students are taught a systematic process for providing MTM and other related clinical services using the Pharmacists' Patient Care Process (PPCP), which involves providing patient-centered, team-based care through a standardized process.[74] In Illustration 12-12, we see a prime opportunity for the community pharmacist to provide MTM services using the PPCP. The patient has returned to the pharmacy with her bilingual son and has brought in all her medications. In this scenario, the pharmacist could now work with the patient to determine if each prescription medication, over-the-counter medicine, and herbal product is safe, indicated, and being optimally used. For more information on community pharmacy-based services, readers are encouraged to explore the illustrated cases "Organized Chaos," "Transformation," and "Breathe" in Chapter 2 Community Pharmacy.

As this final intervention depicted in "Barriers" unfolds, it is likely that the fictional patient will receive the same benefits that scores of real individuals have already experienced due to psychiatric pharmacists using MTM as part of a team-based approach to care. For example, a pharmacy service called Meds-Help has supported individuals at the Department of Veterans Affairs (VA) in correctly and consistently taking antipsychotic medications prescribed to treat bipolar disorder, schizophrenia, or schizoaffective disorder, using unit dose packaging, refill reminders, and individual sessions to review all the patient's medications and provide tailored education.[75] Likewise, at Hennepin County Mental Health Center in Minneapolis, pharmacists are integrated into the health center, providing MTM services to patients with severe mental illness.[76] This includes reviewing medications for efficacy, drug interactions, duplicate therapy, therapeutic dosing, and the development and implementation of a long-term treatment plan. As with the patient depicted in this case, these ongoing efforts of pharmacists integrated across multiple mental health practice settings serve to overcome multiple barriers to patient care, ultimately making positive impacts on the social, psychological, emotional, and physical well-being of their patients.

DISCUSSION QUESTIONS FOR "BARRIERS"

1. Internal thoughts and dialogue in Spanish were used in Illustrations 12-7 through 12-9. How did that impact your understanding and emotional reactions to what was occurring? How do you think that relates to what the patient was feeling during this encounter?

2. Illustrations 12-8 and 12-12 highlight this patient using prescription, over-the-counter, and herbal products together. What are some methods that might be used to communicate this information to the interprofessional team? Who should be responsible for that communication?

3. Collaboration with a medical interpreter is shown in Illustration 12-10, while a bilingual family member is brought along to provide interpretive services in Illustration 12-12. What are the strengths and weaknesses of each approach? Are there other approaches that could be used?

4. In both Illustrations 12-7 and 12-12, lithium is mentioned aloud in relationship to a specifically identifiable patient in the community pharmacy. What, if anything, is the difference between these two scenarios? What methods can you think of to support patient privacy in busy healthcare settings?

5. Within this case, cultural competency training is never explicitly addressed. Which of the depicted members of the mental health team do you think should receive such training? Who should be responsible for providing it?

CHAPTER SUMMARY

- Pharmacists are an integral part of the interprofessional mental health team, tasked with the design, implementation, and monitoring of complex medication regimens.

- Pharmacists can, and do, engage with patients who have mental health concerns on a daily basis, in settings that include community pharmacies, inpatient mental health facilities, and everything in between.

- Approximately 10% of individuals will develop addiction, or substance use disorder, during their lifetime, with common substances ranging from depressants and stimulants to cannabinoids and opiates.

- Opioid use disorder and associated overdose deaths have plagued the United States in recent years, and pharmacists have been on the front lines of this crisis working to reduce illegal opioid use and to promote the use of naloxone (Narcan), an opioid overdose-reversal agent.

- The use of psychotropic medications to treat mental health conditions such as depression, anxiety, schizophrenia, and bipolar disorder is common, making pharmacists key members of interprofessional mental health teams.

- Mental health conditions are often stigmatized; as a result, pharmacists and other health professionals must work diligently to ensure the privacy and confidentiality of their patients. Providing such care in a culturally competent manner when working on behalf of patients from diverse backgrounds is equally important.

- Individuals who desire specific training in mental health beyond the PharmD may choose to pursue a specialty residency, research fellowship, and/or pursue board certification as a psychiatric pharmacist.

- The College of Psychiatric and Neurologic Pharmacists website (cpnp.org) is a great starting point to get more information, find training programs in your area, and contact pharmacists working in this practice area.

REFERENCES

1. MentalHealth.gov. What Is Mental Health? Available at https://www.mentalhealth.gov/basics/what-is-mental-health. Accessed May 31, 2020.

2. Muehsam D, Lutgendorf S, Mills PJ, et al. The embodied mind: a review on functional genomic and neurological correlates of mind-body therapies. *Neurosci Biobehav Rev.* 2017;73:165-181.

3. Office of the Assistant Secretary for Planning and Evaluation. *Innovative Medicaid Managed Care Coordination Programs for Co-Morbid Behavioral Health and Chronic Physical Health Conditions: Final Report.* Washington DC; 2015.

4. Groopman J. The troubled history of psychiatry. Available at https://www.newyorker.com/magazine/2019/05/27/the-troubled-history-of-psychiatry. Accessed May 31, 2020.

5. Rubio-Valera M, Chen TF, O'Reilly CL. New roles for pharmacists in community mental health care: a narrative review. *Int J Environ Res Public Health.* 2014;11(10):10967-10990.

6. American Psychiatric Association. What is psychotherapy? Available at https://www.psychiatry.org/patients-families/psychotherapy. Accessed May 31, 2020.

7. Gillespie SM, Manheim C, Gilman C, et al. Interdisciplinary team perspectives on mental health care in VA home-based primary care: a qualitative study. *Am J Geriatr Psychiatry.* 2019;27(2):128-137.

8. Hesdorffer DC. Comorbidity between neurological illness and psychiatric disorders. *CNS Spectr.* 2016;21(3):230-238.

9. World Health Organization. Depression and other common mental disorders: global health estimates. Available at https://www.who.int/mental_health/management/depression/prevalence_global_health_estimates/en/. Accessed May 31, 2020.

10. Substance Abuse and Mental Health Services Administration. *Key Substance Use and Mental Health Indicators in the United States: Results from the 2017 National Survey on Drug Use and Health.* Rockville, MD; 2018. Available at https://www.samhsa.gov/data/. Accessed May 31, 2020.

11. National Institute of Mental Health. Mental illness. Available at https://www.nimh.nih.gov/health/statistics/mental-illness.shtml. Accessed May 31, 2020.

12. Corrigan PW, Druss BG, Perlick DA. The impact of mental illness stigma on seeking and participating in mental health care. *Psychol Sci Public Interest.* 2014;15(2):37-70.

13. Wu L-T, Blazer DG. Substance use disorders and psychiatric comorbidity in mid and later life: a review. *Int J Epidemiol.* 2014;43(2):304-317.

14. *Medical Expenditure Panel Survey (MEPS).* Rockville, MD; 2017.

15. Greenblatt DJ, Harmatz JS, Shader RI. Update on psychotropic drug prescribing in the United States: 2014–2015. *J Clin Psychopharmacol.* 2018;38(1):1-4.

16. Margineanu DG. Neuropharmacology beyond reductionism—a likely prospect. *Biosystems.* 2016;141:1-9.

17. Panza F, Lozupone M, Stella E, et al. Psychiatry meets pharmacogenetics for the treatment of revolving door patients with psychiatric disorders. *Expert Rev Neurother.* 2016;16(12):1357-1369.

18. Gotlib D, Bostwick JR, Calip S, Perelstein E, Kurlander JE, Fluent T. Collaborative care in ambulatory psychiatry: content analysis of consultations to a psychiatric pharmacist. *Psychopharmacol Bull.* 2017;47(4):41-46.

19. Goldstone LW, Saldana SN, Werremeyer A. Pharmacist provision of patient medication education groups. *Am J Health Syst Pharm.* 2015;72(6):487-492.

20. Chung B, Dopheide JA, Gregerson P. Psychiatric pharmacist and primary care collaboration at a skid-row safety-net clinic. *J Natl Med Assoc.* 2011;103(7):567-574.

21. McLaughlin JE, Kennedy L, Garris S, et al. Student pharmacist experiences as inpatient psychiatry medication education group leaders during an early immersion program. *Curr Pharm Teach Learn.* 2017;9(5):856-861.

22. German A, Johnson L, Ybarra G, Warholak T. Assessment of pharmacists' self-reported preparedness to provide pharmacotherapy services to individuals with psychiatric disorders. *Ment Heal Clin.* 2018;8(1):1-6.

23. College of Psychiatric and Neurologic Pharmacists. Practice settings. Available at https://cpnp.org/career/settings. Accessed May 31, 2020.

24. Martin R. It's the go-to drug to treat opioid addiction. Why won't more pharmacies stock it? Available at https://www.npr.org/templates/transcript/transcript.php?storyId=741113454. Accessed May 31, 2020.

25. Kaiser Health News. In North Carolina, Native Americans take control of their health care. US News and World Report. Available at https://www.usnews.com/news/healthiest-communities/articles/2019-07-22/native-americans-take-control-of-their-health-care-in-north-carolina. Accessed May 31, 2020.

26. Cowan P. Regina pharmacy's dedication to mental health is "a dream come true": psychiatrist. Regina Leader Post. Available at https://leaderpost.com/news/local-news/regina-pharmacys-dedication-to-mental-health-is-a-dream-come-true-psychiatrist. Accessed May 31, 2020.

27. College of Psychiatric and Neurologic Pharmacists. *2018 Residency Program Director Survey Results.* Lincoln, NE; 2019. Available at https://cpnp.org/career/residencies/survey. Accessed May 31, 2020.

28. Board of Pharmacy Specialties. Psychiatric pharmacy. Available at https://www.bpsweb.org/bps-specialties/psychiatric-pharmacy/. Accessed May 31, 2020.

29. Merikangas KR, McClair VL. Epidemiology of substance use disorders. *Hum Genet.* 2012;131(6):779-789.

30. National Institute of Drug Abuse. Drugs, brains, and behavior: the science of addiction. Available at https://www.drugabuse.gov/publications/drugs-brains-behavior-science-addiction. Accessed May 31, 2020.

31. IQVIA Institute for Human Data Science. Medicine use and spending in the US: a review of 2018 and outlook to 2022.

Available at https://www.iqvia.com/insights/the-iqvia-institute/reports/medicine-use-and-spending-in-the-us-review-of-2017-outlook-to-2022. Accessed May 31, 2020.

32. Herndon CM, Strickland JM, Ray JB. Pain Management. In: DiPiro JT, Talbert RL, Yee GC, Matzke GR, Wells BG, Posey LM, eds. *Pharmacotherapy: A Pathophysiologic Approach.* 10th ed. New York, NY: McGraw-Hill Education; 2017.

33. Trang T, Al-Hasani R, Salvemini D, Salter MW, Gutstein H, Cahill CM. Pain and poppies: the good, the bad, and the ugly of opioid analgesics. *J Neurosci.* 2015;35(41):13879-13888.

34. Chen Q, Larochelle MR, Weaver DT, et al. Prevention of prescription opioid misuse and projected overdose deaths in the United States. 2019;2(2):1-12.

35. Center for Disease Control and Prevention. Wide-ranging online data for epidemiologic research (WONDER). Atlanta, GA; 2017. Available at http://wonder.cdc.gov. Accessed May 31, 2020.

36. Jalal H, Buchanich JM, Roberts MS, Balmert LC, Zhang K, Burke DS. Changing dynamics of the drug overdose epidemic in the United States from 1979 through 2016. *Science.* 2018;361(6408):eaau1184.

37. The New York Times. Opioid epidemic. Available at https://www.nytimes.com/spotlight/opioid-epidemic. Accessed May 31, 2020.

38. Legal Science. Naloxone overdose prevention laws. Available at http://pdaps.org/datasets/laws-regulating-administration-of-naloxone-1501695139. Accessed May 31, 2020.

39. Green TC, Case P, Fiske H, et al. Perpetuating stigma or reducing risk? Perspectives from naloxone consumers and pharmacists on pharmacy-based naloxone in 2 states. *J Am Pharm Assoc.* 2017;57(2S):S19.e4-S27.e4.

40. Winstanley EL, Clark A, Feinberg J, Wilder CM. Barriers to implementation of opioid overdose prevention programs in Ohio. *Subst Abus.* 2016;37(1):42-46.

41. Berrettini W. A brief review of the genetics and pharmacogenetics of opioid use disorders. *Dialogues Clin Neurosci.* 2017;19(3):229-236.

42. American Psychiatric Association. *Diagnostic and Statistical Manual of Mental Disorders.* 5th ed. Washington, DC: American psychiatric association; 2013.

43. Strand MA, Eukel H, Burck S. Moving opioid misuse prevention upstream: A pilot study of community pharmacists screening for opioid misuse risk. *Res Social Adm Pharm.* 2019;15(8):1032-1036.

44. Belson K. For N.F.L. Retirees, opioids bring more pain. *The New York Times.* Available at https://www.nytimes.com/2019/02/02/sports/nfl-opioids-.html. Accessed May 31, 2020.

45. U.S. Drug Enforcement Administration. State prescription drug monitoring programs. Available at https://www.deadiversion.usdoj.gov/faq/rx_monitor.htm. Accessed May 31, 2020.

46. Gabay M. The federal controlled substances act: schedules and pharmacy registration. *Hosp Pharm.* 2013;48(6):473-474.

47. Center for Disease Control. Calculating total daily dose of opioids for safer dosage. Available at https://www.cdc.gov/drugoverdose/pdf/calculating_total_daily_dose-a.pdf. Accessed May 31, 2020.

48. Garg RK, Fulton-Kehoe D, Franklin GM. Patterns of opioid use and risk of opioid overdose death among medicaid patients. *Med Care.* 2017;55(7):661-668.

49. US Department of Veterans Affairs. Opioid taper decision tool. Available at https://www.pbm.va.gov/AcademicDetailingService/Documents/Pain_Opioid_Taper_Tool_IB_10_939_P96820.pdf. Accessed May 31, 2020.

50. Sullivan MD, Turner JA, DiLodovico C, D'Appollonio A, Stephens K, Chan Y-F. Prescription opioid taper support for outpatients with chronic pain: a randomized controlled trial. *J Pain.* 2017;18(3):308-318.

51. Krebs EE, Gravely A, Nugent S, et al. Effect of opioid vs nonopioid medications on pain-related function in patients with chronic back pain or hip or knee osteoarthritis pain: the SPACE randomized clinical trial. *JAMA.* 2018;319(9):872-882.

52. Fishman MJ, Gordon A, Oslin D, et al. National practice guideline for the use of medications in the treatment of addiction involving opioid use. Available at https://www.asam.org/docs/default-source/practice-support/guidelines-and-consensus-docs/asam-national-practice-guideline-supplement.pdf. Accessed May 31, 2020.

53. Goundrey-Smith S. The connected community pharmacy: benefits for healthcare and implications for health policy. *Front Pharmacol.* 2018;9:1352.

54. Monico N, Thomas S. Alcoholics anonymous (AA) & The 12 steps. https://www.alcohol.org/alcoholics-anonymous/. Accessed May 31, 2020.

55. McHugh RK, Hearon BA, Otto MW. Cognitive behavioral therapy for substance use disorders. *Psychiatr Clin North Am.* 2010;33(3):511-525.

56. Lipari R, Hughes A. How people obtain the prescription pain relievers they misuse. The CBHSQ report. Available at https://www.samhsa.gov/data/sites/default/files/report_2686/ShortReport-2686.html. Accessed May 31, 2020.

57. Walgreens drug disposal program collects 1.2 million pounds. *Daily Herald.* https://www.dailyherald.com/business/20190424/walgreens-drug-disposal-program-collects-12-million-pounds. Accessed May 31, 2020.

58. Park TW, Lin LA, Hosanagar A, Kogowski A, Paige K, Bohnert ASB. Understanding risk factors for opioid overdose in clinical populations to inform treatment and policy. *J Addict Med.* 2016;10(6):369-381.

59. Webster LR. Risk factors for opioid-use disorder and overdose. *Anesth Analg.* 2017;125(5):1741-1748.

60. Health.gov. Healthy people 2020. Available at https://www.healthypeople.gov/2020/topics-objectives/topic/Access-to-Health-Services. Accessed May 31, 2020.

61. Williams DR, Mohammed SA. Racism and health I: pathways and scientific evidence. *Am Behav Sci.* 2013;57(8).

62. Nelson A. Unequal treatment: confronting racial and ethnic disparities in health care. *J Natl Med Assoc.* 2002;94(8):666-668.

63. National Alliance on Mental Illness. Continuing disparities to access to mental and physical health care. Available at https://www.nami.org/About-NAMI/Publications-Reports/Public-Policy-Reports/The-Doctor-is-Out/DoctorIsOut.pdf. Accessed May 31, 2020.

64. National Alliance on Mental Illness. Bipolar disorder. Available at https://www.nami.org/Learn-More/Mental-Health-Conditions/Bipolar-disorder. Accessed May 31, 2020.

65. Harvard medical school. National comorbidity survey (NCS). Available at https://www.hcp.med.harvard.edu/ncs/index.php. Accessed May 31, 2020.

66. Bobo WV. The diagnosis and management of bipolar I and II disorders: clinical practice update. *Mayo Clin Proc.* 2017;92(10):1532-1551.

67. Herndon CM, Strickland JM, Ray JB. Pharmacotherapy of psychosis and mania. In: Dipiro J, Talbert R, Yee G, Matzke G, Wells B, Posey L, eds. *Pharmacotherapy: A Pathophysiologic Approach.* 10th ed. New York, NY: McGraw-Hill Education; 2017.

68. National Center for Complementary and Integrative Health. Herbs at a glance. Available at https://nccih.nih.gov/health/herbsataglance.htm. Accessed May 31, 2020.

69. Centers for Disease control and Prevention. Cultural competence. Available at https://npin.cdc.gov/pages/cultural-competence#what. Accessed May 31, 2020.

70. American Psychological Association. Statement of APA president in response to mass shootings in Texas, Ohio. Available at https://www.apa.org/news/press/releases/2019/08/statement-shootings. Accessed May 31, 2020.

71. Heathcarecareers.org. Healthcare interpreter. Available at https://explorehealthcareers.org/career/allied-health-professions/health-care-interpreter/. Accessed May 31, 2020.

72. Bluml BM. Definition of medication therapy management: development of professionwide consensus. *J Am Pharm Assoc (2003)*. 2005;45(5):566-572.

73. Medicare prescription drug, improvement, and modernization act of 2003. 2003. Available at www.govtrack.us/congress/bills/108/hr1. Accessed May 31, 2020.

74. Joint Commission of Pharmacy Practitioners. The patient care process. Available at https://jcpp.net/wp-content/uploads/2016/03/PatientCareProcess-with-supporting-organizations.pdf. Accessed May 31, 2020.

75. Valenstein M, Kavanagh J, Lee T, et al. Using a pharmacy-based intervention to improve antipsychotic adherence among patients with serious mental illness. *Schizophr Bull*. 2011;37(4):727-736.

76. McKee JR, Lee KC, Cobb CD. Psychiatric pharmacist integration into the medical home. *Prim Care Companion CNS Disord*. 2013;15(4):PCC.13com01517.

CHAPTER 13

Technology

Featuring the Illustrated Case Studies "Leverage," "Integrated," & "Innovator"

Authors
Natalie S. Schmitz, Daniel J. Ruhland, Kimberly Harrison, & Joseph A. Zorek

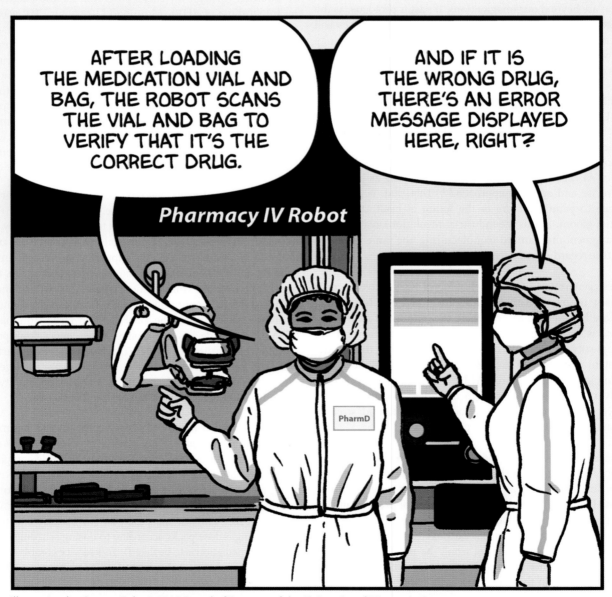

Illustration by George Folz, © 2019 Board of Regents of the University of Wisconsin System

BACKGROUND

Technology has played an integral role in the evolution of modern healthcare, from the development of the first vaccine in 1796 to investigating 3D-printed organs today.[1,2] In recent years, technological advances seem to be accelerating at an exponential rate.[3] Ray Kurzweil, a famous inventor and author, proposed the idea that technological advances extend beyond the mere invention of tools but, in fact, each technological advancement builds upon previous innovations to create an even more powerful technology. The end result is constant acceleration in the speed of innovations. Kurzweil predicts that, in the 21st century, we will see approximately 20,000 years' worth of progress in only 100 years.[4] This phenomenon is easily illustrated through the evolution of the phone. The first telephone, invented in the late 1800s, required a human to operate a switchboard. Nearly a century later, over 5 billion people have a mobile phone, drastically increasing connectivity throughout the world.[5]

New technological developments will likely impact healthcare in ways that are beyond our imaginations. If past is prologue, as the saying goes, what we can be sure of is that these advances will disrupt traditional ways of delivering care. Changes in technology require various professions and specialties to adapt and expand services or pivot to another focus. Just as the industrial revolution displaced many workers, it is predicted that artificial intelligence (AI) will impact nearly every job on the planet. Approximately 25% of US jobs will face high automation exposure, with 70% of current tasks at risk for substitution.[6] Historically, for example, skin cancer has been visually diagnosed by a dermatologist. Now, a technology called deep convolutional neural networks (CNNs), a form of AI called machine learning, is emerging as perhaps a more precise and accurate approach.[7–10] That said, it would be inaccurate to paint a picture of the future of healthcare as all doom and gloom. Just as the industrial revolution created many jobs to augment mechanized manufacturing, the same may very well be true regarding modern automation and AI.

The latest generation of new technologies is expected to produce many innovations that will be integrated into healthcare. Healthcare has entered an era where the amount of data being produced is outpacing our ability to analyze or interpret it. As the complexity and amount of data available within the healthcare system continues to increase, the need and role for AI is becoming increasingly clearer. AI has the potential to enhance the delivery of healthcare through improved diagnoses, treatment recommendations, medication adherence, and streamlined, more efficient administrative activities.[11]

Machine learning, one of the most prevalent forms of AI, is most commonly applied to a healthcare field called precision medicine, which is defined as using an individual's specific genes, environment, and lifestyle to inform disease treatment or prevention.[12] In precision medicine, many factors need to be taken into account including individual attributes and various treatment regimens to predict which treatment protocol would be most successful. In this case, the computer program, or "machine," uses algorithms to identify patterns in the data. With each iteration, the machine "learns" these patterns and what influences certain changes or outcomes. This approach allows it to become more proficient, for example, when identifying optimal treatment protocols using a specific data set.[11] The most well-known machine learning system is IBM's Watson. Watson received significant media attention for its focus on precision medicine of cancer diagnostics and treatment. However, complete, successful integration of such technologies into the healthcare setting has yet to be realized.

Another form of AI is rule-based expert systems, where "if-then" rules are used to control and leverage data. This is prominent in electronic health record (EHR) systems, an example of which is highlighted in the illustrated case "Integrated" later in this chapter.[11] The Health Information Technology for Economic and Clinical Health (HITECH) Act of 2009 sparked a wave of EHR adoption throughout US hospitals.[13] In 2008, under 10% of acute care hospitals had an EHR in place. Following the HITECH Act, EHR adoption rose precipitously to 96% in 2015. To incentivize adoption, HITECH originally designated $36 billion to be awarded through incentive programs for the adoption and meaningful use of EHRs. Meaningful use of an EHR was classified mainly as the exchange of health information. Use of technology such as e-prescribing and prescription drug monitoring programs were measured with subsequent incentives being paid out if threshold utilization levels were met. The Medicare Access and CHIP Reauthorization Act (MACRA) of 2015 continues to incentivize the adoption of EHR technologies with a focus on information exchange and quality of care.[14] MACRA modernized the measures previously implemented by HITECH with the incorporation of direct messaging between patients and providers and the use of patient-generated data within measures of quality.

Several technology giants have recognized opportunities for impact and growth within the healthcare space. For example, in 2018, Apple updated its mobile Apple Health apps to enable the display of electronic health records from 39 hospitals.[15] Other apps are available to optimize clinical research by improving enrollment, informed consent, and data collection, or increasing patient access to their own health records.[15,16] In addition, a new Apple Watch, including advanced heart monitoring through an electrocardiogram, has received clearance from the US Food and Drug Administration (FDA).[15,16] Other devices and applications are under development to monitor chronic diseases outside clinical settings while sharing that data with health professionals to improve disease management.[16] These technologies and advancements have the opportunity to revolutionize not only pharmacy but healthcare as a whole.

Amazon is another major technology company that has migrated into the healthcare space. Since starting as an online book retailer, Amazon has evolved into one of the most valuable companies in the world, with units that focus on their massive online marketplace, a cloud computing platform, AI, groceries, and now medications. PillPack, an online pharmacy, was acquired by Amazon in June 2018.[17] PillPack sorts medications by dose and packages them in single-dose packs according to dosing schedule (i.e., time of day the mediation is to be taken). This service combines the convenience of blister packs with mail-order pharmacy. Other retail pharmacies are now offering similar services.

Impact of Technological Advances on Pharmacy Practice

Many technologies have impacted the practice of pharmacy over the last several decades. The following are noteworthy for the disruptions they caused, which mostly led to positive shifts toward novel professional activities for both pharmacy technicians and pharmacists alike: computers, including EHRs, computerized physician order entry, and remote prescription verification; automated dispensing cabinets; barcode medication administration; telemedicine; and mobile health devices, including wearable technologies.[18,19]

As valued and trusted health professionals, it is crucial for pharmacists to be agile and stay current on developing technologies, including the role technological advances could play to improve patient care and maximize medication therapy. In the past, pharmacists have been able to incorporate new technologies in order to expand their services, increase healthcare access, improve patient outcomes and safety, and reduce the cost of care.[20] For example, automated dispensing gave pharmacists more time to dedicate toward patient counseling and medication therapy management, the combination of which resulted in reductions in medication errors.[21] Technological advances will continue to transform the practice of pharmacy. In response, the profession must continue to rise to this challenge and leverage new technologies, as they emerge, to spur innovation.

PHARMACISTS IN ACTION

Text-Based AI Improves Medication Adherence

Mobile technologies have become progressively more integrated into daily life, with one of the major uses being text messaging. In fact, 97% of smartphone users regularly text, amounting to over five billion texters throughout the world.[22,23] Text messages are now being used to improve communication between patients, health professionals, and healthcare systems, including appointment reminders and improved medication adherence.[24–26] These messages can vary from standard reminders to personalized messages.[27–29] Some studies have combined text messages with other services including electronic pill dispensers, requesting laboratory (i.e., lab) values from patients, and subsequent medication adjustments.[30,31] The impact of text-based refill reminders using AI to mimic human conversation was studied at Kaiser Permanente in Southern California, where 12,272 patients with chronic diseases, all covered by Medicare Part D, were targeted for this intervention.[32] The refill rate for this group was compared to 76,068 patients who did not receive text messages. The group that received tailored text messages had a 14% higher refill rate than the control group, which illustrated the significant impact text messaging solutions can have on medication adherence. Text alerts for medication refill reminders have since become ubiquitous in mainstream pharmacy practice, including at major pharmacy retailers.

Video Telehealth Training Improves Inhaler Technique

Appropriate inhaler technique is critical to manage symptoms of chronic obstructive pulmonary disease (COPD) and asthma. However, poor inhaler technique is common in both of these conditions.[33–35] Inhaler technique should be taught upon therapy initiation and followed by regular retraining to re-evaluate technique and reinforce proper use.[36] However, patient demographics, particularly for patients living in rural settings, can make this difficult if not impossible to carry out. Pharmacists at the Veterans Affairs (VA) Puget Sound Health Care System examined the use of video telehealth to train and retrain patients living in rural communities prescribed one or more inhalers.[37] Pharmacists provided up to four inhaler training sessions using video telehealth.[37] This method significantly improved inhaler technique and was well received by participants of the program, indicating video telehealth training is a promising tool for pharmacists to teach inhaler technique and could be applied to other medication delivery devices.[37]

BECOMING A PHARMACIST WITH TECHNOLOGICAL EXPERTISE

To be on the cutting edge of these new developments, it is imperative for pharmacists to have a growth mindset.[38] Pharmacists should keep an eye out for technologies that could be incorporated into pharmacy practice or other areas of healthcare or even work to identify practice or patient needs that could be addressed by apps, websites, or devices. Pharmacists should also participate in the development of relevant technologies. Developing the habit of lifelong learning and a spirit of curiosity and inquisitiveness is important to all health professionals due to rapid changes in both diagnostics and treatments.[39]

One such advancement is pharmacogenomics, the study of how genes affect an individual's response to a drug.[40] Pharmacogenomic testing is increasingly becoming part of routine patient care. Although it is likely that pharmacogenomics will be incorporated in all forms of pharmacy practice, there are opportunities for pharmacists to specialize. Pharmacogenomics certificates, focused on the integration of pharmacogenomics into pharmacy practice to improve medication use, are available through the American Society of Health-System Pharmacists (ASHP), the American College of Clinical Pharmacy, and some universities and healthcare systems.[41–44]

Electronic health records are becoming increasingly integrated into healthcare and can be leveraged to improve patient care and outcomes. EHR certifications, such as those offered by EPIC, one of the largest EHR companies in the United States, offer training in numerous areas including inpatient and outpatient pharmacy, emergency care, oncology, cardiology, and obstetrics, among many others.[45,46] These certifications demonstrate proficiency within a given area and can be beneficial for a career in health information technology (HIT).

In addition, Doctor of Pharmacy (PharmD) graduates who wish to specialize in specific areas have the opportunity to pursue post-graduate residencies. Typically, post-graduate year 1 (PGY-1) is focused on generalized clinical training and post-graduate year 2 (PGY-2) offers more specialized training. There are several PGY-2 residencies that have technology foci, including pharmacy informatics, medication systems and operations, and clinical pharmacogenomics.[47]

LEVERAGE: An Illustrated Case Study

Story by Kimberly Harrison & Joseph A. Zorek
Illustrations by George Folz, © 2019 Board of Regents of the University of Wisconsin System

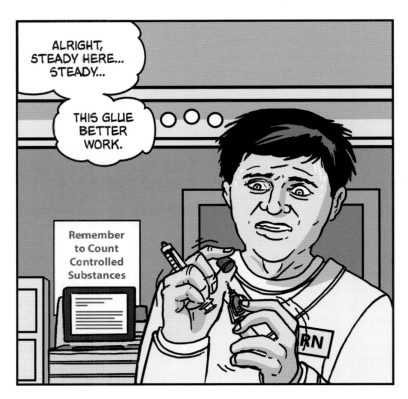

Illustration 13-1

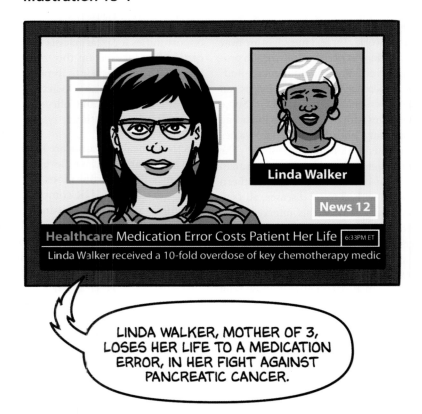

Illustration 13-2

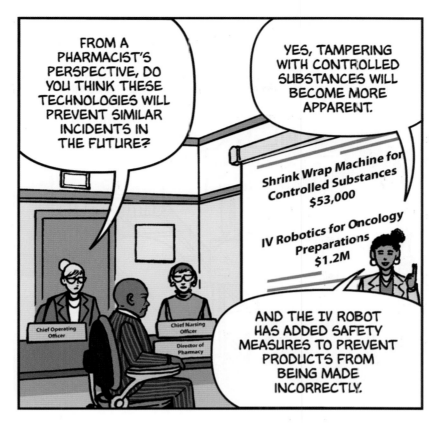

Illustration 13-3

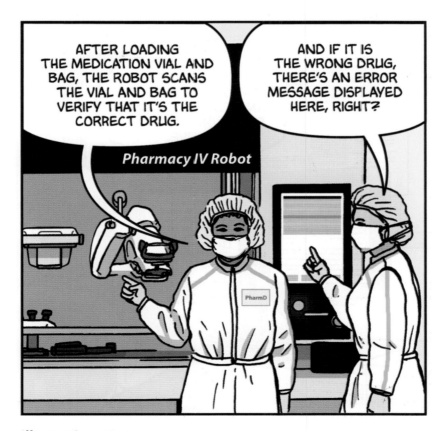

Illustration 13-4

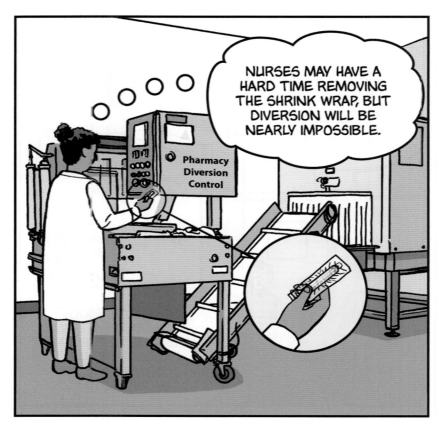

Illustration 13-5

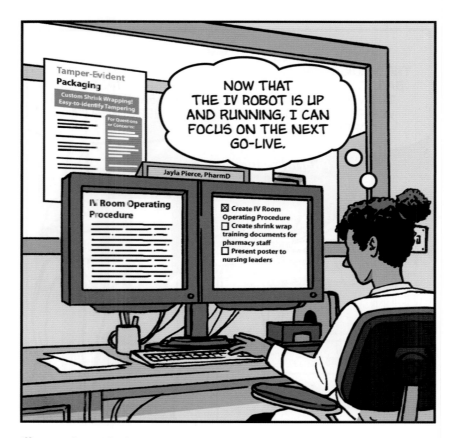

Illustration 13-6

Thoughts on "Leverage"

The use of technology and automation has become common practice in most industries, and healthcare is no exception.[48-50] Broadly speaking, healthcare technologies represent any equipment that facilitates care delivery or the provision of professional services. Within pharmacy, many technological advances have been used to automate repetitive human work.[48] This is beneficial for many reasons, the primary of which is to increase efficiency by decreasing the amount of manual labor needed to prepare, dispense, secure, and administer medications.

One of the most commonly used technologies in hospital settings is the automated dispensing cabinet (ADC).[51,52] ADCs securely store medications, similar in concept to vending machines. They are physically located in a locked medication room on the same hospital floor as the patient. Alternative medication storage on a hospital floor is in less secure cabinets or shelves, referred to as floor stock. Pharmacy staff monitor medication orders placed by providers such as physicians, physician assistants, and nurse practitioners, and proactively verify and send electronic medication orders to the ADC prior to the time they are needed. Once the order is at an ADC on the floor, at or near the administration time, the patient's nurse gains access to the medication by logging into the ADC and selecting the patient's name and needed medication, which triggers the ADC to unlock and open the appropriate medication drawer.

If an ADC is not in use, every medication dose must be dispensed from the pharmacy, which is most often located in the lower levels of the hospital. The medication must be gathered and/or prepared in the pharmacy, labeled with the patient's name and other required information (drug name, dose, instructions, etc.), and delivered to the floor either directly by a pharmacy technician or via the pneumatic tube system. These systems essentially consist of a highway of pressurized tubes inside the hospital's walls capable of sending small containers from one part of the hospital to another. Readers may recognize the same system in use by many drive-through stations at banks. Once the medication is on the floor, it must be placed in the corresponding patient's medication bin. ADCs have proven to improve medication distribution efficiency for over three decades by reducing the number of medication deliveries to a floor by 50% to 75% and by reducing the total amount of time pharmacy spends in dispensing medications by 30%.[53,54] ADCs have allowed pharmacists to focus their time and attention on other clinical and/or professional services. Many of the examples in this book of pharmacists working alongside other health professionals would not have been possible without leveraging this technology.

Hospital pharmacies must store, prepare, and dispense all medications needed for all patients in the hospital, whether using ADCs or not. The ability to do this effectively is often impacted by space limitations; in other words, there simply is not enough room to store the large amount of medications needed to care for all hospitalized patients. Carousel dispensing, a technology adapted from other industries, automates the storage and retrieval process within a pharmacy and provides another example of automation in pharmacy.[55] The carousel is essentially a large storage locker comprised of rows of medications housed within bins, with an electric motor operated by a computer system.[56] Pharmacy staff type the desired medication into the computer, and the carousel spins until the desired medication emerges. Staff either pick the medication from the carousel location or restock it with additional medication. In both cases, the medication is scanned into the computer system to confirm the correct medication is being picked or stored. Without a carousel dispensing technology, pharmacies utilize shelves to store medications and the dispensing or restocking requires pharmacy staff to manually walk to the location. This automation improved the efficiency of dispensing to such an extent that one hospital was able to reallocate the time and effort of two dedicated pharmacy staff members.[57]

Medication-related technologies are leveraged by other health professionals within hospitals, as well. Intravenous (IV) pumps are used primarily by health professionals who administer medications (e.g., nurses, anesthesiologists); however, pharmacists play an important role in managing how medications are given using this automation.[58] As opposed to the oral route of medication administration, with tablets or capsules, for example, the IV route involves administering specially formulated liquid medications directly into a patient's blood. This allows for much more rapid effects. Some IV medications must be given over an extended period of time to prevent the patient from having an adverse reaction. An IV pump can administer these IV medications to patients over a pre-defined time period or at a desired rate based on what is programmed into the pump.[57] If no pump is available, IV medications must be delivered using gravity. This method may require medications to be further diluted and can take much longer to administer. IV pumps decrease the manual workload for nurses.[59] Pumps started out as a basic technology, essentially easing the workload of nurses; however, in recent years, these pumps have evolved to adapt "smart" technologies. A smart pump is one that is capable of storing institution-specific drug libraries.[58] These libraries contain set doses and rates for administration of most IV medications, which further decreases the amount of work required for administering IV medications. With expert knowledge of IV medications, administration rates, etc., pharmacists are typically responsible for maintaining these libraries.[59]

While gained efficiency is the primary benefit from use of technology and automation in pharmacy, there are other benefits, as well. The illustrated case "Leverage," for example, depicts the use of technologies to prevent drug diversion and to decrease life-threatening medication errors. The protagonist of the case, a female pharmacist with expertise in medication systems and operations (MSO), works with her colleagues in pharmacy and other health professions to utilize technology and automation to realize these benefits for the organization.

There has been a 10-fold increase in the use of opioids in the United States in the last 20 years.[60] Opioids are medications intended to treat pain; however, their potential for causing physical and psychological dependence and addiction is high.[61] Once physically and psychologically dependent on opioids, individuals experience intense withdrawal symptoms if they stop taking these medications. As a result, some engage in risky behaviors, including illegal ones, to obtain opioids if they are unable to do so legally. Unfortunately, this situation can lead to diversion, defined as unaccountable loss, theft, use for unintended purposes, or tampering of a drug.[62] Health professionals are not immune to this problem; in fact, it has been estimated that health professionals have similar drug abuse potential as the general population.[63] One US city found that there were 423 documented cases of diversion by health professionals over 10 years. This number is likely a small representation of the true problem as documentation of such cases is low. See the illustrated case "Gasping" in Chapter 12 Mental Health for a more in-depth review of opioids and substance use disorders. Those interested in a pharmacist-led service to help patients quit nicotine-containing products are encouraged to read the illustrated case "Change Talk" in Chapter 4 Prevention & Wellness.

Preventing drug diversion is one of the principle roles of pharmacists within society. Many drugs at risk of diversion are legally classified in the United States as controlled substances.[64] The US Drug Enforcement Administration (DEA) is responsible for ensuring compliance with the Controlled Substance Act. This is a federal law that puts substances controlled under previous law into a classification system called schedules, as explained in Table 13-1. Whether a substance is controlled or not is based on the substance's medical use, potential for abuse, and safety/dependency liability.

Because most controlled substances are medications, it is the responsibility of pharmacies, pharmacy departments within hospitals, and all pharmacists to ensure they are appropriately secured and monitored to prevent diversion. In most settings, pharmacists use technologies and automation to keep controlled substances stored in secured, locked locations.[62] Access to controlled substances is limited and tracked by electronic or paper logs and surveillance cameras in some cases. Electronic or paper records are generated to capture who accesses the medications, when they were accessed, and why they were accessed.

It is speculated that diversion by health professionals is closely linked to having access to such medications.[65,66] Due to this, pharmacy departments implement measures to prevent and detect diversion of controlled substances.[62,65] Since many health professionals are involved, pharmacists must work closely with nurses, physicians, other health professionals, and internal audit departments to prevent diversion. One common method to detect and prevent diversion is to count the controlled substance every time it changes hands.[62] Illustration 13-1 includes a poster in the medication room reminding nurses of this task, providing a good example of interprofessional collaboration between nursing and pharmacy. Auditing is another diversion detection method whereby the use and movement of controlled substances are tracked and accounted for on a regular basis. When counts do not match or there is suspicion of diversion, an investigation is initiated.

The illustrated case "Leverage" begins inside a medication room, where an ADC is being used to store medications, including controlled substances, in a secured fashion to prevent diversion. Unfortunately, a nurse who is struggling with opioid use

Table 13-1. United States Drug Enforcement Administration Schedule of Controlled Substances		
Schedule	**Substance Examples***	**Description**
I	▪ heroin ▪ lysergic acid diethylamide (i.e., LSD) ▪ methylenedioxypyrovalerone (i.e., Bath Salts)	Substances with no medical use and high abuse potential that may lead to severe psychological and physical dependence; Schedule I substances deemed unsafe even under medical supervision
II	▪ cocaine ▪ fentanyl (Duragesic) ▪ hydromorphone (Dilaudid) ▪ methamphetamine ▪ morphine (MS Contin) ▪ oxycodone (OxyContin)	Substances with high abuse potential that may lead to severe psychological and physical dependence; some Schedule II substances are used for medical conditions
III	▪ anabolic steroids ▪ codeine (Tylenol with Codeine #3) ▪ ketamine (Ketalar) ▪ testosterone (Depotest)	Less abuse potential than Schedule I or I substances, with moderate to low risk of psychological and physical dependence; some Schedule III substances are used for medical conditions
IV	▪ alprazolam (Xanax) ▪ carisoprodol (Soma) ▪ lorazepam (Ativan) ▪ tramadol (Ultram) ▪ zolpidem (Ambien)	Low abuse potential, with low risk of psychological and physical dependence; Schedule IV substances are used for medical conditions
V	▪ atropine/diphenoxylate (Lomotil) ▪ cough syrup with codeine (Robitussin AC) ▪ pregabalin (Lyrica)	Less abuse potential than Schedule IV substances, with some combination products containing limited quantities of higher-risk substances; Schedule V substances are used for medical conditions

*Substance examples listed in alphabetical order with prescription medications presented as "generic name (Brand Name)."

disorder has used his login credentials to gain access to one of his patient's fentanyl syringes, a powerful opioid, and he is currently in the act of diverting this medication for personal use.[65]

Several months earlier, this nurse sustained a back injury while helping a family member unload heavy boxes and furniture during a move. Long shifts at the hospital, including limited opportunities to sit and frequent patient bed transfers, exacerbated his injury. When over-the-counter pain medications failed to provide relief, he was prescribed hydrocodone with acetaminophen (Vicodin). This worked for some time, but pain control worsened and he was prescribed oxycodone with acetaminophen (Percocet). Slowly, the nurse developed tolerance to the effects of oxycodone and he began to require escalating doses to obtain the same level of pain control. When requests to refill his oxycodone prescription early were denied, this nurse found himself in a difficult and unfortunate situation. Experiencing debilitating withdrawal symptoms with no mechanism to legally obtain oxycodone, he decided to take a few oxycodone tablets from his patients. After several months of this type of diversion, and with ever-increasing physical and psychological dependence on opioids, Illustration 13-1 captures this nurse in the midst of his first attempt to divert the powerful opioid fentanyl. Clearly distraught by the inherent risks (e.g., job loss, license revocation, imprisonment) and feeling deeply ashamed, this illustration seeks to capture the culmination of a series of unfortunate events, to draw attention to the power of physical and psychological dependence on controlled substances, and to highlight the important role pharmacists must play to ensure such medications remain secured.

Desperate to find something to treat his withdrawal symptoms, the nurse in Illustration 13-1 is shown removing fentanyl from a syringe, intending to replace this with water. A tamper-evident cap is shown in his right hand, which was intentionally added to the syringe by pharmacy to prevent diversion. However, a work-around to bypass detection was found by using glue to re-secure the tamper-evident cap. This behavior is not only illegal, but it is also dangerous for the individual and his patient, who may receive the syringe with water instead of fentanyl.[65,67] One study documented six outbreaks of bloodstream infections over a 10-year span as a result of patients receiving injectable controlled substances that had been tampered with in a manner consistent with the story depicted in the illustrated case "Leverage." One hundred eighteen patients experienced bacterial and viral bloodstream infections, causing patient harm, increased exposure to antimicrobial medications (i.e., antibiotics, antivirals), and increased utilization of healthcare services, including longer hospitalizations.[67] While not explicitly stated, the nurse's diversion in "Leverage" was discovered because the doctored fentanyl caused a pattern of infections in his patients, and nursing colleagues who became suspicious alerted hospital administrators.

Around the same time of this diversion event, a tragic medication preparation error caused the death of a patient already fighting for her life against cancer (Illustration 13-2). The patient, Linda Walker, received what she and her oncology (i.e., cancer) team thought was a regular round of chemotherapy infusion targeting her disease. Instead, the pharmacy technician who prepared the infusion misread the medication order and added 1.91 grams of

gemcitabine to the infusion bag instead of 1.71 grams of gemcitabine. The pharmacy was short-staffed that day, and both the pharmacy technician and the pharmacist responsible for verifying her work were overwhelmed and distracted. The pharmacist failed to catch the error, and Mrs. Walker received this overdose of gemcitabine, a chemotherapy agent used to treat pancreatic cancer.[68] The overdose caused Mrs. Walker to become severely anemic. Coupled with her underlying cancer and immunocompromised state, fatigue from the anemia caused Mrs. Walker to faint when walking down a flight of stairs. She sustained a severe head injury during her fall that resulted in intracranial bleeding and was found unresponsive by her family the next day. Readers interested in learning more about the role of pharmacists in cancer are encouraged to explore the illustrated cases "Compromising" and "Compassion" in Chapter 9 Oncology.

Hospital pharmacies are complex and busy with the responsibility to prepare and dispense all medications needed for all patients. Medication errors like the one experienced by Mrs. Walker, unfortunately, can result from this complexity.[69] A medication error is defined as any failure of a planned action occurring at any step in the medication use process: procurement, storage, compounding, dispensing, and administration.[69-71] Most medication errors do not cause patient harm, but when they do, as highlighted in "Leverage," it can be devastating.[70] The medication error rate has been estimated to be around 5%.[71] In terms of deaths attributable to these errors, an estimated 7000 to 9000 Americans lose their lives each year from medication errors.[72]

In response to these tragic events, a medication systems and operations (MSO) pharmacist named Dr. Jayla Pierce, working in coordination with the Director of Pharmacy, proposed two solutions to minimize future risks to the organization. Both solutions involved the purchase of new equipment leveraging technology and automation.[73,74] Illustration 13-3 depicts Jayla's presentation to administrative leaders in the hospital. The first purchase would automate shrink wrapping every controlled substance syringe, shown in Illustration 13-5, essentially strengthening the current approach by making any tampering more difficult to cover up. The second purchase would minimize human error in chemotherapy preparation via IV robotics (Illustration 13-4). Readers interested in leadership positions, like those held by the Director of Pharmacy, Chief Nursing Officer, and Chief Operating Officer in Illustration 13-3, and career options available within pharmacy administration, are encouraged to explore the illustrated cases "Opportunities" and "Relationships" in Chapter 15 Administration.

Fortunately, the administrative team supported Jayla's proposed solutions and facilitated organizational investment into these two technologies. From that point forward, Jayla is shown taking responsibility for the successful implementation of these technologies within the pharmacy department. This includes training (Illustration 13-4), quality assurance (Illustration 13-5), and alignment with policies and procedures within the department and throughout the organization (Illustration 13-6). While there is much work to be done, Jayla's efforts and expertise will surely have a positive impact on patients and health professionals within this organization well into the future.

1. The illustrated case "Leverage" highlights three main benefits of implementing technology and automation in pharmacy. Can you think of additional benefits that might be realized through this approach?

2. Illustration 13-2 shows the anchor of an evening news program reporting on a tragic medication error that resulted in a patient losing her life. What other types of medication errors can you think of that might occur in a complex organization like a hospital?

3. Diversion of controlled substances is a serious issue. One method for preventing diversion was highlighted in this illustrated case. How might pharmacists or administrative leaders prevent such diversion from occurring?

4. When presenting a business case to a group of people, the presentation must be concise, highlighting the most important details with a clear request. As it relates to the Pharmacy IV Robot, what details do you think the pharmacist would/should have covered in her presentation in Illustration 13-3?

5. Thoughts on "Leverage" describes efficiency gained from the implementation of technology and automation in terms of reducing the number of pharmacy technicians needed. This type of disruption, displacement, or replacement of human workers is controversial. Where do you fall on this issue? Is it a net positive from your perspective? Or a net negative? Why?

INTEGRATED: An Illustrated Case Study

Story by Daniel J. Ruhland & Joseph A. Zorek
Illustrations by George Folz, © 2019 Board of Regents of the University of Wisconsin System

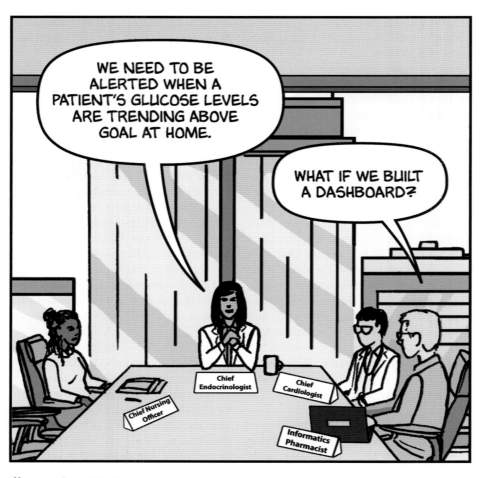

Illustration 13-7

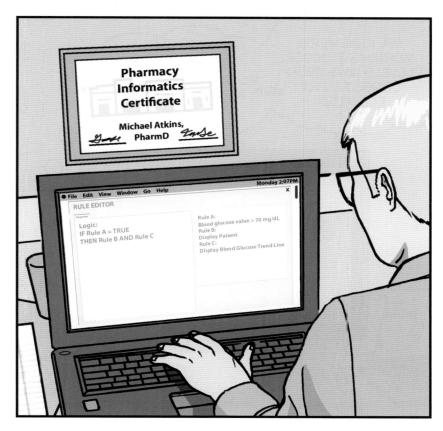

Illustration 13-8

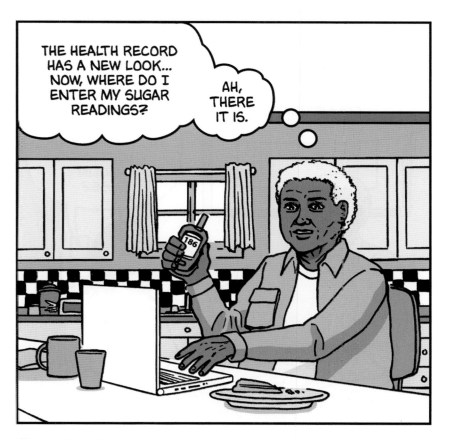

Illustration 13-9

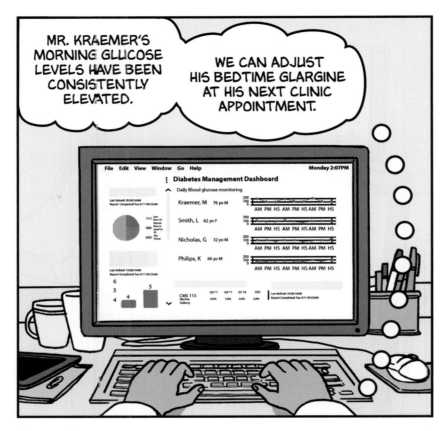

Illustration 13-10

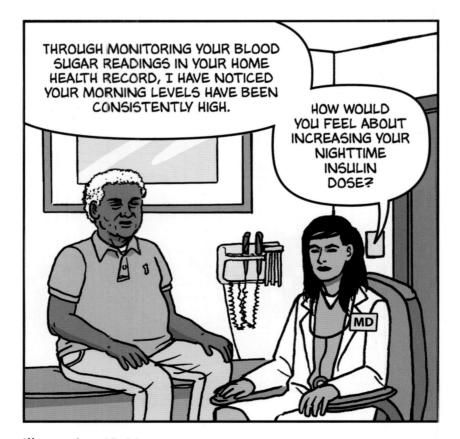

Illustration 13-11

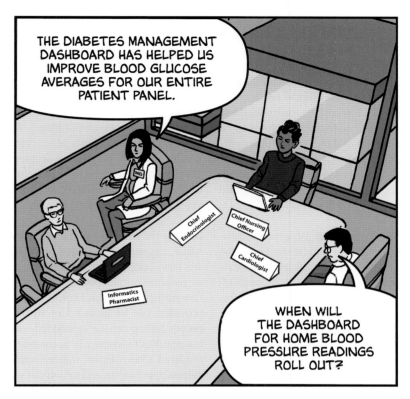

Illustration 13-12

Thoughts on "Integrated"

Electronic health records (EHRs) have ushered in remarkable shifts in healthcare delivery. When utilized to their full potential, EHRs have been shown to increase provider efficiency, reduce costs, and increase patient safety.[75-82] One EHR implementation in a medical intensive care unit (MICU), where the most critically ill adult patients are treated in a hospital, led to significant decreases in mortality (i.e., death) risk and MICU length of stay.[83] Importantly, in this study, the rate of serious medication errors also decreased following EHR implementation. Another study evaluated the impact of an EHR implementation on medication error rates and found a significant decrease in prescribing, dispensing, and administration errors.[84] The EHR improved the quality of care from prescribers, pharmacists, and nursing staff, leading to increased patient safety.

Positive outcomes such as these are realized by all types of clinicians leveraging real-time data and information to support their work. Through EHRs, pharmacists are able to monitor drug use within health systems to an extent that would have seemed utterly implausible 20 years ago. Importantly, EHRs also provide a mechanism to facilitate interprofessional communication when decisions, concerns, updates, etc., cannot be communicated face-to-face. Access to information in EHRs, coupled with the ability to communicate efficiently with co-workers in other professions, are core pillars supporting contemporary interprofessional practice in pharmacy.

The illustrated case "Integrated" is unique, as it does not focus on the activities of a pharmacist leveraging EHR capabilities to do his or her job better. Instead, the protagonist, Dr. Michael Atkins, is a pharmacy informaticist who initiates, as depicted in Illustrations 13-7 and 13-8, use of his unique combination of knowledge and skills to help clinicians in other professions do their jobs better. As such, this case provides a nontraditional example of interprofessional practice. Pharmacists have been utilizing data and analytics for decades to optimize medication dispensing.[55,85,86] EHRs have allowed for more efficient, consistent, and accurate utilization of data and analytics tools across all areas of health care. These parallels make pharmacists ideal candidates to take an expanded role in EHR management and customization within a healthcare setting.[78] Customization of the EHR through the development of health condition-specific dashboards encapsulates Michael's important contribution in "Integrated."

Pharmacy informatics focuses on the effective management and delivery of medication-related data, information, and knowledge across all electronic platforms available within a health system to strengthen the medication use process.[78] Pharmacy informaticists, like Michael, perform a variety of functions in the execution of their work. Three well-documented examples include (1) medication alerts to promote the safe use of medications, (2) order sets to promote use of the most effective medications, and (3) dashboards to monitor patient populations and provide clinicians with in-depth information on the health status of patients for whom they are providing care. Interventions such as these are broadly categorized as clinical decision support (CDS).

CDS provides clinicians with relevant clinical knowledge and/or patient-specific information in a targeted manner at the moment a clinical decision, like the decision of which medication would work best for a patient, is being made. Prior to the existence of EHRs, CDS came in the form of handwritten notes inserted into the patient's medical chart, which was a large binder full of paper health records, or through verbal communication. Providers, such as physicians, physician assistants, and nurse practitioners, would fill out paper order forms that were designed to match the institution's drug formulary, which is a list of medications that are allowed to be used at a given hospital, and meet their clinical needs based on a patient's diagnosis. Additionally, institutions maintained up-to-date paper copies of textbooks and national guidelines to be used as references to support decision making. In this older paradigm, pharmacists generally intervened after the medication orders were received and provided recommendations to avoid adverse drug events, drug interactions, patient allergies, and sub-optimal medication selection.

National guidelines are written by a group of experts, generally convened by a well-respected organization (e.g., the American Heart Association), who evaluate all available evidence for a given disease state (e.g., high blood pressure).[86] Recommendations based on this evidence and expert opinion are then developed, including appropriate medication use at various stages of treatment. EHRs integrate digital copies of textbooks and guidelines, and pharmacy informaticists develop order sets within the EHR to match recommendations within these, and institution-specific, guidelines. When designed correctly, CDS delivers the right information to the right person in the right intervention format, through the right channel, at the right time in their workflow.[87] For more information on drug formularies and evidence-based decision making, see the illustrated cases "Relapse" in Chapter 14 Population Health and "Support" in Chapter 3 Primary Care, respectively.

Medication alerts are a powerful CDS tool to ensure safe medication utilization. Alerts can be displayed in the EHR to a provider placing a medication order, to a pharmacist verifying a medication order, or to a nurse administering a medication to a patient. Medication alerts are utilized to avoid numerous types of dangerous medication errors. Drug interaction alerts are designed to pop up automatically within the EHR if a patient is currently taking a medication that has a dangerous interaction with a medication being ordered. Such alerts typically request that the provider discontinue one or both orders. Allergy alerts display in a similar manner if a patient has a documented allergy within the EHR to the medication being ordered. If a medication is being ordered at a dangerously high dose (or a dose that is outside the normally accepted range), a medication dose alert will display requesting the provider to adjust the order. Pregnancy and lactation alerts are also utilized when teratogenic medications (i.e., medications that have been shown to cause birth defects when taken by pregnant women) and medications expressed in a mother's breast milk are being ordered. Alerts such as these can be displayed in an interruptive manner, similar to the *Would you like to save changes?* pop-up that appears when you close a Microsoft Word document. Interruptive alerts require the user's acknowledgment that they are overriding the alert before they can finalize the order.

A systematic review is a rigorous methodology whereby researchers first identify every study that has been published on a given topic, then evaluate all evidence produced in those studies to identify patterns, trends, and potentially generalizable results.[88]

A systematic review published in 2017 found that 53% of studies on the effectiveness of medication alerts reported significantly improved prescribing behavior.[89] One reason that the benefits of medication alerts are not seen more consistently is because of something called alert fatigue, which is the desensitization providers experience over time as they repeatedly encounter medication alerts. If providers continually encounter alerts they find to be inappropriate or not useful, they begin to lose faith in the value of medication alerts as a tool to help them. In practice, medication alerts are overridden at rates ranging from 49% to 96%.[90] This demonstrates that pharmacy informaticists have much work to do to optimize medication alerts; that said, when configured appropriately, these alerts have the potential to improve care.

Possibly the most influential CDS tools are order sets which, as the name suggests, are groups of orders that are placed together. Order sets can contain medication orders, lab orders, and orders for staff to monitor certain patient matters like pain levels or heart rate. Diagnostic imaging and consult orders for patients to see specialty providers can be included in an order set, as well. Additionally, proper billing can be embedded into an order set to ensure the hospital/health system is accurately reimbursed for the services rendered. Order sets are utilized across all medical specialties, in all patient populations, and in hospital settings as well as clinic settings.

Medication selection can be complicated for providers as they must consider the patient's diagnosis, age, and weight, as well as which medications are on the health system's drug formulary. Order sets are an ideal tool to optimize prescribing patterns. Take, for example, a scenario whereby a physician diagnoses a patient with pneumonia and is sitting down to the computer to place an order for antibiotics. Generally, a sputum sample will be taken and sent to a laboratory within the hospital to identify the cause of the pneumonia (i.e., the exact type of bacteria found in the sputum). The laboratory will also run tests on the bacteria causing the infection to identify antibiotic susceptibilities, which is a list of antibiotics that will kill the bacteria. This knowledge will allow the physician to use targeted therapy she knows will cure the infection; however, these tests take time, and empiric antibiotic therapy (i.e., medication selection based on the physician's best guess) must be started right away. A well-designed order set containing the proper empiric medication options based on different types of pneumonia can help the physician make the best choice in a situation like this. National guidelines, for example, recommend different empiric treatment for community-acquired pneumonia, healthcare-associated pneumonia, and aspiration pneumonia.[91] In one study, an intelligently designed pneumonia order set increased prescriber compliance with national guidelines and decreased in-hospital mortality.[92] In other words, patient lives were saved by leveraging the potential of the EHR. Readers interested in learning more about infections, antibiotics, and the knowledge, skills, and contributions of pharmacists who specialize in this area are encouraged to read the illustrated cases "Wounded" and "Superinfection" in Chapter 8 Infectious Diseases.

Pharmacy informaticists, leveraging their clinical knowledge, play a key role in building order sets within hospital and health system EHRs. In the pneumonia example above, the pharmacy informaticist would ensure inclusion of appropriate antibiotics in the pneumonia order set based on national guidelines and the hospital's drug formulary. Additionally, he would use his knowledge of EHR capabilities to optimize prescribing. Most EHRs allow for defaults to be established within an order set; for example, a default dose for a specific medication can be established. Continuing with the pneumonia example, a dose of azithromycin 500 mg may have been defaulted for the treatment of community-acquired pneumonia, as this is what is currently recommended in national guidelines. Default settings such as this can significantly influence prescribing habits to increase providers' compliance with evidence-based medication use; in turn, this can improve patient care and decrease medication errors.[93]

The CDS tool featured in the illustrated case "Integrated" is a dashboard. Dashboards are versatile tools used to query multiple databases in order to display large amounts of information to users in an easily digestible, visually appealing manner. As the name suggests, dashboards can visually mirror a motor vehicle dashboard with various information displayed in graph, chart, or list format. A well-designed dashboard functions as a centralized location for a provider to find important information. Dashboards can be designed to present patient-specific information, which providers can then use in direct patient care. Additionally, dashboards are useful in presenting trends in medication usage throughout a health system for providers to track patterns.

The Diabetes Management Dashboard in Illustration 13-10 incorporates patient-documented blood glucose readings for providers to monitor. Self-monitoring of blood glucose levels for diabetes patients is considered standard of care.[94] Illustration 13-9 shows a patient with type 2 diabetes doing this; however, instead of keeping that information to himself, he is shown entering his blood glucose reading into a secured database. The data housed in this database is one source of information used to create the dashboard shown in Illustration 13-10. Information from other databases with diabetes-relevant information would also be displayed; for example, hemoglobin A1c levels, patient-reported diet, or blood pressure readings from previous visits.[95] Clinical dashboards can be utilized to display lab results, vital signs, medications, and other patient information to assist providers in their clinical decision making. By presenting patient information in a consolidated, easy-to-interpret fashion, dashboards have become vital tools for provider efficiency and patient safety. Illustration 13-10 shows the physician utilizing the Diabetes Management Dashboard created by Michael to prospectively develop a plan for the patient's insulin therapy ahead of the office visit depicted in Illustration 13-11. Clinical dashboards have proven effective at improving diabetes care, as well as oncology and cardiology care.[95-97] It is revealed in Illustration 13-12 that Michael and the Chief Cardiologist are working on such a dashboard for blood pressure monitoring.

Readers interested in learning more about type 2 diabetes, including monitoring parameters, medication therapies, and complications from uncontrolled diabetes, are encouraged to explore the illustrated cases "Holistic" in Chapter 3 Primary Care and "Screen" in Chapter 4 Prevention & Wellness. To explore the role of pharmacists in the interprofessional care of patients with cancer or cardiovascular disease, see the illustrated cases "Compromising" and

"Compassion" in Chapter 9 Oncology and "Underlying Cause," "Educator," and "Empowerment" in Chapter 5 Cardiology.

Dashboards are also valuable tools for hospital/health system administrators as they can be utilized to monitor patient safety metrics, quality of care indicators, patient throughput, transitions of care, and staff workload and productivity. Pharmacy safety dashboards can display information such as barcode medication administration adherence numbers to ensure nursing staff are using the appropriate safety tools to administer patients' medications. Medication alert override rates can be displayed which, as described above, can indicate sub-optimal medication alerts being presented to providers. Additionally, medication-specific information can be displayed for high risk medications. Frequent use of naloxone, for example, which is a reversal agent used for opioid overdoses, may indicate overprescribing of these medications. See the illustrated case "Gasping" in Chapter 12 Mental Health for a more in-depth discussion of opioids and the role of naloxone as a life-saving measure. For more information on leadership roles, including activities of pharmacy managers, Directors of Pharmacy, and Chief Pharmacy Officers, see the illustrated cases "Opportunities" and "Relationships" in Chapter 15 Administration.

Pharmacy informaticists take an intermediary role when developing dashboards by first, as shown Illustration 13-7, meeting with stakeholders to determine their goals. Aligning stakeholder goals with the technical capabilities of the EHR is critical. Next, as shown in Illustration 13-8, the pharmacy informaticist configures the dashboard to query appropriate information from available databases. Patient-specific data is pulled from the EHR while medication information can be drawn from databases housing historical records of past medication use. This process can take several weeks depending on the complexity of the health condition and the amount of information displayed on the dashboard. Following initial configuration, dashboards are generally refined through repeated testing to ensure established goals of stakeholders are met. Once stakeholders are satisfied with the initial configuration, additional testing is completed with a small group of clinicians, which allows for further refinements and customization based on feedback prior to being implemented for the entire organization. After implementation, the pharmacy informaticist continuously enhances the dashboard as stakeholders submit requests for optimization based on their experiences.

In many ways, the marriage of pharmacy and health informatics is natural and synergistic. Building a useful EHR, for example, requires in-depth knowledge of both hospital/health system operations and clinical practice. Through their education and training, pharmacists develop expertise in both of these areas. Furthermore, pharmacists must be detail-oriented to ensure the safe and effective use of medications. For every patient, this involves checking proper medication selection, dosing, and administration frequency. A similar ability to focus attention on fine details is required in pharmacy informatics; for example, a single incorrect keystroke in a line of computer code can cause major downstream errors and complications. By leveraging EHRs to improve medication use, pharmacy informaticists are playing a critical role increasing the health of patients and populations.

DISCUSSION QUESTIONS FOR "INTEGRATED"

1. The illustrated case "Integrated" depicts several steps undertaken by a pharmacy informaticist in the development of the Diabetes Management Dashboard. What additional, unseen steps must have been taken to ensure the dashboard functioned correctly before it was put to use?

2. In Illustration 13-9, the patient enters his blood glucose reading into the electronic health record from home, providing valuable data for the Diabetes Management Dashboard. What other patient information can you think of that might be self-documented in a similar manner in order to help health professionals make better-informed clinical decisions?

3. Illustration 13-10 shows a physician reviewing the Diabetes Management Dashboard in advance of her scheduled office visits to develop treatment plans, including changes to medication therapy. With the time she saves by using the dashboard, what other patient needs might she engage in to advance the health of her patients?

4. The illustrated case "Integrated" presents positive impacts of leveraging technology to support clinical decision making. What negative impacts might incorporating technology like this into the patient care workflow result in?

5. Clinical decision support tools other than dashboards were discussed in this essay as additional mechanisms to improve care through technology. How might these tools be used to improve the care of patients with diabetes? How about other health conditions like asthma or hypertension (i.e., high blood pressure)?

INNOVATOR: An Illustrated Case Study

Story by Natalie S. Schmitz & Joseph A. Zorek
Illustrations by George Folz, © 2019 Board of Regents of the University of Wisconsin System

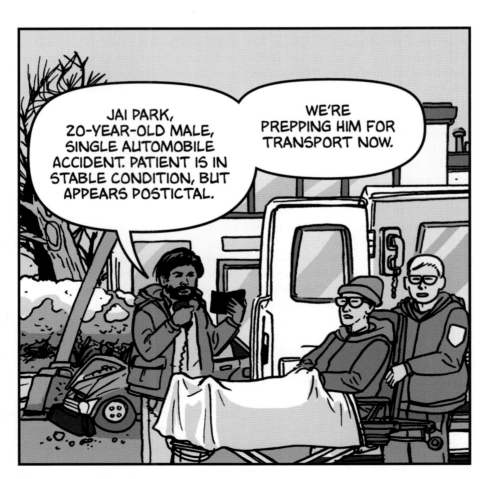

Illustration 13-13

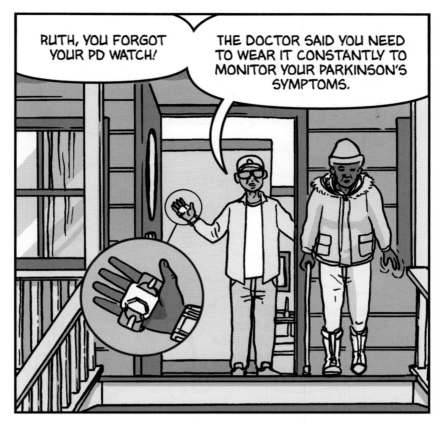

Illustration 13-14

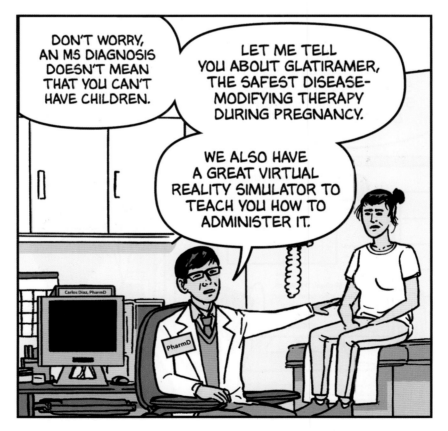

Illustration 13-15

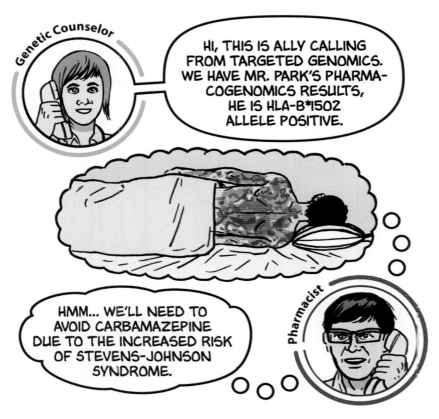

Illustration 13-16

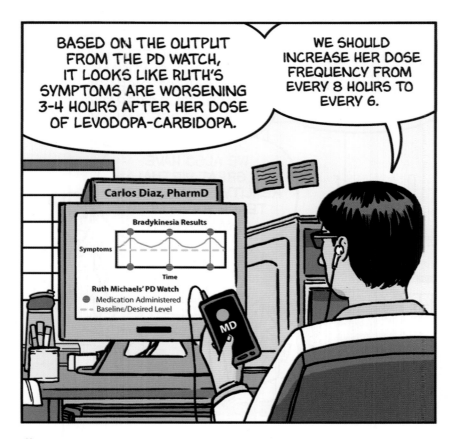

Illustration 13-17

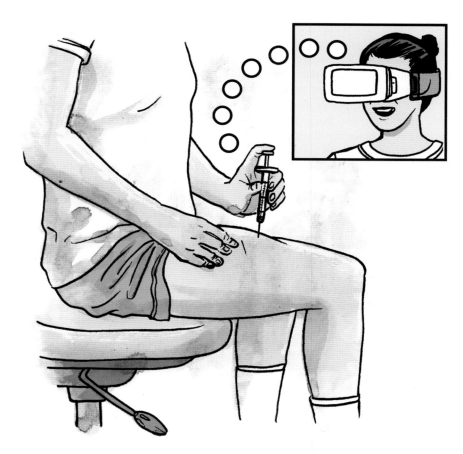

Illustration 13-18

Thoughts on "Innovator"

In the illustrated case "Innovator," a pharmacist uses innovative technologies to monitor drug safety and efficacy and to teach appropriate medication administration. Some of these technologies are becoming widely used in pharmacy, like pharmacogenomic testing, while others, like wearable devices and virtual reality, represent opportunities for more widespread application in the future. "Innovator" highlights the importance for all health professionals, not just pharmacists, to continuously monitor technological advances in society. There are many examples of new technologies completely transforming industries. Mostly, these transformations are positive; however, there are downsides, as well, such as negative impacts on job markets as workers get displaced.[98] In order to guard against this risk, pharmacists must continuously strive to improve their knowledge and skills. Keeping abreast of new technologies that could be incorporated to enhance pharmacy practice and patient care is one mechanism to do that.

The development of video streaming services like those through HBO, Hulu, and Netflix, and their impact on once-popular video rental methods, such as cable providers or brick-and-mortar stores, provides a rich example to highlight this point of disruptive innovation.[99] What began as a low-cost alternative to watch select television shows and movies has rapidly evolved into the most popular way to consume video content in the United States.[99] Interestingly, the companies that became household names by leveraging video streaming technology to deliver content have now begun creating it. Having redefined consumer habits in this part of the entertainment industry, they are now in the process of redefining content production and business platforms, as well.[100] Similarly, the ability of novel technologies to upend the healthcare industry, and pharmacy practice more specifically, is apparent. In fact, there are already many great examples of this in action.

Innovations in drug design and development have had a dramatic impact on traditional roles of pharmacists. For many decades, for example, patients with a heart condition called atrial fibrillation were treated almost exclusively with a drug called warfarin to reduce the risk of blood clots leading to stroke.[101,102] Warfarin is a complicated medication that interacts with a lot of other drugs, as well as many types of food.[103] To be used safely, health professionals must monitor patients diligently, including frequent changes in daily doses based on ever-fluctuating levels of warfarin in their blood. Pharmacists proved themselves to be capable and cost-effective in this role, and management of warfarin patients evolved into a niche practice area over time, complete with pharmacist-run clinics.[104,105] In 2010, however, a new class of drugs to prevent blood clots called Direct Oral Anticoagulants emerged, requiring much less monitoring than warfarin.[101,102] This innovation in drug development spurred changes in prescribing patterns that have reduced the number of patients taking warfarin. As a result, demand for warfarin clinics and pharmacists with specialized knowledge and skills to manage warfarin in this practice area decreased, which has prompted an evolution in services and expertise provided by anticoagulation clinics.[106] For a more in-depth discussion of warfarin, treatment of atrial fibrillation, and this practice evolution, readers are encouraged to explore the illustrated case "Empowerment" in Chapter 5 Cardiology.

Innovations in drug design and development have expanded opportunities for pharmacists in other arenas. For example, many new medications have come to market in recent years representing an entirely new category of drugs called biologics.[107] Biologics are mostly injectable medications that, once in the body, target a specific malfunctioning system (e.g., the immune system).[108] One example of a biologic medication is adalimumab (Humira), which reduces inflammation by interfering with a specific cytokine called tumor necrosis factor alpha (TNF-α).[109] Cytokines are substances secreted by cells in the immune system that have an effect on other cells. TNF-α is a pro-inflammatory cytokine (i.e., it leads to inflammation); therefore, interfering with TNF-α decreases inflammation.

As more biologics enter the market, prescribers may opt to leverage these novel drugs to a greater extent.[110] These medications are expensive, costing an average of $10,000 to $30,000 per year.[111] Spurred in part by the introduction of biologics, and in an effort to control costs and improve adherence rates, specialty pharmacies have emerged in recent years. Pharmacists, with an intimate understanding of drug supply/management, expert knowledge of biologics, and demonstrated ability to improve patient adherence regardless of drug class, have stepped into new roles in specialty pharmacy.[112] Those interested in learning more about biologics are encouraged to explore the illustrated case "Relapse" in Chapter 14 Population Health. For a more in-depth discussion of specialty pharmacy, see the illustrated case "Opportunities" in Chapter 15 Administration.

Pharmacogenomics, a featured technology in "Innovator," is another example highlighting expanded opportunities for pharmacists who develop specialized knowledge. Broadly speaking, this is the science of how a person's genetic makeup, or their genes, affects how he or she will respond to certain drugs.[40] Genes, composed of DNA, vary in terms of form and function. Some are responsible for traits we inherit, like eye color or height, while others make proteins that impact our health. Interestingly, some genes, known as alleles, vary from one person to another. These alleles are responsible for variations in how these genes function, or express themselves. The basic premise of pharmacogenomic testing is that knowledge of an individual's genes and alleles provides health professionals with additional information to make sound decisions regarding medication selection, dosing, and monitoring. If a specific allele is associated with a high risk of a certain side effect, and the patient has this allele, then an alternative medication can be prescribed. Currently, there are over 20 companies and 70 labs that provide pharmacogenomic testing through a healthcare provider.[113]

Pharmacogenomic results can be used to guide and/or inform medication selection, dosing, and potential adverse effects, and it has been shown to reduce sub-optimal outcomes, cost of treatment, and adverse effects.[114] One example of the role of pharmacogenomics in drug dosing is warfarin, the anticoagulant described above. All drugs have a therapeutic range, which is a concentration within the blood that is high enough to produce the desired effect, but low enough to avoid toxicities. Warfarin's therapeutic range is narrow, so small dosing changes in either direction (i.e., more or less drug) can be catastrophic; take too little, and the risk of blood clot and stroke increases, take too much, and uncontrollable bleeding may occur. Variants in two genes called CYP2C9 and VKORC1 have been associated with changes in warfarin metabolism that impact optimal dosing. Genetic testing for warfarin, in addition to routine monitoring, has been shown to help predict effective doses and avoid unwanted effects.[115]

As a result of pharmacists' training, knowledge, and skills, they are uniquely qualified to interpret pharmacogenomic results and apply that information in medication management strategies including optimal drug and dose selection. Pharmacists have expert knowledge, for example, on how drugs are metabolized, or broken down, in the body. This mostly takes place in the liver through biochemical reactions. Patients who have genetic variations in one or more liver enzymes (i.e., proteins that facilitate biochemical reactions in the body) responsible for these biochemical reactions are at a higher risk of certain adverse drug reactions (ADRs). For example, a drug might accumulate to toxic levels if a genetic variation leads to a deficiency in how it is metabolized. See Chapter 11 Critical Care for additional information on how drugs move in the body (i.e., pharmacokinetics). Those interested in ADR identification are encouraged to read the illustrated case "Support" in Chapter 3 Primary Care.

The story of Jai Park in "Innovator," as shown in Illustrations 13-13 and 13-16, highlights the role pharmacogenomics can play in pharmacy practice. In this scenario, it can be deduced from the term "postictal" that Mr. Park's automobile accident was caused by a seizure. This term refers to an altered state of consciousness that follows a seizure where a patient can be disoriented, confused, and/or drowsy.[116,117] Dr. Carlos Diaz, the neurology pharmacist featured in "Innovator," is shown in Illustration 13-16 learning from a genetic counselor at a genomics company that Mr. Park tested positive for the HLA-B*1502 allele, which is a genetic variation that has been associated with increased risk of Stevens-Johnson syndrome (SJS) in patients who take an anti-seizure medication called carbamazepine.[118]

Stevens-Johnson syndrome is a rare, severe condition that causes skin tissue to blister and die.[119] As depicted in Illustration 13-16, SJS can be incredibly painful and debilitating. It is often caused by reaction to medications including some antibiotics, pain medications, and anti-seizure medications. The anti-seizure medication prescribed to Mr. Park upon discharge from the hospital would have been reviewed and optimized during his first visit with the interprofessional neurology team working in the outpatient clinic shown in the illustrated case. While not explicitly described in "Innovator," this first visit included a genetic sample being sent to

Targeted Genomics for analysis. A few weeks later, in preparation for Mr. Park's follow-up visit, Carlos called Targeted Genomics for results and learned of Mr. Park's genetic variation in the HLA-B*1502 allele. Using his knowledge of this ADR, he immediately starts thinking of medication options other than carbamazepine for Mr. Park.

Illustrations 13-14 and 13-17 highlight the emerging role of wearable technologies, which have evolved rapidly in recent years from their origins in fitness tracking to a growing tool for real-time healthcare monitoring.[120,121] Broadly speaking, these are electronic devices that patients wear, such as fitness trackers, smartwatches, electrocardiogram monitors, blood pressure monitors, and biosensors. These devices are designed to collect health and fitness data including physical activity (e.g., number of steps taken), heart rhythm, respiratory rate, temperature, blood glucose, ultraviolet ray exposure, reproductive cycle trackers, and sleep monitoring, among others.[122] If current trends in the United States continue, where use of wearables increased from 9% in 2014 to 33% in 2018,[123] pharmacists and other health professionals will have no choice but to prepare for greater adoption of these technologies within their practices.

Wearable technologies have multiple potential applications in healthcare. Fitness trackers, for example, can increase patient quality of life by encouraging behaviors that improve physical activity, leading to weight loss and potential improvements in chronic conditions.[124-128] Other wearables enable early detection of certain diseases that may otherwise have gone unnoticed, such as arrhythmias, high blood pressure, or sleep apnea.[129-131] Monitoring disease progression, the efficacy of therapeutic approaches, and medication adherence are additional applications.[132] The latter is a primary concern and professional activity for pharmacists. There are several examples of pharmacists impacting medication adherence in this book; those interested in learning more are encouraged to review the illustrated cases "Transformation" and "Breathe" in Chapter 2 Community Pharmacy, "Swish" and "Holistic" in Chapter 3 Primary Care, "Relapse" in Chapter 14 Population Health, and "Opportunities" in Chapter 15 Administration.

Because they are continuously worn, these technologies offer a more accurate view of a patient's health status compared to traditional periodic measurements, such as a single blood pressure reading during an annual visit. Customizing medication therapy based on an average daily blood pressure reading over a period of several weeks, for example, would be desirable compared to determining a medication regimen based on a single data point. The illustrated case "Integrated" in this chapter highlights how greater access to health data can improve medication selection and, as a result, patients' health.

Illustrations 13-14 and 13-17 highlight the role wearable technologies can play in chronic disease management. In this case, a patient named Ruth Michaels uses a wearable device (i.e., her "PD watch") that detects bodily movements associated with Parkinson's disease (PD). PD is a neurodegenerative disorder that primarily effects the neurons that produce a chemical in the brain called dopamine.[133] Decreases in the amount of dopamine in the brain lead to movement (also called "motor") symptoms that are considered the hallmark of the disease, such as tremor of the hands or feet, stiffness/rigidity of the limbs, and a general slowing of movements (e.g., pace of walking, arm swing while walking) referred to as bradykinesia.[133] Non-motor symptoms such as depression, anxiety, and decreases in cognitive abilities (e.g., memory problems) have also been described.[133]

Carbidopa-levodopa is a common medication used in the treatment of PD that increases the amount of dopamine in the brain; in turn, increased dopamine levels lead to reductions in PD symptoms.[134] However, a side effect of this medication is dyskinesia, or involuntary, erratic movements. It is important to monitor the timing of bradykinesia and dyskinesia symptoms, as these symptoms provide valuable clues to optimize the dosing and timing of carbidopa-levodopa. Illustration 13-17 reveals the output from Mrs. Michaels' PD watch. Based on the timing of the bradykinesia she is experiencing, Carlos discovers that the carbidopa-levodopa is wearing off too soon and that the dosing schedule needs to be adjusted. Importantly, we see from his phone that Carlos is communicating this discovery to Mrs. Michaels' physician, which is an excellent example of interprofessional practice to improve health outcomes.

The availability and application of wearable technologies like Mrs. Michaels' PD watch are expected to improve not only healthcare quality, but also, importantly, access to care. This may be particularly important for patients who live in rural areas where access to health professionals may be limited (see "Breathe" in Chapter 2 Community Pharmacy for a more in-depth exploration of this topic). It is also easy to imagine how the utilization of wearable technologies could have improved the health of a variety of characters throughout this book; for suggestions of specific cases, see "Screen" in Chapter 4 Prevention & Wellness (physical activity), "Underlying Cause" and "Empowerment" in Chapter 5 Cardiology (heart rhythm and blood pressure, respectively), and "Integrated" in this chapter (blood glucose).

The final technology highlighted in "Innovator" (Illustrations 13-15 and 13-18) is augmented or visual reality (AR/VR). AR/VR is a computer-generated simulation that either supplements reality (AR) or immerses the user in a visual reality experience (VR).[135] The most widely known applications for AR/VR technologies are in flight simulators and video games; however, this is rapidly expanding to other sectors of the economy, including healthcare.[136,137] The role of AR/VR in pharmacy practice is far from mainstream, but one can easily see potential applications; examples include adjunctive (i.e., supplemental) treatment in pain management or anxiety, patient education, and education/training of pharmacists and pharmacy students.

Virtual reality has been shown to be an effective treatment for distress, anxiety, and acute or chronic pain associated with physical and psychological illnesses.[138] VR has been applied as a distraction technique in adult and pediatric patients receiving vaccinations, intravenous injections, laceration repair, caring for burn wounds, fibromyalgia, phantom limb pain, and bone marrow aspiration or biopsy.[139-141] AR/VR applications are thought to be a reasonable alternative or addition to traditional medication-based approaches. A pharmacy chain in Sweden, for example, implemented VR therapy for patients with acute pain in 2016.[142,143] In this case, a virtual reality app, "Happy Place," was created to distract patients from temporary pain, such as that from vaccine administration. Although there are limited results outside of positive anecdotal reports, there is hope that this technology could be used for other types of pain and as a supplement to pain medications.[144]

Another potential application of AR/VR within pharmacy practice is patient education and training, as demonstrated in Illustrations 13-15 and 13-18.[142] AR/VR could provide audio and visual counseling and instructions for patients receiving new prescriptions. This would be especially useful for medications that require specific administration techniques in order to properly work, including injectables and inhalers. One can also imagine the use of AR/VR to educate patients more generally on their disease states and the way specific drugs work in the body. Increased patient understanding has been shown to lead to better medication adherence and patient satisfaction with the care they receive.[145-147]

The illustrated case "Innovator" highlights how pharmacists can use technology to optimize patient care. Pharmacogenomics, wearables, and AR/VR are just a few of the potential innovations that can and will play a role in the future of pharmacy practice, and in healthcare delivery more generally. Staying abreast of new technologies and being creative and innovative with their applications has the potential to create opportunities for pharmacists to improve the safe and effective use of medications.

DISCUSSION QUESTIONS FOR "INNOVATOR"

1. The illustrated case "Innovator" highlighted the use of pharmacogenomics, wearables, and AR/VR. What other emerging technologies can you think of that might impact pharmacy practice or healthcare delivery?

2. What are some barriers to implementing technological innovations in healthcare? How might they be overcome?

3. The illustrated case "Innovator" portrays positive outcomes associated with adoption of emerging technologies. In what ways might new technologies negatively impact patients or their healthcare experiences?

4. Do you think emerging technologies will make health professionals from different professions (e.g., nurses, pharmacists, physicians) more or less reliant upon one another, and why?

5. Technologies often emerge because they solve, mitigate, or otherwise address a recognized problem. Based on your knowledge of pharmacy, what do you see as the biggest problem waiting for a technological solution?

CHAPTER SUMMARY

- Technological innovations such as computers, electronic health records (EHR), computerized physician order entry, remote prescription verification, automated dispensing cabinets, barcode medication administration, telemedicine, mobile health devices, and wearable technologies have resulted in significant changes in pharmacy and the healthcare industry as a whole.

- Within pharmacy, many technological advances have been used to automate repetitive human work.

- It is crucial for pharmacists to be agile and stay current on developing technologies, including the role technological advances could play to improve patient care and maximize medication therapy.

- One of the most commonly used technologies in hospital settings is the automated dispensing cabinet, which has enabled pharmacists to focus their time and attention on other clinical and/or professional services.

- While gained efficiency is the primary benefit from use of technology and automation in pharmacy, additional benefits exist, such as drug diversion prevention/detection and reductions in medication errors.

- The implementation of EHRs has been shown to increase provider efficiency, reduce costs, and increase patient safety, which has enabled pharmacists to promptly monitor drugs and has provided an important mechanism to facilitate interprofessional communication when decisions, concerns, updates, etc., cannot be communicated face-to-face.

- Pharmacists have been using data and analytics for decades to optimize medication dispensing, which makes them ideal candidates to take an expanded role in EHR management and customization within a healthcare setting as pharmacy informaticists.

- Technological innovations in healthcare have been leveraged to create new areas of emphasis for pharmacists, including pharmacogenomics.

- It will continue to be imperative for pharmacists to stay current on innovations and creatively apply them to pharmacy practice to improve the safe and effective use of medications.

REFERENCES

1. Hajar R. History of medicine timeline. *Heart Views*. 2015;16(1):43-45.

2. Grossman D. Scientists successfully 3D print an organ that mimics lungs. Hearst Magazine Media, Inc. Popular Mechanics Web site. Available at https://www.popularmechanics.com/science/health/a27355578/3d-print-lungs/. Accessed February 26, 2020.

3. Berman AD, Jason. Technology feels like it's accelerating—because it actually is. Singularity Education Group. Available at https://singularityhub.com/2016/03/22/technology-feels-like-its-accelerating-because-it-actually-is/. Accessed February 26, 2020.

4. Kurzweil R. The law of accelerating returns. Kurzweil Network. Available at https://www.kurzweilai.net/the-law-of-accelerating-returns. Accessed February 26, 2020.

5. Silver L. Smartphone ownership is growing rapidly around the world, but not always equally. Pew Research Center. Available at https://www.pewresearch.org/global/2019/02/05/smartphone-ownership-is-growing-rapidly-around-the-world-but-not-always-equally/. Accessed February 26, 2020.

6. Muro MM, Maxim R, Whiton J. Automation and artificial intelligence: how machines are affecting people and places. Available at https://www.brookings.edu/wp-content/uploads/2019/01/2019.01_BrookingsMetro_Automation-AI_Report_Muro-Maxim-Whiton-FINAL-version.pdf. Accessed February 27, 2020.

7. Brinker TJ, Hekler A, Enk AH, et al. Deep neural networks are superior to dermatologists in melanoma image classification. *Eur J Cancer*. 2019;119:11-17.

8. Esteva A, Kuprel B, Novoa RA, et al. Dermatologist-level classification of skin cancer with deep neural networks. *Nature*. 2017;542(7639):115-118.

9. Haenssle HA, Fink C, Schneiderbauer R, et al. Man against machine: diagnostic performance of a deep learning convolutional neural network for dermoscopic melanoma recognition in comparison to 58 dermatologists. *Ann Oncol*. 2018;29(8):1836-1842.

10. Mar VJ, Soyer HP. Artificial intelligence for melanoma diagnosis: how can we deliver on the promise? *Ann Oncol*. 2018;29(8):1625-1628.

11. Davenport T, Kalakota R. The potential for artificial intelligence in healthcare. *Future Healthc J*. 2019;6(2):94-98.

12. US National Library of Medicine. What is precision medicine? Available at https://ghr.nlm.nih.gov/primer/precisionmedicine/definition. Accessed March 16, 2020.

13. Henry J, Pylypchuk Y, Searcy T, Patel V. Adoption of electronic health record systems among U.S. non-federal acute care hospitals: 2008-2015. The office of the national coordinator for health information technology ONC data brief. Available at https://dashboard.healthit.gov/evaluations/data-briefs/non-federal-acute-care-hospital-ehr-adoption-2008-2015.php. Accessed February 27, 2020.

14. The office of the national coordinator for health information technology. Fact sheet: quality payment program and health information technology. Available at https://www.healthit.gov/sites/default/files/factsheets/macra_health_it_fact_sheet_final.pdf. Accessed February 27, 2020.

15. Chen A. As tech companies move into healt care, here's what to watch in 2019. Available at https://www.theverge.com/2019/1/3/18166673/technology-health-care-amazon-apple-uber-alphabet-google-verily. Accessed February 26, 2020.

16. Healthcare. Apple. Available at https://www.apple.com/healthcare/. Accessed February 26, 2020.

17. Garcia A. Amazon rolls out "Amazon Pharmacy" branding to Pill-Pack. Available at https://www.cnn.com/2019/11/15/tech/amazon-pharmacy-pillpack/index.html. Accessed February 26, 2020.

18. Goundrey-Smith S. Examining the role of new technology in pharamcy: now and in the future. The pharmaceutical journal: a royal pharmaceutical society publication. Available at https://www.pharmaceutical-journal.com/examining-the-role-of-new-technology-in-pharmacy-now-and-in-the-future/11134174.article?firstPass=false. Accessed February 26, 2020.

19. Kushan D. Three ways technology has changed pharmacy. Available at https://www.healthcareis.com/blog/three-ways-technology-has-changed-pharmacy. Accessed May 31, 2020.

20. Schueth A, Hein W, Hull J. Five technology trends: changing pharmacy practice today and tomorrow. Available at https://www.pharmacytimes.com/publications/directions-in-pharmacy/2015/august2015/five-technology-trends-changing-pharmacy-practice-today-and-tomorrow. Accessed February 26, 2020.

21. Erickson A. Technology: Will it help or hurt the future of pharmacy practice? Available at https://www.pharmacist.com/article/technology-will-it-help-or-hurt-future-pharmacy-practice. Accessed February 26, 2020.

22. GSMA Asia Pacific. Number of unique mobile subscribers worldwide hits five billion infographics. Available at https://www.gsma.com/asia-pacific/resources/number-of-unique-mobile-subscribers-worldwide-hits-five-billion-infographics/. Accessed May 31, 2020.

23. Burke K. How many texts do people send every day (2018)? Available at https://www.textrequest.com/blog/how-many-texts-people-send-per-day/. Accessed February 26, 2020.

24. Tao D, Xie L, Wang T, Wang T. A meta-analysis of the use of electronic reminders for patient adherence to medication in chronic disease care. *J Telemed Telecare*. 2015;21(1):3-13.

25. Gurol-Urganci I, de Jongh T, Vodopivec-Jamsek V, Atun R, Car J. Mobile phone messaging reminders for attendance at healthcare appointments. *Cochrane Database Syst Rev*. 2013;2013(12):CD007458-CD007458.

26. Wang K, Wang C, Xi L, et al. A randomized controlled trial to assess adherence to allergic rhinitis treatment following a daily short message service (SMS) via the mobile phone. *Int Arch Allergy Immunol*. 2014;163(1):51-58.

27. Strandbygaard U, Thomsen SF, Backer V. A daily SMS reminder increases adherence to asthma treatment: a three-month follow-up study. *Respir Med*. 2010;104(2):166-171.

28. Kim GS, Se-Bum P, Jungsuk Oh. An examination of factors influencing consumer adoption of short message servce (SMS). *Psychology & Marketing*. 2008;25:769-786.

29. Farris KB, Salgado TM, Batra P, et al. Confirming the theoretical structure of expert-developed text messages to improve adherence to anti-hypertensive medications. *Res Social Adm Pharm*. 2016;12(4):578-591.

30. Vervloet M, van Dijk L, Santen-Reestman J, van Vlijmen B, Bouvy ML, de Bakker DH. Improving medication adherence in diabetes type 2 patients through real time medication monitoring: a randomised controlled trial to evaluate the effect of monitoring patients' medication use combined with short message service (SMS) reminders. *BMC Health Serv Res*. 2011;11:5-5.

31. Yoon K-H, Kim H-S. A short message service by cellular phone in type 2 diabetic patients for 12 months. *Diabetes Res Clin Pract*. 2008;79(2):256-261.

32. Brar Prayaga R, Jeong EW, Feger E, Noble HK, Kmiec M, Prayaga RS. Improving refill adherence in medicare patients with tailored and interactive mobile text messaging: pilot study. *JMIR Mhealth Uhealth*. 2018;6(1):e30.

33. Gillette C, Rockich-Winston N, Kuhn JA, Flesher S, Shepherd M. Inhaler technique in children with asthma: a systematic review. *Acad Pediatr*. 2016;16(7):605-615.

34. Melzer AC, Ghassemieh BJ, Gillespie SE, et al. Patient characteristics associated with poor inhaler technique among a cohort of patients with COPD. *Respir Med*. 2017;123:124-130.

35. Sanchis J, Gich I, Pedersen S. Systematic review of errors in inhaler use: has patient technique improved over time? *Chest*. 2016;150(2):394-406.

36. Vogelmeier CF, Criner GJ, Martinez FJ, et al. Global strategy for the diagnosis, management, and prevention of chronic obstructive lung disease 2017 report. GOLD Executive Summary. *Am J Respir Crit Care Med* 2017;195(5):557-582.

37. Locke ER, Thomas RM, Woo DM, et al. Using video telehealth to facilitate inhaler training in rural patients with obstructive lung disease. *Telemed J E Health*. 2019;25(3):230-236.

38. Cooley JH, Larson S. Promoting a growth mindset in pharmacy educators and students *Curr Pharm Teach Learn*. 2018;10(6):675-679.

39. Eckel S. Focus on current thinking: lifelong learning and health-system pharmacists. Available at https://www.pharmacytimes.com/news/focus-on-current-thinking-lifelong-learning-and-health-system-pharmacists. Accessed February 26, 2020.

40. U.S. National Library of Medicine. What is pharmacogenomics? Available at https://ghr.nlm.nih.gov/primer/genomicresearch/pharmacogenomics#:~:targetText=Pharmacogenomics%20is%20the%20study%20of,to%20a%20person's%20genetic%20makeup. Accessed May 31, 2020.

41. Coppock K. New pharmacogenomic certificant program available to pharmacists. Available at https://www.pharmacytimes.com/news/new-pharmacogenomics-certificate-program-available-to-pharmacists. Accessed February 26, 2020.

42. California Society of Health-System Pharmacists. Pharmacogenomics certificate program. Available at https://www.cshp.org/page/CP_PGX. Accessed February 26, 2020.

43. University of Colorado Skaggs School of Pharmaceutical Sciences. Pharmacogenomics certificate program. Available at http://www.ucdenver.edu/academics/colleges/pharmacy/AcademicPrograms/ContinuingEducation/CertificatePrograms/PGXcertificate/Pages/PGXcert.aspx. Accessed February 26, 2020.

44. American College of Clinical Pharmacy. ACCP launches applied pharmacogenomics certificate program. Available at https://www.accp.com/report/index.aspx?iss=0618&art=7. Accessed February 26, 2020.

45. HCi Group. How to become epic certified and why you should do it. Available at https://blog.thehcigroup.com/how-to-become-epic-certified-and-why. Accessed March 19, 2020.

46. University of Wisconsin: Health Information Management & Technology. Epic certification and other healthcare IT certifications. Available at https://himt.wisconsin.edu/about-himt/epic-certification-and-health-it-certifications/. Accessed March 19, 2020.

47. American Society of Health-System Pharmacists. Residency directory. Available at https://accreditation.ashp.org/directory/#!/program/residency. Accessed March 19, 2020.

48. Chui M, James M, Miremaid M. Where machines could replace humans—and where they can't (yet). Available at https://www.mckinsey.com/business-functions/mckinsey-digital/our-insights/where-machines-could-replace-humans-and-where-they-cant-yet. Accessed February 3, 2020.

49. Uzialko A. Workplace automation is everywhere, and it's not just about robots. Available at https://www.businessnewsdaily.com/9835-automation-tech-workforce.html. Accessed February 3, 2020.

50. Radu S. Top industries to be changed by automation. Available at https://www.usnews.com/news/best-countries/slideshows/most-likely-industries-to-be-changed-by-automation. Accessed February 3, 2020.

51. Schneider PJ, Pedersen CA, Scheckelhoff DJ. ASHP national survey of pharmacy practice in hospital settings: dispensing and administration-2017. *Am J Health Syst Pharm*. 2018;75(16):1203-1226.

52. Volpe G, Cohen S, Capps RC, et al. Robotics in acute care hospitals. *Am J Health Syst Pharm*. 2012;69(18):1601-1603.

53. Schwarz HO, Brodowy BA. Implementation and evaluation of an automated dispensing system. *Am J Health Syst Pharm*. 1995;52(8):823-828.

54. Berdot S, Blanc C, Chevalier D, Bezie Y, Lê LMM, Sabatier B. Impact of drug storage systems: a quasi-experimental study with and without an automated-drug dispensing cabinet. *Int J Qual Health Care*. 2019;31(3):225-230.

55. Temple J, Ludwig B. Implementation and evaluation of carousel dispensing technology in a university medical center pharmacy. *Am J Health Syst Pharm*. 2010;67(10):821-829.

56. Carousel product for use in integrated restocking and dispensing system. Available at http://patft.uspto.gov/netacgi/nph-Parser?Sect1=PTO1&Sect2=HITOFF&d=PALL&p=1&u=%2Fnetahtml%2FPTO%2Fsrchnum.htm&r=1&f=G&l=50&s1=6,847,861.PN.&OS=PN/6,847,861&RS=PN/6,847,861. Accessed February 7, 2020.

57. Monahan JJ, Webb JW. Intravenous infusion pumps—an added dimension to parenteral therapy. *Am J Hosp Pharm*. 1972;29(1):54-59.

58. Poppe LB, Eckel SF. Evaluating an approach to improving the adoption rate of wireless drug library updates for smart pumps. *Am J Health Syst Pharm*. 2011;68(2):170-175.

59. Kennerly J, Jenkins A, Lewis AN, Eckel SF. Implementing smart pumps for epidural infusions in an academic medical center. *Am J Health Syst Pharm*. 2012;69(7):607-611.

60. Shipton EA, Shipton EE, Shipton AJ. A review of the opioid epidemic: what do we do about it? *Pain Ther*. 2018;7(1):23-36.

61. Sindt JJ, Nonintravenous RH. Opioids. In: Hemmings HE, TD, ed. *Pharmacology and Physiology for Anesthesia: Foundations and Clinical Application*. 2nd ed. Philadelphia, PA: Elsevier; 2019.

62. Brummond PW, Chen DF, Churchill WW, et al. ASHP guidelines on preventing diversion of controlled substances. *Am J Health Syst Pharm*. 2017;74(5):325-348.

63. Inciardi JA, Surratt HL, Kurtz SP, Burke JJ. The diversion of prescription drugs by health care workers in Cincinnati, Ohio. *Subst Use Misuse*. 2006;41(2):255-264.

64. U.S. Drug Enforcement Administration. A DEA resource guide. Available at https://www.dea.gov/sites/default/files/drug_of_abuse.pdf. Accessed January 2, 2020.

65. The Joint Commission. Drug diversion and impaired health care workers. Available at https://www.jointcommission.org/-/media/tjc/newsletters/quick_safety_drug_diversion_final2pdf.pdf. Accessed January 2, 2020.

66. Berge KH, Dillon KR, Sikkink KM, Taylor TK, Lanier WL. Diversion of drugs within health care facilities, a multiple-victim crime: patterns of diversion, scope, consequences, detection, and prevention. *Mayo Clin Proc*. 2012;87(7):674-682.

67. Berge KH, Lanier WL. Bloodstream infection outbreaks related to opioid-diverting health care workers: a cost-benefit analysis of prevention and detection programs. *Mayo Clin Proc*. 2014;89(7):866-868.

68. Campen CJ, Dragovich T, Baker AF. Management strategies in pancreatic cancer. *Am J Health Syst Pharm*. 2011;68(7):573-584.

69. Kuiper SA, McCreadie SR, Mitchell JF, Stevenson JG. Medication errors in inpatient pharmacy operations and technologies for improvement. *Am J Health Syst Pharm*. 2007;64(9):955-959.

70. Rough S, Shane R, Phelps P, et al. A solution to an unmet need: pharmacy specialists in medication-use systems and technology. *Am J Health Syst Pharm.* 2012;69(19):1687-1693.

71. Wittich CM, Burkle CM, Lanier WL. Medication errors: an overview for clinicians. *Mayo Clin Proc.* 2014;89(8):1116-1125.

72. Tariq RA, Scherbak Y. Medication Errors. In: *StatPearls.* Treasure island (FL): StatPearls Publishing LLC.; 2020.

73. Skibinski KA, White BA, Lin LI, Dong Y, Wu W. Effects of technological interventions on the safety of a medication-use system. *Am J Health Syst Pharm.* 2007;64(1):90-96.

74. Institute for Safe Medication Practices. ISMP guidelines for safe preparatioan of compounded sterile preparations. Available at https://www.ismp.org/sites/default/files/attachments/2017-11/Guidelines%20for%20Safe%20Preparation%20of%20Compounded%20Sterile%20Preperations_%20revised%202016.pdf. Accessed January 3, 2020.

75. King J, Patel V, Jamoom EW, Furukawa MF. Clinical benefits of electronic health record use: national findings. *Health Serv Res.* 2014;49(1 Pt 2):392-404.

76. Cheriff AD, Kapur AG, Qiu M, Cole CL. Physician productivity and the ambulatory EHR in a large academic multi-specialty physician group. *Int J Med Inform.* 2010;79(7):492-500.

77. Howard J, Clark EC, Friedman A, et al. Electronic health record impact on work burden in small, unaffiliated, community-based primary care practices. *J Gen Intern Med.* 2013;28(1):107-113.

78. Zlabek JA, Wickus JW, Mathiason MA. Early cost and safety benefits of an inpatient electronic health record. *J Am Med Inform Assoc.* 2011;18(2):169-172.

79. Adler-Milstein J, Salzberg C, Franz C, Orav EJ, Newhouse JP, Bates DW. Effect of electronic health records on health care costs: longitudinal comparative evidence from community practices. *Ann Intern Med.* 2013;159(2):97-104.

80. Ammenwerth E, Schnell-Inderst P, Machan C, Siebert U. The effect of electronic prescribing on medication errors and adverse drug events: a systematic review. *J Am Med Inform Assoc.* 2008;15(5):585-600.

81. Bates DW, Teich JM, Lee J, et al. The impact of computerized physician order entry on medication error prevention. *J Am Med Inform Assoc.* 1999;6(4):313-321.

82. Bates DW, Cohen M, Leape LL, Overhage JM, Shabot MM, Sheridan T. Reducing the frequency of errors in medicine using information technology. *J Am Med Inform Assoc.* 2001;8(4):299-308.

83. Han JE, Rabinovich M, Abraham P, et al. Effect of electronic health record implementation in critical care on survival and medication errors. *Am J Med Sci.* 2016;351(6):576-581.

84. McComas J, Riingen M, Chae Kim S. Impact of an electronic medication administration record on medication administration efficiency and errors. *Comput Inform Nurs.* 2014;32(12):589-595.

85. Klein EG, Santora JA, Pascale PM, Kitrenos JG. Medication cart-filling time, accuracy, and cost with an automated dispensing system. *Am J Hosp Pharm.* 1994;51(9):1193-1196.

86. Whelton PK, Carey RM, Aronow WS, et al. 2017 ACC/AHA/AAPA/ABC/ACPM/AGS/APhA/ASH/ASPC/NMA/PCNA Guideline for the prevention, detection, evaluation, and management of high blood pressure in adults: a report of the American College of Cardiology/American Heart Association task force on clinical practice guidelines. *Circulation.* 2018;138(17):e484-e594.

87. Campbell R. The five "rights" of clinical decision support. *J ahima.* 2013;84(10):42-47; quiz 48.

88. Annane D, Jaeschke R, Guyatt G. Are systematic reviews and meta-analyses still useful research? Yes. *Intensive Care Med.* 2018;44(4):512-514.

89. Page N, Baysari MT, Westbrook JI. A systematic review of the effectiveness of interruptive medication prescribing alerts in hospital CPOE systems to change prescriber behavior and improve patient safety. *Int J Med Inform.* 2017;105:22-30.

90. van der Sijs H, Aarts J, Vulto A, Berg M. Overriding of drug safety alerts in computerized physician order entry. *J Am Med Inform Assoc.* 2006;13(2):138-147.

91. Kalil AC, Metersky ML, Klompas M, et al. Management of adults with hospital-acquired and ventilator-associated pneumonia: 2016 Clinical practice guidelines by the infectious diseases Society of America and the American Thoracic Society. *Clin Infect Dis.* 2016;63(5):e61-e111.

92. Ballard DJ, Ogola G, Fleming NS, et al. Advances in patient safety—the impact of standardized order sets on quality and financial outcomes. In: Henriksen K, Battles JB, Keyes MA, Grady ML, eds. *Advances in Patient Safety: New Directions and Alternative Approaches (Vol. 2: Culture and Redesign).* Rockville (MD): Agency for Healthcare Research and Quality (US); 2008.

93. Olson J, Hollenbeak C, Donaldson K, Abendroth T, Castellani W. Default settings of computerized physician order entry system order sets drive ordering habits. *J Pathol Inform.* 2015;6:16.

94. Del Valle KL, McDonnell ME. Chronic care management services for complex diabetes management: a Practical Overview. *Curr Diab Rep.* 2018;18(12):135.

95. Dagliati A, Sacchi L, Tibollo V, et al. A dashboard-based system for supporting diabetes care. *J Am Med Inform Assoc.* 2018;25(5):538-547.

96. Hartzler AL, Izard JP, Dalkin BL, Mikles SP, Gore JL. Design and feasibility of integrating personalized PRO dashboards into prostate cancer care. *J Am Med Inform Assoc.* 2016;23(1):38-47.

97. Banerjee D, Thompson C, Kell C, et al. An informatics-based approach to reducing heart failure all-cause readmissions: the Stanford heart failure dashboard. *J Am Med Inform Assoc.* 2017;24(3):550-555.

98. Manyika J, Lund S, Chui M, et al. Jobs lost, jobs gained: What the future of work will mean for jobs, skills and wages. Available at https://www.mckinsey.com/featured-insights/future-of-work/jobs-lost-jobs-gained-what-the-future-of-work-will-mean-for-jobs-skills-and-wages. Accessed May 31, 2020.

99. Moore R. 11 Disruptive innovation examples (and why uber and tesla don't make the cut). https://openviewpartners.com/blog/11-disruptive-innovation-examples-and-why-uber-and-tesla-dont-make-the-cut/#.XfP1zpJKgWo. Accessed May 31, 2020.

100. Alsin A. The future of media: disruptions, revolutions and the quest for distribution. Available at https://www.forbes.com/sites/aalsin/2018/07/19/the-future-of-media-disruptions-revolutions-and-the-quest-for-distribution/#6ee8fe4060b9. Accessed May 31, 2020.

101. Dobesh PP, Fanikos J. Direct oral anticoagulants for the prevention of stroke in patients with nonvalvular atrial fibrillation: understanding differences and similarities. *Drugs.* 2015;75(14):1627-1644.

102. Hoie EB, O'Brien KK, Neighbors K, Castillo SL, Begley KJ. Direct oral anticoagulants for the prevention of stroke in nonvalvular atrial fibrillation. *US Pharm.* 2017;42(2):32-35.

103. Holbrook AM, Pereira JA, Labiris R, et al. Systematic overview of warfarin and its drug and food interactions. *Arch Intern Med.* 2005;165(10):1095-1106.

104. Hou K, Yang H, Ye Z, Wang Y, Liu L, Cui X. Effectiveness of pharmacist-led anticoagulation management on clinical outcomes: a systematic review and meta-analysis. *J Pharm Pharm Sci.* 2017;20(1):378-396.

105. Hosmane SR, Tucker J, Osman D, Williams S, Waterworth P. Inpatient oral anticoagulation management by clinical pharmacists: safety and cost effectiveness. *J Clin Med Res.* 2010;2(2):90-92.

106. Barnes GD, Nallamothu BK, Sales AE, Froehlich JB. Reimagining anticoagulation clinics in the era of direct oral anticoagulants. *Circ Cardiovasc Qual Outcomes.* 2016;9(2):182-185.

107. Kinch MS. An overview of FDA-approved biologics medicines. *Drug Discov Today.* 2015;20(4):393-398.

108. Raychaudhuri SP, Raychaudhuri SK. Biologics: target-specific treatment of systemic and cutaneous autoimmune diseases. *Indian J Dermatol.* 2009;54(2):100-109.

109. Humira (adalimumab) injection, for subcutaneous use. In. Chicago, IL: AbbVie Inc.; 2019.

110. McShea MB, Mark; Pollum, Roy D. Biosimilars and follow-on biologics: a pharmacist opportunity. Available at https://www.pharmacytimes.com/publications/issue/2016/novec mber2016/biosimilars-and-followon-biologics-a-pharmacist-opportunity. Accessed May 31, 2020.

111. Chen BK, Yang YT, Bennett CL. Why biologics and biosimilars remain so expensive: despite two wins for biosimilars, the Supreme Court's recent rulings do not solve fundamental barriers to competition. *Drugs.* 2018;78(17):1777-1781.

112. Ng C. Pharmacists' role in the emerging biosimilar market. Available at https://www.pharmacytimes.com/contributor/charles-ng-pharmd-mba-candidate-2017/2016/09/pharmacists-role-in-the-emerging-biosimilar-market. Accessed May 31, 2020.

113. Bonner L. 23andMe releases pharmacogenomics test that doesn't require prescription. Available at https://www.pharmacist.com/article/23andme-releases-pharmacogenomics-test-doesnt-require-prescription. Accessed May 31, 2020.

114. American Society of Health-System Pharmacists. ASHP statement on the pharmacist's role in clinical pharmacogenomics. *Am J Health-Syst Pharm.* 2015;72:579-581.

115. Ritchie MD. The success of pharmacogenomics in moving genetic association studies from bench to bedside: study design and implementation of precision medicine in the post-GWAS era. *Hum Genet.* 2012;131(10):1615-1626.

116. Remi J, Noachtar S. Clinical features of the postictal state: correlation with seizure variables. *Epilepsy Behav.* 2010;19(2):114-117.

117. Fisher RS, Engel JJJr. Definition of the postictal state: when does it start and end? *Epilepsy Behav.* 2010;19(2):100-104.

118. Tangamornsuksan W, Chaiyakunapruk N, Somkrua R, Lohitnavy M, Tassaneeyakul W. Relationship between the HLA-B*1502 allele and carbamazepine-induced Stevens-Johnson syndrome and toxic epidermal necrolysis: a systematic review and meta-analysis. *JAMA Dermatol.* 2013;149(9):1025-1032.

119. Cekic S, Canitez Y, Sapan N. Evaluation of the patients diagnosed with Stevens Johnson syndrome and toxic epidermal necrolysis: a single center experience. *Turk Pediatri Ars.* 2016;51(3):152-158.

120. Dias D, Paulo Silva Cunha J. Wearable health devices—vital sign monitoring, systems and technologies. *Sensors.* 2018;18(8):2414.

121. Liao Y, Thompson C, Peterson S, Mandrola J, Beg MS. The future of wearable technologies and remote monitoring in health care. *Am Soc Clin Oncol Educ Book.* 2019;39:115-121.

122. Phaneuf A. Latest trends in medical monitoring devices and wearable health technology. Available at https://www.businessinsider.com/wearable-technology-healthcare-medical-devices. Accessed February 26, 2020.

123. Francis J. Accenture study finds growing demand for digital health services revolutionizing delivery models: patients, doctors + machines. Available at https://newsroom.accenture.com/news/accenture-study-finds-growing-demand-for-digital-health-services-revolutionizing-delivery-models-patients-doctors-machines.htm. Accessed February 26, 2020.

124. Cadmus-Bertram LA, Marcus BH, Patterson RE, Parker BA, Morey BL. Randomized trial of a fitbit-based physical activity intervention for women. *Am J Prev Med.* 2015;49(3):414-418.

125. Tedesco S, Barton J, O'Flynn B. A review of activity trackers for senior citizens: research perspectives, commercial landscape and the role of the insurance industry. *Sensors.* 2017;17(6):1277.

126. Heale LD, Dover S, Goh YI, Maksymiuk VA, Wells GD, Feldman BM. A wearable activity tracker intervention for promoting physical activity in adolescents with juvenile idiopathic arthritis: a pilot study. *Pediatr Rheumatol Online J.* 2018;16(1):66.

127. Valle CG, Deal AM, Tate DF. Preventing weight gain in African American breast cancer survivors using smart scales and activity trackers: a randomized controlled pilot study. *J Cancer Surviv.* 2017;11(1):133-148.

128. Buckingham SA, Williams AJ, Morrissey K, Price L, Harrison J. Mobile health interventions to promote physical activity and reduce sedentary behaviour in the workplace: A systematic review. *Digit Health.* 2019;5:2055207619839883.

129. Tison GH, Singh AC, Ohashi DA, et al. Cardiovascular risk stratification using off-the-shelf wearables and a multi-task deep learning algorithm. *Circulation.* 2017;136:A21042.

130. Koshy AN, Sajeev JK, Nerlekar N, et al. Smart watches for heart rate assessment in atrial arrhythmias. *Int J Cardiol.* 2018;266:124-127.

131. Giebel GD, Gissel C. Accuracy of mHealth devices for atrial fibrillation screening: systematic review. *JMIR Mhealth Uhealth.* 2019;7(6):e13641.

132. Burns M. Current and future role of wearables in healthcare. Available at https://www.digitalistmag.com/customer-experience/2019/06/04/current-future-role-of-wearables-in-healthcare-06198759. Accessed February 26, 2020.

133. Reich SG, Savitt JM. Parkinson's Disease. *Med Clin North Am.* 2019;103(2):337-350.

134. Tarakad A, Jankovic J. Diagnosis and management of Parkinson's disease. *Semin Neurol.* 2017;37(2):118-126.

135. PC Mag. Encyclopedia: Definition of AR/VR. Available at https://www.pcmag.com/encyclopedia/term/69784/ar-vr. Accessed May 31, 2020.

136. LaValle S. *Virtual Reality.* University of Oulu; 2019.

137. Eckert M, Volmerg JS, Friedrich CM. Augmented reality in medicine: systematic and bibliographic review. *JMIR Mhealth Uhealth.* 2019;7(4):e10967.

138. Ventola CL. Virtual reality in pharmacy: opportunities for clinical, research, and educational Applications. *PT*. 2019;44(5):267-276.

139. Pourmand A, Davis S, Marchak A, Whiteside T, Sikka N. Virtual reality as a clinical tool for pain management. *Curr Pain Headache Rep*. 2018;22(8):53.

140. Glennon C, McElroy SF, Connelly LM, et al. Use of virtual reality to distract from pain and anxiety. *Oncol Nurs Forum*. 2018;45(4):545-552.

141. Arane K, Behboudi A, Goldman RD. Virtual reality for pain and anxiety management in children. *Can Fam Physician*. 2017;63(12):932-934.

142. Fox BI, Felkey BG. Virtual reality and pharmacy: opportunities and challenges. *Hosp Pharm*. 2017;52(2):160-161.

143. Ergurel D. Swedish pharmacy chain launches virtual reality experience for pain relief. Available at https://haptic.al/ virtual-reality-pain-relief-8d366d3bf91e#.mjxtzca57. Accessed February 26, 2020.

144. Swetlitz I. Swedish clinics use virtual reality to reduce the sting of shots. Available at https://www.statnews.com/2016/10/27/ virtual-reality-pain-app/. Accessed May 31, 2020.

145. Schoenthaler AM, Butler M, Chaplin W, Tobin J, Ogedegbe G. Predictors of changes in medication adherence in blacks with hypertension: moving beyond cross-sectional data. *Ann Behav Med*. 2016;50(5):642-652.

146. Salvo MC, Cannon-Breland ML. Motivational interviewing for medication adherence. *J Am Pharm Assoc (2003)*. 2015;55(4):e354-e361; quiz e362-353.

147. Tiao DK, Chan W, Jeganathan J, et al. Inflammatory bowel disease pharmacist adherence counseling improves medication adherence in Crohn's disease and ulcerative colitis. *Inflamm Bowel Dis*. 2017;23(8):1257-1261.

CHAPTER 14

Population Health

Featuring the Illustrated Case Studies "Unsung Hero," "Relapse," & "Interconnected"

Authors
Laurel M. Legenza, Trisha M. Seys Rañola, Natalie S. Schmitz, & Joseph A. Zorek

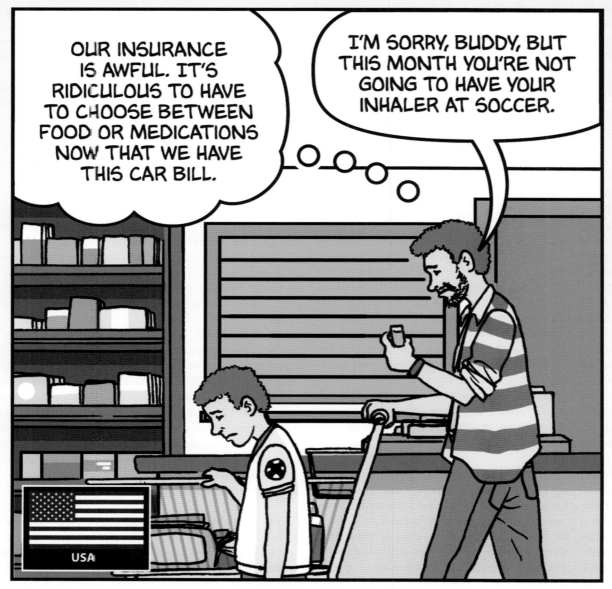

Illustration by George Folz, © 2019 Board of Regents of the University of Wisconsin System

BACKGROUND

Population health aims to improve the health of an entire population and reduce health inequities between population groups.[1] This includes policies and interventions that impact the underlying social causes of health conditions, as well as the study of health outcome distributions within a group. Well-known public health activities, including the promotion of preventive health measures (e.g., hand washing, immunizations, use of bicycle helmets) are population health initiatives. Population health, in other words, is a broad framework that encompasses efforts to leverage governmental, business, non-profit, and community-based entities to improve health.[2]

The Let's Move! campaign initiated by former First Lady of the United States Michelle Obama took a population health approach to the problem of childhood obesity.[3] Campaign officials were successful in making changes across industries, economic sectors and Congress, passing the Healthy, Hunger-Free Kids Act. Schools offered healthier meals. Only snacks and beverages meeting the new nutrition standards could be marketed and sold at schools, meaning there were more fruits and vegetables available. Large chain restaurants reduced portion sizes and replaced french fries with fruits and vegetables in kids' meals. Combined, all of these changes impacted the availability, quality, and marketing of food products to children and their families, while simultaneously encouraging greater exercise. Childhood obesity rates declined in the last decade, and many credit Let's Move! as an important contributing factor.[4]

Based in Oakland, California, Kaiser Permanente provides an example of a health system that has embraced population health. Broadly speaking, a health system is a healthcare organization that includes at least one hospital and one physician group that work in tandem to provide comprehensive care to a defined patient population. Many health systems are comprised of hospitals, clinics, and pharmacies owned and operated by a single entity. These can be for-profit or non-profit organizations, as well as governmental health systems such as the Veterans Health Administration or academic health systems that have an association with a university. Kaiser Permanente is a non-profit health system combined with a managed care organization that serves approximately 9 million members across nine states.[5] The managed care component, as in other health systems, focuses on cost-effective solutions to the provision of care.[6] Examples of managed care solutions include requiring patients to only see providers within an approved network or allowing out-of-network visits with a higher co-payment.

Kaiser Permanente's model incentivizes population health management with high quality affordable care provided to its members, individuals, and employer groups. One such approach was initiated in response to high rates of homelessness observed in service areas.[7] Recognizing that stable housing is essential to good health, Kaiser Permanente began housing initiatives to address the issue of housing insecurity. This included investing in apartment buildings to support upgrades and ensure affordable rents. This initiative is also partnering across city, county, and non-profit sectors to find housing for homeless Oakland residents, as well as creating and preserving existing housing for low-income residents nationally.

An intentional focus on improving the health of populations is a welcomed shift within the United States. Unfortunately, compared to Australia, Canada, France, Germany, the Netherlands, New Zealand, Norway, Sweden, Switzerland, and the United Kingdom, healthcare in the United States was found to be the most expensive and the least effective.[8] This comparison highlighted that the United States had the highest burden of chronic diseases, the highest rates of suicide and avoidable death, and the lowest life expectancy of all 11 countries. In terms of cost, the United States spent nearly twice as much on healthcare compared to the average healthcare expenditure of our peers (16.9% vs. 8.8%).

Healthcare reform initiatives for many years have aimed to simultaneously improve patient and population health outcomes while reducing costs.[9] A basic value equation (Value = Quality/Cost) demonstrates the need to both increase quality and reduce costs to provide better value to populations.[10,11] The Patient Protection and Affordable Care Act of 2010 provides a robust example of such reform.[12] This law encouraged the formation of accountable care organizations (ACOs) as a mechanism to incentivize value. ACOs are voluntarily formed groups of physicians and other health professionals, hospitals, and/or health systems that join together to take responsibility for specific patient populations. More than 1000 ACOs have formed since 2011.[13,14] ACOs are eligible for financial rewards for meeting quality metrics established by insurers. They are also subject to penalties for missing established quality metrics.

Multiple ACO payment structures exist with various levels of financial risk and reward.[15,16] The US Centers for Medicare and Medicaid Services (CMS) administers the governmental insurance program Medicare, which covers adults 65 years of age and older. Medicare offers several ACO programs to incentivize care coordination in an effort to increase value.[17] Medications bring their own level of complexity regarding risk, costs, and value. Many health insurance plans utilize pharmacy benefit management companies (PBMs) to optimize medication use across populations and to improve outcomes and reduce unnecessary costs.[18] The illustrated case "Relapse" in this chapter provides more information on PBMs. Readers are also encouraged to explore the illustrated case "Relationships" in Chapter 15 Administration for additional information. While substantial progress has been made in moving toward value-based delivery of healthcare, many health systems are still somewhere in a transition phase and continue to operate outside of a population health management paradigm.

Global health extends the population health view worldwide, and is a recognition that all populations, regardless of political borders, are interconnected and interdependent.[19] No single stakeholder can address all of the world's health threats alone.[20] This fact was exemplified by the deadly virus SARS-CoV-2, which infected large swaths of the world's population and wreaked havoc on health and economic indicators alike during the COVID-19 pandemic.[21] The United Nation's Sustainable Development Goals embody transforming global population health through 17 interconnected factors including, for example, poverty, hunger, health and well-being, education, and work and economic growth.[22] Pharmacists, with expert knowledge and skills related to the development, manufacturing, acquisition, management, distribution, and use of medications play a vital role in the health of patients and populations, both within the United States and globally.

Health and Other Professionals Who Contribute to Population Health Initiatives

Public health programs, and the professionals who lead them, serve as a foundation for the health of populations. For example, many public health programs exist to ensure that water is safe to drink and that infectious diseases are kept under control.[23] Dedicated professionals working within the city or local public health departments driving such efforts typically have a public health background; that is, they have earned an advanced degree in public health (e.g., Master of Public Health [MPH], Doctor of Public Health [DrPH]).[24] Such degrees prepare individuals to develop solutions to population health problems from the view of the whole country, state, city, or even neighborhood.[25]

The list of collaborators to public health professional-led initiatives is dependent on the initiative itself; generally speaking, it is more expansive than the health professionals who have appeared throughout this book as interprofessional collaborators. Returning to the water quality and sanitation example, preventing contamination or the spread of infectious diseases may require partnership and teamwork with the individuals who ensure those systems operate effectively; this can include city planners, architects, engineers, plumbers, and waste management professionals.[25] Public health professionals also contribute to emergency preparedness and response initiatives.[27] The types of collaborators or contributing professionals in that setting can vary widely and may involve interface with state and federal officials. For an example, readers are encouraged to explore the illustrated case "Mobilized" in Chapter 4 Prevention & Wellness.

The US Surgeon General is considered the most trusted and respected federal authority on public health in America.[28] The Surgeon General provides the best scientific information available on how to improve health and reduce risk of illness and injury. More than 6500 public health professionals work under the direction of the Surgeon General as members of the US Public Health Service Commissioned Corps.[29] The Commissioned Corps employs an array of health professionals, such as dentists, dietitians/nutritionists, nurses, pharmacists, physicians, and a host of therapists from different professions.[29] Large organized governmental programs work toward reducing health disparities and employ a variety of health professionals. Nationally, the US Department of Health and Human Services (HHS) also employs health professionals. The Indian Health Service (IHS) is an agency within HHS that employs frontline and managerial health professionals to provide care to federally recognized Native American Tribes and Alaska Natives. Pharmacy officers in the Commissioned Corps are often appointed to serve within IHS. Federally Qualified Health Centers serve as an important population health backstop, employing a host of health professionals to provide care to vulnerable populations regardless of an individual's ability to pay.[30,31]

Role of Pharmacists in Population Health Initiatives

Pharmacists can specialize in managing the health of populations in a variety of settings, such as health systems, managed care organizations, PBMs, governmental and nongovernmental organizations, and within global organizations like the World Health Organization (WHO). Opportunities also exist within more traditional pharmacist roles to practice through the lens of population health. For an example of this, readers are encouraged to explore the illustrated case "Unsung Hero" in this chapter.

Pharmacists serve as medication experts within managed care organizations, PBMs, and insurance companies.[32] When the results of new large-scale drug trials are published, for example, pharmacists review these critically to inform recommendations as to whether changes should be made to policies or drug formularies. Thus, pharmacists contribute to decisions that affect entire populations of patients regarding the coverage of high cost medications by PBMs or insurance companies. Pharmacists are also involved in providing prior authorizations to individual patients for medications otherwise not covered. Population health management programs with pharmacist involvement such as these are impactful. For example, one organization sought to identify actionable interventions to improve the health of patients with heart conditions.[33] They leveraged the knowledge and skills of advanced pharmacy students, who reviewed patients' records for adherence to critical medications and the need for dose adjustments based on kidney function. This effort resulted in nearly 1400 actionable interventions for patients within this population.

Population health services have also been developed to manage high-risk populations within health systems and across pharmacy settings. Pharmacists play key roles within these services, including leadership roles. Pharmacists have been managing populations taking high-risk medications like anticoagulants (i.e., blood thinners) for many years.[34–36] These programs make a difference at the population level, as they have been found to reduce mortality and length of hospital stay compared to hospitals without pharmacist-led services.[36] Pharmacists also continue to be involved in managing populations taking newer anticoagulation medications and testing algorithms for identifying patients needing anticoagulation; for example, patients with a heart condition called atrial fibrillation that increases the risk of stroke.[37–39]

Across the United States, pharmacists design and provide population health-focused programs to manage a large swath of health conditions.[40,41] A large systematic review that explored the impact of pharmacist-led chronic disease management programs found that such programs improved key indicators/goals for patients with diabetes, high blood pressure, and high cholesterol.[42] Community pharmacists are also making a positive impact on the health of populations. A review of research on community pharmacist-led interventions found associated improvements in clinical outcomes for patients with diabetes, heart disease, high cholesterol, respiratory diseases, and Human Immunodeficiency Virus (HIV).[43] Community pharmacists are also well positioned to expand public health roles in the management and use of HIV medications.[44] The value of pharmacists in population health management is poised to grow well into the future.

POPULATION HEALTH PHARMACISTS IN ACTION

Native Land

Native American populations in the United States experience disproportionate social and health disparities compared to other populations, including rates of chronic diseases.[45] For example, Native Americans are twice as likely to have diabetes compared to white populations, and they are also disproportionally at risk for mental health conditions, such as depression, post-traumatic stress disorder, and substance use disorders. The complex history of Native Americans and the resulting historical trauma must be recognized within these statistics. Red Lake IHS, like many health systems, was experiencing a shortage of primary care providers in 2012.[46] They responded by incorporating pharmacists into the primary care setting with a patient-centered, team-based care approach. The Red Lake IHS program aims were decidedly aligned with population health: expanding access to care, meeting facility quality indicators, and improving health outcomes. Over time, as population health quality metrics improved, pharmacists' activities expanded from anticoagulation into medication-assisted treatment of substance use disorders and behavioral health medication management clinics. As a result, Red Lake IHS has begun formally recognizing pharmacists as members of the primary care medical staff.[47]

Partners for Kids

Pharmacists at Partners For Kids (PFK) have been called the "Next Big Thing" in population health management.[48] PFK is one of the oldest and largest pediatric ACOs in the United States, and it represents a partnership between Nationwide Children's Hospital and more than 1000 physicians.[49] Nationally, Medicaid provides health coverage for the most economically disadvantaged children.[50] In central and southeastern Ohio, PFK has brought together five Medicaid managed care plans; collectively, PFK provides approximately 330,000 children with high-quality care and care coordination at a low cost. The program has achieved impressive goals, such as reducing the amount of hospital admissions and readmissions.[51] Two PFK pharmacists have been successfully integrated with a population health focus. Key contributions include developing prescribing resources, providing medication-related education, developing clinical decision support for providers, and providing disease-specific medication therapy management recommendations.[11] The pharmacists also manage a preferred drug list, which has reduced disruptions created by medications being prescribed that are not covered by Medicaid. PFK pharmacists also partner with state Medicaid payors to implement cost-effective and clinically appropriate therapies.[52,53] For example, when an inhaler was modified by the manufacturer and became difficult for children to use, the PFK pharmacists were able to successfully influence drug formulary changes to ensure that patients were able to maintain control of their asthma. These efforts have led to improvements in asthma control and reductions in emergency department visits.

BECOMING A POPULATION HEALTH PHARMACIST

While the path to a career as a population health pharmacist is not as direct as other pharmacy practice areas, there are a number of training opportunities that provide essential knowledge and skills to succeed in this area. Some academic training opportunities that align with pillars of population health can be completed in conjunction with pre-pharmacy coursework, during, or after pharmacy school. Opportunities available during pharmacy school include: (1) elective population health-focused experiential education rotations, (2) international elective experiential education rotations, and (3) global health certificate programs and/or global/population health coursework. Students may also engage in population health research with faculty inside and outside pharmacy. Dual degree programs can be completed during pharmacy school. Many pharmacy programs offer a combined Master of Public Health (MPH) and Doctor of Pharmacy (PharmD) degree. Master's degrees in Public Affairs or Public Policy also support successful careers dedicated to advancing population health.

Post-graduate residency training programs after completion of the PharmD degree can provide additional opportunities to develop population health-relevant skills.[40] After finishing a general post-graduate year 1 residency, specialty post-graduate year 2 residencies especially helpful to population health careers are available; these include drug information, managed care, pharmacy outcomes/analytics, and health system pharmacy administration.[54] The American Society of Health-System Pharmacists maintains a directory of accredited pharmacy residencies.[54] Of note, IHS also has residency programs. Research fellowships in global health, population health, or public health provide additional avenues for early career pharmacists to develop additional knowledge and skills in this field. The US Centers for Disease Control and Prevention also have training programs for health professionals, including pharmacists, to specialize in population health and public health fields.

UNSUNG HERO: An Illustrated Case Study

Story by Trisha M. Seys Rañola & Joseph A. Zorek
Illustrations by George Folz, © 2019 Board of Regents of the University of Wisconsin System

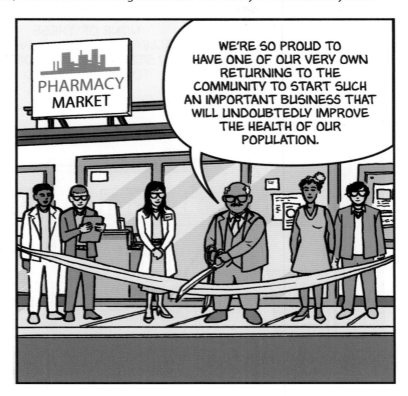

Illustration 14-1

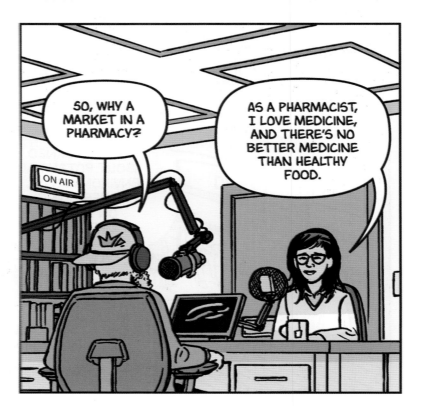

Ilustration 14-2

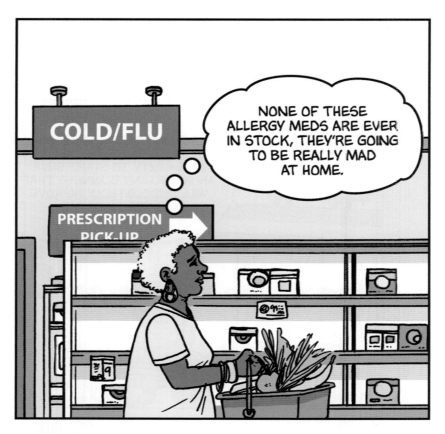

Illustration 14-3

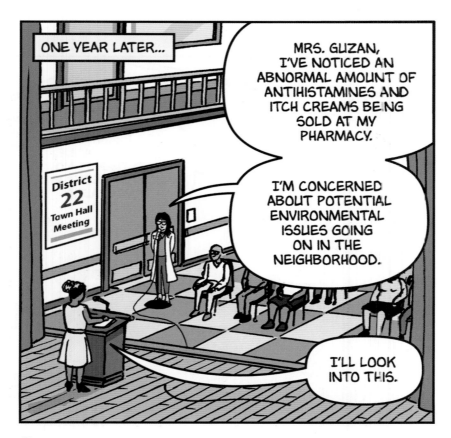

Illustration 14-4

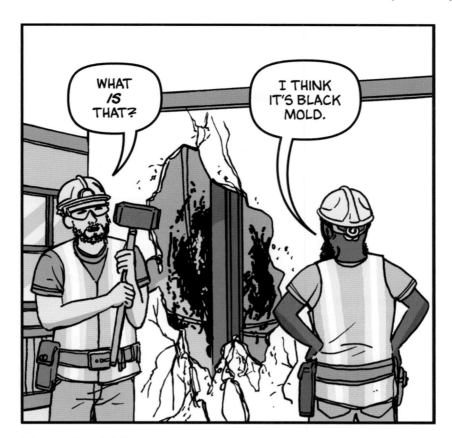

Illustration 14-5

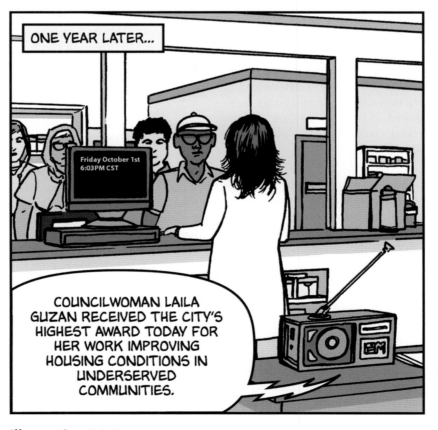

Illustration 14-6

Thoughts on "Unsung Hero"

The illustrated case "Unsung Hero" emphasizes connections between health and many factors that, up until recently, have not been at the forefront for many health professionals. Examined through the lens of a pharmacist with an entrepreneurial spirit, this story illustrates the complex interconnections between physical well-being, nutrition, housing, environment, political advocacy, and government policy. Exploring this complex web leads to an understanding that no decision, large or small, should be taken without first considering potential impacts on health. Indeed, the World Health Organization (WHO), through its Health in All Policy campaign, urges governments around the globe to consider the health of all people when making new policy, whether it relates to a new bike path around a lake, gas emission standards, or how much corn to grow.[55]

The pharmacist in this illustrated case, intentionally unnamed, is a humble person focused on making positive change; hence, the title. She grew up in the lower-resourced neighborhood to which she is returning, as shown in Illustration 14-1. While not described, her backstory includes witnessing the impact of local businesses relocating to more profitable communities throughout her childhood and adolescence. Determined to make a difference in her community, and undeterred by the inherent risks, she opens a pharmacy with a fresh food market in a community that has neither. The ceremonial ribbon-cutting in Illustration 14-1 demonstrates the value of this decision to her community, and foreshadows how important Pharmacy Market will become. This pharmacist addresses issues of food security, access to primary care and health education, and advocates for politicians to solve problems affecting her neighbors. First-hand knowledge of how social determinants of health (SDH) impact well-being set her down a path as an entrepreneurial pharmacist determined to improve health by all means necessary, not just through medication use. Readers interested in primary care are encouraged to explore the illustrated cases "Support," "Swish," and "Holistic" in Chapter 3 Primary Care.

SDH are defined as "conditions in the environments in which people are born, live, learn, work, play, worship, and age that affect a wide range of health, functioning, and quality of life outcomes and risks."[56] Examples of SDH include safe and affordable housing, and access to healthy food and education.[56] Americans spend about two-thirds of their life in their own home, making it a resource for both healing properties and, conversely, a potential source of environmental toxins, like lead.[57] Sadly, the Robert Wood Johnson Foundation noted in 2017 that over 500,000 children under the age of 5 had elevated lead blood levels attributable to unsafe housing, placing them at high risk of developmental issues such as stunted growth, lower IQ, learning disabilities, and long-term consequences like lower educational obtainment, anemia, hypertension, and toxicity to reproductive organs.[57-59] Similar to safe housing, good nutrition and access to healthy food is important for staying healthy over the course of a lifespan.[60] Interestingly, this SDH is not just focused on lack of food, but on the quality of food available. In terms of opportunity, education, and especially early childhood education, has been shown to improve health outcomes for the entire family.[61] When a child is enrolled in school, this allows for increased maternal employment and income, decreased healthcare costs, reduction in crime, and increased future income of the child.

In addition to focusing on traditional health interventions, like improving blood pressure control, health professionals from all professions are increasingly being encouraged to devote their attention to addressing SDH. Traditional healthcare delivery approaches, like 15-minute visits to the physician followed by monthly visits to the pharmacy to pick up medication refills, will not suffice in many cases. Research has evolved in this area, and we now know that a person's whole health cannot be addressed by simply treating the symptoms of a problem. See the illustrated case "Holistic" in Chapter 3 Primary Care for a compelling example.[62-64] Revisiting blood pressure to highlight this issue, prescribing medications as a singular intervention does not address lack of access to healthy foods and safe spaces to exercise. These upstream issues at the root of health problems must be addressed alongside their physical manifestations. For an example of upstream issues, see the illustrated case "Screen" in Chapter 4 Prevention & Wellness.

A consensus paper published by the National Academies of Sciences, Engineering, and Medicine (NASEM) provides a framework for practicing health professionals to address these issues.[65] This framework encourages health professionals to view SDH through the lens of individual patients by incorporating the following five activities into healthcare delivery: awareness, adjustment, assistance, alignment, and advocacy. The first three apply to interactions with individual patients, while the last two involve activities that health professionals or organizations can engage in to address SDH at a population level. Awareness, adjustment, and assistance involve identifying social risks, adjusting healthcare interventions based on them, and leveraging known resources in the community; for example, during a patient visit. Opening a pharmacy with an emphasis on fresh foods in a neighborhood that does not have easy access to either demonstrates alignment, where resources are invested to address known SDH in a community. The last activity, advocacy, deals with promoting action in public policy to improve identified SDH within communities. The protagonist in "Unsung Hero" is shown advocating in Illustration 14-4 for her patients at an elected official's town hall meeting (Councilwoman Laila Guzan), an act that ultimately sets the dominoes in motion for the identification and mitigation of a health issue related to safe and affordable housing.

In Illustration 14-2, the pharmacist is shown promoting her new store at a local radio station and discussing the similarities between medications and food, and why she sees the combination as a natural fit to promote health. Food is a basic resource that all people need to function, live, work, and thrive. Without food, we live in a state of food insecurity, which is more than just the physical sensation of hunger. The US Department of Agriculture (USDA) provides the following distinction:

"Hunger refers to a personal, physical sensation of discomfort, while food insecurity refers to a lack of available financial resources for food at the level of the household."[66]

Unfortunately, millions of Americans are affected by food insecurity; roughly 1 in 8 according to 2017 survey data.[66] Poverty is the main contributing factor to food insecurity. However, it can affect those living above the poverty line and is, in fact, related to interconnected policies on education, income levels, and food deserts. A food desert is defined by the USDA as a community where at least 500 people or a third of the population live a mile from a supermarket or large grocery store in urban areas, or more than 10 miles in rural parts of the country.[66]

Differences in health between communities that arise from SDH are called health disparities. For example, the 2016 Community Health Needs Assessment for San Antonio, Texas indicated a 20-year difference in life expectancy between two neighborhoods; residents in one area were expected to live 70 to 74 years, while those in another part of the city were expected to live 90 to 94 years.[67] This dramatic difference was correlated in the report to the SDH of having a safe community and housing and access to grocery stores.[67] Health disparities can also be seen between racial and ethnic groups, with one dramatic example being infant mortality rates. Even when matched for educational achievement and income, babies born to Black, non-Hispanic women are twice as likely to die before reaching their first birthday than babies born to White women.[68,69] While income and education are important factors, other SDH are contributing factors, including access to primary care and chronic stress related to discrimination.[69,70]

Pharmacists are well-positioned within the healthcare system to address health disparities, and not just those tied to food as described in "Unsung Hero." Pharmacists are the most accessible health professionals in the United States, and in recent decades the profession has been organizing itself to improve the health of patients and communities through this accessibility.[60,64,71,72] Importantly, improving access to primary care services is a United Nations health priority.[22] Vaccine administration is perhaps the most publicized example, where patients can now bypass a multitude of barriers and receive many types of vaccines by simply walking into their local pharmacy. See the illustrated case "Organized Chaos" in Chapter 2 Community Pharmacy for an example. Pharmacists also contribute their expertise associated with vaccine administration in response to disease outbreaks through large-scale immunization efforts. An example of this activity can be seen in the illustrated case "Mobilized" in Chapter 4 Prevention & Wellness.

Similar to in-store vaccine administration, some pharmacies have begun offering walk-in services for many basic primary care needs, thus eliminating the challenges associated with taking time off work, arranging for child care, and figuring out how to get from home to the appointment.[73,74] Examples of these services include treatment for a variety of common non-life-threatening illnesses such as bronchitis, pink eye, and strep throat. Additionally, pharmacies may offer basic physicals for school-aged sports teams or blood pressure checks.[73] Analyses of outcomes from these services have shown them to be as effective, yet less expensive, than traditional care.[74] These services are offered mostly through collaborative practice agreements with physicians, which is another incredible facilitator of interprofessional practice. For more on this topic, see the illustrated case "Breathe" in Chapter 2 Community Pharmacy.

As demonstrated in "Unsung Hero," patterns of medication use can reveal patterns of disease within a community.[75] The study of these patterns is called epidemiology, and researchers in this field often track medication use through prescription and controlled substance databases. Readers are encouraged to explore the illustrated case "Gasping" in Chapter 12 Mental Health for an example. Over-the-counter medication use is trickier to track because it takes place without a prescription or insurance claim. Fortunately, the protagonist in this illustrated case recognizes a pattern of higher-than-expected allergy medication sales. Searching for clues, she relates this back to her knowledge of SDH; in particular, the potential perils associated with housing insecurity.

Medications to treat allergy symptoms typically follow seasonal patterns of use tied to naturally occurring environmental allergens, such as pollen. These include oral medications to treat symptoms such as itchy eyes and runny noses, as well as topical medications applied to the skin as creams or ointments for mild rashes, which can occur through contact with something in the environment that the body sees as foreign. Overwhelmingly, sales of allergy medications ebb and flow based on the time of the year, with heavier sales when allergens in the environment are high, such as in the spring and fall. In the illustrated case "Unsung Hero," the pharmacist cannot keep these products in stock, creating a shortage. This is noticeable not only in purchasing data, but also in customer feedback, as evidenced in Illustration 14-3.

While the pharmacist is uncertain as to the specific cause, she understands that this trend is likely attributable to something environmental within her community. By reporting the unusual pattern of medication use to her local Councilwoman, Ms. Laila Guzan (Illustration 14-4), she set into motion an investigation that uncovered low-income housing units contaminated with black mold (Illustrations 14-5 and 14-6). The protagonist's advocacy can be linked back to the NASEM framework, and highlights that pharmacists have a pivotal role to play providing data for population health systems, including the identification and sharing of medication use trends that may influence public policy.[75]

While the illustrated case "Unsung Hero" is hypothetical, there are many real-world examples of pharmacists impacting their communities in similar ways.[21] The city of Flint, Michigan was faced with a public health crisis caused by lead-contaminated drinking water, and pharmacists in the community rallied to respond. Community members were in need of lead blood level testing, but were wary of government responses to the crisis. To engage community members, public health officials tapped into the trust community pharmacists have established with their neighbors.[76,77] With guidance from the Michigan Pharmacists Association, the Michigan Department of Health and Human Services, and the Genesee County Health Department, participating pharmacists provided point-of-care lead testing for community members. For more on point-of-care testing, see the illustrated case "Empowerment" in Chapter 5 Cardiology. Lead testing in Flint was coupled with patient education on the meaning of results and ways to minimize lead exposure. All results were sent to appropriate state and local health professionals for additional services, if needed.[76] Additionally, pharmacies donated tens of thousands of bottles of water to local food banks and relief organizations and provided education on safe lead-free drinking water.[78]

Another real-world example involves a partnership between CVS Health, home to the largest network of retail pharmacies in the United States, and Aetna, one of the nation's largest health insurance providers, to develop effective population health interventions based on aggregated health insurance data on SDH.[79]

Professional pharmacy organizations around the country are increasingly promoting the role of pharmacists to minimize the negative consequences of SDH.[80] Many states also have pharmacy organizations that allow a platform for advocacy on this topic.[81] These organizations facilitate the sharing of pharmacists' daily practice observations to connect with state and national policymakers charged with addressing SDH. Examples of this include safe medication drop-off locations and community naloxone standing use orders for pharmacists, which have been offered to address the scourge of opioid-related overdoses. See the illustrated case "Gasping" in Chapter 12 Mental Health for more details on naloxone. Pharmacists engaged in these advocacy efforts protect the environment, increase health education, and create access to healthcare for those in need.

DISCUSSION QUESTIONS FOR "UNSUNG HERO"

1. In Illustration 14-2, the pharmacist gives an interview highlighting the fresh produce she is selling at Pharmacy Market, addressing one aspect of social determinants of health (SDH). What other SDH needs might Pharmacy Market address?

2. The pharmacist in "Unsung Hero" identifies a pattern of medication use that exposes an environmental issue in her neighborhood. Can you think of other medication use patterns that might indicate an issue related to social determinants of health?

3. The illustrated case "Unsung Hero" highlights the important contributions of pharmacists, many of which go unrecognized or uncelebrated. Have you ever helped others without being recognized or receiving credit? If so, how did it make you feel?

4. Altruism, as demonstrated in "Unsung Hero," is obviously a positive attribute for a health professional. What other attributes, personality traits, etc., are important for health professionals to possess?

5. Think about pharmacists you have encountered in your life. What barriers might prevent these individuals from practicing pharmacy with a focus on social determinants of health in addition to medication use and clinical care?

RELAPSE: An Illustrated Case Study

Story by Natalie S. Schmitz & Joseph A. Zorek
Illustrations by George Folz, © 2020 McGraw-Hill Education

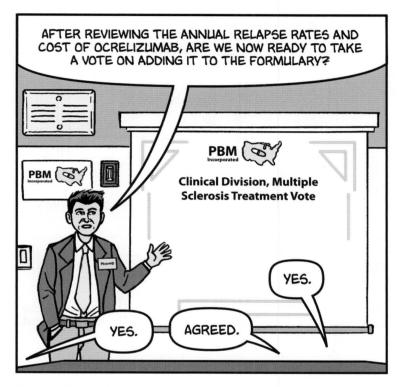

Illustration 14-7

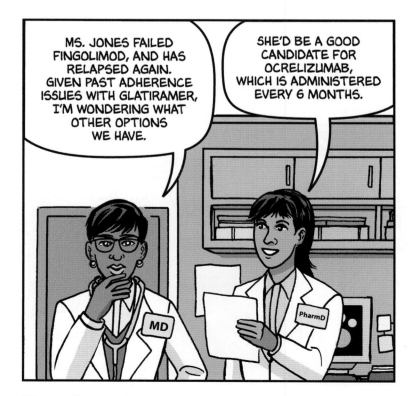

Illustration 14-8

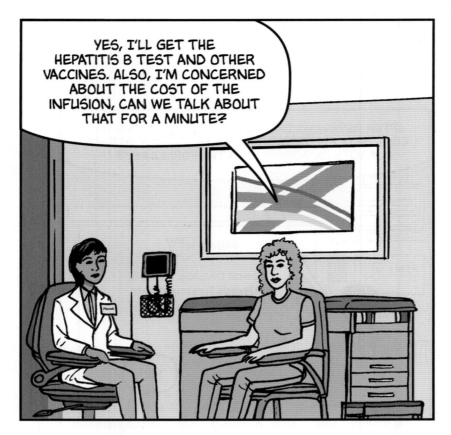

Illustration 14-9

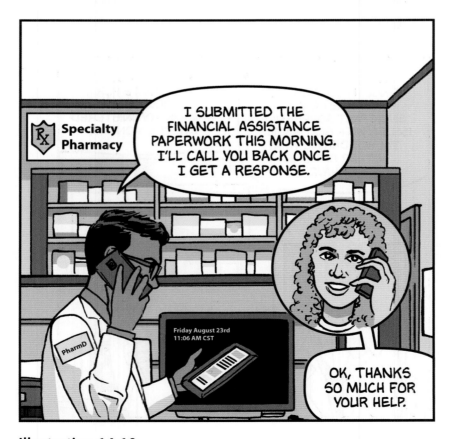

Illustration 14-10

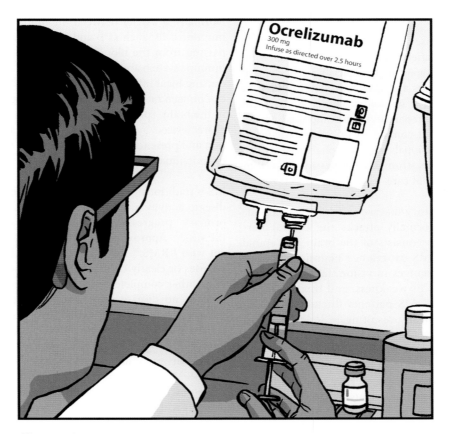

Illustration 14-11

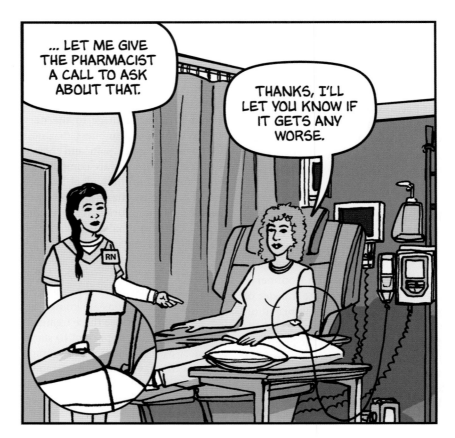

Illustration 14-12

Thoughts on "Relapse"

The illustrated case "Relapse" highlights the importance of pharmacists in the lives of patients with multiple sclerosis (MS). The roles of three different types of pharmacists are portrayed: one who manages formularies and access to medications at a PBM, another employed in a neurology clinic, and a third engaged in sterile products preparation and compounding at a specialty pharmacy. Given the complexity of MS and the number of different health professionals involved, pharmacists in all of these settings must possess strong interprofessional collaboration skills to optimize patient care.

MS is a chronic, inflammatory disease in which an individual's immune system abnormally attacks the central nervous system (CNS), which consists of the brain and spinal cord.[82] Most people with MS experience neurologic symptoms as a result, such as changes in vision, fatigue, walking difficulties, muscle spasms or weakness, and tingling of the face, body or extremities.[83] MS patients fluctuate between relapse and remission, typically resulting in long-term disability primarily characterized by the inability to work due to vision changes, fatigue, cognitive deterioration, or difficulty walking.[84] This disease affects over 2.3 million people worldwide and is the most prevalent cause of disability in young adults.[85,86] While the primary cause of MS is not fully understood, scientists believe that a combination of factors increase risk of developing the disease; examples include gender, age, geography, ethnic background, genetics, and an abnormal immune response to an infection.

MS is typically diagnosed in young adulthood, between 20 and 40 years of age, and it is two to three times more common in women than in men.[87] Although MS occurs in most racial/ethnic groups, Caucasians and those of northern European ancestry are more likely to develop it than others.[87] Historically, geographic location has also been associated with MS, where a pattern has been observed linking increased incidence with increased distance from the equator.[88,89] Additionally, those who have had Epstein Barr Virus, which is the virus that causes mononucleosis, are thought to be at an increased risk for developing MS.[90]

The underlying cause of MS is thought to be immune-mediated demyelination of the CNS.[82] A substance called myelin coats nerve cells, and this enables nerve impulses, or signals carrying messages/information, to be rapidly transferred from one nerve cell to another. Demyelination strips myelin from nerve cells, causing lesions that lead to problems with the transfer of these impulses. Demyelination causes message/information transfer to slow down or to be disrupted completely. As a result, the flow of signals within the brain and between the brain and the body gets disrupted. MS patients experience symptoms that coincide with the location of their lesions. These can include, but are not limited to, decreases in mobility and cognition, depression, anxiety, and fatigue, all of which greatly impact quality of life.

Normally, a barrier between the brain and the blood prevents immune cells, such as B and T cells, and other infiltrates from passing from the blood into the CNS. In MS, cells from the immune system are able to pass through the blood-brain barrier, causing local inflammation and demyelination. Demyelination can be seen on MRI scans as lesions or plaques that are located in the brain, spinal cord, and nerves of the eye. This disease is characterized by progressively deteriorating clinical presentation and presence of lesions in the CNS that vary over time and by individual.[91,92]

MS is traditionally categorized into three subtypes that describe disease activity and progression: relapsing remitting (RRMS), primary progressive (PPMS), and secondary progressive (SPMS).[93] Approximately 85% of individuals initially present with RRMS.[94] Relapsing forms of MS are characterized by relapses or clearly defined attacks and worsening of symptoms with either complete or incomplete recovery. RRMS has minimal or no disease progression during the periods between relapses. Some patients with RRMS go on to develop SPMS, which is characterized by initial presentation of RRMS followed by progressive, gradual worsening of symptoms over time. Conversely, about 15% of patients are initially diagnosed with PPMS.[94] PPMS is characterized by gradual worsening of symptoms and disability from disease onset that occasionally presents with minor improvements or plateauing of disease progression. Exacerbations, known as relapses or flares, can cause worsening of old symptoms, as well as the appearance of new symptoms. These range from mild to severe, the latter of which can even interfere with activities of daily living such as eating, bathing, and getting dressed.[95,96] Several triggers can lead to MS flares, including disease progression, stress, increased body heat, and infection.

Symptoms of MS can be divided into three categories: primary, secondary, and tertiary.[97] Primary symptoms are those that are related to direct damage to the nervous system and include fatigue, weakness, numbness, dizziness, difficulty walking, spasticity, vision changes, pain, and changes in mood and cognition. Secondary symptoms are complications of primary symptoms. For example, if an individual has difficulty walking, is experiencing numbness, dizziness, and weakness, they are at a higher risk for falls and injuries. Tertiary symptoms are social, psychological, and vocational complications of the disease, such as loss of employment and impact on interpersonal relationships.

Although there is no cure for MS, available treatments can modify the course of disease and delay the onset of disability; thus, these medications are known as disease modifying therapies (DMTs).[97] Because these treatments can change the course of the disease, it is important to start as soon as there is a suspicion of MS. The number of therapies available for relapsing forms of MS has grown considerably since the introduction of DMTs in the 1990s. These therapies, listed in Table 14-1, differ in efficacy, side effects, prerequisite safety procedures, and route of administration.

Table 14-1. Categories and Examples of Medications Commonly Used in the Treatment of Multiple Sclerosis		
Category	**Medication Examples***	**Physiologic Effect**
Injectable disease modifying therapies	▪ glatiramer (Copaxone, Glatopa)	Reduces demyelination of nerves by activating cells that suppress T lymphocytes**
	▪ interferon beta-1a (Avonex, Rebif)	Reduce immune cell trafficking across the blood-brain barrier and neuron demyelination by decreasing expression of inflammatory cytokines*** and increasing expression of anti-inflammatory cytokines
	▪ interferon beta-1b (Betaseron, Extavia)	
	▪ peginterferon beta-1a (Plegridy)	
Oral disease modifying therapies	▪ cladribine (Mavenclad)	Impairs DNA synthesis, causing B**** and T lymphocyte death, which reduce nerve demyelination
	▪ dimethyl fumarate (Tecfidera)	Activate a specific pathway to promote anti-inflammatory effects and reduce nerve demyelination
	▪ diroximel fumarate (Vumerity)	
	▪ fingolimod (Gilenya)	Prevent lymphocyte migration into the CNS by blocking lymphocyte excretion from the lymph nodes*****
	▪ siponimod (Mayzent)	
	▪ teriflunomide (Aubogio)	Reduces nerve demyelination and increases anti-inflammatory effects by blocking pyrimidine synthesis and inhibiting rapidly diving cells such as T and B lymphocytes
Infused disease modifying therapies	▪ alemtuzumab (Lemtrada)	Binds to specific receptors on several immune cells, reducing lymphocyte and immune cell activity to reduce nerve demyelination
	▪ natalizumab (Tysabri)	Blocks T lymphocyte migration into the CNS
	▪ ocrelizumab (Ocrevus)	Binds to a specific receptor on B lymphocytes to promote cell death and decrease nerve demyelination

*Medication examples presented in alphabetical order as "generic name (Brand Name)."
**T lymphocytes are a type of white blood cell that help fight off infections.
***Cytokines are a type of protein secreted by specific cells to modulate the immune system.
****B lymphocytes are a type of white blood cell that are responsible for producing antibodies.
*****Lymph nodes are small glands throughout the lymphatic system that filter lymph fluid and build lymphocytes.

Selecting drug therapy should be based on the patient's disease activity, other health conditions or comorbidities, and the patient's personal values and preferences. Despite growing options of DMTs for relapsing forms of MS, therapies for progressive subtypes of the disease are lacking. Ocrelizumab, the medication referred to throughout "Relapse," was the first drug approved for PPMS and is also indicated for RRMS. In Illustration 14-8, the physician and pharmacist are depicted considering which medication options are most efficacious and would improve medication adherence. For example, glatiramer is self-injected into the subcutaneous layer of the skin every day or three times a week depending on the formulation. Fingolimod is a capsule that is taken every day. Both of these medications require self-administration of the drug. Alternatively, ocrelizumab is typically infused by a clinician every 6 months. Due to the infusion duration, this may require time off work, which may not be feasible for some patients. Yet for others, this treatment regimen may be preferable compared to having to manage self-administration of medications on a daily or variable weekly basis.

Management of patients' health conditions can be improved by interventions to address non-adherence or by switching to alternative therapies.[98] Using a shared decision-making approach by involving the patient in medication selection is significantly associated with improved adherence rates.[99,100] While not explicitly shown, this strategy was used in the management of Ms. Jones' MS therapeutic plan. As it relates to ocrelizumab, the safety risks, necessary blood tests, vaccines prior to therapy initiation, possible side effects, and unique drug administration make patient-specific medication counseling essential. Illustration 14-9 depicts this counseling by the pharmacist, where we learn of Ms. Jones' concern regarding the affordability of her new medication.

PBMs, like the one where the pharmacist in Illustration 14-7 is employed, play a vital role in medication access and affordability questions. PBMs are often viewed as an intermediary between health insurance plans, which provide prescription drug coverage, and their members who access prescription drugs through that coverage.[101-103] PBMs manage medication access for populations of insured patients, and their role is generally viewed as one aimed at optimizing clinical outcomes while minimizing costs.[102] To meet this objective, PBMs offer many programs and services to assist health plans; examples include managing drug formularies, a list of medications covered, at least in part, by the insurance plan, and negotiating with drug manufacturers and pharmacies to optimize services and value.[102,103] PBMs also work with pharmaceutical companies to establish rebates or discounts to make medications more affordable for populations of patients.[102,103] In addition, some PBMs offer mail-order pharmacy services, provide specialty pharmacy services, and perform drug utilization reviews.[103]

Retail and community pharmacies are highly impacted by the actions of PBMs. The high costs associated with medications has been under considerable scrutiny, and some have called into question the practices of PBMs that may be contributing to this issue.[104,105] PBMs, for example, have the ability to decide how much pharmacies will be reimbursed for their services. Because PBMs are highly integrated in nearly every step of the chain of prescription medication distribution, their practices impact pharmacists, healthcare providers, and patients.

In recent years, several populations of patients have been negatively impacted by what some have described as skyrocketing costs of prescription medications. For example, between 2007 and 2016, the list price of epinephrine auto-injectors (EpiPen), a life-saving medication, increased by 500%. From 2002 to 2013, the cost of insulin increased by more than 300%, and from 2012 to 2019, the cost of adalimumab (Humira), a medication for rheumatoid arthritis, increased by more than 200%.[106] Overall costs are impacted by pharmaceutical manufacturers, who set initial drug prices, and entities within the medication distribution chain. The role of a PBM is to help manage drug costs by negotiating payment rates with drug manufacturers using drug formularies, drug utilization reviews, and rebates. However, the lack of transparency from both drug manufacturers and PBMs has spurred a debate regarding the cause of rising prescription drug costs.[106]

Ms. Jones' concerns about the affordability of the new MS medication she is being recommended, expressed in Illustration 14-9, are justified. Lifetime costs for an individual patient with MS, some of which are borne by patients, but most of which are covered by health insurance plans, can exceed $4 million with a large portion of that directed toward medications.[107,108] DMTs cost, on average, more than $70,000 per year.[107,109–111] Due to the cost and complexity of MS therapies, PBMs and specialty pharmacies are becoming increasingly involved in the treatment of patients with MS.

Pharmacists perform important roles in nearly every function of a PBM. This career path is particularly appealing to those interested in the economic and business aspects of medication use. One of the best-known roles for a pharmacist at a PBM is within mail order processes, many of which are directly managed by PBMs. Many employers require employees to obtain chronic medications through a mail-order service. Mail-order pharmacists typically work in large settings, filling prescriptions, performing drug utilization reviews and calling prescribers to clarify certain medication orders. Another common role for pharmacists in the PBM setting is to provide services and support to patients or providers by phone; this includes medication therapy management, disease management programs, patient consultations, and prior authorization requests to facilitate patients' access to certain medications. PBM pharmacists can also work directly with clients (i.e., health insurance plans) to design prescription benefits that would provide the best value for members of that health insurance plan.

Another responsibility of a PBM pharmacist is formulary management. This includes creating and updating the drug formulary for health insurance plans. A drug formulary is a list of drugs that the insurance company or PBM agrees to cover and how much that entity will pay for them. Establishing and maintaining this list requires a thorough understanding of current and emerging therapies and their corresponding safety and efficacy profiles. In Illustration 14-7, we see a PBM pharmacist proposing adding a new drug for MS, ocrelizumab, to the formulary based on a detailed analysis of efficacy, evaluated by annual relapse rates, and a comparative analysis of the costs of other medications on the market.

Specialty pharmacies primarily focus on high-cost medications for rare or complex health conditions, such as cancer, rheumatoid arthritis, HIV, Crohn's disease, hepatitis C, and MS.[112] The key features that determine whether a medication fits the "specialty" definition include treatment of a complex or rare condition, high cost, limited distribution, special storage or handing requirements, and ongoing safety or efficacy monitoring.[112] Specialty medications may be made from living cells (i.e., biologics), or may need to be injected or infused. Other medications in this category may only be available through a limited distribution network. Patients with health conditions involving specialty medications often need to obtain prior authorization (i.e., approval) from their insurance company or PBM, may require financial assistance due to the high costs, and generally need thorough education to facilitate medication adherence and to appropriately manage/minimize side effects.

Considering these criteria, many MS medications qualify as specialty drugs. Illustrations 14-10, 14-11, and 14-12 highlight three of the many services provided by specialty pharmacists. Illustration 14-10 shows the pharmacist working with the patient to submit required documentation to apply for financial assistance with the drug manufacturer. In Illustration 14-11, the specialty pharmacist is shown preparing ocrelizumab for infusion. Illustration 14-12, which takes place during Ms. Jones' first infusion, provides a great example of interprofessional practice between the specialty pharmacist and nurse, who will work collaboratively to troubleshoot Ms. Jones' emerging adverse drug reaction.

MS is a complex, chronic disease that is often debilitating and greatly impacts quality of life. There are many opportunities for pharmacists to positively impact the care of patients with MS through both traditional and non-traditional roles. In the illustrated case "Relapse," three different types of pharmacists contributed to Ms. Jones' care through drug formulary management, medication selection, patient counseling and education, completing a financial assistance application, preparation of medications, and side effect monitoring and evaluation. Management of complex conditions like MS requires an interprofessional team to optimize therapeutic efficacy and safety and, as demonstrated throughout "Relapse," pharmacists of many stripes play an integral role on that team. This illustrated case also highlights unique contributions pharmacists make to population health initiatives.

DISCUSSION QUESTIONS FOR "RELAPSE"

1. Illustration 14-7 depicts a pharmacist at a Pharmacy Benefit Management (PBM) company leading a discussion and vote to add a medication to treat multiple sclerosis (MS) to the PBM's formulary. How might this decision impact the health of an entire population of patients?

2. Ms. Jones' physician and pharmacist in the neurology clinic are shown discussing alternative medication therapies for Ms. Jones in Illustration 14-8. After reading Thoughts on "Relapse," what additional concerns or ideas might you raise in this discussion if you were the pharmacist?

3. Ms. Jones expresses her concerns about the price of the newly prescribed medication in Illustration 14-9. What factors do you think impact the cost of this medication for Ms. Jones and other patients with MS? Who controls these factors and how might they be modified?

4. What other health professionals, not represented in "Relapse," might have a positive impact on patients with MS? How specifically would these health professionals contribute to the interprofessional care of Ms. Jones? What would the pharmacist need to know, or do, to coordinate her activities with these individuals?

5. The illustrated case "Relapse" highlights the rising cost of medications, particularly those categorized as specialty medications for specific patient populations, and the strain/burden this places on patients. What role do you think pharmacists can play to minimize this impact on patients?

INTERCONNECTED: An Illustrated Case Study

Story by Laurel M. Legenza & Joseph A. Zorek
Illustrations by George Folz, © 2019 Board of Regents of the University of Wisconsin System

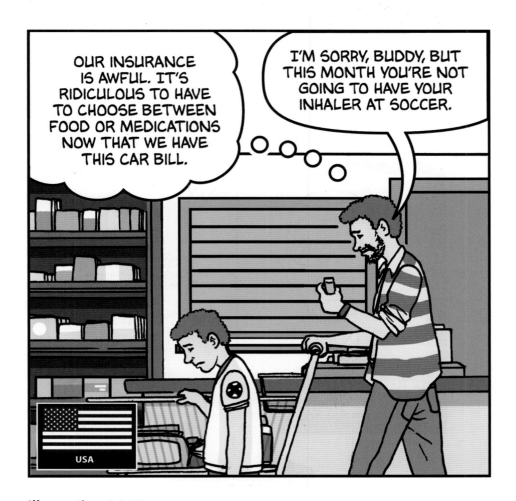

Illustration 14-13

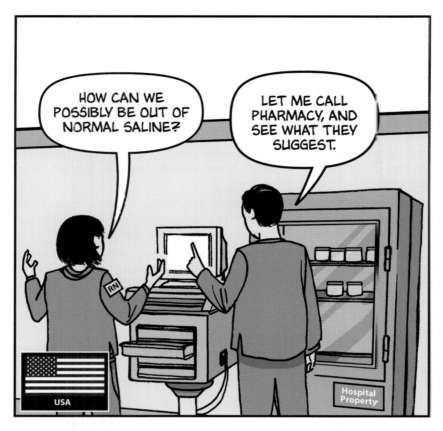

Illustration 14-14

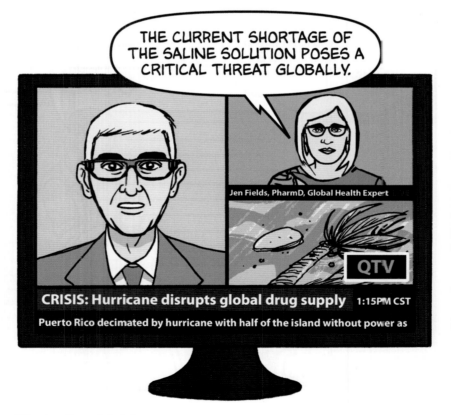

Illustration 14-15

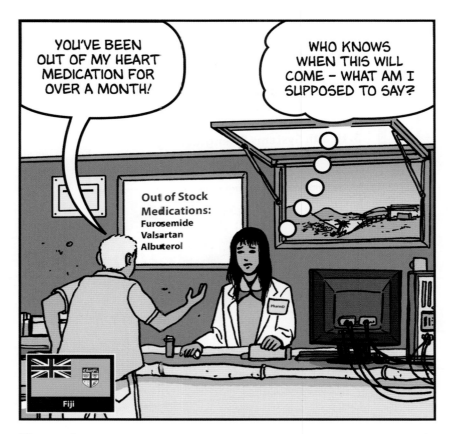

Illustration 14-16

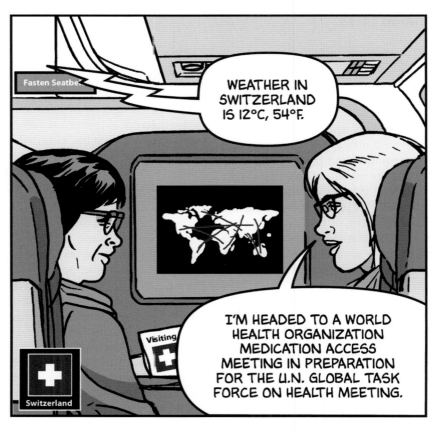

Illustration 14-17

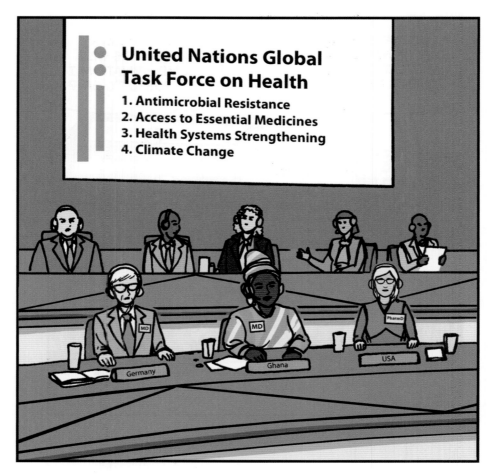

Illustration 14-18

Thoughts on "Interconnected"

The health of individuals, nationally and internationally, is much more interconnected than it may appear when you visit a pharmacy. Pharmacists must understand these interconnections because the medications they manage are part of a complex global system. Drug shortages due to interruptions in the supply of raw materials, manufacturing problems, and company mergers have impacted the availability of medications in the United States.[113] Similarly, extreme weather-related events have disrupted the global supply chain for some of the most essential medications used around the world.[114-116] The illustrated case "Interconnected" highlights the essential role of pharmacists as positive contributors to the global medication use system and, as a result, population health.

Presented earlier in this chapter, the illustrated case "Unsung Hero" explores how social determinants can affect an individual's health, quality of life, and health risks.[117] Lack of access to medications for uninsured or underinsured individuals is one vitally important contributor. Recent studies estimate that nearly a quarter of Americans experience difficulty affording the medications they need, while nearly three-quarters of Americans think prescription drug costs are unreasonable.[118,119] Non-adherence to medications due to cost affects millions of Americans, and unfortunately this problem has increased over the last two decades.[120] Pharmacists, by virtue of their education, training, and position within the healthcare system, are frequently frontline providers helping patients tackle medication access issues.

In the United States, drug coverage is determined by patients' health insurance plans, and individuals with limited or no prescription insurance may have to pay the majority or all of their drug costs out-of-pocket; meaning, the full retail price. Pharmacists help patients understand the complex systems that impact their drug coverage, including topics such as prior authorization and formulary management. See the illustrated case "Relapse" in this chapter for a more in-depth exploration of prescription insurance coverage. Importantly, pharmacists connect patients to available resources when prescribed medications are unaffordable, or to other members of the interprofessional team, like social workers, who can provide more specialized assistance.[121] See the illustrated case "Holistic" in Chapter 3 Primary Care for more information on interprofessional practice with social workers.

The illustrated case "Interconnected" opens with a medication access issue experienced by an uninsured family in the United States (Illustration 14-13), which has put a father in the unenviable position of having to choose between food and his son's asthma medication due to an unexpected bill. Appropriate treatment of asthma often requires two different types of inhalers; one as "controller," used daily to prevent asthma attacks, and another as a "reliever" or "rescue," either used prior to exposure to a known asthma trigger, or when an asthma attack is actively happening.[122] Readers are encouraged to explore the illustrated case "Swish" in Chapter 3 Primary Care for a more detailed discussion of asthma, including different types and treatment modalities. While not explicitly stated, the backstory of this family is one of constant compromises, where financial difficulties are directly, and negatively, impacting their health. This can be inferred by the fact that the son, who needs both controller and reliever inhalers, sporadically gets access to just one.

Worldwide, the prevalence of asthma is 4.3% in adults, while in the United States it is 7.7%.[123,124] Although diagnosed asthma rates are higher in high-rescurce countries, most asthma-related deaths occur in low-income countries.[125] With so many individuals affected, the ability to access a reliever inhaler, such as albuterol, is critical. As the American family shown in Illustration 14-13 is struggling with access to albuterol due to financial hardship, asthma patients thousands of miles away in the South Pacific island country of Fiji are experiencing access issues due to an entirely different reason; namely, a drug shortage (Illustration 14-16). These two illustrations highlight the expansive nature and global impact of medication access issues, regardless of whether patients live in high- or low-resource settings. The drug shortage in Fiji also serves to introduce the complex and interconnected systems that make up the global drug supply. Drug shortages result in increased costs, medication errors, and adverse clinical outcomes (including death), as well as other negative consequences such as delays in medication treatment and needed surgeries.[126,127] A detailed understanding of this system enables pharmacists to provide the best possible care to the patients and populations they serve.

Unfortunately, disruptions in the global drug supply chain have become routine, and they frequently appear in the media.[114,128,129] For example, epinephrine, which is used to reverse anaphylaxis during severe drug allergies, is a life-saving medication that has been on shortage due to manufacturing issues.[130] It is a key component of emergency medical kits required on airplanes. Airlines in recent years have been granted exemptions from this requirement to allow them to fly with incomplete kits, which is a terrifying prospect for some.[131] The causes of these disruptions are multifaceted, including natural disasters. The shortage of normal saline depicted in Illustrations 14-14 and 14-15 was inspired by a real drug shortage caused by Hurricane Maria in 2017, which destroyed a key manufacturing plant in Puerto Rico.[3] This particular plant produced many small intravenous solution products used in the United States, including normal saline.

Normal saline is a sterile solution of sodium chloride in water at a concentration of 0.9%, which makes it compatible with blood. It is used to restore fluid balance for a vast range of patient conditions from mild dehydration to trauma situations involving massive blood loss. It is also used as a diluent to administer intravenous medications; for example, antibiotics and chemotherapy medications may be diluted in normal saline so they can be administered into a patient's vein. This book is replete with illustrations of patients receiving intravenous medicines and/or fluid support using normal saline. Its use in hospitalized patients is ubiquitous, and pharmacists manage normal saline like any other drug product through the stages of acquisition, storage, and distribution.[132] Saline shortages are not uncommon and, unfortunately, such shortages impact our healthcare system on a regular basis.[133]

A normal saline shortage inspired by Hurricane Maria, as depicted in Illustration 14-15, created the confusion shown in Illustration 14-14. Here, two nurses in the medication room of a hospital ward in the United States are attempting to obtain normal saline for their patients. Puzzled and frustrated, they decide to contact the hospital pharmacy for guidance, highlighting how important it is for pharmacists to understand the complexities of the drug supply chain. Pharmacists tap into several resources to assist them, including up-to-date lists of products on shortage. Some of these lists, incredibly, can grow to be larger than 400 products long.[134]

There are many linkages in the global drug supply chain that make it susceptible to disruption. For example, a medication tablet can contain active and inactive ingredients that are manufactured in multiple countries, and some ingredients are produced by a single manufacturer or supplier.[135,136] Meanwhile, per US Food and Drug Administration (FDA) requirements, the country of origin label, which all drugs must include, is the location where the final manufacturing step takes place. As a result, the origin of the active ingredient is considered proprietary and rarely disclosed.[136,137] If production by the sole manufacturer of any of the needed ingredients ends, the entire global system is affected.[127] There are many reasons production such as this may end, or be stalled. Extreme weather events are highlighted in the illustrated case; however, according to the FDA, quality and manufacturing problems are the main cause of shortages (37% of shortages).[138] The FDA works with manufacturers to address these issues, and production may be halted while issues are resolved.[137,139,140] Production of newer, more profitable drugs can also lead to shortages of older drugs, which may be discontinued (2% of shortages).[137-139]

When a manufacturer files a patent for a novel medication, they are granted protection in the United States for 20 years that ensures it can be sold without competition.[141] As soon as this patent protection expires, additional manufacturers are allowed to produce and sell generic versions of that medication. Competition in this new marketplace can result in low profitability, so there may be little incentive for companies to continue producing and selling generic medications when market conditions become unfavorable.[137] Furosemide is an example of a generically available medication that has been on shortage lists recently, including our fictional drug shortage list in Fiji

(Illustration 14-16). The importance of furosemide to patients around the world with cardiovascular issues such as hypertension or heart failure cannot be overstated. For more information on these disease states, see the illustrated cases "Underlying Cause" and "Educator," respectively, in Chapter 5 Cardiology.

Manufacturing plants can also be closed for regulatory issues, such as poor conditions resulting from noncompliance with accepted manufacturing standards, known as Current Good Manufacturing Practice (CGMP) regulations. Drug-quality-related regulations, in fact, are included in parts of the US Code of Federal Regulations and apply to drugs made in the United States, as well as imported drugs.[142,143] This is important because 80% of active ingredients in both brand and generic drugs are currently made in China or India, due to lower production costs and environmental standards.[144] Poor manufacturing can have serious consequences due to the introduction of impurities, which can change important properties of the drug. For example, a drug might degrade too quickly in the heat and not deliver its intended purpose when taken, or it might be released too quickly in the body and result in adverse effects. Impurities themselves can be dangerous, even carcinogenic (i.e., cancer-causing).[135] In 2018, a probable carcinogenic chemical called n-Nitrosodimethylamine, or NDMA, was found in valsartan, a common blood pressure medication, and resulted in a massive global recall that included 24 European countries and the United States.[145] The recall was expanded over 50 times since it was initially announced to include additional products and similar medications, highlighting the scope of this issue.[146,147]

The book *Bottle of Lies* has drawn attention to poor drug manufacturing practices in India and repeated noncompliance with CGMP regulations.[22] The FDA inspects drug manufacturing production in the United States and globally. Language barriers and outdated training have been shown to complicate international efforts and reduce the quality of inspections.[135,144] Despite this, deceptive and illegal activities tied to generic drug manufacturing have been identified; for example, laboratory results have been hidden or masked, and data reported to the FDA has been falsified.[135] Legal action is taken when inspections turn up such behavior.[135,148] This is reassuring, yet the existence of such problems in the first place highlight the inherent challenges and risks associated with such a complex and interconnected global system.

Pharmacists serve as trusted experts within health systems domestically and internationally. Pharmacy departments play a vital role managing drug shortages, and the level of strategic planning required rivals that of emergency preparedness for natural disasters and infectious disease outbreaks.[127,133] Management strategies during drug shortages also parallel emergency management approaches. For example, early notification of stakeholders can help limit the impact of drug shortages.[133] During a shortage, pharmacists educate affected health professionals and administrators about relevant issues, including action plans in place, therapeutic alternatives available, and temporary guidelines that limit use to only specific evidence-based indications. Managing shortages and making alternative recommendations are complex and time-intensive activities. The nurses in Illustration 14-14 call the pharmacy for such recommendations, highlighting the critical role of pharmacists. Alternative options may include leveraging the knowledge and skills pharmacists have regarding drug compounding; however, this can be time- and cost-intensive.[149] For a more in-depth exploration of compounding, including legal and regulatory issues, see the illustrated case "Transformation" in Chapter 2 Community Pharmacy. Those interested in administrative leadership to solve complex medication access issues are encouraged to read the illustrated case "Opportunities" in Chapter 15 Administration, while those interested in pharmacists' contributions to an emergency response are encouraged to read the illustrated case "Mobilized" in Chapter 4 Prevention & Wellness.

National news media sources interview pharmacists for their expert insights on drug shortages and solutions to associated crises.[114,150–152] Dr. Jen Fields, the protagonist introduced in Illustration 14-15, provides an example of this. She first appears on a nationally syndicated television show as a global health expert to comment on drug shortages. Illustrations 14-17 and 14-18 reveal that recognition of Jen's expertise is such that she has been selected to represent the United States at a WHO meeting and also on a United Nations Task Force addressing, among other related topics, access to essential medicines.

Global organizations like the WHO, an agency of the United Nations, and the International Pharmaceutical Federation (FIP) create policies and recommendations for access to medications. FIP represents more than four million pharmacists, pharmaceutical scientists, and pharmacy educators globally and provides recommendations to guide and inform the WHO. For example, leaders within FIP co-authored a WHO bulletin dedicated to medication shortages.[153] Additionally, FIP produces global statements to inform policy development within individual countries, such as therapeutic interchange and the role of pharmacists in treating non-communicable diseases.[154,155] FIP members also actively contribute to global research, such as evaluating the cost of providing essential medicines.[156] Every 2 years, FIP members contribute to the WHO publication "Model Lists of Essential Medicines."[157–159] These documents provide guidance to more than 150 countries on which medicines and products to prioritize for wide availability and affordability throughout health systems. The WHO and FIP also jointly produce global practice guidelines for pharmacy, and the illustrated case "Interconnected" shines a spotlight on the indispensable contributions of pharmacists to this effort.[160]

Domestically, pharmacists use their expertise and knowledge of global health and medication use to shape legislative, regulatory, and marketing policies.[161] The American Society of Health-System Pharmacists (ASHP) and organizations such as the American Hospital Association, the FDA, the Institute for Safe Medication Practices and others in the United States, for example, work collectively to provide consensus recommendations for mitigating risk associated with drug shortages.[140,161]

Interestingly, drug information pharmacists lead the team behind ASHP's current drug shortages list, which is a key resource pharmacists use to support the work of other health professionals, like the nurses depicted in Illustration 14-14, through interprofessional practice.[162] Those interested in learning more about drug information pharmacy are encouraged to read the illustrated case "Support" in Chapter 3 Primary Care.

The illustrated case "Interconnected" highlights the complex global system that generates, at times, incredible challenges to ensuring the safe and effective use of medications. Pharmacists, by virtue of their training, expertise, and position within the healthcare system, are frequently called upon to solve problems originating from this complexity. Dr. Jen Fields, the protagonist in "Interconnected," encapsulates the inspirational work done by many pharmacists who have established themselves as global health experts. These pharmacists help shape domestic and international policies and contribute to the development of resources that strengthen the health and well-being of our entire population. Such efforts support the work of frontline health professionals, including pharmacists, who benefit from, and leverage, the recommendations and resources created through engagement with international organizations such as the World Health Organization and United Nations to improve health outcomes for populations. Given the complexity and challenges associated with our globally interconnected drug supply, it is reassuring to know that pharmacists have stepped into important roles as global health experts.

DISCUSSION QUESTIONS FOR "INTERCONNECTED"

1. The father depicted in Illustration 14-13 is unable to afford his son's asthma inhaler. Have you or someone you know ever had trouble affording medications? What steps could, or should, pharmacists take to help families in this situation?

2. Illustrations 14-13 and 14-16 highlight the global nature of medication access and supply issues. If the child in America has an asthma attack and is hospitalized, who should be held responsible for that? What about the man in the pharmacy in Fiji? Who should be held accountable if he were to have a heart attack and pass away because his heart medication was out of stock?

3. Some politicians have argued that all Americans, regardless of income level, should have access to healthcare and needed medications. Other politicians have argued that the costs associated with providing such access make this idea impractical, and even irresponsible. Which side of this argument do you fall on, and why?

4. Illustration 14-15 draws attention to the fragile nature of the global drug supply through a fictitious extreme weather event inspired by Hurricane Maria. What are your thoughts about relying on a single manufacturer for critical medications? What steps might be taken to guard against such risks?

5. The importance of pharmacists engaging in prominent organizations with a stake in globally relevant medication issues, such as the World Health Organization and the United Nations, was highlighted in the illustrated case "Interconnected." Did the portrayal of pharmacists engaging in global health issues surprise you, and why?

CHAPTER SUMMARY

- Population health encompasses all social determinants of health and aims to improve the well-being of people by reducing health inequality and inequity through policy and health systems strengthening.

- Social determinants of health provide a lens through which to view the whole health of an individual, including the impact of factors such as nutrition, housing, education, neighborhoods, and health system processes and structures, as equally important to health outcomes.

- Pharmacists can incorporate social determinants of health questions into individual patient care plans to optimize well-being.

- Pharmacists contribute meaningfully to population health in a multitude of ways, such as medication management of chronic conditions like diabetes, reviewing safety and efficacy of new drug therapies on the market, and managing critical drug shortages.

- Private and public healthcare entities, including accountable care organizations, have responded to value-based reimbursement models for delivery of health services, which represents a population health approach to the payment for health services rendered.

- Pharmacists work to shape domestic and international policy through organizations like the American Society of Health-System Pharmacists, the International Pharmaceutical Federation, and the World Health Organization.

- Opportunities for pharmacists to engage in population health management services are expected to increase well into the future.

REFERENCES

1. Kindig D, Stoddart G. What is population health? *Am J Public Health*. 2003;93(3):380-383.
2. Institute of Medicine (U.S.). Committee on quality measures for the healthy people leading health indicators, institute of

medicine (U.S.). Board on population health and public health practice. Toward quality measures for population health and the leading health indicators. In: Washington, District of Columbia: The National Academies Press,; 2013. Available at http://www. nap.edu/catalog.php?record_id=18339. Accessed May 31, 2020.

3. Obama M. *Becoming*. 1st ed. New York: Crown, an imprint of the Crown Publishing Group; 2018.

4. Wenig S. Obesity rate for young children plummets 43% in a decade. Available at https://www.nytimes.com/2014/02/26/health/obesity-rate-for-young-children-plummets-43-in-a-decade.html?_r=2. Accessed March 25, 2020.

5. Kaiser Permanente. Health care model. Available at https://thrive.kaiserpermanente.org/care-near-you/northern-california/santarosa/about-us/health-care-model/. Accessed March 25, 2020.

6. Managed Care. MedlinePlus. Available at https://medlineplus.gov/managedcare.html. Accessed March 29, 2020.

7. Kaiser Permanente. Improving health through stable housing. Available at https://about.kaiserpermanente.org/community-health/news/improving-health-through-stable-housing. Accessed March 25, 2020.

8. Tikkanen R, Abrams MK. U.S. health care from a global perspective, 2019: higher spending, Worse Outcomes? Available at https://www.commonwealthfund.org/publications/issue-briefs/2020/jan/us-health-care-global-perspective-2019. Accessed March 26, 2020.

9. Bodenheimer T, Sinsky C. From triple to quadruple aim: care of the patient requires care of the provider. *Ann Fam Med*. 2014;12(6):573-576.

10. Wegner SE. Measuring value in health care: the times, they are a changin'. *N C Med J*. 2016;77(4):276-278.

11. Kuhn C, Groves BK, Kaczor C, et al. Pharmacist involvement in population health management for a pediatric managed medicaid accountable care organization. *Children*. 2019;6(7):82.

12. Public Law 111-148 to be codified as amended in various sections of Title 42 of the U.S.C. and the Internal Revenue Code, 26 U.S.C. Available at https://www.congress.gov/111/plaws/publ148/PLAW-111publ148.pdf. Accessed May 31, 2020.

13. Miller J. The state of ACOs. Medical economics. Available at https://www.medicaleconomics.com/article/state-acos. Accessed March 26, 2020.

14. Muhlestein D, Robert S. Saunders RS, Richards R, McClellan MB. Recent progress in the value journey: growth of ACOs and value-based payment models in 2018. Available at https://www.healthaffairs.org/do/10.1377/hblog20180810.481968/full/. Accessed March 26, 2020.

15. Committee on Geographic Variation in Health Care Spending and Promotion of High-Value Care; Board on Health Care Services; Institute of Medicine; Newhouse JP, Garber AM, Graham RP, et al., editors. Variation in health care spending: target decision making, not geography. Washington (DC): National Academies Press (US); 2013 Oct 1. 4, Payment and organizational reforms to improve value. Available at https://www.ncbi.nlm.nih.gov/books/NBK201643/. Accessed May 31, 2020.

16. Centers for Medicare and Medicaid Services. Next generation ACO model. Available at https://innovation.cms.gov/innovation-models/next-generation-aco-model. Accessed March 29, 2020.

17. Centers for Medicare and Medicaid Services. Accountable care organizations (ACOs): General information. Available at https://innovation.cms.gov/innovation-models/aco. Accessed March 29, 2020.

18. Arnold J. Are pharmacy benefit managers the good guys or band guys of drug pricing? Available at https://www.statnews.com/2018/08/27/pharmacy-benefit-managers-good-or-bad/. Accessed March 11, 2020.

19. Koplan JP, Bond TC, Merson MH, et al. Towards a common definition of global health. *Lancet*. 2009;373(9679):1993-1995.

20. Frenk J, Gomez-Dantes O, Moon S. From sovereignty to solidarity: a renewed concept of global health for an era of complex interdependence. *Lancet*. 2014;383(9911):94-97.

21. Coronavirus disease 2019 (COVID-19) Situation Report – 69. WHO. Available at https://www.who.int/docs/default-source/coronaviruse/situation-reports/20200329-sitrep-69-covid-19.pdf?sfvrsn=8d6620fa_2. Accessed March 29, 2020.

22. United Nations. United Nation's sustainable development goals. Available at https://www.un.org/sustainabledevelopment/sustainable-development-goals/. Accessed May 31, 2020.

23. American Public Health Association. Public health vs. clinical health professions: what's the difference? Available at https://www.apha.org/professional-development/public-health-careermart/careers-in-public-health-newsletter/job-searching-salaries-and-more/public-health-vs-clinical-health-professions-whats-the-difference. Accessed March 24, 2020.

24. Gebbie KM, Potter MA, Quill B, Tilson H. Education for the public health profession: a new look at the Roemer proposal. *Public Health Rep*. 2008;123(Suppl 2):18-26.

25. Colgrove J, Fried LP, Northridge ME, Rosner D. Schools of public health: essential infrastructure of a responsible society and a 21st-century health system. *Public Health Rep*. 2010;125(1):8-14.

26. Rietveld LC, Siri JG, Chakravarty I, Arsenio AM, Biswas R, Chatterjee A. Improving health in cities through systems approaches for urban water management. *Environ Health*. 2016;15(Suppl 1):31.

27. Rose DA, Murthy S, Brooks J, Bryant J. The evolution of public health emergency management as a field of practice. *Am J Public Health*. 2017;107:S126-S133.

28. U.S. Department of Health and Human Services. Office of the Surgeon General. Available at https://www.hhs.gov/surgeongeneral/index.html. Accessed March 24, 2020.

29. U.S. Public Health Service Commissioned Corps. Careers and benefits. Available at www.usphs.gov/profession/. Accessed March 23, 2020.

30. Jones EB, Ku L. Sharing a playbook: integrated care in community health centers in the United States. *Am J Public Health*. 2015;105(10):2028-2034.

31. Davis MM, Balasubramanian BA, Cifuentes M, et al. Clinician staffing, scheduling, and engagement strategies among primary care practices delivering integrated care. *J Am Board Fam Med*. 2015;28(Suppl 1):S32-S40.

32. Academy of Managed Care Pharmacy. Formulary Management. Available at https://www.amcp.org/about/managed-care-pharmacy-101/concepts-managed-care-pharmacy/formulary-management. Accessed March 29, 2020.

33. Cannon EC, Zadvorny EB, Sutton SD, et al. Value of pharmacy students performing population management activity

interventions as an advanced pharmacy practice experience. *Am J Pharm Educ.* 2019;83(5):6759.

34. Smythe MA. Advances in anticoagulation management: the role of pharmacy. *Ann Pharmacother.* 2007;41(3):493-495.

35. Miller RR. History of clinical pharmacy and clinical pharmacology. *J Clin Pharmacol.* 1981;21(4):195-197.

36. Bond CA, Raehl CL. Pharmacist-provided anticoagulation management in United States hospitals: death rates, length of stay, Medicare charges, bleeding complications, and transfusions. *Pharmacotherapy.* 2004;24(8):953-963.

37. Wang SV, Rogers JR, Jin Y, et al. Stepped-wedge randomised trial to evaluate population health intervention designed to increase appropriate anticoagulation in patients with atrial fibrillation. *BMJ Qual Saf.* 2019;28(10):835-842.

38. Ashjian E, Kurtz B, Renner E, Yeshe R, Barnes GD. Evaluation of a pharmacist-led outpatient direct oral anticoagulant service. *Am J Health Syst Pharm.* 2017;74(7):483-489.

39. Jones AE, King JB, Kim K, Witt DM. The role of clinical pharmacy anticoagulation services in direct oral anticoagulant monitoring. *J Thromb Thrombolysis.* 2020. Online ahead of print.

40. American Society of Health-System Pharmacists. ASHP statement on the role of health-system pharmacists in public health. *Am J Health Syst Pharm.* 2008;65(5):462-467.

41. Jones LK, Greskovic G, Grassi DM, et al. Medication therapy disease management: Geisinger's approach to population health management. *Am J Health Syst Pharm.* 2017;74(18):1422-1435.

42. Greer N, Bolduc J, Geurkink E, et al. Pharmacist-led chronic disease management: a systematic review of effectiveness and harms compared with usual care. *Ann Intern Med.* 2016;165(1):30-40.

43. Newman TV, San-Juan-Rodriguez A, Parekh N, et al. Impact of community pharmacist-led interventions in chronic disease management on clinical, utilization, and economic outcomes: An umbrella review. *Res Social Adm Pharm.* 2020. Online ahead of print.

44. Farmer EK, Koren DE, Cha A, Grossman K, Cates DW. The pharmacist's expanding role in HIV pre-exposure prophylaxis. *AIDS Patient Care STDS.* 2019;33(5):207-213.

45. Weinstein JN, Amaro HD, Baca E, et al. The state of health disparities in the United States. In: Weinstein JN, Geller A, Negussie Y, Baciu A, eds. *Communities in Action: Pathways to Health Equity.* Washington: Natl Academies Press; 2017 57-97.

46. Berg S. How embedded pharmacists improve care for Native American patients. Available at https://www.ama-assn.org/practice-management/payment-delivery-models/how-embedded-pharmacists-improve-care-native-american. Accessed March 27, 2020.

47. Svingen CG. Clinical pharmacist credentialing and privileging: a process for ensuring high-quality patient care. *Federal Practitioner for the Health Care Professionals of the VA, DoD, and PHS.* 2019;36(4):155-157.

48. Brind Amour K. Pharmacists: The "Next Big Thing" in population health management. Available at https://pediatricsnationwide.org/2019/09/25/pharmacists-the-next-big-thing-in-population-health-management/. Accessed March 27, 2020.

49. Nationwide Children's. Partners for kids: pediatric accountable care. Available at https://www.nationwidechildrens.org/impact-quality/partners-for-kids-pediatric-accountable-care. Accessed May 31, 2020.

50. Centers for Medicare and Medicaid Services. Medicaid. Available at https://www.medicaid.gov/medicaid/index.html. Accessed March 29, 2020.

51. Weier RC, Gardner W, Conkol K, Pajer K, Kelleher KJ. Partners for kids care coordination: lessons from the field. *Pediatrics.* 2017;139(Suppl 2):S109-S116.

52. Small L. Pediatric managed medicaid ACO leverages pharmacists to improve care. Available at https://aishealth.com/drug-benefits/pediatric-managed-medicaid-aco-leverages-pharmacists-to-improve-care/. Accessed March 27, 2020.

53. Small L. Pediatric Managed Medicaid ACO Touts crucial role of its pharmacists. Available at https://www.mmitnetwork.com/member-content/pediatric-managed-medicaid-aco-touts-crucial-role-of-its-pharmacists/. Accessed March 27, 2020.

54. American Society of Health-System Pharmacists. Residency Directory. Available at https://accreditation.ashp.org/directory/#/program/residency. Accessed March 30, 2020.

55. World Health Organization. Health in all policies. Available at https://apps.who.int/iris/bitstream/handle/10665/112636/9789241506908_eng.pdf. Accessed May 31, 2020.

56. HealthyPeople.gov. Healthy people 2020. Available at https://www.healthypeople.gov/2020/topics-objectives/topic/social-determinants-of-health. Accessed March 25, 2020.

57. Wahowiak L. Healthy, safe housing linked to healthier, longer lives: Housing a social determinant of health. The Nation's Health. A Publication of the American Public Health Association. Available at http://thenationshealth.aphapublications.org/content/46/7/1.3. Accessed May 31, 2020.

58. Robert Wood Johnson Foundation. Comments from Donald Schwarz, MD, on a new federal strategy to reduce childhood lead exposure and impacts. Available at https://www.rwjf.org/en/library/articles-and-news/2017/11/comments-from-donald-schwarz-on-federal-strategy-to-reduce-childhood-lead-exposure.html. Accessed May 31, 2020.

59. World Health Organization. Lead poisoning and health. Available at https://www.who.int/news-room/fact-sheets/detail/lead-poisoning-and-health. Accessed May 31, 2020.

60. Stephen J, Hawley L, Kramer R, et al. The health equity resource toolkit for state practitioners. Available at https://www.cdc.gov/nccdphp/dnpao/state-local-programs/health-equity/index.html. Accessed May 31, 2020.

61. Ramon I, Chattopadhyay SK, Barnett WS, Hahn RA, Community Preventive Services Task Force. Early childhood education to promote health equity: a community guide economic review. *J Public Health Manag Pract.* 2018;24(1):E8-E15.

62. Rakel D, Sakallaris B, Jonas W. Creating optimal healing environments. In: Rxxakel D, ed. *Integrative Medicine.* 4th ed. Philadelphia, PA: Elsevier, Inc.; 2018:12-19.

63. Schroeder SA. Shattuck lecture—We can do better—improving the health of the American people. *N Engl J Med.* 2007;357(12):1221-1228.

64. Woolf SH, Glasgow RE, Krist A, et al. Putting it together: finding success in behavior change through integration of services. *Ann Fam Med.* 2005;3(Suppl 2):S20-S27.

65. National Academies of Sciences, Engineering, and Medicine. Integrating social care into the delivery of health care: moving upstream to improve the nation's health. Washington, DC: The National Academies Press; 2019.

66. Coleman-Jensen A, Matthew R, Christian G, et al. Household food security in the United States in 2017. U.S. Department of Agriculture, Economic Research Service. Available at https://www.ers.usda.gov/webdocs/publications/90023/err-256.pdf?v=0. Accessed May 31, 2020.

67. Schrank A. Available at https://www.tpr.org/post/health-report-shows-life-expectancy-disparities-across-san-antonio-neighborhoods. Accessed May 31, 2020.

68. Kung HC, Hoyert DL, Xu J, et al. Deaths: final data for 2005. Hyattsville, MD: Centers for Disease Control and Prevention, National Center for Health Statistics, 2008.

69. Robert Wood Johnson Foundation. Issue Brief #6: Exploring the social determinates of health. Race, socioeconomic factors and health. April 2011.

70. Braveman P, Egerter S. Overcoming obstacles to health: report from the Robert Wood Johnson Foundation to the Commission to Build a Healthier America. Robert Wood Johnson Foundation; University of California, San Francisco, Center on Social Disparities in Health, 2008.

71. Meyerson BE, Ryder PT, Richey-Smith C. Achieving pharmacy-based public health: a call for public health engagement. *Public Health Rep*. 2013;128(3):140-143.

72. Kelly C. Paving the way: pharmacists as health care providers. Available at https://www.pharmacytimes.com/publications/directions-in-pharmacy/2014/december2014/paving-the-way-pharmacists-as-health-care-providers. Accessed May 31, 2020.

73. Hamilton M. Why walk-in health care is a fast-growing profit center for retail chains. Available at https://www.washingtonpost.com/business/why-walk-in-health-care-is-a-fast-growing-profit-center-for-retail-chains/2014/04/04/a05f7cf4-b9c2-11e3-96ae-f2c36d2b1245_story.html. Accessed May 31, 2020.

74. Mehrotra A, Liu H, Adams JL, et al. Comparing costs and quality of care at retail clinics with that of other medical settings for 3 common illnesses. *Ann Intern Med*. 2009;151(5):U321-U350.

75. Benjamin GC. Ensuring population health: an important role for pharmacy. *Am J Pharm Educ*. 2016;80(2):19.

76. Balick R. Pharmacists step up to help in Flint, MI. Available at https://www.pharmacytoday.org/article/S1042-0991(17)30241-4/fulltext. Accessed May 31, 2020.

77. Crossley K. Public Perceives Pharmacists as some of the most trusted professionals. Available at https://www.pharmacytimes.com/publications/career/2019/careerswinter19/public-perceives-pharmacists-as-some-of-the-most-trusted-professionals. Accessed May 31, 2020.

78. Ross M. Pharmacies rally for Flint's water crisis. Available at https://www.pharmacytimes.com/week-in-review/pharmacy-week-in-review-march-11-2016. Accessed May 31, 2020.

79. Levy S. CVS Health, Unite Us launch platform to address social determinants of health. Available at https://www.pharmacist.com/article/cvs-health-unite-us-launch-platform-address-social-determinants-health. Accessed May 31, 2020.

80. Pharmacy Quality Alliance. https://www.pqaalliance.org/pqa-caring-for-the-whole-patient. Accessed May 31, 2020.

81. Pharmacy Society of Wisconsin. Available at http://www.pswi.org. Accessed May 31, 2020.

82. Lassmann H. Multiple sclerosis pathology. *Brain Pathol*. 2018;28(5):721-722.

83. Calabresi PA. Diagnosis and management of multiple sclerosis. *Am Fam Physician*. 2004;70(10):1935-1944.

84. National Multiple Sclerosis Society. Private disability claims: a guide for people with MS. Available at https://www.nationalmssociety.org/NationalMSSociety/media/MSNationalFiles/Brochures/Guidebook-Private-Disability-Insurance-Claims-A-Guide-for-People-with-MS.pdf20. Accessed March 22, 2020.

85. Browne P, Chandraratna D, Angood C, et al. Atlas of multiple sclerosis 2013: a growing global problem with widespread inequity. *Neurology*. 2014;83(11):1022-1024.

86. Berman AD, Jason. Technology feels like it's accelerating—because it actually is. Available at https://singularityhub.com/2016/03/22/technology-feels-like-its-accelerating-because-it-actually-is/. Accessed February 26, 2020.

87. Evans C, Beland SG, Kulaga S, et al. Incidence and prevalence of multiple sclerosis in the Americas: a systematic review. *Neuroepidemiology*. 2013;40(3):195-210.

88. Simpson S Jr, Wang W, Otahal P, Blizzard L, van der Mei IAF, Taylor BV. Latitude continues to be significantly associated with the prevalence of multiple sclerosis: an updated meta-analysis. *J Neurol Neurosurg Psychiatry*. 2019;90(11):1193-1200.

89. Simpson S Jr, Blizzard L, Otahal P, Van der Mei I, Taylor B. Latitude is significantly associated with the prevalence the multiple sclerosis: a meta-analysis. *J Neurol Neurosurg Psychiatry*. 2011;82(10):1132-1141.

90. Langer-Gould A, Wu J, Lucas R, et al. Epstein-Barr virus, cytomegalovirus, and multiple sclerosis susceptibility: A multiethnic study. *Neurology*. 2017;89(13):1330-1337.

91. Lublin FD. The diagnosis of multiple sclerosis. *Curr Opin Neurol*. 2002;15(3):253-256.

92. Belbasis L, Bellou V, Evangelou E, Ioannidis JP, Tzoulaki I. Environmental risk factors and multiple sclerosis: an umbrella review of systematic reviews and meta-analyses. *Lancet Neurol*. 2015;14(3):263-273.

93. Katz Sand I. Classification, diagnosis, and differential diagnosis of multiple sclerosis. *Curr Opin Neurol*. 2015;28(3):193-205.

94. McKay KA, Kwan V, Duggan T, Tremlett H. Risk factors associated with the onset of relapsing-remitting and primary progressive multiple sclerosis: a systematic review. *Biomed Res Int*. 2015;2015:817238.

95. California Society of Health-System Pharmacists. Pharmacogenomics Certificate Program. Available at https://www.cshp.org/page/CP_PGX. Accessed February 26, 2020.

96. Buzaid A, Dodge MP, Handmacher L, Kiltz PJ. Activities of daily living: evaluation and treatment in persons with multiple sclerosis. *Phys Med Rehabil Clin N Am*. 2013;24(4):629-638.

97. Ben-Zacharia AB. Therapeutics for multiple sclerosis symptoms. *Mt Sinai J Med*. 2011;78(2):176-191.

98. Costello K, Kennedy P, Scanzillo J. Recognizing nonadherence in patients with multiple sclerosis and maintaining treatment adherence in the long term. *Medscape J Med*. 2008;10(9):225.

99. Ben-Zacharia A, Adamson M, Boyd A, et al. Impact of shared decision making on disease-modifying drug adherence in multiple sclerosis. *Int J MS Care*. 2018;20(6):287-297.

100. Koudriavtseva T, Onesti E, Pestalozza IF, Sperduti I, Jandolo B. The importance of physician-patient relationship for improvement of adherence to long-term therapy: data of survey in a cohort of multiple sclerosis patients with mild and moderate disability. *Neurol Sci*. 2012;33(3):575-584.

101. Becker C. Prescribing a pharmacy benefits manager. The shadowlands of PBMs. Seek out the experts to navigate the

gray territory of drug-benefits managing. *Mod Healthc.* 2004;34(45):S4.

102. Arnold J. Are pharmacy benefit managers the good guys or band guys of drug pricing? Available at https://www.statnews.com/2018/08/27/pharmacy-benefit-managers-good-or-bad/. Accessed March 11, 2020.

103. Hoffman-Eubanks B. The role of pharmacy benefit managers in American Health Care: pharmacy concerns and perspectives: Part 1. Available at https://www.pharmacytimes.com/news/the-role-of-pharmacy-benefit-mangers-in-american-health-care-pharmacy-concerns-and-perspectives-part-1. Accessed March 11, 2020.

104. Nabhan C, Phillips EG Jr, Feinberg BA. How pharmacy benefit managers add to financial toxicity: The Copay Accumulator Program. *JAMA Oncol.* 2018;4(12):1665-1666.

105. Drettwan JJ, Kjos AL. An ethical analysis of pharmacy benefit manager (PBM) practices. *Pharmacy.* 2019;7(2):65.

106. Entis L. Why does medicine cost so much? Here's how drug prices are set. Available at https://time.com/5564547/drug-prices-medicine/. Accessed March 23, 2020.

107. Owens GM. Economic burden of multiple sclerosis and the role of managed care organizations in multiple sclerosis management. *Am J Manag Care.* 2016;22(6 Suppl):s151-158.

108. O'Brien JA, Ward AJ, Patrick AR, Caro J. Cost of managing an episode of relapse in multiple sclerosis in the United States. *BMC Health Serv Res.* 2003;3(1):17.

109. Ernstsson O, Gyllensten H, Alexanderson K, Tinghog F, Friberg E, Norlund A. Cost of illness of multiple sclerosis—a systematic Review. *PLoS One.* 2016;11(7):e0159129.

110. Hartung DM. Economics and cost-effectiveness of multiple sclerosis therapies in the USA. *Neurotherapeutics.* 2017;14(4):1018-1026.

111. Hartung DM, Bourdette DN, Ahmed SM, Whitham RH. The cost of multiple sclerosis drugs in the US and the pharmaceutical industry: too big to fail? *Neurology.* 2015;84(21):2185-2192.

112. Hagerman JF, Stephanie; Rice, Gary. Specialty pharmacy: a unique and growing industry. Available at https://www.pharmacist.com/specialty-pharmacy-unique-and-growing-industry. Accessed March 20, 2020.

113. Ventola CL. The drug shortage crisis in the United States: causes, impact, and management strategies. *PT.* 2011;36(11):740.

114. McGinley L. Hospitals scramble to avert saline shortage in wake of Puerto Rico disaster. Available at https://www.washingtonpost.com/news/to-your-health/wp/2017/10/09/hospitals-scramble-to-avert-saline-shortage-in-wake-of-puerto-rico-disaster/. Accessed January 3, 2020.

115. Jarvis LM. Hurricane Maria's lessons for the drug industry. American Chemical Society. Available at https://cen.acs.org/pharmaceuticals/biologics/Hurricane-Marias-lessons-drug-industry/96/i37. Accessed January 3, 2020.

116. Aton A. Hurricane Maria takes a toll on global medical supplies. Available at https://www.scientificamerican.com/article/hurricane-maria-takes-a-toll-on-global-medical-supplies/. Accessed January 3, 2020.

117. HealthyPeople.gov. Healthy People 2020. Available at https://www.healthypeople.gov/2020/topics-objectives/topic/social-determinants-of-health. Accessed January 5, 2020.

118. Kirzinger A, Lopes L, Wu B, Brodie M. Tracking Poll—February 2019: Prescription drugs. Available at https://www.kff.org/health-reform/poll-finding/kff-health-tracking-poll-february-2019-prescription-drugs/. Accessed January 8, 2020.

119. DiJulio B, Firth J, Brodie M. Kaiser health tracking poll: August 2015. Available at https://www.kff.org/health-costs/poll-finding/kaiser-health-tracking-poll-august-2015/. Accessed January 8, 2020.

120. Kennedy J, Wood EG. Medication costs and adherence of treatment before and after the Affordable care act: 1999–2015. *Am J Public Health.* 2016;106(10):1804-1807.

121. Aldridge Young C. Helping patients find and use prescription assistance programs. Available at https://www.pharmacist.com/article/helping-patients-find-and-use-prescription-assistance-programs. Accessed January 5, 2020.

122. Mayo Clinic. Asthma medications: know your options. Available at https://www.mayoclinic.org/diseases-conditions/asthma/in-depth/asthma-medications/art-20045557. Accessed January 5, 2020.

123. To T, Stanojevic S, Moores G, et al. Global asthma prevalence in adults: findings from the cross-sectional world health survey. *BMC Public Health.* 2012;12:204.

124. Centers for Disease Control and Prevention. Asthma. Available at https://www.cdc.gov/nchs/fastats/asthma.htm. Accessed January 10, 2020.

125. World Health Organization. Asthma. Available at https://www.who.int/news-room/fact-sheets/detail/asthma. Accessed January 5, 2020.

126. Phuong JM, Penm J, Chaar B, Oldfield LD, Moles R. The impacts of medication shortages on patient outcomes: a scoping review. *PLoS One.* 2019;14(5):e0215837.

127. Fox ER, McLaughlin MM. ASHP guidelines on managing drug product shortages. *Am J Health Syst Pharm.* 2018;75(21):1742-1750.

128. Goodwyn, Wade. Doctors raise alarm about shortages of pain medications. Available at https://www.npr.org/2018/07/20/629942414/doctors-raise-alarm-about-shortages-of-pain-medications. Accessed January 4, 2020.

129. A dire scarcity of drugs is worsening, in part, because they are so cheap. Available at https://www.economist.com/international/2019/09/14/a-dire-scarcity-of-drugs-is-worsening-in-part-because-they-are-so-cheap. Accessed January 4, 2020.

130. US Food and Drug Administration. Current and resolved drug shortages and discontinuations reported to FDA. Epinephrine. Available at https://www.accessdata.fda.gov/scripts/drugshortages/dsp_ActiveIngredientDetails.cfm?AI=Epinephrine%20Injection,%20Auto-Injector&st=c. Accessed January 3, 2019.

131. Caryn Rabin R. Why lifesaving drugs may be missing on your next flight. Available at https://www.nytimes.com/2019/10/03/health/drugs-airplanes-faa.html. Accessed January 4, 2020.

132. Tonog P, Lakhkar AD. Normal Saline. In: StatPearls. Treasure Island, FL: StatPearls Publishing; 2019. Available at https://www.ncbi.nlm.nih.gov/books/NBK545210/. Accessed January 4, 2020.

133. Hick JL, Hanfling D, Courtney B, Lurie N. Rationing salt water--disaster planning and daily care delivery. *N Engl J Med.* 2014;370(17):1573-1576.

134. Shaban H, Maurer C, Willborn RJ. Impact of drug shortages on patient safety and pharmacy operation costs. *Fed Pract.* 2018;35(1):24-31.

135. Eban K. *Bottle of Lies: The Inside Story of the Generic Drug Boom.* New York, NY, USA: Harper Collins; 2019.

136. Lazarus D. Column: Where do prescription drugs come from? Good luck answering that question. Available at https://www.latimes.com/business/lazarus/la-fi-lazarus-drugs-country-of-origin-20180515-story.html. Accessed January 8, 2020.

137. Fox ER, Birt A, James KB, Kokko H, Salverson S, Soflin DL. ASHP guidelines on managing drug product shortages in hospitals and health systems. *Am J Health Syst Pharm.* 2009;66(15):1399-1406.

138. US Food and Drug Administration. Drug shortages infographic. Available at https://www.fda.gov/media/91517/download. Accessed January 3, 2020.

139. US Food and Drug Administration. Frequently asked questions about drug shortages. Available at https://www.fda.gov/drugs/drug-shortages/frequently-asked-questions-about-drug-shortages#q4. Accessed January 3, 2020.

140. Drug shortages roundtable: Minimizing the impact on patient care. *Am J Health Syst Pharm.* 2018;75(11):816-820.

141. US Food and Drug Administration. Frequently asked questions on patents and exclusivity. Available at https://www.fda.gov/drugs/development-approval-process-drugs/frequently-asked-questions-patents-and-exclusivity. Accessed January 5, 2020.

142. US Food and Drug Administration. Current good manufacturing practice (CGMP) regulations. Available at https://www.fda.gov/drugs/pharmaceutical-quality-resources/current-good-manufacturing-practice-cgmp-regulations. Accessed January 4, 2020.

143. US Food and Drug Administration. Human drug imports. Available at https://www.fda.gov/drugs/guidance-compliance-regulatory-information/human-drug-imports. Accessed January 10, 2020.

144. Eban K. These pills could kill you. Available at https://www.bostonglobe.com/ideas/2019/05/24/ideas-katherine-eban-these-pills-could-kill-you/d4gYXkoMR24n1ucLUkbnqJ/story.html. Accessed January 4, 2020.

145. Farrukh MJ, Tariq MH, Malik O, Khan TM. Valsartan recall: global regulatory overview and future challenges. *Ther Adv Drug Saf.* 2019;10:2042098618823458.

146. Edney A, Berfield S, Yu E. Carcinogens have infiltrated the generic drug supply in the U.S. Available at https://www.bloomberg.com/news/features/2019-09-12/how-carcinogen-tainted-generic-drug-valsartan-got-past-the-fda. Accessed January 4, 2019.

147. US Food and Drug Administration. FDA updates and press announcements on angiotensin II receptor blocker (ARB) recalls (Valsartan, Losartan, and Irbesartan). Available at https://www.fda.gov/drugs/drug-safety-and-availability/fda-updates-and-press-announcements-angiotensin-ii-receptor-blocker-arb-recalls-valsartan-losartan. Accessed January 4, 2019.

148. Generic drug manufacturer ranbaxy pleads guilty and agrees to pay $500 million to resolve false claims allegations, cGMP violations and false statements to the FDA. US Department of Justice Press Release. Available at https://www.justice.gov/opa/pr/generic-drug-manufacturer-ranbaxy-pleads-guilty-and-agrees-pay-500-million-resolve-false. Accessed January 4, 2020.

149. Mazer-Amirshahi M, Fox ER. Saline shortages—many causes, no simple solution. *N Engl J Med.* 2018;378(16):1472-1474.

150. A dire scarcity of drugs is worsening, in part, because they are so cheap. Available at https://www.economist.com/international/2019/09/14/a-dire-scarcity-of-drugs-is-worsening-in-part-because-they-are-so-cheap. Accessed January 4, 2020.

151. McGinley L. Low prices of some lifesaving drugs make them impossible to get. Available at https://www.washingtonpost.com/national/health-science/low-prices-of-some-lifesaving-drugs-make-them-impossible-to-get/2019/06/18/abd03190-66bb-11e9-82ba-fcfeff232e8f_story.html. Accessed January 3, 2020.

152. Thomas K. A vital drug runs low, though its base ingredient is in many kitchens. Available at https://www.nytimes.com/2017/05/21/health/sodium-bicarbonate-solution-critical-shortage-hospitals.html. Accessed January 5, 2020.

153. Gray A, Manasse HR. Shortages of medicines: a complex global challenge. *Bull World Health Organ.* 2012;90(3):158-158A.

154. Pharmacist's authority in pharmaceutical product selection: therapeutic interchange and substitution. FIP Statement of Policy. 2018. Available at https://www.fip.org/file/2086. Accessed January 5, 2020.

155. The roles of pharmacists in non-communicable diseases. FIP Statement of Policy. 2019. Available at https://www.fip.org/file/4338. Accessed January 5, 2019.

156. Wirtz VJ, Hogerzeil HV, Gray AL, et al. Essential medicines for universal health coverage. *The Lancet.* 2017;389(10067):403-476.

157. World Health Organization. WHO model lists of essential medicines. Available at https://www.who.int/medicines/publications/essentialmedicines/en/. Accessed January 5, 2020.

158. World Health Organization. The selection and use of essential medicines: report of the WHO Expert Committee, 2013 (including the 18th WHO model list of essential medicines and the 4th WHO Model list of essential medicines for children). Technical report series 985. World Health Organization: 2014. Available at https://apps.who.int/iris/handle/10665/112729. Accessed January 5, 2020.

159. World Health Organization. The selection and use of essential medicines. Report of the WHO expert committee, 2009 (including the 16th WHO Model List of Essential Medicines and the 2nd WHO model list of essential medicines for children). Technical report series 958. World Health Organization: 2009. Available at https://apps.who.int/iris/bitstream/handle/10665/44287/WHO_TRS_958_eng.pdf. Accessed January 5, 2020.

160. Joint FIP/WHO guidelines on good pharmacy practice: standards for quality of pharmacy services. Forty-fifth report of the WHO expert committee on specifications for pharmaceutical preparations. WHO technical report series. 2011;961:310-23.

161. Drug shortages as a matter of national security: improving the resilience of the nation's healthcare critical infrastructure. Recommendations from September 20, 2018 Summit. Available at https://www.ashp.org/~/media/assets/advocacy-issues/docs/Recommendations-Drug-Shortages-as-Matter-of-Natl-Security. Accessed January 5, 2020.

162. American Society of Health-System Pharmacists. Current drug shortages. Available at https://www.ashp.org/Drug-Shortages/Current-Shortages. Accessed January 4, 2020.

CHAPTER 15

Administration

Featuring the Illustrated Case Studies "Opportunities" & "Relationships"

Authors

David R. Hager, Steve Rough, & Joseph A. Zorek

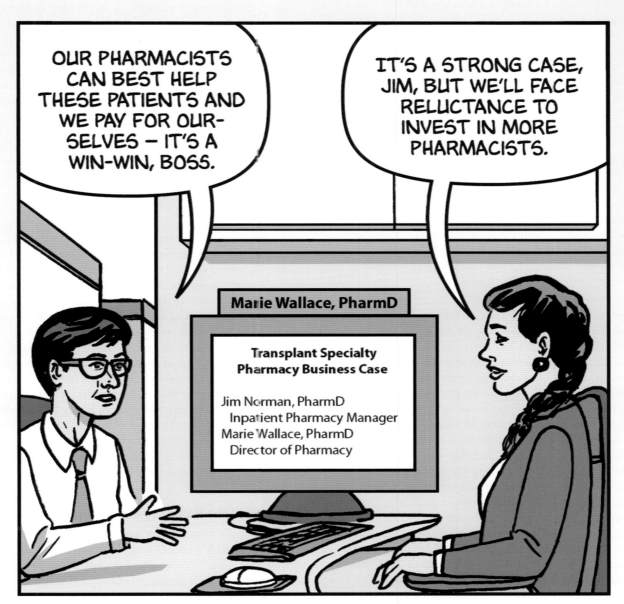

Illustration by George Folz, © 2019 Board of Regents of the University of Wisconsin System

BACKGROUND

Administration in healthcare is focused on creating an environment where health professionals can practice effectively and efficiently. Healthcare administrators' goals are to improve the quality of care provided while managing the business aspects associated with making that possible. This field has evolved significantly as hospitals have grown and expanded into health systems.[1] The first formal healthcare administrator education program was offered in 1934 and has expanded to more than 100 programs.[2] Growth of positions in this field has been significant. While the number of physicians in the United States grew by 150% between 1975 and 2010, for example, the number of healthcare administrators during the same period increased by 3200%.[3]

There are many challenges within the US healthcare system. In 2016, the United States spent 17.8% of its gross domestic product on healthcare, while the average spending in similar high-income countries was much lower, at 11.5%.[4] Despite this high degree of spending, life expectancy in the United States is 78.8 years, nearly 3 years less than the average life expectancy in other high-income countries.[4] Recent efforts focused on combating billing fraud, implementing electronic health records, and adopting evidence-based practices have neither improved outcomes nor lowered costs, at least on a large scale across the entire country.[5] Several reasons have been identified for this disproportionate spending compared to other high-income countries; these include (1) higher salaries for health professionals, (2) greater use and cost of pharmaceuticals, and (3) higher administrative costs. The latter are largely comprised of healthcare administrator positions, which are considered essential due to the rapid pace of change in healthcare associated with regulations and accelerating technological advances.[3] For more information and examples of the impact of technology on pharmacy practice, and healthcare more generally, readers are encouraged to explore the illustrated cases "Leverage," "Integrated," and "Innovator" in Chapter 13 Technology.

Effective healthcare administrators maintain a razor-sharp focus on value, ensuring every dollar spent results in improvements in health outcomes.[6] This has been challenging as measuring costs accurately, and defining appropriate health outcomes, have proven elusive. Advances in treatments for cancer highlight this challenge well. The average price of new cancer medications increased 10% per year between 1995 and 2013.[7] These increasing costs have outpaced associated improvements in health outcomes: for example, the median improvement in survival has been 2.1 months in patients with solid tumors over a similar time period.[8] Measuring the amount of time added to cancer patients' lives is a common health outcome measure, and comparing this to the cost of cancer treatments (including medications) provides useful information to make judgments regarding value. The average cost of cancer medications for each additional year of life those medications provide has increased from $54,000 in 1995 to $207,000 in 2013.[9] Many of these medications were approved by the US Food and Drug Administration (FDA) based on data demonstrating what some

consider modest clinically significant improvements, which has led stakeholders (e.g., professional cancer societies) to question whether health outcomes used to justify FDA approval of cancer therapies need to be redefined.[10] Patient advocacy groups, oncologists (i.e., physicians who specialize in treating cancer), and healthcare administrators have struggled to justify large financial investments based on such outcomes, and there have been calls for large-scale reforms as a result, including using value within clinical guidelines.[11] Healthcare administrators need to help members of interprofessional teams understand these issues, as it falls on those health professionals to communicate the complexities, including financial ramifications, of treatment options to patients in a manner that facilitates development of shared goals.[12]

Another focus of healthcare administrators is reducing error by improving systems of care. Medical errors are estimated to cause 44,000 to 98,000 deaths each year in US hospitals.[13] These errors also constitute a total annual cost of approximately $17 billion.[14] Fundamental changes in healthcare delivery have been proposed to prevent these errors; as a result, the need for leadership has never been greater.[15] Healthcare administrators must marshal resources, forge consensus, and experiment with potential interventions or innovations in care delivery to address these pressing issues. One solution that has been suggested is to organize health professionals into interprofessional teams, with clear roles established for each team member to maximize their contribution to patient care and the health of populations.[5] This book is replete with examples of pharmacists contributing to the interprofessional care of patients. See Chapter 1 Interprofessional Practice in Pharmacy for a more in-depth exploration of this topic.

Concrete measures have emerged in recent years to help stakeholders evaluate the impact of various interventions and innovations in care delivery. Several of these, like 30-day hospital readmission rates and surveys capturing patients' experiences (e.g., Hospital Consumer Assessment of Healthcare Providers and Systems surveys, or HCAHPS for short), have begun to drive how administrative decisions are made.[16] This has been reinforced as payment models for healthcare delivery have begun shifting toward rewarding value; many stakeholders believe this evolution must continue.[17] Improving the quality of care delivered in a manner that adds value to the US healthcare system poses a complex challenge for healthcare administrators. To contribute to solutions, effective pharmacy leaders will need skills and expertise in the areas of human resource management, financial management, project and team leadership, data analysis, business planning, strategic planning, ethics, negotiation, and interprofessional collaboration.[1]

Members of the Health System Leadership Team

Most healthcare organization mission statements are similar; namely, to provide patients with easy access to cost-effective, high-quality care.[18] Variability between these organizations comes from how each decides to accomplish that mission. Two healthcare organizations in the same city may, for example, focus on completely different types of care. That difference will drive the need for specialized healthcare administrators in various areas. These administrators, in turn, are often organized in a hierarchical structure with a single leader at the top who oversees the efforts of multiple healthcare administrators with specialized knowledge and goals specific to a well-defined area within the organization (see Figure 15-1).[19]

The extent and quality of collaboration of various administrators across all levels within a healthcare organizations have been associated with better problem solving and innovation.[20] There are administrators at multiple levels of management within healthcare organizations: lower-level management, mid-level management, and upper-level or senior management. Senior management might include a chief operating officer (COO), a chief medical officer (CMO), or a chief nursing officer (CNO) (see Figure 15-1). Members of this group are often referred to as the "C-suite" in healthcare because they often have the term "Chief" in their title. C-suite administrators are responsible for entire areas of organizational performance, and they typically report directly to the chief executive officer (CEO), the top person in the healthcare organization.

The composition of C-suite administrators evolves in concert with changes in healthcare, and not all organizations have the same C-suite titles.[21] Common C-suite members include a chief financial officer (CFO), who is responsible for ensuring a positive financial future; a chief information officer (CIO), who may decide the future of technology within the organization; and a chief pharmacy officer (CPO), who may be responsible for medication use wherever it occurs.[22] An interprofessional group of senior leaders from the C-suite might come together to set the strategy for the entire organization by analyzing the health needs in their community, or they might work to identify trends within the workforce to determine where to invest resources in training and education.

Another level of healthcare administrators, generally referred to as mid-level managers, are in place to help C-suite administrators execute organizational strategies and deliver results for organizational initiatives. Examples of mid-level managers include a director of compliance, who would report to the COO, and a director of inpatient operations within a pharmacy department, who would report to the CPO (see Figure 15-2). Generally, these individuals conduct strategic planning for their specific service line/unit, provide leadership development opportunities for employees, and ensure resources are aligned with the goals of the organization. These individuals are typically responsible for larger units within their departments, and related activity within the organization tied directly to those units; for example, the director of patient care services in a pharmacy department would ensure all transplant patients receive high quality care, while the director of inpatient operations in a pharmacy department, on the other hand, would ensure all employees follow state and federal regulations related to medication use. Mid-level managers representing different parts of the organization might collaborate to meet common challenges, such as maximizing medication use to improve transplant outcomes.

Finally, lower-level managers are in place to help mid-level managers successfully execute organizational strategies that fall under their purview. Examples of lower-level managers include a nurse manager or a pharmacy manager. The scope of responsibility for these individuals is more targeted, such as nursing or pharmacy services provided on a selection of hospital floors or wards. Lower-level managers are often responsible for overseeing staffing decisions, improving employee performance, and designing how patient care in that area is conducted for their profession. These individuals might work interprofessionally to create a new care transition system for discharging a patient from the hospital more safely and efficiently. Readers interested in care transitions are encouraged to explore the illustrated cases "Breakdown" in Chapter 1 Interprofessional Practice in Pharmacy and "Support" in Chapter 3 Primary Care.

Role of Pharmacy Administrators within Health System Leadership Teams

Overall, pharmacy administrators are responsible for both the clinical and financial outcomes related to medication use.[22,23] Pharmacy administrators make sure that medications are provided and used in a consistent and evidence-based manner that maximizes value. At the top of the pharmacy administrative team is the CPO (see Figures 15-1 and 15-2). The CPO is a relatively new title that demonstrates the need for healthcare organizations to engage the pharmacy profession proactively in strategic decision making.[22] This raises the stature/standing of the pharmacy profession within the organization, placing it on par with medicine and nursing, two professions that commonly

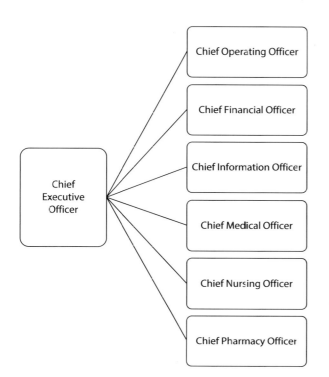

Figure 15-1. Example of an Executive Leadership Structure within a Healthcare Organization

Chief Executive Officer

Chief Operating Officer

Chief Financial Officer

Chief Information Officer

Chief Medical Officer

Chief Nursing Officer

Chief Pharmacy Officer

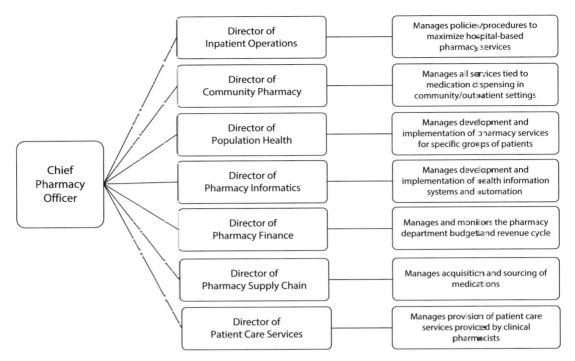

Figure 15-2. Example of a Pharmacy Department Administration Leadership Structure

have representation in the form of a CMO or CNO. Within many healthcare organizations, the Director of Pharmacy is still the highest position/title, with designated responsibility to lead all pharmacy operations akin to a CPO, yet reporting directly to the CMO, CNO, or COO rather than the CEO.

The CPO is responsible for overseeing pharmacy patient care services, medication safety, medication preparation and delivery services, medication purchasing and inventory systems, regulatory compliance for medications, medication expenses, medication reimbursement, and technology systems related to obtaining, dispensing, or clinically reviewing medications. The CPO must be competent in time management, strategic thinking, execution, consensus building, healthcare finances, decision making, leading and developing people, advocacy, regulatory compliance, technology deployment and business development. These individuals often feel satisfied in their work because of their ability to influence the profession of pharmacy, the sense of accomplishment associated with leading large-scale improvements in medication use, the level of autonomy they have within their positions, and the relationships they have with other leaders across the organization.[24]

The CPO directs a mid-level management team of pharmacists empowered to lead specialized areas within the pharmacy department.[25] These mid-level managers, who often hold a title of Director, oversee core specialties of the department. The number of Directors and their specific titles vary depending on the size of the organization and the number of sites of care covered. Some typical pharmacy specialties that would report to the CPO include inpatient operations, community pharmacy, population health, informatics, pharmacy finance, pharmacy supply chain, and patient care services (see Figure 15-2).[26,27] In addition to interprofessional collaboration, these pharmacy administrators need to demonstrate skills in teambuilding, data analytics, systems thinking, change management, and performance improvement to contribute meaningfully.[28] These individuals often feel rewarded because of their ability to make an impact and improve services, solve problems, help develop others, and be involved with large scale organizational priorities.[24] Pharmacy administrators of all levels work collaboratively within their areas of training and expertise to achieve the mission of the pharmacy department; usually, improving the health of patients and populations through optimal medication use.

As a career path, pharmacy administration is not only available in healthcare organizations; it is also a career option in community pharmacy, managed care pharmacy, the pharmaceutical industry, and academia. A 10-year shortage in pharmacy leaders was predicted in 2013, driven by a lack of available pharmacists with administrative experience, belief that administrative positions are tougher now than in the past, and a lack of interest.[24,29] Those perceptions may be unfounded, as current leaders have rising job satisfaction and are less likely to leave their positions.[24]

HEALTH SYSTEM PHARMACY LEADERS IN ACTION

Leading in Drug Shortage Mitigation and Advocacy

Drug shortages occur when a commonly used medication becomes unavailable or is in short supply. They can impact how pharmacists prepare or dispense medications and also influence patient care by postponing the usual course of care or requiring use of alternative medications, thus increasing costs and the potential to harm patients.[30] The drug shortage situation in the United States has never been worse than it is today; there were 238 documented occurrences in 2018, up from 61 in 2005.[31,32] Patients in need of medications, including life-saving ones for diseases like cancer, are being forced to sometimes go without. One survey of oncologists found that 83% were unable to use preferred medication regimens due to pervasive shortages of cancer drugs like vincristine, a drug used for multiple types of childhood cancers.[33] A drug shortage team, spearheaded by a pharmacist, was developed in Utah to respond to shortages and, importantly, advocate for legislative changes to fundamentally address the issue.[32] This team developed mechanisms to identify alternative products, make changes to drug preparations, implement systems to allocate medications, and advance communication strategies to ensure all members of the interprofessional team were informed and updated on a regular basis. A 2019 study estimated that $230 million each year is spent on alternative drugs due to shortages, highlighting the importance of pharmacists engaging in this manner.[34] Those interested in a more in-depth exploration of drug shortages are encouraged to read the illustrated case "Interconnected" in Chapter 15 Population Health.

Stemming the Rising Tide of Drug Costs

Drug costs have risen substantially in recent years, which has presented a real challenge for pharmacy administrators in leadership positions throughout the US healthcare system. For example, the cost of epinephrine auto-injectors (EpiPen), a life-saving product used to treat severe allergic reactions, increased by 461% over an 8-year period from $56.64 to $317.82.[35,36] The cost of pyrimethamine, a drug used to treat an infection associated with Human Immunodeficiency Virus (HIV), increased by over 5000% from $13.50 to $750 per pill.[36,37] Insulin, a life-saving medication for patients with diabetes, provides another example of escalating costs putting patients in precarious situations; some simply cannot afford it, and medication adherence, and health outcomes, suffer as a result.[38] The impact of cost increases on hospitals and pharmacy departments is also staggering. From 2015 to 2017, there was an 18.5% average increase in prescription drug spending per adjusted hospital admission, from $468.50 to $555.40 per admission. Pharmacy administrators have advocated for aggressive measures within their organizations to curb skyrocketing costs, such as creating mechanisms to identify commonly used high-cost medications and discontinuing or optimizing treatments as soon as possible.[39] Other pharmacy administrators are advocating for systematic change through legislative measures leading to legal changes to bring more competition for single source products.[40] Pharmacists across the profession have brought attention to this critical issue through presentations, newspaper articles, television appearances, and radio interviews.[41–46]

BECOMING A HEALTH SYSTEM PHARMACY LEADER

All graduates of accredited doctor of pharmacy (PharmD) programs receive education in leadership. This is a required component of the curriculum and is a part of the Accreditation Council for Pharmacy Education (ACPE) standards that all schools of pharmacy must meet. This requirement was added in recent years to guard against a potential leadership gap within the profession, as previously mentioned.[29] While leadership development offerings have expanded since its inclusion in the ACPE standards, many schools do not have required coursework in this area and it may be taught through elective courses or experiential activities.[47] While not all pharmacy school graduates will pursue formal leadership roles, it is important that all pharmacists have leadership skills to be effective in whatever professional role they ultimately assume.[48]

For those who do desire a formal leadership role, one of the surest paths to a position in pharmacy administration is the completion of a Health System Pharmacy Administration and Leadership (HSPAL) residency program.[49] This residency training follows the completion of the PharmD degree, where pharmacists commit to either a 2-year program at a single training site (a combined post-graduate year 1 [PGY-1]/post-graduate year 2 [PGY-2] program) or elect after a PGY-1 residency to complete a 1-year PGY-2 program. Many of these programs include the opportunity to obtain master's degrees, usually in health system pharmacy administration. The goal of these programs is to prepare pharmacists for success in pharmacy administration through hands-on learning. Most residents who complete these programs enter the workforce as pharmacy managers (e.g., lower-level administrators).

While completing a HSPAL residency program is an option for pharmacy graduates, it is not the only path to a career in pharmacy administration. For some, the pathway to administration is gradual and occurs after practicing clinically.[50,51] Recent surveys indicate that up to 45% of current pharmacists intend to take a leadership position at some point in their career.[24] These individuals often practice clinically for years and take on more projects and responsibilities over time. As a result, they garner respect as an informal clinical leader in their practice area, which results in opportunities for formal leadership. In order to gain credentials that may be expected for pharmacists within leadership positions, such individuals may elect to pursue formal leadership education and training through a graduate degree program.[52] Alternatively, training programs, continuing education, and certificates focused on developing leadership skills are available to experienced pharmacists through many pharmacy professional organizations.[24] While pathways into pharmacy administration differ, those who succeed often share similarities; these include passion for improving patient care, a strong desire to lead, and effective leadership skills.

OPPORTUNITIES: An Illustrated Case Study

Story by David R. Hager, Steve Rough, & Joseph A. Zorek
Illustrations by George Folz, © 2019 Board of Regents of the University of Wisconsin System

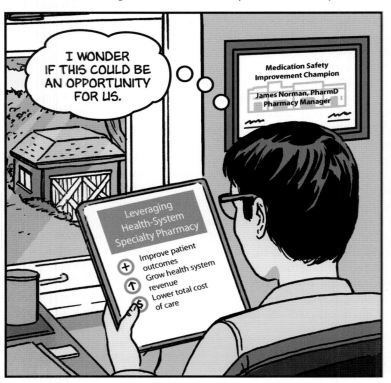

Illustration 15-1

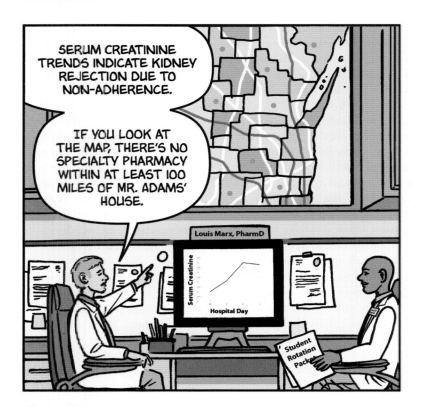

Illustration 15-2

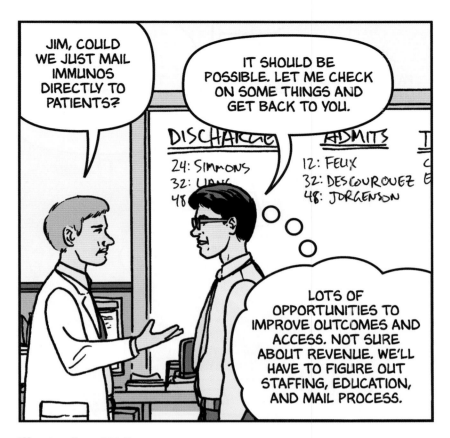

Illustration 15-3

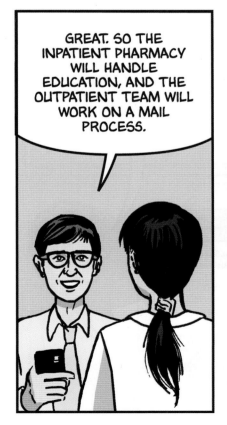
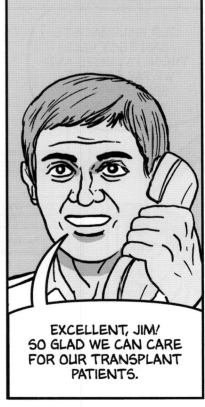

Illustration 15-4

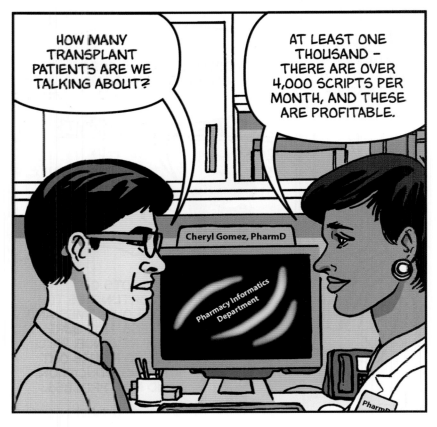

Illustration 15-5

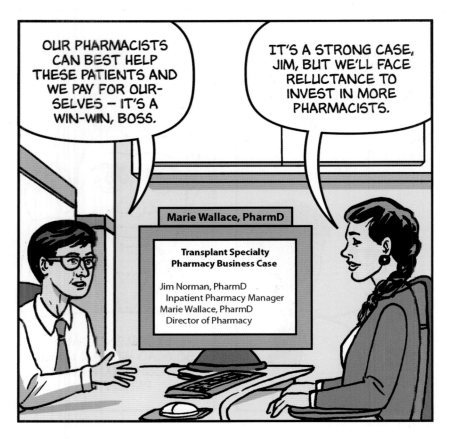

Illustration 15-6

Thoughts on "Opportunities"

Medication non-adherence, a term used to describe when a patient does not take medications as prescribed, is a major problem in the United States.[53] Studies show that non-adherence leads to increased rates of death, hospitalization, and significant cost to the healthcare system.[54-58] Researchers have estimated that $100 to $289 billion a year is spent in the United States as a result of this problem.[54]

There are several key barriers that have been linked to non-adherence, including many that are highlighted throughout this book: motivation or ability (see the illustrated cases "Transformation" in Chapter 2 Community Pharmacy and "Swish" in Chapter 3 Primary Care), memory (see "Burden" in Chapter 7 Geriatrics), understanding (see "Breakdown" in Chapter 1 Interprofessional Practice in Pharmacy, "Breathe" in Chapter 2 Community Pharmacy, and "Educator" in Chapter 5 Cardiology), and issues, like financial barriers, that lead to an inability to access medications (see "Holistic" in Chapter 3 Primary Care, and "Interconnected" in Chapter 14 Population Health).[59] Access to medications is cited as perhaps the most significant contributor to medication non-adherence, and this is particularly true for transplant recipients.[60,61] For some patients who have organs that do not function well enough, such as their kidneys, pancreas, liver, heart, or lungs, the best option to improve quality of life, or to extend life, is to surgically add or replace a healthy organ from a living or deceased donor.[62,63] This transplanted organ is called a graft. Our immune systems are trained to attack what enters our body that does not belong to us, or is otherwise recognized as foreign, such as bacteria or viruses. As a result, a graft that previously belonged to another person will be attacked, damaged, and ultimately fail if this predictable immune response, called rejection, is not prevented.

Anti-rejection medications (i.e., immunosuppressives or "immunos") are vital to preserving graft function and, ultimately, patient survival. As their name implies, these medications suppress the immune response to attack the graft and thus maximize the likelihood of successful transplantation. The most common and evidence-based immunosuppressive regimen contains three medications, each from a different category.[64,65] While this combination significantly decreases the risk of rejection, it also leads to side effects that can be debilitating. Common examples include diarrhea, tremor, mood swings, insomnia, and increased risk of infection or cancer. The complexity of the anti-rejection regimen and the side effects combine to create a real challenge to medication adherence. When additional barriers are added to the equation, such as high medication costs, limited distribution of immunosuppressives to local pharmacies, and stringent insurance requirements, rates of non-adherence ranging from 15% to 55% are reported even though these are lifesaving medications.[66,67]

Non-adherence matters more to healthcare organizations than ever before due to evolving payment models. Payment mechanisms for the provision of healthcare have shifted in recent years from being focused on the services provided (e.g., physician visits, laboratory tests ordered, medication doses administered, procedures completed) to the quality of patient outcomes (e.g., prevention of hospital-acquired infections, hospital readmissions, mortality).[68,69] This is commonly referred to as "pay for performance" or "value-based payment." For example, the US Centers for Medicare and Medicaid Services (CMS) introduced a value-based payment system in 2008 in response to the Medicare Improvements for Patients and Providers Act that was expanded in 2010 under the Patient Protection and Affordable Care Act.[70] Incentives were provided for healthcare organizations to achieve the Triple Aim; specifically, improving population health and individual patient experiences with care while reducing costs.[17,71] Value-based payment models are intended to reward healthcare organizations for improving the quality of care they provide, as opposed to rewarding the shear amount of care provided. This shift toward quality has sparked incredible changes in the healthcare landscape over the last decade; chief among them being the proliferation of health systems. Broadly speaking, a health system is a healthcare organization that includes at least one hospital and one physician group that work in tandem to provide comprehensive care to a defined patient population.

Another outcome of the move to value-based care was the expansion of quality measures and associated regulations. The illustrated case "Opportunities" focuses on the transplant setting because it is one of the most regulated fields in healthcare, and the need for strong pharmacy leaders in this area has been recognized.[72,73] Multiple regulatory bodies monitor the quality, and hence value, of the care delivered in transplant programs. As a result, transplant programs must demonstrate high quality outcomes for their entire patient population; failure to do so is a justifiable reason for a regulatory body to close the program. Ensuring this population is adherent to their medications is vital to demonstrating quality and value. CMS, for example, requires that an interprofessional team manages transplant patient populations, and one required member of that team must be an individual with transplant pharmacology qualifications, training, and experience.[74] This is often interpreted as a pharmacist, although having a pharmacist in this role is not explicitly required.[73] These transplant pharmacists, then, must be supported by an administrative leader who understands their needs and can help them succeed in this interprofessional environment.

Pharmacist administrators (e.g., supervisors, managers, directors, chief pharmacy officers) are responsible for collaborating with others to ensure patient care is delivered effectively. Oftentimes, pharmacist administrators are relied upon for their understanding of medications and the medication use process, which is highly complex within health systems. These individuals contribute to each step of the process, which ranges from formulary decision-making (to determine which medications will be available for use in the health system) and how selected medications will be administered to monitoring medication use patterns and the systematic evaluation of their utility, efficacy, and value.[75] Effective pharmacist administrators improve the medication use systems and processes around them, leading to a better environment for patient care.[76] Beyond technical skills, pharmacist administrators must be self-aware leaders capable of vision setting, networking, professional growth, and mentoring.[23]

The illustrated case "Opportunities" describes some of the activities that an inpatient pharmacy manager working in a health system might engage in. In this case, Dr. Jim Norman, the manager, is responsible for the pharmacy services provided to transplant patients. Illustration 15-1 shows Jim searching for mechanisms to leverage specialty pharmacy within his management role. Specialty pharmacy is a rapidly expanding part of pharmacy practice, particularly at healthcare organizations that deliver specialized care.[77] Broadly speaking, specialty pharmacy operates as an extension of community pharmacy practice, including the dispensing of medications in patient populations that have multiple chronic diseases and where the medications are either potentially toxic, restricted in terms of their sale/use, or costly.[78] Transplant patients and transplant-associated medications fall within this category. Other health conditions where use of specialty medications is prevalent include hepatitis C, cancer, multiple sclerosis, and rheumatoid arthritis.[79]

Well-run specialty pharmacies help improve population health outcomes and the patient experience of care while lowering total healthcare costs.[80-82] This may seem counterintuitive based on the high cost of specialty medications. For example, in both multiple sclerosis and rheumatoid arthritis, despite the high drug expense, the improved adherence to these medications slows disease progression, thereby reducing emergency department visits, hospitalizations, and need for physician office visits.[81,82] Even in hepatitis C, where high treatment costs were decried by patients and patient advocacy groups, treatment of hepatitis C with these high cost drugs, on average, pay for themselves within 16 months. Expanded patient access to the high cost drugs, thus, would lead to greater savings to the healthcare system by preventing cirrhosis, or liver failure, and the need for liver transplants.[82-84] Pharmacists who specialize in these high cost, high-risk drugs focus on adherence, ensuring anticipated benefits are materializing, and managing medication side effects. Health systems benefit from specialty pharmacies because the medications can produce new revenue streams, usually in the hundreds of millions of dollars.[79] On average, a community pharmacy generates $55 in revenue per prescription filled. Revenue generated from specialty medications, in contrast, can reach $2100 per prescription filled, on average.[79,85]

In his management role, Jim oversees a transplant pharmacist named Dr. Louis Marx, who is depicted in Illustration 15-2 discussing a patient case with a student pharmacist. Louis is reviewing the patient's serum creatinine, which is one way to measure how well kidneys are working.[86] Creatinine is a protein made in the body when muscle is broken down, and it is removed from the body through the kidneys. Serum creatinine increases when the kidneys are not working well; hence, high levels of serum creatinine indicate poor kidney function or kidney damage. The graph Louis and his student are discussing in Illustration 15-2 shows an alarming increase in the patient's serum creatinine, and thus a worsening of kidney function that may represent the early stages of graft rejection. While there are several potential causes for increased serum creatinine in a kidney transplant recipient, Louis has discovered through interviewing the patient that medication access issues have led to non-adherence of immunosuppressive medications. This is troublesome for Louis, because facilitating medication adherence is an increasingly core function of transplant pharmacists working in both hospital and clinic settings.[73]

Particularly in rural parts of the United States, access to healthcare may be limited (for a more in-depth discussion of rural pharmacy, see the illustrated case "Breathe" in Chapter 2 Community Pharmacy). With immunosuppressives being high cost and high risk to patients, they are considered specialty medications as defined above, and access to these medications is often restricted to specialty pharmacies.[87] For a patient who lives a great distance from a specialty pharmacy, simply obtaining the medications can be an insurmountable barrier, especially when other social and economic variables are taken into account. See the illustrated case "Unsung Hero" in Chapter 14 Population Health for a more in-depth exploration of these variables. Pharmacists like Louis, who have a detailed understanding of patient, health system, and financial considerations for transplant medications, are needed to help patients navigate the complexities associated with accessing their life-saving medications.[73] Illustration 15-3 shows Louis advocating with his supervisor, Jim, to address the access issues he and his student identified in Illustration 15-2.

Illustration 15-3 depicts Jim's attempt to connect the dots between Louis' description of the medication access issues he is facing and the research article he read over the weekend (Illustration 15-1). Jim's thoughts demonstrate the potential benefits and challenges to setting up a specialty pharmacy focused on immunosuppressives. Realigning workflow and responsibilities to coordinate across multiple teams within the pharmacy department would be required. For most specialty pharmacies, this includes pharmacy personnel to perform clinical, billing, and insurance processing duties, phone systems to effectively contact patients, and mailing systems for medication delivery. Louis' idea of mailing prescriptions from the health system's pharmacy seems like a small request compared to the alternative; namely, graft rejection.

As an administrative leader with a vision, Jim recognizes that it could also be the start of something much larger for the health system.

Jim continues to pursue this specialty pharmacy idea by collaborating with leaders of other units within the pharmacy department. He begins by focusing on logistics, as demonstrated in the first half of Illustration 15-4. Best practice in pharmacy dictates that every patient should receive education and counseling about their medications.[88,89] Typically, this occurs at the pickup window of an outpatient pharmacy. Within healthcare, outpatient is a general term used to describe healthcare encounters that take place outside of a hospital; conversely, inpatient is used to describe activities that take place inside a hospital. Illustration 15-4 shows Jim figuring out which pharmacy team will handle specific duties. The inpatient transplant pharmacy team will provide patients with education on each transplant medication, and the outpatient pharmacy team will handle the complex billing and mailing to make sure patients can access (i.e., afford) their medications and that the medications arrive to patients' homes unaltered by conditions in transit.

Having established that the pharmacy department is equipped to handle the logistics associated with this new specialty pharmacy service, Jim must next effectively demonstrate its future profitability. To create new programs, pharmacist administrators need to account for risks and benefits, including new expenses and projected new revenue. Considering the complexities associated with value-based payments and the many realignments taking place with health system formation, expansion, and consolidation, which impact care for patients and populations, pharmacist administrators like Jim must be able to financially justify new patient care services. Illustrations 15-5 and 15-6 detail Jim's efforts to create a business plan and to win the support of key leaders within the pharmacy department; perhaps most importantly the director of pharmacy, Dr. Marie Wallace.

Return-on-investment (ROI) is a key aspect of business plans utilized to inform and persuade health system leaders. In essence, ROI accounts for all new expenses and revenue, and shows over time what the financial impact would be for the organization.[90] To develop an accurate ROI projection, Jim starts by exploring how many patients within the health system might use the new specialty pharmacy transplant service, how many prescriptions might be filled, and the revenue that would be generated with each transplant medication filled. Jim turns to Dr. Cheryl Gomez for help, depicted in Illustration 15-5, who is a pharmacy informaticist with specialized training in computer systems, medication reimbursement, and data generation. Pharmacy informaticists are increasingly in demand as the amount of data generated by health systems continues to expand.[91] For a more in-depth exploration of pharmacy informatics, see the illustrated case "Integrated" in Chapter 13 Technology.

Having established the feasibility and profitability of the new specialty pharmacy transplant service, Jim takes the business case to Marie in an effort to procure necessary resources (Illustration 15-6). Marie's perspective and training are different from that of Jim's. Marie not only has the clinical training of the doctor of pharmacy degree, but she has also completed a Health System Pharmacy Administration and Leadership residency program. This has prepared her to run a pharmacy department within a health system and to know what types of opportunities are likely to be successful in meeting the goals of the organization. Marie knows that the chief executive officer, or CEO, will require a strong defense of the proposal to justify increased resource allocation to the pharmacy department. With a strong business case demonstrating improvements in population health and the patient care experience while reducing health expenditures, and support from across her pharmacy leadership team, Marie makes the decision that this new pharmacy service is worth pursuing. It remains to be seen whether Marie's relationships with other key leaders in the health system are strong enough to make this program a reality.

DISCUSSION QUESTIONS FOR "OPPORTUNITIES"

1. Illustration 15-2 shows a student pharmacist learning from an experienced pharmacist in a unique clinical environment. What would be the opportunities and challenges of that type of learning? How might it be different from classroom-based learning?

2. Non-adherence to immunosuppressive medications is shown to be a complex problem to solve within the transplant setting. Why might a patient skip taking medications she/he has been told are essential to saving her/his life? What factors can you think of that make taking medications so complex?

3. Illustration 15-5 introduces pharmacy informatics. Where is health data being generated today and how might that be different than in the past? In what ways might health data be used to improve care? In what ways might health data be misused?

4. Specialty pharmacy medications are costly and must be closely monitored. How should pharmacists approach these medications? Should they be treated differently than non-specialty medications?

5. Throughout the case, the pharmacy manager Jim is shown collaborating with several other leaders within the pharmacy department who have specialized roles (e.g., outpatient pharmacy manager, pharmacy informatics specialist). What are the advantages of having an administrative team with specialized roles? Can you think of disadvantages to this approach?

RELATIONSHIPS: An Illustrated Case Study

Story by David R. Hager, Steve Rough, & Joseph A. Zorek
Illustrations by George Folz, © 2019 Board of Regents of the University of Wisconsin System

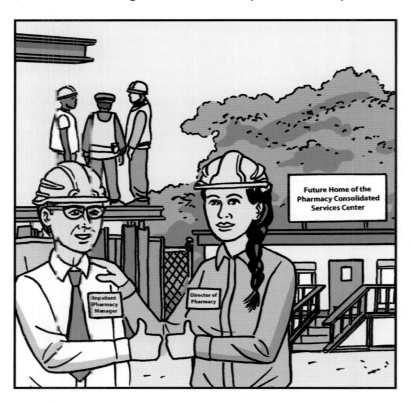

Illustration 15-7

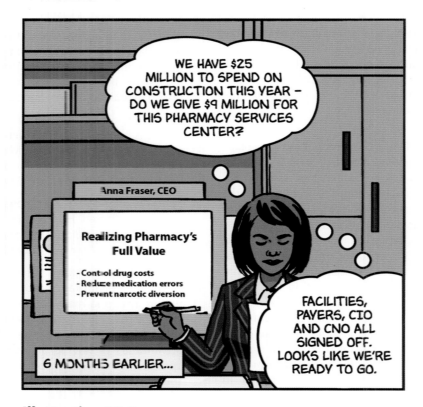

Illustration 15-8

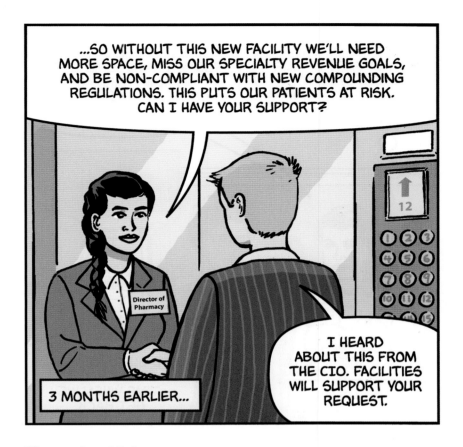

Illustration 15-9

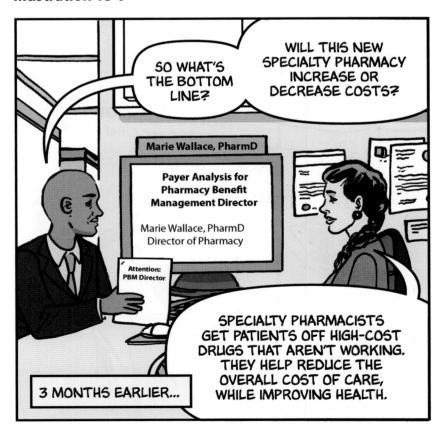

Illustration 15-10

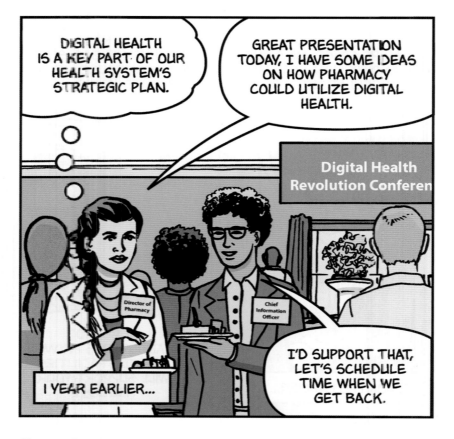

Illustration 15-11

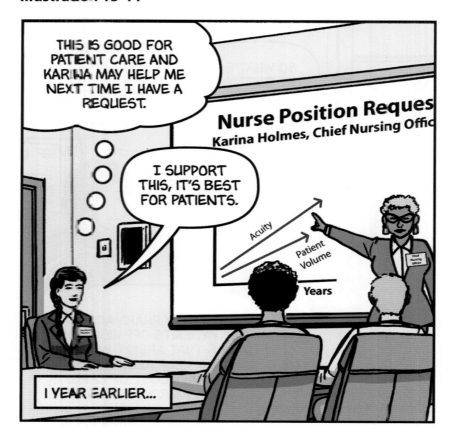

Illustration 15-12

Thoughts on "Relationships"

Peter Drucker, considered by many to be the 20th-century's leading expert on administration, stated that hospitals are "the most complex human organization ever devised."[92] Drucker split the workforce into two groups: manual workers who performed physical tasks; and knowledge workers who, leveraging specialized training, produced knowledge, ideas, and information. The complexity of hospitals is driven, in large part, by the interplay of these manual and knowledge workers. A vast array of unique specialties of knowledge workers must coordinate their efforts for the hospital to run and for patients to receive adequate care. These coordinated efforts must also interface seamlessly with essential tasks performed by manual workers.

To highlight this complexity, consider the fact that patients being treated for cancer often develop infections that can be life-threatening. Physicians with specialized knowledge in oncology (to treat the cancer) and infectious diseases (to treat the infection) must coordinate not only amongst themselves, but also with other knowledge workers involved in caring for the patient. This may include, for example, and depending on the situation, pharmacists, nurses, counseling psychologists, and social workers. Additionally, coordination with manual workers would also be essential; for example, with housekeeping staff who clean and disinfect the facility to prevent the spread of infectious microorganisms or pharmacy technicians to prepare medication infusions. Each of these groups of workers expects to have a leader who understands their unique needs; someone equipped to manage the group's relationships with others throughout the hospital. A cadre of competent administrators, therefore, is essential for the hospital to achieve its objectives and to reach its potential.

The Healthcare Leadership Alliance (HLA) describes itself as a consortium of major professional associations in the United States, each dedicated to advancing best practices in healthcare management and leadership in their respective profession/discipline.[93] As a result, the HLA represents over 140,000 healthcare management professionals in the United States. The HLA has identified the following five competencies as critical for administrators in healthcare settings: communication and relationship management; leadership; professionalism; knowledge of the healthcare environment; and business skills and knowledge.[93]

The illustrated case "Relationships" is a fictional account of how many of these competencies can be demonstrated by pharmacy administrators to improve patient care in the complex environment of a health system. The case opens at the end of a 3-year journey where Dr. Jim Norman, an inpatient pharmacy manager, and Dr. Marie Wallace, the Director of Pharmacy, are congratulating themselves on a job well done (Illustration 15-7). They have shared a vision for several years to improve medication use and management within the health system by consolidating space and resources within a pharmacy consolidated services center (PCSC).[94,95] Buildings such as these have become increasingly common within health systems for reasons that are as diverse as they are compelling. This begins with the need to demonstrate compliance with a large number of federal and state laws and regulations that govern medication use. In addition to compliance, another driver of this trend is financial; namely, increased standardization, enhanced efficiency, and better inventory management lead to appreciable cost savings.[96,97] The PCSC in "Relationships" is separate from the hospitals or clinics and serves as a central hub for pharmacy services that can be completed off-site and are better managed centrally. This often includes specialty pharmacy services, digital health services, batch production of sterile products, administrative staff, pharmacy financial services, and pharmacy supply chain activities.

Getting to a multimillion-dollar capital investment is not something that happens quickly; hence, the extended timeline of this illustrated case. Along the way, Marie and her team demonstrated each of the common competencies of healthcare managers described above, beginning with professionalism. Some have argued that professionalism in healthcare is beginning to erode as changes in the way healthcare is delivered is putting pressure on health professionals.[98] The Code of Ethics for Pharmacists outlines eight principles to guide how pharmacists interact with patients, other health professionals, and society.[99] One of the principles is lifelong learning and a duty to maintain professional competence.[100]

To be effective as a knowledge worker, as Drucker put it, pharmacists and pharmacy administrators must continually develop their knowledge, skills, and abilities. This is particularly true in healthcare because new information and technological advances are generated at a rapid pace, creating an environment where one can quickly fall behind in the absence of continually striving for improvement. Both illustrated cases in this chapter highlight professionalism and professional development well. The illustrated case "Opportunities" opens with Jim reading an article on specialty pharmacy in his free time to identify new ideas for how to care for his patients (Illustration 15-1). In "Relationships," Marie is shown attending a conference on digital health to better understand this field (Illustration 15-11).

Continuous professional development is an expectation of all healthcare administrators. In fact, the chief executive officer (CEO), Anna Fraser, is also shown reviewing an article on "Realizing Pharmacy's Full Value" as she deliberates whether to invest in the PCSC (Illustration 15-8). If she funds the $9 million pharmacy project, which represents a large portion of the budget for such expenditures, requests from other departments will inevitably be declined. To inform her decision, Anna is relying on the level of support from other leaders within the organization, such as the head of facilities, the pharmacy benefit management group (i.e., "Payers"), the chief information officer (CIO), and the chief nursing officer (CNO). It is impractical for the CEO of a large health system to fully understand the intricacies, nuances, or impact of every single request on frontline employees. However, her relationships with key administrative leaders, and the ability to rely on their in-depth understanding of the departments they lead, provides invaluable perspective on the strength of one request compared to another. The strength of these relationships, in other words, will play a key role in her decision-making process. Similarly, relationships are equally important to pharmacy leaders advocating for funding of new pharmacy programs and services.

This scenario highlights why communication and relationship management represent one of the five common competencies of healthcare administrators. The ability to communicate clearly and concisely is essential to success as every interaction, whether informal or formal, provides opportunities to advance an idea or cause. Take, for example, the informal interaction Marie has with the head of facilities during a chance encounter in an elevator (Illustration 15-9), which takes place 3 months prior to the CEO's decision regarding whether to invest in the PCSC. While not explicitly shown, Marie has prepared for this moment by honing her argument and practicing its delivery. She has thought through how to get the head of facilities interested in the building by highlighting overlap with facilities' needs and/or priorities (e.g., space, fines associated with improper compounding facilities). Importantly, Marie presents a clear vision for the future and directly asks for support.[101]

A key part of Marie's request in Illustration 15-9 relates to compliance with federal and state regulations, many of which involve proper facilities to intake, store, and compound medications. Pharmacy is one of the most regulated professions in modern healthcare, with accountability to more than 55 external entities.[102] These entities include the United States Pharmacopeia (USP), The Joint Commission, CMS, state Boards of Pharmacy, the US Drug Enforcement Administration, and the FDA. As a result, pharmacy administrators must constantly monitor changes in the healthcare environment because regulations frequently evolve in response. Recently, regulatory bodies have been focused on methods to reduce opioid abuse, lower the rising cost of prescription drugs, and improve the safety of patients and health professionals associated with compounding sterile products (intravenous drug preparations) and hazardous medications (chemotherapy or other medications that may have genotoxic or teratogenic effects).[104]

Many pharmacy clean rooms, where sterile compounding of intravenous products takes place, are not up to revised USP standards.[103] These standards have been updated recently, and are increasingly being enforced by regulatory bodies in response to several highly publicized examples of substandard compounding that put patients' health and lives at risk. One example includes the New England Compounding Center outbreak of 2012.[104] As a result of unethical leadership and improper facilities and procedures, drug products for administration into the spinal column of patients were not prepared in a sterile fashion. This led to 793 patients across 20 states contracting fungal meningitis, an infection that causes inflammation in the brain and spinal cord.[104] Of the 793 patients who contracted fungal meningitis in this outbreak, 64 lost their lives as a result. To avoid harming patients and to meet regulatory requirements, many pharmacy departments within health systems need to upgrade their compounding facilities. Those interested in exploring compounding pharmacy in more depth, including different types of compounding and the legal and regulatory environment, are encouraged to read the illustrated case "Transformation" in Chapter 2 Community Pharmacy.

Due to the significant costs associated with these upgrades, and the effect those costs would have on other priorities or needs within the organization, it is understandable that decision makers like the CEO in "Relationships" may demonstrate a degree of skepticism, scrutiny, or hesitancy. Understanding these complexities, Marie builds the case for this large organizational investment steadily and strategically over the course of several years. Marie appreciated that support from an administrative leader in one department would impact the degree of support from administrative leaders in other departments. This is demonstrated in Illustration 15-9, where the head of facilities reveals that his support for Marie's proposal had already begun to develop in a conversation with the CIO.

Marie's participation in a digital health conference, depicted in Illustration 15-11, was referenced earlier in relation to professionalism. Fortunately, Marie's colleague, the health system's CIO, was also in attendance. This provided an opportunity to discuss various projects; importantly, one of these was the PCSC. Marie was able to use her skills in relationship management to develop the trust and credibility with the CIO required to move her agenda forward. Networking is an aspect of relationship management, and it should not be confused with socializing. Networking is an intentional process through which someone builds connections with others to gain access to skills or information, or to people (e.g., key decision makers) they are not in a position to meet with or influence.[105] Often these connections develop through shared activities or common interests. In Marie's case, she has been taking the opportunity to connect with the CIO over both; her attendance at his presentation (a shared activity), and digital health (a common interest). While not explicitly stated, networking in this manner allowed Marie to set up a follow-up meeting with the CIO, where she was able to solidify his support by effectively communicating the value of the PCSC to the organization; this includes, importantly, helping the CIO reach organizational digital health goals. Based on the head of facilities' response in the elevator and the CEO's mental checklist, we know Marie's work in relationship management paid off and that the CIO turned out to be a key ally.

All healthcare organizations are under financial pressure to minimize costs to patients and to the US economy. Healthcare insurers have also been challenged to increase efficiencies and innovations in an attempt to lower costs.[106] Pharmacy benefits have been separated from healthcare benefits by many insurers as a result.[107] When a patient picks up a prescription, drug insurance claims are electronically processed in real time by a Pharmacy Benefit Management company, or PBM, of that patient's insurance company or health plan. This outside company, the PBM, determines the amount of reimbursement the pharmacy will receive for the product dispensed, as well as how much money the patient will pay as an out-of-pocket expense. Since specialty pharmacy medications are expensive, and Marie's proposal includes a new specialty pharmacy, it appears to the director of the health system's PBM at first to be a threat to his ability to control medication costs.

The health system's PBM director must be responsive to the needs and goals of the health insurer, which is going to hold him and his team accountable for achieving cost efficiencies. Marie must get the support of the PBM director in Illustration 15-10 or her proposal will fail. Again, we see that Marie is up to the challenge and has prepared for this meeting, as she had for meetings with other administrative leaders. Marie emphasizes that the expanded specialty pharmacy will not increase spending on high-cost medications; rather, she shows him an analysis of how expanded pharmacy services within the proposed specialty pharmacy will, in fact, lower costs. The PCSC specialty pharmacy will reduce costs by closely monitoring patient response to therapy, supporting efforts to improve medication adherence, and providing a hub for interprofessional communication back to physicians and other prescribers when medications are not producing desired effects. High-quality, interprofessional care such as this promises to lower cost while improving health outcomes.[108]

One of the ways that chief pharmacy officers or directors of pharmacy work to build relationships is through active participation in stakeholders' meetings. The final illustration of the case (Illustration 15-12) depicts Marie doing just this, approximately 2.5 years before her request for the PCSC is under consideration by the CEO. The CNO, Dr. Karina Holmes, is presenting her case for additional nursing resources due to the strains that have been placed on her department from increasing patient volumes in addition to higher patient acuity (i.e., degree of illness). It is clear to Marie that patients and the organization will benefit, including financially, from additional nursing resources. Voicing this support for a critical cause, thinks Marie, may also help build an ally in Karina who, one day, may support a proposal for additional pharmacy resources. While the idea for the PCSC had yet to be born, the important relationship building that took place this day laid the foundation for its ultimate approval years later.

The illustrated case "Relationships" tells the story of Dr. Marie Wallace, a pharmacy administrator who, after years of strategic decisions and actions, is able to enact a shared vision for a PCSC that will benefit patients, her pharmacy department, and the financial well-being of her employer, a large health system. Marie accomplishes this by mastery of essential leadership competencies in healthcare; namely, effective communication and relationship management, effective advocacy and leadership, professionalism through lifelong learning, expertise in the healthcare system and business skills. With this new facility and the effective pharmacy administration team that contributed to its creation, the pharmacy department is poised for a bright future.

DISCUSSION QUESTIONS FOR "RELATIONSHIPS"

1. Think about three individuals in your life who you consider strong leaders. What are the defining qualities or characteristics that make them stand out? Do any of these align with the five common competencies described in this illustrated case?

2. How does the picture of leadership painted by this story align with your notion of effective leadership in healthcare?

3. Maintaining up-to-date knowledge about the healthcare environment, including one's own profession, requires a commitment to lifelong learning. What tools or resources help you learn best? When you enter your career, how might understanding your learning preferences influence whether you succeed or fail?

4. Asking for help and support from others can be intimidating, and it is depicted in this case as one behavior associated with relationship building. Do you consider this a strength or a weakness in a leader? Why?

5. How might convincing your colleagues and supervisors to invest $9 million in an initiative be risky? Think of an example of when you took a risk to achieve something that seemed out of reach, or that maybe did not have a clear or guaranteed outcome. What drove you to take that risk?

CHAPTER SUMMARY

- Given rising complexity and significant challenges to the US healthcare system, healthcare administration, including pharmacy leadership, is a rapidly expanding field.

- Rising healthcare costs for patients and society have focused healthcare administrators, pharmacy leaders, professional organizations, and politicians on finding sustainable solutions to lower costs and improve care.

- Health systems are often led by a single leader, the chief executive officer, or CEO, who is advised by the "C-suite." Increasingly, the C-suite includes a chief pharmacy officer, or CPO, who advises on overall medication use strategy.

- Pharmacy administrative leadership teams are composed of individuals with different backgrounds, each bringing their unique talents, strengths, and training to the task of improving patient outcomes through the safe and effective use of medications.

- Completion of a Health System Pharmacy Administration and Leadership residency program is an effective way to prepare for a career in pharmacy administration and may facilitate career advancement.

- Because of a shift in reimbursement from volume to value, and with patient care complexities on the rise, health systems have become the dominant way healthcare is delivered in the United States.

- Pharmacist administrators collaborate interprofessionally to ensure care is provided in the most effective manner possible.

- Managing high-cost, high-risk medications through a specialty pharmacy provides a unique opportunity for pharmacists to improve care, lower costs, and generate new revenue for health systems.

- Professionalism as a pharmacist includes a lifelong dedication to continued learning.

- Effective pharmacy administrators can clearly and concisely articulate a vision and a message.

- Building a professional network with a strong set of relationships facilitates a leader's ability to effect positive change.

ACKNOWLEDGMENT

The authors would like to acknowledge Dr. Joelle Hall, PharmD, Health System Pharmacy Administration Resident at UW Health in Madison, Wisconsin, for her assistance with background research and the generation of Figures 15-1 and 15-2.

REFERENCES

1. What is Health and Medical Administration? HealthcareAdministrationEDU. Available at https://www.healthcareadministrationedu.org/what-is-health-and-medical-administration/. Accessed May 30, 2020.

2. About CAHME. Commission on accreditation of healthcare management education. Available at https://cahme.org. Accessed May 30, 2020.

3. The rise (and rise) of the healthcare administrator. AthenaInsight. Available at https://www.athenahealth.com/insight/expert-forum-rise-and-rise-healthcare-administrator. Published November 6, 2017. Accessed May 30, 2020.

4. Health Care Spending in US, Other High-Income Countries. Available at https://www.commonwealthfund.org/publications/journal-article/2018/mar/health-care-spending-united-states-and-other-high-income. Accessed May 30, 2020.

5. Porter ME, Lee TH. The strategy that will fix health care. *Harvard Business Review*. Available at https://hbr.org/2013/10/the-strategy-that-will-fix-health-care. Accessed May 30, 2020.

6. Stremikis DB and K. Getting real about health care value. *Harvard Business Review*. Available at https://hbr.org/2013/09/getting-real-about-health-care-value. Accessed May 30, 2020.

7. Howard DH, Chernew ME, Abdelgawad T, Smith GL, Sollano J, Grabowski DC. New anticancer drugs associated with large increases in costs and life expectancy. *Health Aff*. 2016;35(9):1581-1587.

8. Fojo T, Mailankody S, Lo A. Unintended consequences of expensive cancer therapeutics—the pursuit of marginal indications and a Me-Too mentality that stifles innovation and creativity: The John Conley lecture. *JAMA Otolaryngol Head Neck Surg*. 2014;140(12):1225-1236.

9. Howard DH, Bach PB, Berndt ER, Conti RM. Pricing in the market for anticancer drugs. *J Econ Perspect*. 2015;29(1):139-162.

10. Kumar H, Fojo T, Mailankody S. An appraisal of clinically meaningful outcomes guidelines for oncology clinical trials. *JAMA Oncol*. 2016;2(9):1238-1240.

11. Tefferi A, Kantarjian H, Rajkumar SV, et al. In support of a patient-driven initiative and petition to lower the high price of cancer drugs. *Mayo Clin Proc*. 2015;90(8):996-1000.

12. Harrington SE, Smith TJ. The role of chemotherapy at the end of life. *JAMA*. 2008;299(22):2667-2678.

13. Leape LL. Institute of Medicine Medical Error Figures Are Not Exaggerated. *JAMA*. 2000;284(1):95-97.

14. Van Den Bos J, Rustagi K, Gray T, Halford M, Ziemkiewicz E, Shreve J. The $17.1 billion problem: the annual cost of measurable medical errors. *Health Aff*. 2011;30(4):596-603.

15. Institute of Medicine (US) Committee on quality of health care in America. *Crossing the Quality Chasm: A New Health System for the 21st Century*. Washington (DC): National Academies Press (US); 2001. Available at http://www.ncbi.nlm.nih.gov/books/NBK222274/. Accessed January 2, 2020.

16. Berwick DM, James B, Coye MJ. Connections between quality measurement and improvement. *Med Care*. 2003;41(Supplement):I-30-I-38.

17. Berwick DM, Nolan TW, Whittington J. The triple aim: care, health, and cost. *Health Aff*. 2008;27(3):759-769.

18. Bolon DS. Comparing mission statement content in for-profit and not-for-profit hospitals: does mission really matter? *Hosp Top*. 2005;83(4):2-9.

19. Introduction to Health Care Management. Available at https://www.jblearning.com/catalog/productdetails/9781284156560#productInfo. Accessed May 30, 2020.

20. Kinnaman ML, Bleich MR. Collaboration: Aligning resources to create and sustain partnerships. *J Prof Nurs*. 2004;20(5):310-322.

21. Dyrda L. 38 hospital and health system C-level roles, defined. Available at https://www.beckershospitalreview.com/hospital-management-administration/38-hospital-and-health-system-c-suite-executive-positions.html. Accessed May 30, 2020.

22. Ivey MF. Rationale for having a chief pharmacy officer in a health care organization. *Am J Health Syst Pharm*. 2005;62(9):975-978.

23. Zilz DA, Woodward BW, Thielke TS, Shane RR, Scott B. Leadership skills for a high-performance pharmacy practice. *Am J Health Syst Pharm*. 2004;61(23):2562-2574.

24. White SJ, Enright SM. Is there still a pharmacy leadership crisis? A seven-year follow-up assessment. *Am J Health Syst Pharm*. 2013;70(5):443-447.

25. American College of Clinical Pharmacy. Career opportunities in clinical pharmacy. Available at https://www.accp.com/stunet/compass/career.aspx#leadership. Accessed January 2, 2020.

26. Pharmacy Administration: the intersection of business and pharmacy. Pharmacy times. Available at https://www.pharmacytimes.com/contributor/the-nontraditional-pharmacist/2018/10/pharmacy-administration-is-the-intersection-of-business-and-pharmacy. Accessed January 2, 2020.

27. Magrum B, Weber RJ. Restructuring a pharmacy department: leadership strategies for managing organizational change. *Hosp Pharm*. 2018;53(4):225-229.

28. Zilz DA, Woodward BW, Thielke TS, Shane RR, Scott B. Leadership skills for a high-performance pharmacy practice. *Am J Health Syst Pharm*. 2004;61(23):2562-2574.

29. White SJ. Will there be a pharmacy leadership crisis? An ASHP Foundation Scholar-in-Residence report. *Am J Health Syst Pharm*. 2005;62(8):845-855.

30. American Society of Health-System Pharmacists. Drug shortages FAQs. Available at https://www.ashp.org:443/Drug Shortages/Current Shortages/Drug Shortages FAQs. Accessed May 30, 2020.

31. McGinley L. Low prices of some lifesaving drugs make them impossible to get. Washington post. Available at https://www.washingtonpost.com/national/health-science/low-prices-of-some-lifesaving-drugs-make-them-impossible-to-get/2019/06/18/abd03190-66bb-11e9-82ba-fcfeff232e8f_story.html. Accessed May 30, 2020.

32. Coppock K. Pharmacists play a role in responding to drug shortages. Available at https://www.pharmacytimes.com/conferences/ashpmidyear2018/pharmacists-play-a-role-in-responding-to-drug-shortages. Accessed May 30, 2020.

33. Rabin RC. Faced with a drug shortfall, doctors scramble to treat children with cancer. Available at https://www.nytimes.com/2019/10/14/health/cancer-drug-shortage.html. Accessed May 30, 2020.

34. Hernandez I, Sampathkumar S, Good CB, Kesselheim AS, Shrank WH. Changes in drug pricing after drug shortages in the United States. *Ann Intern Med.* 2019;170(1):74.

35. Mylan CEO salary rose by 600 percent as EpiPen price rose 400 percent. NBC News. Available at https://www.nbcnews.com/business/consumer/mylan-execs-gave-themselves-raises-they-hiked-epipen-prices-n636591. Accessed May 30, 2020.

36. Saltiel M, Finnefrock M. Hyperinflation—definitions and causes. *J Pharm Pract.* 2018;31(4):370-373.

37. Long H. What happened to AIDS drug that spiked 5,000%. Available at https://money.cnn.com/2016/08/25/news/economy/daraprim-aids-drug-high-price/index.html. Accessed May 30, 2020.

38. Fralick M, Kesselheim AS. The U.S. Insulin Crisis—rationing a lifesaving medication discovered in the 1920s. *N Engl J Med.* 2019;381(19):1793-1795.

39. Paavola A. 11 healthcare pharma leaders offer advice on controlling drug spend. Available at https://www.beckershospitalreview.com/pharmacy/11-healthcare-pharma-leaders-offer-advice-on-controlling-drug-spend.html. Accessed May 30, 2020.

40. Knoer S. Antidote to rising drug prices languishes on the Hill. Available at https://thehill.com/blogs/congress-blog/healthcare/412830-antidote-to-rising-drug-prices-languishes-on-the-hill. Accessed May 30, 2020.

41. Knoer S. How to reduce medical drug prices at a stroke. Available at https://www.newsweek.com/how-reduce-medical-drug-prices-stroke-730638. Accessed May 30, 2020.

42. Knoer S. What does PBM stand for? In many states, it's programs bilking millions. Available at https://www.statnews.com/2018/06/29/pharmacy-benefit-managers-profits-ohio/. Accessed May 30, 2020.

43. Hospitals are playing Gotcha! with big pharma, at last. Available at https://roundtables.abl.org/hospitals-playing-gotcha-with-big-pharma-at-last/. Accessed May 30, 2020.

44. Lupkin S. Hospitals say they're being slammed by drug price hikes. Available at https://khn.org/news/hospitals-say-theyre-being-slammed-by-drug-price-hikes/. Accessed May 30, 2020.

45. Kacik A. Health system-led drug company unlikely to make a dent in drug prices, shortages. Available at https://www.modernhealthcare.com/article/20180118/NEWS/180119905/health-system-led-drug-company-unlikely-to-make-a-dent-in-drug-prices-shortages. Accessed May 30, 2020.

46. American Society of Health-System Pharmacy. ASHP presents Knoer with 2019 John W. Webb Lecture Award. Available at https://www.ashp.org:443/News/2019/10/21/ASHP-Presents-Knoer-with-2019-John-W-Webb-Lecture-Award. Accessed May 30, 2020.

47. Feller TT, Doucette WR, Witry MJ. Assessing opportunities for student pharmacist leadership development at schools of pharmacy in the United States. *Am J Pharm Educ.* 2016;80(5).

48. White SJ. Leadership: successful alchemy. *Am J Health Syst Pharm.* 2006;63(16):1497-1503.

49. Gazda NP, Griffin E, Hamrick K, et al. Development and implementation of a combined master of science and PGY1/PGY2 health-system pharmacy administration residency program at a large community teaching hospital. *Hosp Pharm.* 2018;53(2):96-100.

50. Mark SM. Things I wish I had known before becoming a pharmacy leader. *Hosp Pharm.* 2013;48(1):68-76.

51. Pollard SR, Clark JS. Survey of health-system pharmacy leadership pathways. *Am J Health Syst Pharm.* 2009;66(10):947-952.

52. Wiley F. Pharmacists step into leadership roles. Available at https://www.drugtopics.com/article/pharmacists-step-leadership-roles. Accessed May 30, 2020.

53. Brody JE. The cost of not taking your medicine. Available at https://www.nytimes.com/2017/04/17/well/the-cost-of-not-taking-your-medicine.html. Accessed May 30, 2020.

54. Rosenbaum L, Shrank WH. Taking our medicine — improving adherence in the accountability era. *N Engl J Med.* 2013;369(8):694-695.

55. Ho PM, Rumsfeld JS, Masoudi FA, et al. Effect of medication nonadherence on hospitalization and mortality among patients with diabetes mellitus. *Arch Intern Med.* 2006;166(17):1836-1841.

56. Vestbo J, Anderson JA, Calverley PMA, et al. Adherence to inhaled therapy, mortality and hospital admission in COPD. *Thorax.* 2009;64(11):939-943.

57. Fitzgerald AA, Powers JD, Ho PM, et al. Impact of medication nonadherence on hospitalizations and mortality in heart failure. *J Card Fail.* 2011;17(8):664-669.

58. Kim S, Shin DW, Yun JM, et al. Medication adherence and the risk of cardiovascular mortality and hospitalization among patients with newly prescribed antihypertensive medications. *Hypertension.* 2016;67(3):506-512.

59. Sabaté E, World Health Organization, eds. *Adherence to Long-Term Therapies: Evidence for Action.* Geneva: World Health Organization; 2003.

60. Patzer RE, Serper M, Reese PP, et al. Medication understanding, non-adherence, and clinical outcomes among adult kidney transplant recipients. *Clin Transplant.* 2016;30(10):1294-1305.

61. Nevins TE, Nickerson PW, Dew MA. Understanding medication nonadherence after kidney transplant. *J Am Soc Nephrol.* 2017;28(8):2290-2301.

62. Port FK, Wolfe RA, Mauger EA, Berling DP, Jiang K. Comparison of survival probabilities for dialysis patients vs cadaveric renal transplant recipients. *JAMA.* 1993;270(11):1339-1343.

63. National Kidney Foundation. Kidney transplant. Available at https://www.kidney.org/atoz/content/kidney-transplant. Accessed May 30, 2020.

64. Ekberg H, Tedesco-Silva H, Demirbas A, et al. Reduced exposure to calcineurin inhibitors in renal transplantation. *N Engl J Med.* 2007;357(25):2562-2575.

65. Halloran PF. Immunosuppressive drugs for kidney transplantation. *N Engl J Med.* 2004;351(25):2715-2729.

66. Medicare pays for a kidney transplant, but not the drugs to keep it viable. Available at https://www.npr.org/sections/health-shots/2016/12/22/506319553/medicare-pays-for-a-kidney-transplant-but-not-the-drugs-to-keep-it-viable. Accessed May 30, 2020.

67. Zhu Y, Zhou Y, Zhang L, Zhang J, Lin J. Efficacy of interventions for adherence to the immunosuppressive therapy in kidney transplant recipients: a meta-analysis and systematic review. *J Investig Med.* 2017;65(7):1049-1056.

68. What is pay for performance in healthcare? Available at https://catalyst.nejm.org/pay-for-performance-in-healthcare/. Accessed May 30, 2020.

69. Agency for Healthcare Research and Quality. Defining health systems. Available at https://www.ahrq.gov/chsp/chsp-reports/resources-for-understanding-health-systems/defining-health-systems.html. Accessed May 30, 2020.

70. Centers for Medicare & Medicaid Services. Value based programs. Available at https://www.cms.gov/Medicare/Quality-Initiatives-Patient-Assessment-Instruments/Value-Based-Programs/Value-Based-Programs.html. Accessed May 30, 2020.

71. Galvin G. Population Health: The 'North Star' of the triple aim. Available at https://www.usnews.com/news/healthiest-communities/articles/2018-05-25/a-decade-later-triple-aim-health-care-framework-offers-lessons-promise. May 30, 2020.

72. Woodside KJ, Sung RS. Do federal regulations have an impact on kidney transplant outcomes? *Adv Chronic Kidney Dis.* 2016;23(5):332-339.

73. Alloway RR, Dupuis R, Gabardi S, et al. Evolution of the role of the transplant pharmacist on the multidisciplinary transplant team. *Am J Transplant.* 2011;11(8):1576-1583.

74. Centers for Medicare & Medicaid Services. Transplant. Available at https://www.cms.gov/Medicare/Provider-Enrollment-and-Certification/GuidanceforLawsAndRegulations/Transplant-Laws-and-Regulations.html. Accessed May 30, 2020.

75. American Society of Health-System Pharmacists. ASHP Guidelines on preventing medication errors in hospitals. Available at https://www.ashp.org/-/media/assets/policy-guidelines/docs/guidelines/preventing-medication-errors-hospitals.ashx. Accessed May 30, 2020.

76. American Society of Health-System Pharmacists. ASHP discussion guide on the pharmacist's role in quality improvement. Available at https://www.ashp.org/-/media/assets/pharmacy-practice/resource-centers/leadership/leadership-of-profession-pharmacists-role-quality-improvement-guide.ashx. Accessed May 30, 2020.

77. Rim MH, Smith L, Kelly M. Implementation of a patient-focused specialty pharmacy program in an academic healthcare system. *Am J Health Syst Pharm.* 2016;73(11):831-838.

78. Colgan K. Specialty pharmacy in the limelight. *Am J Health Syst Pharm.* 2016;73(11):743-743.

79. Bagwell A, Kelley T, Carver A, Lee JB, Newman B. Advancing patient care through specialty pharmacy services in an academic health system. *J Manag Care Spec Pharm.* 2017;23(8):815-820.

80. Tang J, Bailey J, Chang C, et al. Effects of specialty pharmacy care on health outcomes in multiple sclerosis. *Am Health Drug Benefits.* 2016;9(8):420-429.

81. Barlow JF, Faris RJ, Wang W, Verbrugge RR, Garavaglia SB, Aubert RE. Impact of specialty pharmacy on treatment costs for rheumatoid Arthritis. Available at https://www.pharmacytimes.com/publications/ajpb_2012/ajpb_2012_nov/impact-of-specialty-pharmacy-on-treatment-costs-for-rheumatoid-arthritis. Accessed May 30, 2020.

82. Roebuck MC, Liberman JM. Assessing the burden of illness of chronic hepatitis C and the impact of direct-acting antiviral use on healthcare costs in Medicaid. *Am J Manag Care.* 2019;25 (8 Suppl):S131-S139.

83. Rattay T, Dumont IP, Heinzow HS, Hutton DW. Cost-effectiveness of access expansion to treatment of hepatitis C virus infection through primary care providers. *Gastroenterology.* 2017;153(6):1531-1543.e2.

84. Fox M. Hepatitis C cure eludes patients as states struggle with costs. Available at https://www.nbcnews.com/health/health-news/hepatitis-c-cure-eludes-patients-states-struggle-costs-n870846. Accessed May 30, 2020.

85. Fein AJ. Pharmacy owners' profits fall as industry competition rises. Available at https://www.drugchannels.net/2018/01/new-data-pharmacy-owners-profits-fall.html. Accessed May 30, 2020.

86. Gowda S, Desai PB, Kulkarni SS, Hull VV, Math AAK, Vernekar SN. Markers of renal function tests. *N Am J Med Sci.* 2010;2(4):170-173.

87. Hlubocky JM, Stuckey LJ, Schuman AD, Stevenson JG. Evaluation of a transplantation specialty pharmacy program. *Am J Health Syst Pharm.* 2012;69(4):340-347.

88. Gu NY, Gai Y, Hay JW. The effect of patient satisfaction with pharmacist consultation on medication adherence: an instrumental variable approach. *Pharm Pract.* 2008;6(4):201-210.

89. ASHP guidelines on pharmacist-conducted patient education and counseling. *Am J Health Syst Pharm.* 1997;54(4):431-434.

90. Sherman E. How to calculate return on investment for your business. Available at https://www.inc.com/erik-sherman/how-to-calculate-return-on-investment-for-your-bus.html. Accessed May 30, 2020.

91. ASHP statement on the pharmacist's role in informatics. *Am J Health Syst Pharm.* 2016;73(6):410-413.

92. Drucker PF. They're not employees, they're people. Available at https://hbr.org/2002/02/theyre-not-employees-theyre-people. Accessed May 30, 2020.

93. Stefl ME. Common competencies for all healthcare managers: the healthcare leadership alliance model. *J Healthc Manag.* 2008;53(6):360-373; discussion 374.

94. Abdulsalam Y, Gopalakrishnan M, Maltz A, Schneller E. The emergence of consolidated service centers in health care. *J Bus Logist.* 2015;36(4):321-334.

95. New data shows many health system pharmacies considering consolidated distribution models to address medication management challenges. Available at https://www.prnewswire.com/news-releases/new-data-shows-many-health-system-pharmacies-considering-consolidated-distribution-models-to-address-medication-management-challenges-300749101.html. Accessed May 30, 2020.

96. Visante Business of Pharmacy Forum Report. Available at https://www.visanteinc.com/wp-content/uploads/2018/05/Visante-Business-of-Pharmacy-Forum-Report.pdf. Accessed May 30, 2020.

97. Candy TA, Schneider PJ, Pedersen CA. Impact of United States Pharmacopeia chapter 797: results of a national survey. *Am J Health Syst Pharm.* 2006;53(14):1336-1343.

98. ABIM Foundation. American Board of Internal Medicine; ACP-ASIM Foundation. American College of Physicians-American Society of Internal Medicine; European Federation of Internal Medicine. Medical professionalism in the new millennium: a physician charter. *Ann Intern Med.* 2002;136(3):243-246.

99. American Society of Health-System Pharmacists. Code of Ethics for Pharmacists. Available at https://www.ashp.org/-/media/assets/policy-guidelines.docs/endorsed-documents/code-of-ethics-for-pharmacists.ashx. Accessed May 30, 2020.

100. American Society of Health-System Pharmacists. ASHP Statement on Professionalism. Available at https://www.ashp.org/-/media/assets.policy-guidelines/docs/statements/professionalism.ashx. Accessed May 30, 2020.

101. Meltzer D. 3 Components of the perfect elevator pitch. Available at https://www.entrepreneur.com/article/313574. Accessed May 30, 2020.

102. Pharmacy law matters: legal and regulatory developments affecting pharmacy in 2018. *Pharmacy Today.* 2019;25(1):39-57.

103. Barlas S. Deaths from contaminated methylprednisolone highlight failures of compounding pharmacies: less hospital access to outside vendors and more visits from state pharmacy boards. *P T.* 2013;38(1)27-57.

104. Food and Drug Administration Office of Criminal Investigations. January 31, 2018: New England compounding center pharmacist sentenced for role in nationwide fungal meningitis outbreak. Available at http://www.fda.gov/inspections-compliance-enforcement-and-criminal-investigations/press-releases/january-31-2018-new-england-compounding-center-pharmacist-sentenced-role-nationwide-fungal. Accessed May 30, 2020.

105. Uzzi B, Dunlap S. How to build your network. Available at https://hbr.org/2005/12/how-to-build-your-network. Accessed May 30, 2020.

106. Fitch: Healthcare pricing, profit margin pressure will persist in 2019. Modern healthcare. Available at https://www.modernhealthcare.com/article/20181130/NEWS/181139995/fitch-healthcare-pricing-profit-margin-pressure-will-persist-in-2019. Published November 30, 2018. Accessed December 30, 2019.

107. Fein AJ. CVS, Express scripts, and the evolution of the PBM business model. Available at https://www.drugchannels.net/2019/05/cvs-express-scripts-and-evolution-of.html. Accessed May 30, 2020.

108. Pulvermacher A, Nelson C. Benefits of developing a collaborative, outcomes-based specialty pharmacy program. *Am J Health Syst Pharm.* 2016;73(11):839-843.

Index